Anxiety Disorders in Children and Adolescents

Second Edition

Edited by

Wendy K. Silverman

Professor of Psychology and Director of the Child Anxiety and Phobia Program,
Florida International University, Miami, Florida, USA

Andy P. Field

Professor of Child Psychopathology at the University of Sussex, Brighton, UK

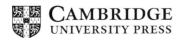

CAMBRIDGE
UNIVERSITY PRESS

CAMBRIDGE UNIVERSITY PRESS
Cambridge, New York, Melbourne, Madrid, Cape Town,
Singapore, São Paulo, Delhi, Tokyo, Mexico City

Cambridge University Press
The Edinburgh Building, Cambridge CB2 8RU, UK

Published in the United States of America by Cambridge University Press, New York

www.cambridge.org
Information on this title: www.cambridge.org/9780521721486

First edition published in 2001 by Cambridge University Press
Second edition published in 2011 by Cambridge University Press

Printed in the United Kingdom at the University Press, Cambridge

A catalog record for this publication is available from the British Library

Library of Congress Cataloging in publication data
Anxiety disorders in children and adolescents / edited by Wendy K. Silverman, Andy Field. – 2nd ed.
p.   ;   cm. – (Cambridge child and adolescent psychiatry)
Includes bibliographical references and index.
ISBN 978-0-521-72148-6 (pbk.)
1. Anxiety in children.   2. Anxiety in adolescence.   3. Child psychotherapy.
4. Adolescent psychotherapy.   I. Silverman, Wendy K.   II. Field, Andy P.   III. Title.
IV. Series: Cambridge child and adolescent psychiatry series.
[DNLM: 1. Anxiety Disorders – diagnosis.   2. Anxiety Disorders – therapy.   3. Adolescent
Development.   4. Adolescent.   5. Child Development.   6. Child. WM 172]
RJ506.A58A585   2011
618.92′8522 – dc23   2011017972

ISBN 978-0-521-72148-6 Paperback

Anxiety Disorders in Children and Adolescents

201|

Second Edition

X

**This book is to be returned on or before
the last date stamped below.**

Cambridge Child and Adolescent Psychiatry

Child and adolescent psychiatry is an important and growing area of clinical psychiatry. The last decade has seen a rapid expansion of scientific knowledge in this field and has provided a new understanding of the underlying pathology of mental disorders in these age groups. This series is aimed at practitioners and researchers both in child and adolescent mental health services and in developmental and clinical neuroscience. Focusing on psychopathology, it highlights those topics where the growth of knowledge has had the greatest impact on clinical practice and on the treatment and understanding of mental illness. Individual volumes benefit from both the international expertise of their contributors and also from a coherence generated through a uniform style and structure for the series. Each volume provides, first, a historical overview and a clear descriptive account of the psychopathology of a specific disorder or group of related disorders. These features then form the basis for a thorough critical review of the etiology, natural history, management, prevention, and impact on later adult adjustment. While each volume is therefore complete in its own right, volumes also relate to each other to create a flexible and collectable series that should appeal to students as well as experienced scientists and practitioners.

Already published in this series:

Autism and Pervasive Developmental Disorders, Second edition edited by Fred R. Volkmar
9780521549578 paperback

Eating Disorders in Children and Adolescents edited by Tony Jaffa and Brett McDermott
9780521613125 paperback

Cognitive Behaviour Therapy for Children and Families, Second edition edited by Philip Graham
9780521529921 paperback

Suicide in Children and Adolescents edited by Robert A. King and Alan Apter
9780521622264 paperback

Hyperactivity and Attention Disorders of Childhood, Second edition edited by Seija Sandberg
9780521789615 paperback

Outcomes in Neurodevelopmental and Genetic Disorders edited by Patricia Howlin and Orlee Udwin
9780521797214 paperback

Practical Child and Adolescent Psychopharmacology edited by Stan Kutcher
9780521655422 paperback

Specific Learning Disabilities and Difficulties in Children and Adolescents: Psychological Assessment and Evaluation edited by Alan Kaufman and Nadeen Kaufman
9780521658409 paperback

Psychotherapy with Children and Adolescents edited by Helmut Remschmidt
9780521576727 paperback

The Depressed Child and Adolescent, Second edition edited by Ian M. Goodyer
9780521775588 paperback

Schizophrenia in Children and Adolescents edited by Helmut Renschmidt
9780521794282 paperback

Conduct Disorders in Childhood and Adolescence edited by Jonathan Hill and Barbara Maughan
9780521786393 paperback

This book is dedicated to Daniel and Rachel
WKS

Dedicated to Grandad Alf and Grandad Harry, to whom I aspire to be
APF

Contents

Contributors

Nicholas P. Allan
Department of Psychology, Florida State University, Tallahassee, FL, USA

Adrian Angold
Duke University Medical Center, Durham, NC, USA

Caroline L. Bokhorst
Leiden University Institute of Psychology, Leiden, the Netherlands

Sam Cartwright-Hatton
School of Psychology, University of Manchester, UK

Peter Cooper
School of Psychology and Clinical Language Sciences, University of Reading, UK

William Copeland
Duke University Medical Center, Durham, NC, USA

E. Jane Costello
Duke University Medical Center, Durham, NC, USA

Cathy Creswell
School of Psychology and Clinical Language Sciences, University of Reading, UK

Helen L. Egger
Duke University Medical Center, Durham, NC, USA

Thalia C. Eley
Social, Genetic and Developmental Psychiatry Centre, Institute of Psychiatry, King's College, London, UK

Alaattin Erkanli
Duke University Medical Center, Durham, NC, USA

Andy P. Field
School of Psychology, University of Sussex, Brighton, UK

Antonio Castro Fonseca
Faculty of Psychology and Educational Sciences, University of Coimbra, Portugal

Alice M. Gregory
Department of Psychology, Goldsmiths, University of London, UK

Julie A. Hadwin
Developmental Brain–Behaviour Laboratory, University of Southampton, UK

Annette M. La Greca
Department of Psychology, University of Miami, Coral Gables, FL, USA

Ryan R. Landoll
Department of Psychology, University of Miami, Coral Gables, FL, USA

Kathryn J. Lester
Child Anxiety Theory and Treatment
Laboratory, School of Psychology,
University of Sussex, Brighton,
UK

Christopher J. Lonigan
Department of Psychology, Florida State
University, Tallahassee, FL, USA

Heidi J. Lyneham
Department of Psychology, Macquarie
University, NSW, Australia

Katharina Manassis
Anxiety Disorders Program, Hospital for
Sick Children, Toronto, Ontario,
Canada

Luci M. Motoca
Florida International University, Miami,
FL, USA

Peter Muris
Erasmus University Rotterdam Institute of
Psychology, Woudestein, Rotterdam,
the Netherlands

Lynne Murray
School of Psychology and Clinical
Language Sciences, University of Reading,
UK

Laurel Pelligrino
Weill Cornell Medical College and
New York Presbyterian Hospital,
New York, NY, USA

Sean Perrin
Department of Psychology, Institute of
Psychiatry, London, UK

Beth M. Phillips
Department of Educational
Psychology and Learning Systems, Florida
State University, Tallahassee, FL,
USA

Courtney Pierce
Weill Cornell Medical College and New
York Presbyterian Hospital, New York, NY,
USA

Daniel S. Pine
Mood and Anxiety Disorders Program,
National Institute of Mental Health
Intramural Research Program, Bethesda,
MD, USA

Helena M. Purkis
School of Psychology, University of
Queensland, Brisbane, QLD,
Australia

Ron M. Rapee
Department of Psychology, Macquarie
University, NSW, Australia

Shirley Reynolds
School of Medicine, Health Policy and
Practice, University of East Anglia,
Norwich, UK

Wendy K. Silverman
Department of Psychology, Florida
International University, Miami, FL,
USA

Patrick Smith
Department of Psychology, Institute of
Psychiatry, London, UK

James Stacey
Department of Clinical Psychology, Oxford
University, UK

Philip D. A. Treffers
Lieu dit Boulen, Mahalon, France

John T. Walkup
Weill Cornell Medical College and New
York Presbyterian Hospital, New York, NY,
USA

P. Michiel Westenberg
Leiden University Institute of Psychology,
Leiden, the Netherlands

Charlotte Wilson
School of Medicine, Health Policy and
Practice, University of East Anglia,
Norwich, UK

Shauna B. Wilson
Department of Psychology, Florida
State University, Tallahassee, FL,
USA

William Yule
Department of Psychology, Institute of
Psychiatry, London, UK

Preface

This book began life in 1997 at an international research conference on anxiety disorders in children and adolescents hosted by CURIUM, Academic Centre of Child and Adolescent Psychiatry, Leiden University. Up until that time, child and adolescent anxiety disorder research was largely consumed within treatment and research initiatives aimed at anxiety generally (and typically in adult populations). In fact, a web of knowledge (http://wok.mimas.ac.uk/) search for "child anxiety" or "adolescent anxiety" up to the year 1997 reveals only 30 articles in peer-review journals with those terms as their main topic. This published output does not imply that clinicians and researchers had no interest in child and adolescent anxiety, but that it was finding its feet as a discipline in its own right. The meeting in Leiden was a response to the need to get clinicians and researchers together to discuss the emerging wisdom on theory, assessment, and intervention of child and adolescent anxiety.

Professor Philip Treffers, along with Wendy, organized the Leiden conference while she was on sabbatical there. The resulting first edition of this text contained chapters predominantly based on presentations given at the conference. In the four years between the meeting and the publication of the book in 2001, a further 88 papers had been published with child or adolescent anxiety as their core topic; three times as many as had been published in the 100 or so years before the Leiden meeting. These data show that the book came out at a time when the field was expanding; it represented an important snapshot of this emerging field.

This meeting in Leiden was also the first time that we met. Andy presented a paper co-authored by himself and his Ph.D. supervisor, Professor Graham Davey, and also contributed a chapter to the first edition based on this paper. The next time we met was in 2006 at the Anxiety Disorders Association of America Annual Conference in Maimi. In this five years a great deal had changed in the field: child and adolescent anxiety had established itself as a burgeoning scientific discipline. Our meeting in Miami was in a symposium dedicated to child and adolescent anxiety. During the course of our conversation, Andy told Wendy that he would really like to see an updated version of this book, and Wendy suggested that he might join her and Philip as an editor. He agreed. As we initiated the project, Philip graciously gave the two of us the green light to produce the second edition as the volume's co-editors. We hope that he takes pride in what we have done to extend and update his initial book.

Thus, the desire to update this book emanated from the rapid expansion of research and treatment practice. In the years since the first edition came out and now (2001–2010) another 347 papers have been published with child and adolescent anxiety at their core. Again, this represents a three-fold increase in research output in the last nine years compared to before that time.

This version of the book bears only slight resemblance to its predecessor because the field has changed so much in the past decade. To reflect these changes we went back to the drawing board and the book is now divided into four sections that we believe reflect the broad themes of research over the past 10 years. We will outline these specific developments below, but one global theme is a growing appreciation of the need to consider the social, cognitive, and emotional development of the child/adolescent when thinking about psychopathology. We have several chapters that specifically address this issue but have also asked contributors to consider developmental issues in their chapters.

Section 1: Historical and conceptual issues

This section retains an updated version of the last edition's overview of the historical development (Treffers and Silverman) and clinical phenomenology (Fonseca and Perrin) of child and adolescent anxiety research. This volume adds chapters that look at the developmental epidemiology of anxiety disorders (Costello, Egger, Copeland, Erkanli, and Angold) and at the normal developmental pattern of fears generally (Muris and Field) and social anxiety disorder specifically (Bokhorst and Westenberg). The last 10 years has seen a burgeoning interest in information processing in child and adolescent anxiety and two new chapters explore the role of development in information processing biases (Field, Hadwin, and Lester) and the success of adult models of anxiety when applied downward to child samples (Cartwright-Hatton, Reynolds, and Wilson).

Section 2: The biology of child and adolescent anxiety

The past 10 years has seen an exponential increase in our understanding of both the genetic contribution (Gregory and Eley) to child and adolescent anxiety and the brain structures that underlie it (Pine). Therefore, we have added two new chapters on these topics. In the previous edition, we had a chapter on behavioral inhibition, but for this edition we expanded this topic to discuss temperament more generally and with specific emphasis on the links between temperament, brain, and genetics (Lonigan, Phillips, Wilson, and Allan).

Section 3: Environmental influences on child and adolescent anxiety

We now know that environmental factors explain around two-thirds of the variance in childhood and adolescence and in this part of the book we have tried to focus on the main environmental factors. We have retained expanded and updated chapters on the role of learning (Field and Purkis), traumatic experiences (Smith, Perrin, and Yule), attachment (Manassis), and peer influences (La Greca and Landoll). In addition, we have added a chapter on parental influence because of the surge of interest in the intergenerational transmission of anxiety (Creswell, Murray, Stacey, and Cooper).

Section 4: Prevention and treatment of child and adolescent anxiety

There have been significant developments in prevention and treatment of child and adolescent anxiety disorders since the last edition. This final section retains an updated chapter on psychotherapy (Silverman and Motoca), but adds completely new chapters that describe the state-of-the art knowledge on pharmacological management (Pelligrino, Pierce, and Walkup) and prevention (Lyneham and Rapee) of child and adolescent anxiety disorders.

Our work on this book together has been a long but fulfilling road for us both. It has been an enormous amount of work not just for us but also for all of our contributors. Our biggest debt of gratitude is to these people. We are proud to have assembled a stellar cast of authors in this edition; we feel much like a movie director might if she had assembled the entire Hollywood A-list as the cast of her film. All of our contributors have taken time out of very demanding jobs to write for us, and we are very grateful for their belief, commitment, and dedication to the project.

Wendy would like to thank once again, Philip, for giving her the honor and pleasure to work with him in the first place on the first edition back in Leiden in 1997. She also wants to thank her many students she has worked with over the years (you all know who you are!) who have worked so tirelessly with her in research, as well as in helping the families learn how to handle the problem of childhood anxiety and its disorders. She also thanks the families – from whom she and her students too have learned so much.

Andy would like to thank Wendy for giving him the opportunity to work with her on this project; he has learnt an enormous amount from her mentoring. In an attempt to maximize his stress levels he left writing his chapters until the last minute; he is hugely indebted to Zoë for her miraculous stress-reducing abilities, love, support, and tea-making skills.

Historical and conceptual issues

Anxiety and its disorders in children and adolescents in historical perspective

Philip D. A. Treffers and Wendy K. Silverman

Introduction

Much has been written over time about children and adolescents who are so much troubled by anxieties and fears that they are totally put off their stroke. The conceptualization of these anxieties and fears, and the ideas about their origins, have changed over time. In this chapter, using primary sources wherever possible, we trace how anxiety and its disorders in childhood and adolescence have been described and explained in the literature, especially prior to the twentieth century. By so doing, the historical record is being preserved – something that we believe is important to do as we are of the view (held by many) that our futures are generally better off when they are informed by our pasts.

Knowledge of the history of our disciplines is important. Neve and Turner (2002) point out that history shows "how all medical practices have their rationality and their purpose, even when seeming outdated to the modern mind. The most modern of therapies and the most sophisticated of disease entities will share in that fate, and history can . . . teach the need for modesty . . . " (Neve & Turner, 2002, p. 382). Historical research also teaches us that professionals can deny the impact of even extreme situations. It is not common knowledge for example that in 1855 a French physician Maxime Durand-Fardel supplied data on suicide in French children. He concluded that from the period 1836 to 1844, 132 children in France had committed suicide in relation to maltreatment. Two years later Ambrose Tardieu (1857; in Labbé, 2005), a professor in legal medicine in Paris, published a monograph about sexual abuse, followed three years later by an article containing detailed data about 32 cases of child maltreatment (Tardieu, 1860; see also Roche, Fortin, Labbé, Brown, & Chadwick, 2005). At the time, however, Durand-Fardel and Tardieu did not succeed in bringing the miserable circumstances in which so many children grew up to the notice of physicians. It was generally accepted that children did not have rights, and that parents could determine how they punished their children (Labbé, 2005). Only thanks to the introduction of X-rays in diagnostic procedures could Kempe and his colleagues, a century later, be successful in bringing child maltreatment to the attention of professionals (Kempe, Silverman, Steele, Droegemueller, & Silver, 1962).

Another, more recent example of the "blind spots" of even distinguished professionals appeared in the discussion about the question whether there exists specific, trauma-related psychopathology in children. Garmezy and Rutter (1985) concluded, in spite of convincing evidence to the contrary, that "the form of acute stress reactions in childhood is not

Anxiety Disorders in Children and Adolescents, 2nd edn, ed. W. K. Silverman and A. P. Field. Published by Cambridge University Press. © Cambridge University Press 2011.

markedly different from other emotional disorders not precipitated by severely traumatic experiences" (Garmezy & Rutter, 1985, p. 169).

Currently, the prescription of huge amounts of psychotropic drugs to children, even very young children, and adolescents, appears to reflect another blind spot in professionals (e.g., Zito, Safer, dosReis, Gardner, Boles, & Lynch, 2000). Despite disasters in the past in connection with the careless use of medicines, and notwithstanding the general plea in favor of evidence-based treatment, most of the prescriptions are not justified by empirically based data on effectiveness, side effects, long-term effects, and possible effects of the drugs for the next generation (e.g., Farwell, Lee, Hirtz, Sulzbacher, Ellenberg, & Nelson, 1990; Vitiello & Jensen, 1995; Whittington, Kendall, Fonagy, Cottrell, Cotgrove, & Boddington, 2004). This overuse of prescriptions may be related to the desire of the doctor to "do something": "Leaving the office without a prescription is thought to be 'doing nothing', no matter how much explanation and education about the illness may have taken place" (Pellegrino, 1996, p. 106).

Some pitfalls in historical research in child and adolescent psychiatry

When one studies sources from the past, it can be complicated, and sometimes impossible, to understand the nature of the described problems of the children. Probably this is because, in part, information on the child's developmental history and the child's specific behavioral problems, nowadays considered as essential in considering a diagnosis, are missing in these early descriptions. It is possible too that the meaning of certain behaviors in different periods differs, just as in a certain period the meaning of behavior in diverse cultures can differ (e.g., Van Widenfelt, Treffers, de Beurs, Siebelink, & Koudijs, 2005; Weisz, Suwanlert, Chaiyasit, Weiss, Achenbach, & Walter, 1987). It is plausible too that under different societal circumstances in history the phenomenology of disturbances was not the same as in current times (Berrios, 1999).

For a correct interpretation of problem behavior one should be aware of the position of children in a certain period in a certain country. It can be hard to form an image thereof. Due to several influential authors such as Ariès and DeMause it was long thought, for example, that in the Middle Ages children were perceived as adults in miniature (Ariès, 1960) and were treated in a cruel way (DeMause, 1974). Child abuse and infanticide were thought to have been present on a large scale. More recently, however, others (Kroll & Bachrach, 1986; Pollock, 1983; Shahar, 1990) have presented a more balanced picture. For example, on the basis of extensive source research, Shahar (1990) concluded that in the Middle Ages, authors of medical works, "like most didactic writers, favour[ed] essentially lenient education and granting the child freedom to act in accordance with his natural tendencies" (Shahar, 1990, p. 98).

Terminology too can complicate the correct interpretation of historical texts (Parry-Jones, 1994). The reference to developmental phases, e.g., *infancy* and (in French literature) *puberté* are not unequivocal. This holds as well, if not even more so, for the content of diagnostic categories. Through the years, the meaning of terms such as *melancholia* has changed fundamentally (Berrios, 1996). Several other diagnostic categories, such as *pantophobia* and *lypemania*, and more recently, *hysteria* have disappeared. Problems with terminology in diverse countries especially complicate research in the history of anxiety and anxiety disorders. Berrios (1996, 1997) has charted the different connotations of anxiety-related words in different countries in adult psychiatry, like in France *angoisse, anxiété, craintes, frayeurs*, and in Germany *Shrecken* and *Angst*.

Neve and Turner (2002) base their review on the history of child and adolescent psychiatry almost exclusively on English-language sources. They do not explain why they leave most of the French and German language sources unmentioned. Consequently, their review is somewhat unbalanced. However, in many countries there still is hardly any knowledge in the area at all. Contributions written in such languages as Hungarian, Russian, Swedish, or Arabic, reflecting psychiatry in the countries in which these languages are spoken, have not been discovered. This imbalance in the literature makes it difficult to generalize conclusions, because most of the literature is based almost exclusively on British, American, French, and German sources.

History of anxiety disorders in children and adolescents: general line of development

Attempts made to chart the history of psychiatric and psychosocial approaches to anxiety and anxiety disorders in children and adolescents are scarce. Even in publications on the history of child and adolescent psychiatry (e.g., Parry-Jones, 1994) anxiety disorders are only sparsely mentioned. The general line of development is as follows. Until the nineteenth century anxiety in children was a focus of attention mainly in the field of education. At the beginning of the nineteenth century – the period in which psychiatry developed into an independent discipline – anxiety in children was primarily regarded as a "vulnerability factor," which could later lead to the development of psychiatric problems. In the second half of the nineteenth century the contours of child and adolescent psychiatry became clearly defined. In this period, anxiety in children acquired the status of a psychiatric symptom and "disorder."

In the review that follows, which has no pretensions to exhaustiveness (though we tried our best to be as comprehensive as possible), we hope to shed light on the early history of conceptualizations of anxiety and its disorders in youth. In so doing, the review touches on conceptualizations of child and adolescent psychiatric disorders in general. We present these conceptualizations, because they appear relevant for anxiety disorders, which as such were described for the first time in the second half of the nineteenth century. Also worth noting is that during the times when these writings appeared, it was customary to use the masculine "he" or "his" only. To keep the original flavor of the writings we therefore retained this usage.

Literature up to the nineteenth century

The first set of writings that we could locate where mention was made of anxiety in children was in Hippocrates' (460–370 BC) *Aphorismes*. In his *Aphorismes*, Hippocrates reported fears as being among the illnesses of newborns and infants, as well as aphthae, vomiting, and night fears (*Aphorismes* 24). It would take a long time before anxiety in children would again come to be regarded as an "illness."

It was not until the Middle Ages that anxiety in children was again the focus of attention. Numerous "books of nurture" for parents and children remain from the Middle Ages. Wardle (1991) reported that on the basis of such "books of nurture," he was able to isolate descriptions of 108 child behavioral and emotional problems, including timidity, school refusal, and anxiety. There is no reason to suppose that education was generally hard in the Middle Ages. The following conclusion drawn by Shahar (1990) probably represents a reasonably accurate summary statement about the views of child-rearing in those times: "Since fear and dread cause melancholy, one should refrain, when rearing a child, from angering or saddening him. Nor should one act with excessive merriment. Everything should be done with moderation and in the proper proportion." (Shahar, 1990, p. 98).

This does not mean that there were no harsh measures used in child-rearing, such as physical punishment and frightening. DeMause (1974) and Shahar (1990) provide examples of the use of fearsome masked creatures or drawings as child-rearing techniques during this time. It is unlikely, though, that such practices were widespread, bearing in mind that approaches to child-rearing in the Middle Ages varied considerably, depending in large part on the period and the region. "Frightening" one's children could be a necessity in child-rearing, especially where religious education was involved, as fear was an important concept within the context of religious education. It is understandable that parents adhered strictly to the mores of the day, especially in times when "non-adherence to the teachings" was severely punished by the religious authorities.

In terms of care, in the Middle Ages the care of children with disorders was mainly in the hands of the Church. But also doctors were involved in treating illness in children and adolescents: there are numerous sources in Middle Ages literature, which could be regarded as the "first pediatric publications," such as *The Boke of Children* by the father of English pediatrics, Thomas Phaer (1545). In these publications sleep disorders, nightmares, enuresis, hysteria, and melancholia were treated (see reviews by Ruhräh [1925] and Demaitre [1977]). One of the few publications in which "fear" was addressed was the treatise on stammering by the Italian doctor Hieronymus Mercurialis (1583) in *De morbis puerorum*. The reason for stammering, in his opinion, could often be found in "affections of the mind." One of these affections was fear, as "is both clear from experience and confirmed by Aristotle and Galen . . . " (p. 227).

In the Middle Ages, psychiatric disorders were not viewed as diseases, but as manifestations of the works of the devil. Psychiatric patients were consigned to exorcists and many were burned as witches or wizards. These burnings also included psychiatrically disturbed children (Wessely & Wardle, 1990). The Dutchman Johann Weyer (1515–1588), the father of modern psychiatry (Stone, 1973), and one of the first authors in child psychiatry (e.g., Wier, 1563) played an important role in bringing the care of mental illness away from the clergy and back to the domain of doctors. He illustrated that what was considered as work of the devil was in fact illness or factitious disorder. In the seventeenth century, the idea that psychiatric disturbances were caused by satanic forces lost ground, although the Englishman Robert Burton, in his famous dissertation on melancholy (in that time referring to psychiatric illness in general), named "the power of Divels" as one of the causes of melancholy (Burton, 1621). Burton adopted a multicausal position, pointing to the role of inheritance, which was also manifested in the workings of the mind:

That other inbred cause of Melancholy, is our temperature [temperament] in whole or part, which wee receive from our parents . . . Such as the temperature of the fathers is, such is the sonnes; and looke what disease the father had when he begot him, such his son will have after him . . . Now this doth not so much appeare in the composition of the Body . . . but in manner and condition of the Minde . . . (pp. 96–97)

In addition, Burton identified education as a cause of melancholy:

Parents and such as have the tuition and oversight of children, offend many times in that they are too sterne, always threatening, children, brawling, whipping, or striking; by meanes of which their poore children are so disheartned & cowed that they never have any courage, or a merry houre in their lives, or take pleasure in any thing. . . . Others againe in that other extreame do as much harme. . . Too much indulgence causeth the like . . . (p. 97)

Thanks to the influence of the philosophers of the Enlightenment demonology lost influence. The burning of witches was forbidden in France by royal decree in 1680. Other countries followed in the eighteenth century (Ackerknecht, 1957). Gradually, the approach toward psychiatric patients became more humane. Impressive shifts also occurred in eighteenth-century psychiatry on a conceptual level. Specifically, Hippocratic explanations of psychiatric disorders in terms of disturbances of humoral equilibrium made way to explanations wherein the nervous system was at the center. Of particular note are the ideas of Franz Joseph Gall (1758–1828). This German scholar studied in Vienna, and later in Paris, the localization of psychic functions in brains and skulls. Gall also was interested in the brains and skulls of psychiatric patients. His most well-known pupil was Johann Spurzheim (1776–1832) who published a great deal about his *phrenological* investigations of psychiatric disorders.

At the same time psychological explanations for mental illness were gaining ground. In this context, much significance was attached to the *passions*, because *passions* – on the authority of the French doctor and philosopher Pierre Cabanis (1757–1808) in his *Rapports du physique et du moral de l'homme* (1802) – could have consequences in the physiological domain. Accordingly, the repertory of treatment modalities, in which bleeding still had an important position, was extended to *traitement moral* (moral treatment), a predecessor of psychotherapy. This initiative was especially stimulated by the French psychiatrist Philippe Pinel (1745–1826). It is said that he released the insane in the Bicêtre from their chains in 1795. In fact, Pinel himself notes that this was the idea of another psychiatrist in the hospital, Jean Baptiste Pussin (Harris, 2003). That does not alter the fact that Pinel played an important role in the humanization of psychiatry.

Another milestone around 1800 was the publication of a book wherein Jean Itard (1775–1838) gave an account of his endeavors to educate an *enfant sauvage* (feral child) (Itard, 1801). This description contributed to the identification of mentally handicapped children apart from psychiatrically disordered children and to the development of special facilities for mentally handicapped children in the nineteenth century.

Next we discuss the history of child and adolescent psychiatry in general in the first half of the nineteenth century, followed by a description of anxiety in this period. Next we discuss child and adolescent psychiatry and anxiety in the second half of the nineteenth century.

The first half of the nineteenth century

The contours of child and adolescent psychiatry

From around 1800 the first descriptions were published of children with "moral insanity," where "moral" may usually be interpreted as "psychic." Most case studies appeared in books on general psychiatry. Alexander Crichton (1798) published in his *An Inquiry into the Nature and Origin of Mental Derangement* the translation of a case study, published originally in 1781 by Johann Ernst Greding in Germany. The case concerned a boy, who at the age of 4 days:

Possessed so much strength in his legs and arms, that four women could, at times, with difficulty restrain him. These paroxysms either ended with an indescribable laughter, for which no evident reason could be observed, or else he tore in anger every thing near him; cloaths, linen, bed furniture, and even thread when he could get hold of it. We durst not allow him to be alone, otherwise he would get on the benches and tables, and even attempt to climb up the walls. Afterwards, however, when he began to have teeth, he fell into a general wasting or decline, and died. (in Crichton, 1798, pp. 354–356)

The case study of this little boy with its mythological forces would become the most quoted case in nineteenth-century child psychiatric literature.

Other early descriptions were published by Haslam in his *Observations on Madness and Melancholy* (1798; we unfortunately only got hold of the second edition in 1809), Pinel (1801) in *Traité médico-philosophique sur l'aliénation mentale, ou la manie*, and Perfect (1809) in *Annals of Insanity*. Perfect described an 11-year-old boy who in a short time developed many symptoms:

When spoken to, his answers were vague and inapposite; he seemed agitated at the sight of strangers; turned pale and trembled; had an angry, acute staring, look, with dilated pupils, and dreadful apprehensions that hurried him to examine every part of the room, as if he expected to find some person concealed who intended to do him a mischief. He sometimes appeared timid and distressed, sighed, shed tears, and had not a quarter of an hour's sleep throughout the night. (Perfect, 1809, p. 253)

Perfect gives an impression of the possible causes of the boy's symptoms:

And in this instance it is as singular, that there seems to have been no predisposing cause to insanity; no translation of diseased matter to the membranes of the brain, or any external cause that could mechanically operate to produce delirium; no diffusion of bile, sudden distention of cutaneous eruptions, absorption of matter from abscesses, wounds, or ulcers; no scrophulous or cancerous state of the juices; no worms, no deleterious medicine, nor mercurial preparations; no mental cause; nor could any hereditary claim be adduced of the patient's family, either on the father or mother's side, having ever been remembered to have been subject to maniacal affections. (Perfect, 1809, pp. 251–252)

Causes of psychiatric disturbance in children and adolescents

As illustrated by Perfect's considerations, organic causes, especially *brain disease*, was at the top of considered potential causes of psychiatric disturbance in children. There was general agreement in these days that *inheritance* played an important role in psychiatric problems. Adams (1814) showed a remarkable appreciation of the nuances involved. "*Madness*," he claimed, "as well as *gout*, is never *hereditary*, but in *susceptibility*" (cited in Hunter & Macalpine, 1963, p. 692). When a disposition was involved, only a trivial cause was needed to elicit the mental irritation for the outbreak of the disease:

But when the susceptibility amounts only to a predisposition, requiring the operation of some external cause to produce the disease, there is every reason to hope, that the action of the disease may be for the most part much lessened, if not prevented altogether. (Adams, 1814, cited in Hunter & Macalpine, 1963, p. 692)

Esquirol (1838), similarly, regarded heritability as the most general cause to mental illness. To underline this, he informed his readers that at the time he wrote *Des maladies mentales* he gave attention to several children whose parents he had treated in the first years of his career as a psychiatrist. In Esquirol's opinion, the disease could nevertheless be transferred in another way, from mother to child; that is, mothers who experienced strong emotions during pregnancy had children who at the slightest cause could become insane. Esquirol cited the French Revolution as an example of a time when this was a common phenomenon.

A relation also was drawn between insanity and upbringing. The Englishman James Parkinson, in his short paper on the excessive indulgence of children (Parkinson, 1807), illustrated the far-reaching effects that education and inconsistent child-rearing style could have:

On the treatment the child receives from his parents during the infantile stage of his life, will, perhaps, depend much of the misery or happiness he may experience, not only in, his passage through this, but through the other stages of his existence. (Parkinson, 1807, p. 468)

Another "mental cause" of mental disease in children mentioned in the literature of these days was education: the view that *schooling* – if begun too early or if too intensive – could be harmful to mental health was popular in the nineteenth century (e.g., Adams, 1814). Esquirol (1830) regarded excessive study as one of the causes of the supported increase in diseases of the mind: "The advance of civilization leads to a multiplicity of the insane" (p. 332). He was later more nuanced in his view, remarking that "it is not civilization, that we are to accuse, but the errors and excesses of all sorts, which it enables us to commit" (Esquirol, 1838, p. 42). Jarvis (1852) linked the presumed increase in mental illness in this period to "the improvements in the education of children and youth":

There are more and more of those whose love of knowledge, whose sense of duty, whose desire of gratifying friends, and whose ambition, impel them to make their utmost exertions, to become good scholars. Thus they task their minds unduly, and sometimes exhaust their cerebral energies and leave their brains a prey to other causes which derange them afterwards. (Jarvis, 1852, pp. 358–359)

Masturbation was another factor that was increasingly cited as a cause of psychiatric symptoms in both adults and youth (Hare, 1962; Neuman, 1975). The notion that masturbation was an important cause of mental illness was introduced in the eighteenth century and especially propagated by the Swiss doctor Tissot (1760). The explanation offered by Griesinger (1845) too mentions masturbation as a cause of insanity in children: on the link between masturbation and psychiatric symptoms was both succinct and "state of the art":

The cases of real mental disease in children appear to depend in part on an original irritability of the brain, or produced and maintained by injudicious treatment, partly on deeper organic diseases, partly from sympathetic irritation of the brain transmitted from the genital organs (onanism, approach and entrance of puberty). (Griesinger, 1845, pp. 108–109)

Assumptions about the limited prevalence of child psychiatric disturbances

In the first half of the nineteenth century, numerous authors discussed causes of the supposed limited prevalence of psychiatric disturbances in children. The American Benjamin Rush (1812), for example, had a clear standpoint:

The reason why children and persons under puberty are so rarely affected with madness must be ascribed to mental impressions, which are its most frequent cause, being too transient in their effects, from the instability of their minds, to excite their brains into permanently diseased actions. (Rush, 1812, p. 57)

The French phrenologist Spurzheim (1818), on the other hand, attributed the limited prevalence to the "extreme delicacy of their [children's] cerebral organization which would tend not to tolerate a serious illness without total loss of psychical faculties, or without grave danger to life itself" (p. 114). Esquirol (1838) also believed that mental illness had limited prevalence in childhood, "unless at birth the child suffers from some vice of conformation or convulsions, which occasion imbecility or idiocy" (p. 33). Although Esquirol had this view, he described a number of exceptions. Unlike Spurzheim, Esquirol regarded the limited prevalence of psychiatric disturbances in children as being due to the absence of passions in children:

Infancy, exempt from the influence of the passions, is almost a stranger to insanity; but at the epoch of puberty, the sentiments, unknown until this period, cause new wants to arise. Insanity then appears, to trouble the first moments of the moral existence of man. (Esquirol, 1838, p. 46)

The important role that Esquirol (1838) ascribed to the passions in psychiatric problems is clear in the following statement: "One of the moral causes pointed out by Pinel, and which is frequently met with in practice, is the conflict which arises between the principles of religion, morality, education and the passions" (p. 47). Internal conflict as a cause of mental illness had made its debut!

Course of illness

Occasionally a writer commented on the course of psychiatric illness in children. Adams (1814) suggested that some disturbances were "phase-related": "Sometimes we find the disease cease, as the changes of the constitution during that period are compleated" (p. 692). Esquirol (1838) approached the subject from a retrospective perspective: "Almost all the insane, presented before their sickness, certain functional changes; which extended back many years, even to earliest infancy" (p. 54). In the second edition of his *Mental Pathology and Therapeutics* Griesinger (1861), on the other hand, took a prospective approach: "Also after recovery such patients are much disposed to relapse; their mental health continues in danger during the whole of their lives, or they occasionally become, without being actually insane, owing to an unfavourable change in their whole character, useless for the world" (p. 144). Commenting on the influence of mental disorders on the psychological development of the child in general, Griesinger (1861) claimed: "It is a general characteristic of the mental disorders of childhood that they limit further mental development" (p. 143).

Anxiety

At the close of the eighteenth century, the article "On the different species of phobia" written by Benjamin Rush was published (Rush, 1798). In this ironic essay, Rush defined phobia as "a fear of an imaginary evil, or an undue fear of a real one" (p. 177). Rush not only discussed phobias in adults, but also referred to phobias in children, citing for example thunder phobia as one type ("This species is common to all ages, and to both sexes: I have seen it produce the most distressing appearances and emotions upon many people": p. 179) and ghost phobia ("This distemper is most common among servants and children . . .": p. 180). Rush's writing contains, to our knowledge, the first written description of phobic anxiety in children.

In 1812, Rush's *Medical Inquiries and Observations upon the Diseases of the Mind* was published. The wide fame this book enjoyed was probably due to a section on depression, in which Rush stated "depression of mind may be induced by causes that are forgotten, or by the presence of objects which revive the sensation of distress with which it was at one time associated, but without reviving the cause of it in the memory" (Rush, 1812, p. 46). The book also contained an extensive discussion of fear. In the section "On fear," Rush wrote: "There are so much danger and evil in our world, that the passion of fear was implanted in our minds for the wise and benevolent purpose of defending us from them" (p. 325). Rush distinguished between "reasonable" objects of fear, such as death, and "unreasonable" objects of fear, such as "thunder, darkness, ghosts, speaking in public, sailing, riding, certain animals, particularly cats, rats, insects, and the like" (p. 325). He offered several remedies for the fears found in childhood. For example, Rush's remedy for the fear of death was not to talk about it: "Boys obviate fear in like manner, by silence in passing by a grave-yard, or by conversing upon subjects unconnected with death" (p. 328).

Regarding remedies for unreasonable objects of fear, Rush focused on the importance of education and early preventive measures: "The fear which is excited by darkness may easily be overcome by a proper mode of education in early life. It consists in compelling children to go to bed without a candle, or without permitting company to remain with them until they fall a sleep" (p. 321). And the "fear from certain animals and insects, may all be cured by resolution. It should be counteracted in early life" (p. 332). In the discussion of treatment Rush joins the theory of associationism, which was widespread during that period (Murphy, 1949). Foreshadowing learning theory (see Field & Purkis, Chapter 11, this volume), associationism posited that mental and behavioral phenomena can be explained by means of the association of ideas.

Great advantages may likewise be derived for the cure of fear, by a proper application of the principle of association. A horse will seldom be moved by the firing of a gun, or the beating of a drum, if he hear them for the first time while he is eating; nor will he start, or retire from a wheelbarrow, or a millstone, or any object of that kind, after being once or twice led upon them. The same law of association may be applied in a variety of instances to the human mind, as well to the prevention, as cure, of fear. (Rush, 1812, p. 333)

Rush's interest in phobic fears is not representative: generally anxiety did not occupy a prominent place in the literature on psychiatry in the first half of the nineteenth century.

In a review of the history of anxiety in adult psychiatry, Berrios (1999) concluded that before the late nineteenth century symptoms of anxiety were found in accounts of diseases of the heart, ear, gut, and brain. Anxiety symptoms were treated as real physical complaints and were not part of psychiatry until the end of the nineteenth century. In child and adolescent psychiatry anxiety also had not attracted much attention in this era. Esquirol (1838) emphasized that the upbringing of children should not be fearful. He referred to strong impressions as a cause of disturbances in children, describing the intense fears that could be aroused. He did not regard the fear itself as a disturbance, but fear could form the basis of a mental illness that could arise later, at puberty. Esquirol (1838) described several cases to illustrate this view, including a 3-year-old boy who was:

> . . . frightened at the bears, exhibited . . . as a curiosity. From that time, he was subject to frightful dreams, and at seventeen years of age, he was seized with mania. A girl, six years of age, sees her father massacred, and has since been subject to panic terrors. At fourteen . . . she becomes a maniac. She wishes to rush upon every body. The sight of a knife or a weapon, or of many men assembled, excites her to the most violent fury. (Esquirol, 1838, p. 50)

Anxiety was thus viewed by Esquirol as a vulnerability, that is, as a point from which psychopathology could develop. Griesinger (1861) referred to anxiety in relation to melancholy in children in a similar way: "Simple melancholic states also present themselves, whose foundation is a general feeling of anxiety" (p. 143).

In the first half of the nineteenth century we find the first descriptions of obsessive compulsive symptoms in adults, by Esquirol (1838). The understanding and classification of obsessive disorder was a problem for alienists, the designation of psychiatrists at the time, as this disorder did not fit well with concepts of insanity at the time (Berrios, 1985, 1989). This applied especially for the patients' awareness that their symptoms were bizarre. The disorder was placed under different headings, depending on the authors' view whether obsessions were primarily a volitional, intellectual, or emotional disorder. We did not identify descriptions of obsessive disorder in children and adolescents before 1850.

The second half of the nineteenth century

The birth of child and adolescent psychiatry as a discipline

Although small in number, the pages in Griesinger's handbook devoted to psychiatric disturbances in youth served as the impetus for a growing number of case studies, articles, and chapters on the topic in the second half of the nineteenth century. In these decades, child and adolescent psychiatry began to acquire the form of a specific discipline. Authors were generally familiar with the work of their predecessors, which they used as a springboard for their own ideas. Articles appeared in which current knowledge was brought together. In 1860, a young medical student, James Crichton-Browne, published a review of the state of the art in child and adolescent psychiatry at that moment. The British doctor Charles West, regarded as the founder of modern pediatrics, contributed to child and adolescent psychiatry. It is likely that both Crichton-Browne (Wardle, 1991) and West were a source of inspiration for Maudsley, who, in 1867, published *The Physiology and Pathology of the Mind*. This handbook contained a separate chapter on child and adolescent psychiatry.

Another landmark in the history of child psychiatry was a comprehensive chapter by the German psychiatrist Hans Emminghaus devoted entirely to child and adolescent psychiatry, which appeared in an 1887 handbook on pediatrics. A monograph by the Frenchman Moreau (de Tours) (1888) followed a year later. In 1890, the American Spitzka included a chapter on "insanity" in a pediatric manual. This was followed by another comprehensive publication by Manheimer (1899), who in the title of his book was the first to refer to *child psychiatry*: "*Les Troubles mentaux de l'enfance: précis de psychiâtrie infantile*" (cf. Walk, 1964).

Based on our reading of these publications, we offer the following general summary. First, views on the causes of psychiatric problems in children and adolescents began to be more finely differentiated. The importance attached to *hereditary factors*, referred to by Mannheimer as the "cause of causes," continued to be strong. However, in views on the contribution of hereditary factors, the emphasis shifted away from the hereditary determination of illness to the hereditary determination of temperament. For example, in terms of a "nervous temperament" or a "neuropathic temperament," almost all of the authors treated heredity not as a single entity but in relation to environmental influences. Only in exceptional cases was the influence of heredity as such considered inescapable, for example, when the mother was mentally ill during pregnancy (e.g., Savage, 1881).

Many authors were inspired by the pessimistic view set forth by Morel (1857) in his *Traité des dégénérescences physiques, intellectuelles et morales de l'espèce humaine*. According to Morel, many circumstances could induce degeneration, which by inheritance in a few generations could result in the extinction of the line. So we read in Maudsley's *The Physiology and Pathology of the Mind*:

> . . . *in the child born with a strong predisposition to insanity there is a want of [the] pre-established harmony between the individual constitution and external nature: the morbid creature devours with eager appetite the greatest trash, and rakes out the fire with its fingers; it desires passionately and frantically struggles for what is detrimental to it, and rejects or destroys what is suitable, and should, were it rightly constituted, be agreeable; it loves nothing but destructive and vicious acts, which are the expressions of an advanced degradation, and hates what would further its development, and is necessary to its existence as a social being.* (Maudsley, 1867, pp. 289–290)

In addition to hereditary factors, an *illness in one of the parents* (e.g., lead poisoning, alcoholism, syphilis) (Clevenger, 1883), drunkenness in the parents at conception (Mannheimer, 1899), *illness in the mother during pregnancy and obstetric complications* (e.g., use of forceps) (Clevenger, 1883) were described as causes of child psychiatric problems. Under the influence of developments in pediatrics, the number of descriptions of psychiatric disturbances in relation to *pediatric illnesses* increased (Cohn, 1883; Emminghaus, 1887).

Intensive schooling continued to be regarded as a factor contributing to mental illness: "Education conducted with school honors as the object to be worked for, causes mental overstrain, and is a potent exciting cause" (Clevenger, 1883, p. 600) (cf. Hurd, 1894; Manheimer, 1899). Likewise for upbringing: "Insanity in children [is] practically always hereditary, though bad bringing up might largely conspire with [the] original tendency to produce the result" (Albutt, 1889, p. 131).

In this period, there were two British authors who we believe were ahead of their time in terms of their ideas about the *interaction between parents and child* in relation to child psychiatric problems: West and Savage. Some of their views foreshadow a number of the ideas expressed by Creswell, Murray, Stacey, and Cooper (Chapter 14, this volume). West's (1860, 1871) fame was partly due to his description of "the contribution of the parents" in the continuation of "feigned diseases" (we would probably today speak of somatoform diseases in these cases), and to his recognition of the inability of the parents of these children to provide limits. Perhaps even more advanced was Savage's (1881) hypothesis that "parental style" was partially influenced by the temperament of the child:

I would most emphatically state my belief that very many so-called spoiled children are nothing more or less than children who are morally of unsound mind, and that the spoiled child owes quite as much to his inheritance as to his education. In many cases, doubtless, the parent who begets a nervous child is very likely to further spoil such child by bad or unsuitable education. (Savage, 1881, p. 148)

As in the first half of the nineteenth century, *masturbation* was often cited in the second half of the century as a cause of psychiatric problems in youth. An independent disorder was even suggested, namely "masturbatory insanity" (Maudsley, 1868), which refers probably to hebephrenic dementia praecox or schizophrenia (Hare, 1962). A few decades later, however, authors began to have reservations about the feasibility of a relation between masturbation and mental illness. The German doctor Cohn (1883) remarked that "onanism in a moderate degree is such a widespread ill, especially during puberty, that if it really did have a seriously dangerous influence, the number of mentally ill would take on enormous proportions" (p. 41). At the end of the nineteenth century European authors began to expressly avoid a too rigorous position on the matter (e.g., Maudsley, 1895). In the United States, however, the "masturbatory hypothesis" continued to hold ground for a longer time (e.g., Spitzka, 1890). In 1924 G. Stanley Hall devoted in his opus magnum *Adolescence* 39 pages to masturbation, "one of the very saddest of all the aspects of human weakness and sin . . ." (Hall, 1924, p. 432).

Anxiety and anxiety disorders in child and adolescent psychiatry

Charles West's *On the Mental Peculiarities and Mental Disorders of Childhood* can be viewed as revolutionary. In this essay he gave a central position to the experiential world of the child, and, in particular, to the "imagination" (West, 1860). He illustrated his claims with a realistic description of the experience of anxiety in children:

The child lives at first in the external world, as if it were but a part of himself, or he a part of it . . . The child who dreads to be alone, and asserts that he hears sounds or perceives objects, is not expressing merely a vague apprehension of some unknown danger, but often tells a literal truth. The sounds have been heard; in the stillness of its nursery, the little one has listened to what seemed a voice calling it; or, in the dark, phantasms have risen before its eyes, and the agony of terror with which it calls for a light, or begs for its mother's presence betrays an impression far too real to be explained away, or to be suitably met by hard words or by unkind treatment. (West, 1860, p. 133)

It is likely that Maudsley's (1895) later description of childhood anxiety was inspired by West's writings:

It is difficult for grown-up persons, unless perchance helped by a hateful memory of their own terrors in childhood, to realise the terrible agonies of fright and anguish, which seize some nervous children when they are alone in the dark, or are left by themselves in a large room, or have to pass a room or closet of which they have conceived some formless dread, or are sent alone on a strange errand. (Maudsley, 1895, p. 375)

To the best of our knowledge we owe the first description of anxiety disorders in children to James Crichton-Browne (1860):

Pantophobia is another form of mental disease common in infancy and childhood. It is usually associated with, perhaps dependent upon, cardiac disease. It consists in an exalted or diseased state of the instinct of self-preservation, is often accompanied by delusions, and may occasion such intense misery, that suicide is resorted to as a means of relief. Night terrors, so common young children, are a transient species of pantophobia.... We are acquainted with a boy, who, during infancy, was subject to night terrors, and who, at the age of twelve, and for many succeeding years, was frequently attacked by pantophobia. The attacks were always introduced by palpitation, and characterized by the most intense, yet unaccountable, dread, by loss of identity, and by trembling over the whole body. (Crichton-Browne, 1860, pp. 312–313)

A few years later, Strack (1863) published a description of a 13-year-old girl in whom "precordial anxiety" was brought to the fore as a psychiatric symptom. A number of other case studies followed in which anxiety was a prominent symptom of the children (King, 1880; Savage in the discussion of Albutt, 1899; von Rinecker, 1876). (In scientific literature of these days it was usual to publish the papers in journals with a report of the discussion by the audience.)

As far as we can surmise, Emminghaus (1887) was the first to suggest a relation between anxiety and temperament characteristics – a prelude to the "behavioral inhibition" concept described by Lonigan, Phillips, Wilson, and Allan (Chapter 10, this volume). He wrote of "fearfulness and anxiety as individual predispositions to emotional disorders . . . " (p. 53). Fright, which he regarded as the most common psychic cause of mental disturbances, only led to mental illness if such a predisposition was present. Maudsley (1895), too, drew links between anxiety in children and a "neuropathic temperament":

One little creature used to shriek in an ecstasy of fright whenever another child or dog approached it in the street, yet exulted with a frenzy of delight in a strong wind, no matter how violent; another would go straight up to any strange dog which it met and take instant hold of it, without the least apprehension, never coming to harm by its fearless behavior. (Maudsley, 1895, p. 370)

In his systematic discussion of symptomatology in child psychiatry, *Anomalies of the Feelings*, Emminghaus (1887) also became the first to afford anxiety (*Angor*) a significant role in mental illness. He regarded anxiety, cowardice, and nervousness as pathological only "if they were present as new behavior in the child in addition to other signs of a psychic disorder . . . " (p. 70). One symptom of anxiety was "fear of being alone, especially in the dark, of sleeping alone." This fear, which mainly occurred in young children, by such events as hearing terrifying stories by servants, could continue through childhood. Emminghaus (1887) called anxiety "practically the most common elementary, psychic symptom," because it was characteristic of so many diseases, including "both organic and functional brain diseases" (p. 70).

Emminghaus further noted that milder forms of anxiety in children could be manifested in a number of forms, consisting mainly of impulsive actions, such as apparently cheerful whistling, the imitation of animal noises, naughty behavior, and over-affectionate behavior, especially towards the mother. He called these types of behavior "the masks of anxiety," a concept derived from a publication by the adult psychiatrist Dick (1877). Dick's statement that anxiety "could hide behind a thousand masks," led Emminghaus to the astute observation that "accurate evidence for this will probably be difficult to produce" (Emminghaus, 1887, p. 72).

Finally, Emminghaus (1887) referred to "spontaneous anxiety," which, he said, arose without any recognizable cause, and in the absence of any psychic indications. In describing this form of anxiety, which in his opinion was always pathological, he probably gave the first description of a panic attack. Maudsley (1895) also described panic attacks in adolescents:

. . . singular nervous crises which befall persons who cannot cross an open place or square, being seized with an overwhelming panic of impotence at the bare thought or attempt to cross . . . a reeling of thought and feeling, an indescribable anguish, as if the foundation of self were sinking away . . . (Maudsley, 1895, pp. 409–410)

One finds descriptions of obsessive compulsive symptoms in children in the second half of the nineteenth century (e.g., Moreau (de Tours), 1888). Maudsley's exhaustive description of these symptoms in adolescents (Maudsley, 1895, pp. 407–409) would not be out of place in a modern handbook! Maudsley (1895) attributed (both) panic attacks (and obsessive–compulsive symptoms) to "self-abuse" in adolescents who had a "high-strung neurotic temperament"; at the same time though he was able to place the role of masturbation within a reasonable better perspective: "To conclude self-abuse to be the exciting cause in every case would be to conclude wrongly and to do wrong to the sufferer" (p. 411).

Other opinions also were formulated on the pathogenesis of panic disorders. Emminghaus (1887) took as his starting point the notion of the adult psychiatrist Arndt. Arndt (1874) suggested that the feeling of anxiety could be traced to an abnormal movement of the heart, which, due to abnormally sensitive sensory nerves, was able to be perceived and brought to consciousness. Emminghaus argued differently, claiming that heart activity could remain unchanged with anxiety and that sometimes anxiety could occur with heart disease, and sometimes not. He had no doubt that the root cause of anxiety lay in processes in the cerebral cortex. Maudsley (1895), taking a comparable standpoint, formulated a type of "cognitive hypothesis" about panic attacks:

. . . children of four or five years, sprung from a very neurotic stock, may have fits of moaning melancholy and apprehensive fears which, but for their neuropathic inheritance, might seem quite out of keeping with their tender age and to be inexplicable aberrations of nature. (Maudsley, 1895, p. 379)

In melancholic adolescents, also:

. . . morbid suspicions and fears ensue: fears and fancies of having done something wrong or of being suspected of wrong-doing, of not being loved by parents, of being disliked and spoken ill of by companions, or being watched and followed in the streets . . . (Maudsley, 1895, pp. 393–394)

Classification

The professionalization taking place in the field of child and adolescent psychiatry also was evident in the first attempts at classification (Cohn, 1883; Emminghaus, 1887; Maudsley, 1867; Moreau (de Tours), 1888). Anxiety disorders were included for the first time in the classificatory system of child psychiatry of Cohn (1883). In Cohn's system obsessive–compulsive disorders were given a relatively minor place. Under the heading "real psychoses," beside categories such as melancholy and mania, Cohn included the category "madness" (*Verrücktheit*), which referred to delusional disorders. Obsessions and compulsive behavior were seen as an "abortive form" of these disorders.

Moreau (de Tours) (1888), in his "Etude des formes" (under "Exaltation psychique," which was part of "Formes purement morales") gave anxiety the status of a disorder: "Like all psychic disturbances, and in certain cases, anxiety must be regarded as a real sickness" (p. 191). The "spores of devastation [of anxiety attacks in children] may remain up to an advanced age, and sometimes throughout the person's entire life" (p. 192).

Treatment

The main method advocated in the treatment of psychiatric disorders was pharmacotherapy. On the whole psychiatrists prescribed to children the medicines that were in use for adults. Some of these medicines were not harmless at all (e.g., morphine, hyoscamine). Psychiatrists sometimes report their experience with specific medicines in more or less circumscribed groups of patients. But generally the medicines were widely used. So it is not astonishing that Clevenger (1883) in his survey of the etiology of psychiatric disorders in non-adults remarked: "The toxicants, stramonium, opium, chloral, hyoscamus, santonin, and alcohol, produce acute curable disorders" (p. 601). Some authors specifically mentioned how they treated children with likely anxiety disorders. For example, the persistent anxiety attacks of the girl described by Strack (1863) disappeared after a lengthy treatment with opium. von Rinecker (1876) treated his patient with cannabis. His experience led him to conclude that "Indian hemp as a medicinal remedy has a future in psychiatry" (p. 565).

Occasionally, an anxiety disorder necessitated residential treatment. Clevenger (1883) reported the case of a 10-year-old boy who was admitted to an asylum for "pyrophobia." Manheimer (1899) presented the most detailed description of the time of treatment of anxiety, agitation, and insomnia in children. He mentioned pharmacological remedies, such as linden-blossom tea and orange-blossom water, hypnotics, the various bromides, ether syrup, laurel cherry water, belladonna tincture, chloral and trional, and hydrotherapy (e.g., tepid baths, or bran baths, preferably just before retiring). He also pointed out that psychological treatment – verbal suggestion, reasoning (*raisonnement*), and persuasion – can be effective, as well as hypnotic suggestion in severe cases.

Contributions from psychology and other sciences

In his *Historical Introduction to Modern Psychology* Murphy (1949) concluded that the final decades of the nineteenth century witnessed the appearance of the first systematic and serious publications in the field of child psychology. Interest in child development was strongly influenced by Darwin's theory of evolution. In 1877, Darwin published the observations he had made 37 years earlier on one of his children. On the basis of his observation on fear he remarked:

May we not suspect that the vague but very real fears of children, which are quite independent of experience, are the inherited effects of real dangers and abject superstitions during ancient savage times? It is quite conformable with what we know of the transmission of formerly well-developed characters, that they should appear at an early period of life, and afterwards disappear. (Darwin, 1877, p. 285)

Darwin had a strong influence on Preyer, whose publication *Die Seele des Kindes* (The Mind of the Child) (Preyer, 1882) described development during the early years of life. In the section on fear (*Furcht*) Preyer reflected on why young children were afraid of unfamiliar things: "Why is it that many children are afraid of cats and dogs, before they are aware of the dangerous qualities of these animals?" (p. 104). (It is interesting that Tiedemann

[1787], in his first known "baby biography" [*Beobachtungen über die Entwickelung der Selenfähigkeiten bei Kindern*] made no mention of anxiety.) Following Darwin, Preyer attributed the many fears of children to an "inherited fearfulness," or an "inborn memory," a kind of an ethological explanation. Sully (1895), professor in London and the first scholar to conduct systematic research on the development of normal children, did not share this viewpoint of an "inborn memory." With respect to his observation that very young children were generally afraid of noises, he took a physiological viewpoint, describing the fear as "an organic phenomenon, with a sort of jar to the nervous system" (p. 197). Later in development, he argued, the fear of visual impression arose, but this was "Called forth by the presentation of something new and strange, especially when it involves a rupture of customary arrangements" (p. 199). In his referral to the balance between fear and curiosity Sully adopted a "modern" ethological approach: "It is only . . . when attachment to human belongings has been developed, that the approach of a stranger, especially if accompanied by a proposal to take the child, calls forth clear signs of displeasure and the shrinking away of fear" (p. 201). However, "the most prolific excitant of fear, the presentation of something new and uncanny, is also provocative of another feeling, that of curiosity, with its impulse to look and examine" (p. 224).

At the end of the nineteenth century, two pioneers in psychological research, Alfred Binet and Stanley Hall, conducted several studies on anxiety in children (Binet, 1895; Hall, 1897). These studies were mainly based on information obtained from a large number of checklists. Respondents included for the most part teachers (Binet), and children and adolescents (Hall) about sources of children's anxiety. Seen through a modern lens, the methodology of these studies is of course "loose." Binet (1895) sent about 250 questionnaires to teachers – not at random but only to an élite of the most intelligent and diligent teachers. He also interviewed acquaintances and observed the children in their families and his own family. Hall (1897) published a syllabus in several educational journals. To give an example of his material ("the records of the chief fears of 1,701 people," p. 151) the next quote is illustrative:

Miss Lillie A. Williams, head of psychology at the Trenton, N.J., Normal School, sent reports by 461 persons, of which 118 were original, 163 reminiscence, 75 hearsay. The reminiscences averaged six or seven pages of note paper each. The other 105 were compositions on their fears, past and present, by girls from 5 to 18. (Hall, 1897, p. 150)

More important than these studies' results were their conclusions and the ideas they generated. Both Binet and Hall noted individual differences among children in the degree to which they developed anxious behavior. In regard to the heritability of anxiety, Binet concluded, that it was difficult to reach a conclusion! Specifically, he wrote:

. . . there have been various examples reported of anxious parents having children who are just as anxious as the parents. In the absence of careful observations these reports do not prove much because it is possible that the parents have transferred their own characteristics to their children by means of another route than inheritance, for example through upbringing. (Binet, 1895, p. 244)

Binet discussed in detail the anxiety resulting from poor treatment from parents and how parents may react to their child's anxiety, emphasizing the importance of instilling self-confidence in children. In contrast, Hall (1897) claimed that "a childhood too happy and careless and fearless is a calamity so great that prayer against it might stand in the old service book beside the petition that our children be not poltroons" (Hall, 1897, p. 243).

Hall explained the capacity for fear in evolutionary terms:

As infants, although they cannot speak, yet, unlike apes, have a capacity to be taught language, so we must assume the capacity to fear or to anticipate pain, and to associate it with certain objects and experiences, as to an inherited *Anlage*, often of a far higher antiquity than we are wont to appeal to in psychology. (Hall, 1897, p. 245)

He placed the anxiety study in the context of "exploring feelings, instinct and the rich mines of unconsciousness just opening" (p. 246) and "the full scope of the more basal fears rarely come to expression in consciousness, but only partial aspects of them" (p. 247). This quotation reflects Hall's strong interest in the ideas of European psychiatrists such as Charcot, Bernheim, and Janet (Ross, 1972), who also were all sources of inspiration for Freud. In 1909, at the invitation of Hall, Freud made a visit to the United States. In the same year, with the publication of "Little Hans," an influential chapter was added to the literature on anxiety disorders in children.

Concluding comments

Before the nineteenth century, scant attention was paid to fear and anxiety in children in the psychological and medical literature. This scant attention was probably related in part to the high degree of social cohesion that existed prior to the nineteenth century, with religion playing a particularly prominent role. This social cohesion also helped to contribute to enhanced feelings of self-confidence and certainty among individuals. The emphasis on individualization that followed from the Industrial Revolution, which took place during the course of the nineteenth century, contributed however to heightened sensibilities concerning anxiety. A generalized image of the self disappeared, and individual experience received a new meaning: experienced reality was also reality. It was in this climate that Kierkegaard, in 1844, published his essay *The Concept of Anxiety* (Kierkegaard, 1844). The emphasis on individual experience was reflected as well in how anxiety began to be viewed with respect to mental health: articles appeared in which anxiety as a symptom of disorder was the focus (Flemming, 1848).

In the medical literature on childhood anxiety, West (1860) describing anxiety from the perspective of the individual child, constituted a turning point. The fact that anxiety was now "discovered" in children was probably also related to rising concern about the position of the child. One avenue of expression for this concern was in legislation in the area of child labor (Parry-Jones, 1994). Increasing attention for the position of children also was reflected in the establishment of children's hospitals. In 1860 the first report of non-phobic anxiety disorder in a child was published (Crichton-Browne, 1860).

In the last decades of the nineteenth century tremendous strides were made with respect to thinking about anxiety. Concepts that had been touched on by individual authors in previous centuries – heredity and temperament, upbringing, masturbation, learning at school, and life events – became the subject of careful and systematic thought. Also, thinking about these concepts began to move away from relatively simple views to more complex views – views in which the complex interplay of the various concepts was emphasized. For example, anxiety and its disorders began to be viewed as the result of interaction between life events and temperamental factors (e.g., Emminghaus, 1887).

In other respects too behavior was increasingly approached in a scientific way. Ideas on the "pathogenesis" of anxiety disorders were a prelude to the first scientific conceptualizations of the emotions (e.g., James, 1884). Another example of a scientific approach is the developments of the first systems of diagnostic classification in psychiatry, and child and adolescent psychiatry. In the descriptions of anxiety disorders, phobias can be recognized, as well as indications of generalized anxiety disorders and avoidance disorders. It is notable that in the literature prior to 1900 there were no strong indications of separation anxiety disorders. Bowlby (1973) pointed out that Freud's first mention of separation disorder was not until 1905; and it was not until 1926 that he devoted systematic attention to the subject. Bowlby further pointed out that Freud (1909) gave little consideration to the "true" fear of little Hans, namely, that his mother might desert the family.

Only about half a century after its entrance in psychiatry and psychology, anxiety became a central concept in psychoanalytic theory, which influenced psychiatry and psychology in the twentieth century deeply for decades. In psychoanalytic theory interest in manifest anxiety receded into the background: the interest was especially in anxiety as the supposed mediator for psychopathology in general. In the words of Klein (1981): "The predominant American psychiatric theory in 1959 was that all psychopathology was secondary to anxiety, which in turn was caused by intrapsychic conflict" (p. 235).

Since the 1960s, with the emergence of scientific research in psychopharmacology, neurobiology, and behavioral sciences interest in observable anxiety and anxiety disorders returned. It is fascinating that after such a long interruption the "old" issues (e.g., the significance of heredity, temperament, upbringing) have been put back on the scientific agenda by these disciplines. Thus, insofar as areas of scientific attention are inspired by world-views (Reese & Overton, 1970), it would seem that our world-views in about 100 years have changed less than one might suspect. However, there are some important differences that have come about. The view of masturbation as a "cause" of psychopathology has been abandoned totally, as has the view that learning at school generally contributes to the occurrence of psychopathology.

Moreover, "newer" concepts or issues appear to have come more to the forefront in the last decades of the twentieth century. For example, the meaning of "cognition" in emotion and in emotional disorders, touched upon at the end of the nineteenth century, was articulated much more in the last decades. Bowlby took up the thread of ethology, and placed the significance of experiences in early childhood for later development in a completely different perspective than had been done by Freud. Thinking in terms of causality made room for transactional or contextual processes. Further, the context has been extended to include not only familial but also the child within the context of his peer group.

References

Ackerknecht, E. H. (1957). *Kurze Geschichte der Psychiatrie*. Stuttgart: Ferdinand Enke Verlag.

Adams, J. (1814). *A Treatise on the Supposed Hereditary Properties of Diseases, Particularly in Madness and Scrofula*. London: Callow. [In Hunter & Macalpine, 1963, pp. 691–692.]

Albutt, C. (1889). Insanity of children. *Journal of Mental Science*, **35**, 130–135.

Ariès, P. (1960). *L'Enfant et la vie familiale sous l'Ancien Régime*. Paris: Editions du Seuil.

Arndt, R. G. (1874). Über den melancholischen Angstanfall. *Allgemeine Zeitschrift für Psychiatrie*, **30**, 88–99.

Berrios, G. E. (1985). Obsessional disorders during the nineteenth century: terminological and classificatory issues. In: **W. F. Bynum, R. Porter, & M. Shepard** (eds.) *Anatomy of Madness*, vol. 1, pp. 166–187. London: Tavistock.

Berrios, G. E. (1989). Obsessive–compulsive disorder: its conceptual history in France during the nineteenth century. *Comprehensive Psychiatry*, **30**, 282–295.

Berrios, G. E. (1996). *The History of Mental Symptoms: Descriptive Psychopathology since the Nineteenth Century*. Cambridge, UK: Cambridge University Press.

Berrios, G. E. (1997). History of treatment options for anxiety disorders. In: **J. A. den Boer** (ed.) *Clinical Management of Anxiety*, pp. 1–21. New York: Marcel Dekker.

Berrios, G. (1999). Anxiety disorders: a conceptual history. *Journal of Affective Disorders*, **56**, 83–94.

Binet, A. (1895). La peur chez les enfants. *L'Année Psychologique*, **2**, 223–254.

Bowlby, J. (1973). *Separation: Anxiety and Anger*. London: Hogarth Press.

Burton, R. (1621). *The Anatomy of Melancholy, What It Is, With All the Kinds, Causes, Symptomes, Prognostickes, and Several Cures of It*. Oxford, UK: Cripps. [In Hunter & Macalpine, 1963, pp. 94–99.]

Cabanis, P. (1802). *Rapports du physique et du moral de l'homme*. Paris: Crapart, Caille et Ravier.

Clevenger, S. V. (1883). Insanity in children. *American Journal of Neurology and Psychiatry*, **2**, 585–601.

Cohn, M. (1883). Über die Psychosen im kindlichen Alter. *Archiv für Kinderheilkunde*, **4**, 28–64; 101–107.

Crichton, A. (1798). *An Inquiry into the Nature and Origin of Mental Derangement, Comprehending a Concise System of the Physiology and Pathology of the Human Mind*. London: T. Cadell, junior, and W. Davies.

Crichton-Browne, J. (1860). Psychical diseases of early life. *Journal of Mental Science*, **6**, 284–320.

Darwin, C. (1877). A biographical sketch of an infant. *Mind*, **2**, 285–294. (Supplement no. 24 to *Developmental Medicine and Child Neurology*, **13**, 1971.)

Demaitre, L. (1977). The idea of childhood and child care in medical writings of the Middle Ages. *Journal of Psychohistory*, **4**, 461–491.

DeMause, L. (1974). The evolution of childhood. In **L. DeMause** (ed.) *The History of Childhood*, pp. 1–73. London: Souvenir Press.

Dick, H. (1877). Die Angst der Kranken. *Allgemeine Zeitschrift für Psychiatrie*, **33**, 230–235.

Durand-Fardel, M. (1855). Etude sur le suicide chez les enfants. *Annales Médico-Psychologiques*, **1**, 61–79.

Emminghaus, H. (1887). *Die psychische Störungen des Kindesalters*. Tübingen: Verlag H. Laupp'schen.

Esquirol, J. E. D. (1830). Remarques sur la statistique des aliénés. *Annales de Hygiène*, **4**, 332–359.

Esquirol, J. E. D. (1838). *Des maladies mentales, considérées sous les rapports médical, hygiénique et médico-légal*. Paris: Baillière. [English translation: *Mental Maladies: A Treatise on Insanity*, a facsimile of the English edition of 1845 with an introduction by Raymond de Saussure. New York: Hafner, 1965.]

Farwell, J. R., Lee, Y. J., Hirtz, D. G., Sulzbacher, S. I., Ellenberg, J. H., & **Nelson, K. B.** (1990). Phenobarbital for febrile seizures: effects on intelligence and seizure recurrence. *New England Journal of Medicine*, **322**, 364–369.

Flemming, C. F. (1848). Über Precordialangst. *Allgemeine Zeitschrift für Psychiatrie*, **5**, 341–361.

Freud, S. (1909). Analysis of a phobia in a five-year-old boy. In: *The Standard Edition of the Complete Works of Sigmund Freud*, 7th edn, vol. 10, pp. 5–149. London: Hogarth Press.

Garmezy, N. & **Rutter, M.** (1985). Acute reactions to stress. In: **M. Rutter** & **L. Hersov** (eds.) *Child and Adolescent Psychiatry*, 2nd edn, pp. 152–176. Oxford, UK: Blackwell Scientific Publications.

Griesinger, W. (1845). *Die Pathologie und Therapie der psychischen Krankheiten*. Stuttgart: Adolph Krabbe.

Griesinger, W. (1861). *Die Pathologie und Therapie der psychischen Krankheiten*, 2nd edn. Braunschweig: Friedrich Wreden. [English edition (1867) *Mental Pathology and Therapeutics*. London: The New Sydenham Society; facsimile edition New York: Hafner, 1965.]

Hall, G. S. (1897). A study of fears. *American Journal of Psychology*, **8**, 147–249.

Hall, G. S. (1924). *Adolescence: Its Psychology and Its Relations to Physiology, Anthropology, Sociology, Sex, Crime, Religion, and Education*. New York: Appleton.

Hare, E. H. (1962). Masturbatory insanity: the history of an idea. *Journal of Mental Science*, **108**, 1–25.

Harris, J. C. (2003). Pinel orders the chains removed from the insane at Bicêtre. *Archives of General Psychiatry*, **60**, 442.

Haslam, J. (1809). *Observations on Madness and Melancholy: Including Practical Remarks on those Diseases, together with Cases, and an Account of the Morbid Appearances on Dissection*, 2nd edn. London: J. Callow. [Reprinted New York: Arno Press, 1976.]

Hippocrates (1844). *Aphorisms*, trans. E. Littré. Paris: J.-B. Baillière.

Hunter, R. & Macalpine, I. (1963). *Three Hundred Years of Psychiatry 1535–1860*. London: Oxford University Press.

Hurd, H. M. (1894). Some mental disorders of childhood and youth. *Boston Medical and Surgical Journal*, **131**, 281–285.

Itard, J. M. G. (1801). *De l'éducation d'un homme sauvage, ou, des premiers développements physiques et moreaux du jeune sauvage de l'Aveyron*. Paris: Goujon Fils.

James, W. (1884). What is an emotion? *Mind*, **9**, 188–205.

Jarvis, E. (1852). On the supposed increase of insanity. *Journal of Insanity*, **8**, 333–364.

Kempe, C. H., Silverman, F. N., Steele, B. F., Droegemueller, W., & Silver, H. K. (1962). The battered-child syndrome. *Journal of the American Medical Association*, **181**, 17–24.

Kierkegaard, S. (1844). *The Concept of Anxiety: A Simple Psychologically Orienting Deliberation on the Dogmatic Issue of Hereditary Sin*. [Reprinted Princeton, NJ: Princeton University Press, 1980.]

King, W. P. (1880). Case of morbid juvenile pyrophobia caused by malarial toxhaemia. *The Alienist and Neurologist*, **1**, 345–347.

Klein, D. F. (1981). Anxiety reconceptualized. In: D. F. Klein & J. Rabkin (eds.) *Anxiety: New Research and Changing Concepts*, pp. 235–263. New York: Raven Press.

Kroll, J. & Bachrach, B. (1986). Child care and child abuse in early medieval Europe. *Journal of the American Academy of Child Psychiatry*, **25**, 562–568.

Labbé, J. (2005). Ambroise Tardieu: the man and his work on child maltreatment a century before Kempe. *Child Abuse and Neglect*, **29**, 311–324.

Manheimer, M. (1899). *Les Troubles mentaux de l'enfance: précis de psychiâtrie infantile, avec les applications pédagogiques et médico-légales*. Paris: Société d'éditions scientifiques.

Maudsley, H. (1867). *The Physiology and Pathology of the Mind*. London: Macmillan.

Maudsley, H. (1868). Illustrations of a variety of insanity. *Journal of Mental Science*, **14**, 149–162.

Maudsley, H. (1895). *The Pathology of Mind: A Study of its Distempers, Deformities, and Disorders*. London: Macmillan.

Mercurialis, H. (1583). *De morbis puerorum*. Venice. [In Ruhräh, 1925, pp. 221–236.]

Moreau (de Tours), P. (1888). *La Folie chez les enfants*. Paris: J.-B. Baillière.

Morel, B. A. (1857). *Traité des dégénérescences physiques, intellectuelles et morales de l'espèce humaine et des causes qui produisent ces variétés maladaptives*. Paris: J.-B. Baillière.

Murphy, G. (1949). *Historical Introduction to Modern Psychology*, 5th edn. London: Routledge & Kegan Paul.

Neuman, R. P. (1975). Masturbation, madness, and the modern concepts of childhood and adolescence. *Journal of Social History*, **8**, 1–27.

Neve, M. & **Turner, T.** (2002). History of child and adolescent psychiatry. In: **M. Rutter** & **E. Taylor** (eds.) *Child and Adolescent Psychiatry*, 4th edn, pp. 382–395. Oxford, UK: Blackwell Scientific Publications.

Parkinson, J. (1807). Observations on the excessive indulgence of children, particularly intended to show its injurious effects on their health, and the difficulties it occasions in their treatment during sickness. In: *Medical Admonitions to Families*, 5th edn, pp. 467–473. London: Symonds.

Parry-Jones, W. L. (1994). History of child and adolescent psychiatry. In: **M. Rutter, E. Taylor,** & **L. Hersov** (eds.) *Child and Adolescent Psychiatry: Modern Approaches*, 3rd edn, pp. 794–812. London: Blackwell.

Pellegrino, E. D. (1996). Clinical judgment, scientific data, and ethics: antidepressant therapy in adolescents and children. *Journal of Nervous and Mental Illness*, **184**, 106–108.

Perfect, W. (1809). *Annals of Insanity, Comprising a Selection of Curious and Interesting Cases in the Different Species of Lunacy, Melancholy, or Madness, with the Modes of Practice in the Medical and Moral Treatment, as Adopted in the Cure of Each*, 5th edn. London: Chalmers. [Reprinted New York: Arno Press, 1976.]

Phaer, T. (1545). *The Boke of Children*. [In Ruhräh, 1925, pp. 147–195.]

Pinel, P. (1801). *Traité médico-philosophique sur l'aliénation mentale, ou la manie*. Paris: Caille et Ravier. [English translation: *A Treatise on Insanity*, trans. D. D. Davis, London, 1806. Reprinted New York: Hafner, 1962.]

Pollock, L. A. (1983). *Forgotten Children: Parent–Child Relations from 1500 to 1900*. Cambridge, UK: Cambridge University Press.

Preyer, W. (1882). *Die Seele des Kindes: Beobachtungen über die geistige Entwickelung des Menschen in den ersten Lebensjahren*. Leipzig: T. Grieben.

Reese, H. W. & **Overton, R. B.** (1970). Models of development and theories of development. In: **L. R. Goulet** & **P. B. Baltes** (eds.) *Life-Span Developmental Psychology: Theory and Research*, pp. 115–145. New York: Academic Press.

Roche, A. J., Fortin, G., Labbé, J., Brown, J., & **Chadwick, D.** (2005). The work of Ambrose Tardieu: the first definitive description of child abuse. *Child Abuse and Neglect*, **29**, 325–334.

Ross, D. (1972). *G. Stanley Hall: The Psychologist as Prophet*. Chicago, IL: University of Chicago Press.

Ruhräh, J. (1925). *Pediatrics of the Past*. New York: Hoeber.

Rush, B. (1798). On the different species of phobia. *Weekly Magazine of Original Essays, Fugitive Pieces, and Interesting Intelligence*, **1**, 177–180.

Rush, B. (1812). *Medical Inquiries and Observations upon the Diseases of the Mind*. Philadelphia: Kimber & Richardson. [Reprinted New York: Hafner, 1962.]

Savage, G. H. (1881). Moral insanity. *Journal of Mental Science*, **27**, 147–155.

Shahar, S. (1990). *Childhood in the Middle Ages*. London: Routledge.

Spitzka, E. C. (1890). Insanity. In: **J. M. Keating** (ed.) *Cyclopaedia of the Diseases of Children, Medical and Surgical*, vol. 4, pp. 1038–1053. Philadelphia, PA: J.B. Lippincott.

Spurzheim, G. (1818). *Observations sur la folie, ou sur les dérangemens des fonctions morales et intellectuelles de l'homme*. Paris: Treuttel et Würtz.

Stone, M. H. (1973). Child psychiatry before the twentieth century. *International Journal of Child Psychotherapy*, **2**, 264–308.

Dr. Strack (1863). Seelenstörung bei einem Kinde. *Correspondenz-Blatt der deutschen Gesellschaft für Psychiatrie und Gerichtliche Psychologie*, **10**, 76–78.

Sully, J. (1895). *Studies of Childhood*. London: Longmans, Green, & Co.

Tardieu, A. (1857). *Etude médico-légale sur les attentats aux mœurs*. Paris: J.-B. Baillière.

Tardieu, A. (1860). Etude médico-légale sur les sévices et mauvais traitements exercés sur des enfants. *Annales d'Hygiène Publique et de Médecine Légale*, **13**, 361–398.

Tiedemann, D. (1787). *Beobachtungen über die Entwickelung der Selenfähigkeiten bei Kindern*. [In Chr. Ufer (1897) *Dietrich Tiedemanns Beobachtungen über die Entwickelung der Selenfähigkeiten bei Kindern*. Altenburg: Oskar Bond. English translation in Murchison, C. & Langer, S. (1927) Tiedemann's observations on the development of the mental faculties of children. *Pedagogical Seminary and the Journal of Genetic Psychology*, **34**, 205–230.]

Tissot, S. A. (1760). *L'Onanisme: dissertation sur les maladies produites par la masturbation*. Paris: Libraire Chez le Dentu, 1834. [Reprinted Paris: Le Sycomore, 1980. English translation: *Onanism: or, a Treatise upon the Disorders Produced by Masturbation*, translated from the last Paris edition by A. Hume. London, 1781.]

Van Widenfelt, B. M., Treffers, P. D. A., de Beurs, E., Siebelink, B. M., & **Koudijs, E.** (2005). Translation and cross-cultural adaptation of assessment instruments used in psychological research with children and families. *Clinical Child and Family Psychology Review*, **8**, 135–147.

Vitiello, B. & **Jensen, P. S.** (1995). Developing clinical trials in children and adolescents; developmental perspectives in pediatric psychopharmacology. *Psychopharmacology Bulletin*, **31**, 75–81.

von Rinecker, D. (1876). Über Irresein der Kinder. *Allgemeine Zeitschrift für Psychiatrie*, **32**, 560–565.

Walk, A. (1964). The pre-history of child psychiatry. *British Journal of Psychiatry*, **110**, 754–767.

Wardle, C. J. (1991). Historical influences on services for children and adolescents before 1900. In: **G. E. Berrios** & **H. Freeman** (eds.) *150 Years of British Psychiatry, 1841–1991*, pp. 279–293. London: Gaskell.

Weisz, J. R., Suwanlert, S., Chaiyasit, W., Weiss, B., Achenbach, T. M., & **Walter, B. R.** (1987). Epidemiology of behavioural and emotional problems among Thai and American children: parent reports for ages 6 to 11. *Journal of the American Academy of Child and Adolescent Psychiatry*, **26**, 890–897.

Wessely, S. & **Wardle, C. J.** (1990). Mass sociogenic illness by proxy: parentally reported epidemic in an elementary school. *British Journal of Psychiatry*, **157**, 421–424.

West, C. (1860). On the mental peculiarities and mental disorders of childhood. *Medical Times and Gazette*, Feb. 11, 133–137.

West, C. (1871). *On Some Disorders of the Nervous System in Childhood: being the Lumleian Lectures delivered at the Royal College of Physicians of London in March 1871*. London: Longmans, Green, & Co.

Whittington, C. J., Kendall, T., Fonagy, P., Cottrell, D. F., Cotgrove, A., & **Boddington, E.** (2004). Selective serotonin reuptake inhibitors in childhood depression: systematic review of published versus unpublished data. *The Lancet*, **363**, 1341–1345.

Wier, J. (= Johann Weyer) (1563). Histoires de quelques ieunes enfans demionaques. [In: *De praestigiis daemonum, histoires disputés et discours des illusions et impostures des diables, des magiciens infames etc*, vol. I, bk III, pp. 521–523. Paris: Delahay et Lecrosnier, 1885.]

Zito, J. M., Safer, D. J., dosReis, S., Gardner, J. F., Boles, M., & **Lynch, F.** (2000). Trends in the prescribing of psychotropic medications to preschoolers. *Journal of the American Medical Association*, **283**, 1025–1030.

2

The clinical phenomenology and classification of child and adolescent anxiety

Antonio Castro Fonseca and Sean Perrin

Introduction

Anxiety problems have been recognized and discussed throughout the ages under various expressions and from different perspectives. Yet, their study as a specific form of childhood and adolescence psychopathology was largely neglected prior to the second half of the twentieth century. Only during the last 50 years have consistent efforts been made in psychology and psychiatry towards a better understanding of child and adolescent anxiety and its disorders (see Treffers & Silverman, Chapter 1, this volume). The amount of information that has accumulated is now considerable, and shows that anxiety disorders in young people are one of the most common and debilitating forms of psychopathology, constituting a heavy social and economic burden (Bodden, Dirksen, & Bögels, 2008). Children and adolescents with these conditions are at an increased risk of future depression, poor school adjustment, substance abuse, and other problems in adulthood, including anxiety disorders (Kim-Cohen, Caspi, Moffitt, Harrington, Milne, & Poulton, 2003).

The conceptualization and diagnosis of these disorders have typically relied on theories, methods, and instruments designed for adults. However, new advances in developmental psychology and psychopathology highlighted the plasticity and individual variation in the patterns of anxiety across life as well as the existence of multiple factors contributing to their continuities and discontinuities (Feng, Shaw, & Silk, 2008; Sweeney & Pine, 2004). This has led to the development of new instruments and strategies, more appropriate to account for the special features of anxiety disorders in children and adolescents.

The aim of this chapter is to provide an overview of the scope of these advances as well as of the main challenges that clinicians and researchers are often confronted with in this field. Special attention is devoted here to the distinction between normal and abnormal anxieties, to the logic underlying traditional diagnostic systems of mental disorders as well as its limitations, and to the psychometric properties or clinical relevance of the methods and instruments currently used to assess and diagnose youth's anxiety disorders.

Defining clinical anxiety in children

Anxiety can be defined as a set of emotional reactions arising from the anticipation of a real or imagined threat to the self. In the literature it is often used interchangeably with fear although there are important differences between them (Barlow, 2002). Fears are usually

Anxiety Disorders in Children and Adolescents, 2nd edn, ed. W. K. Silverman and A. P. Field. Published by Cambridge University Press. © Cambridge University Press 2011.

described as reactions, involving avoidance and discomfort, to very specific stimuli (e.g., spiders or blood) whereas anxiety is characterized by a more diffuse type of reaction to less specific stimuli (e.g., apprehension regarding the future).

Despite its manifestations across different ages and contexts, anxiety is generally conceptualized as involving three main components: a motor response, a subjective or cognitive response, and a physiological response, each of them in turn encompassing a greater number of reactions (Lang, 1968). At the behavior or motor level, and usually in the presence of the anxiety-provoking stimulus or situation, anxiety is characterized by escape or avoidance behaviors, enduring the situation with distress, restlessness (e.g., pacing, hand-wringing), and clinging to caregivers or loved ones. Immobility or urgent pleas for assistance may also be seen. At the subjective or cognitive level, anxiety is characterized by fearful apprehension, worries, or perception of uncontrollability over aversive events. Finally, at the somatic or physiological level, anxiety is defined by heightened autonomic arousal (e.g., increased heart rate, skin conductance, and perspiration), which is often reflected in the self-report of multiple somatic complaints.

Lang (1968) first conceptualized anxiety and fear by this three-response system to account for the low to moderate correlations among the multiple measures of this construct. Despite some proposed changes and criticisms (Cone, 1998; Zinbarg, 1998), it is a popular framework within the field (Barlow, 2002; Rachman, 1978, 1990), became the model upon which the DSM-IV anxiety disorders were organized, and has received empirical support in both adult and child research (Austin & Chorpita, 2004; Brown & Barlow, 2002).

One important aspect to consider when diagnosing and treating anxiety manifestations in childhood and adolescence is that mild to occasionally moderate levels of anxiety are part of "normal" human development: they change as children, with age, are confronted with new challenges or situations (see Muris & Field, Chapter 4, and Bokhorst & Westenberg, Chapter 5, this volume), and they present with similar characteristics and developmental trends in different parts of the world, despite some variations (Canino *et al.*, 2004; Mellon & Moutavelis, 2007; Ollendick, Yang, King, Dong, & Akande, 1996). These manifestations of anxiety are believed to constitute adaptive responses to a world not fully understood, which is replete with situations, objects, and events that seem uncontrolled, dangerous, or unpredictable. Naturally, their correct identification may have important implications for the process of assessment and diagnostic classification. So, when do these normative fears become a disorder?

One way of answering this question would be to invoke the concept of *harmful dysfunction* introduced by Wakefield (1992) to define mental disorder. According to it, there is a mental disorder when an internal mechanism is not performing its functions as designed by nature and, as a result, there is harm on the person's well-being as defined by social values or meanings. Regarding anxiety disorders, the first part of that definition – *harmful* – is relatively consensual because anxiety symptoms often cause enormous suffering and impairment. But, when it comes to the second part – *dysfunction* – in many cases it is hard to decide whether those symptoms reflect a fear mechanism that is unable to accomplish its biological function or whether they simply reflect a poor fit of that mechanism with a current environment that may be different from those for which it was originally designed (Wakefield, Horwitz, & Schmitz, 2004, 2005).

Despite these difficulties in establishing clear criteria for the definition of mental disorder, there is relatively broad consensus among researchers and clinicians on the distinction between "normal" and abnormal anxieties (Barlow, 2002). In contrast to normal anxiety, pathological anxiety is seen as being beyond what is expected for a youth's developmental level, disproportionate to the threat posed, persistent, irrational, not transient, and impairing one or more areas of the youth's functioning or psychosocial development (Foley, Pickles, Maes, Silberg, & Eaves, 2004; Kessler, Berglund, Demler, Jin, Merikangas, & Walters, 2005; Moffitt *et al.*, 2007). Further, these extreme manifestations are often accompanied by other psychiatric problems, and have a rather poor prognosis. For example, there is evidence that depression is more than eight times as likely in anxious youths than in their non-anxious counterparts (Costello, Egger, & Angold, 2004), and the negative effects of extreme anxiety often may last into adulthood (Roza, Hofstra, van der Ende, & Verhulst, 2003). On the grounds of these serious psychological and social "dysfunctions," such children and adolescents are generally regarded as having an "anxiety disorder."

In a review of the main studies carried out in the general population, Twenge (2000) concluded there had been a one standard deviation increase in rates of anxiety, in children, adolescents, and young adults. It was shown that "anxiety is so high now that normal samples of children from the 1980's outscore psychiatric populations from the 1950's" (p. 1018). In a later cohort analysis of anxiety in adults, Twenge and colleagues (Twenge *et al.*, 2010) found that increases in anxiety scores as measured by the MMPI between 1989 and 2005 were associated with a shift to extrinsic (materialistic) goals and away from intrinsic values such as community, meaning, and affiliation. This apparent increase in rates of anxiety across the lifespan may help explain the increased research attention that has focused on anxiety and its disorders in children and adolescents (Rapee, Schniering, & Hudson, 2009).

However, there are also studies pointing in a different direction. Canino *et al.* (2004) examined the prevalence rates of separation anxiety disorder in Puerto Rico at two time points separated by 20 years, and found the same prevalence rates of 2% in a large community sample of 4–17-year-olds. This was consistent with the findings reported in another investigation conducted by Achenbach, Dumenci, and Rescorla (2003) in the United States. Comparing data from three large community studies, collected at three time periods over 20 years (i.e., between 1978 and 1999), with the same instruments, these authors found considerable stability in the prevalence rates of anxiety disorders also in three large samples of 4–16-year-olds. It seems, therefore, that if modern living, on the one hand, originates new extreme fears and anxieties (e.g., AIDS, religious terrorism, nuclear war, or violent crime), it may also, on the other hand, reduce these fears through the reorganization of the contexts in which youths live (Grinde, 2005). Naturally, the prevalence of these disorders also depends on the criteria and instruments used to screen them, which may vary from me classification system to the other and change from time to time within the same system (Beesdo, Knappe, & Pine, 2009).

Diagnostic criteria

To account for the diversity of child and adolescent anxiety disorders and to provide guidelines to group them, several classifications schemes have been proposed. The most influential, both in clinical and research settings, have been the categorical systems. According to them, a disorder is identified on the basis of clinical and empirical information about the relationship among symptoms and then one decides if it applies to each individual case, even before their actual cause is known. This approach has a very long history in psychiatry and is well illustrated in the successive editions of *Diagnostic and Statistical Manual of Mental Disorders* (DSM: American Psychiatric Association [APA], 1994, 2000) and the *International Classification of Diseases* (ICD-10: World Health Organization [WHO], 1992), both currently under revision. The underlying assumption is that anxiety-disordered people differ qualitatively from those who do not have such a condition. It is an "either–or" decision with no middle term. In this process, diagnosticians are helped by a set of inclusion and exclusion rules, clearly specified a priori, which establish the criteria for each diagnosis. Such rules are usually set by a committee of experts and are tested through empirical research and clinical work.

In the last version of DSM (APA, 1994, 2000), there is only one anxiety disorder specific to childhood and adolescence: separation anxiety disorder. The remaining disorders are listed in the adult section of the same manual but may be applied to children, as appropriate. They include panic disorder, agoraphobia, specific and social phobia, obsessive–compulsive disorder, post-traumatic stress disorder, acute stress disorder, generalized anxiety disorder, anxiety disorder due to general medical condition, substance-induced anxiety disorder, and anxiety disorder not otherwise specified. Compared with previous editions of the DSM, the current edition had some important changes. For instance, overanxious disorder and avoidant disorder were eliminated as separate categories in the child section of the manual, given their lack of reliability and validity, and included in the adult equivalents of these disorders – generalized anxiety and social phobia, respectively. However, separation anxiety disorder has remained largely unchanged in the various editions of the DSM, and is expected to continue so in its forthcoming revision.

Separation anxiety disorder (SAD) includes excessive worry about separation from the home or major attachment figures, sleep disturbances and nightmares involving separation, crying and pleading when parents do leave, clinging to caregivers or persistent tracking of major attachment figures, disruptions in behavior and/or somatic complaints during separation, persistent fears of being alone, and avoidance of separation from caregivers (e.g., in school refusal behavior). To qualify for this diagnosis, children must have at least three of eight symptoms, onset of the disorder prior to 18 years old, duration of at least 4 weeks, and clinically significant impairment in their functioning, all of which cannot be explained by the presence of other disorders (DSM-IV: APA, 2000). In addition, these symptoms should be in excess of what is typical for a given developmental stage. Accordingly, one would expect a 2-year-old but not an adolescent to demonstrate anxiety on separation from caregivers. Prevalence estimates of SAD in community samples range from 1.8% to 12.9% (Campbell, 2006), and are generally higher among children than among adolescents. For example, Costello, Egger, Copeland, Erkanli, and Angold (Chapter 3, this volume) report, from a meta-analysis, a prevalence rate of 3.9% in 6–12-year-olds compared to only 2.35% in 12–18-year-olds. According to Costello *et al.* (Figure 3.2 in Chapter 3), SAD has the earliest age of onset (a median of 6 years), although it may continue well into adulthood.

Generalized anxiety disorder (GAD) has been less studied in children and early adolescence, as it is a relatively recent category in DSM-IV. It is characterized by excessive and poorly controlled child or adolescent worry about multiple situations and activities (e.g., the future) accompanied by several other problems, including restlessness, poor concentration, sleep disturbance, and somatic complaints. Some of the symptoms (e.g., excessive worry about school achievement or being bullied) may be typical of childhood, and should occur frequently, during at least 6 months. Epidemiological studies on this disorder are still scarce, which has led reviewers to merge studies that use DSM-III-R (overanxious disorder) and DSM-IV criteria, thus producing a wide variation of prevalence rates in the community. In Chapter 3, Costello *et al.*'s meta-analysis suggests similar prevalence rates in 6–12-year-olds (1.7%) and 12–18-year-olds (1.9%). The age of onset for GAD is at around 8 years, but is hugely variable (see Costello *et al.*, Chapter 3, this volume, Figure 3.2).

Social phobia (SOP) is characterized by an intense and persistent fear of social or public situations in which scrutiny from others is anticipated and results in irrational expectations of humiliation or embarrassment. Exposure to these situations or events provokes anxiety to such an extent that they are avoided or endured with great suffering. In children the anxiety may also be manifested through crying, tantrums, or avoiding situations with unfamiliar people, whereas adolescents may present more externalizing problems, suicidal ideation, alcohol abuse, and excessive self-focused attention in social situations (Kashdan & Herbert, 2001). Based on Costello *et al.*'s meta-analysis (see Chapter 3, this volume), social phobia has a lower prevalence rate in 6–12-year-olds (2.2%) compared to 12–18-year-olds (5%). They also report an average age of onset of around 8–9 years old.

Panic disorder (PD) is mainly characterized by discrete but recurrent periods of intense fear (*panic attacks*) that are followed by worry about additional attacks. These discrete episodes are accompanied by cognitive and physiological symptoms (e.g., dizziness, trembling, tachycardia, fear of dying) that may reach a peak within a short period of time. The panic attacks may or may not be associated with situational triggers. Panic disorder is considered a low prevalent condition in childhood, with rates of 1.5% in 6–12-year-olds and 1.1% in 12–18-year-olds (Costello *et al.*, Chapter 3, this volume). Interestingly, some earlier studies did not find any cases of panic disorder in samples from the community (Anderson, Williams, McGee, & Silva, 1987), while others have even questioned its occurrence in children, due to their limited cognitive capacities (see Nelles & Barlow, 1988; Schniering, Hudson, & Rapee, 2000). Nevertheless, the prevalent view is that panic disorders can be found prior to adulthood and that for most cases the age of onset is likely to fall between 15 and 19 years (e.g., Costello *et al.*, Chapter 3, this volume) with a mean of around 19 and an interquartile range of 15 to 20) years of age. However, earlier onset is clearly possible (Ollendick, Birmaher, & Matis, 2004).

Often associated with panic disorders, **agoraphobia** (AG) is characterized by intense anxiety in situations from which escape may seem difficult or in which help may not be available when panic suddenly appears. The occurrence of AG is well documented in late adolescence but less so in childhood (Cartwright-Hatton, McNicol, & Doubleday, 2006). Ford, Goodman, and Meltezer (2003) reported a prevalence rate of 0.07%, whereas in their review of the literature Costello *et al.* (2004) mentioned a prevalence rate of 1.5%. The age of onset of AG is believed to be in adolescence or early adulthood (e.g., around 12 years old in Costello *et al.*, Chapter 3, this volume). Further, Wilson and Hayward (2005) showed that there was a clear link between panic attacks and agoraphobia in adolescents.

Specific phobias (SP), also called simple phobia in previous editions of DSM, have as their core feature an excessive and persistent fear of specific situations, beings, or objects (e.g., insects, loud noises, heights). The expression of SP in children and adolescents may take various forms: running away, clinging behaviors, crying, freezing, or situationally cued panic attacks. These reactions are different from the normal fears in the intensity of the physiological and behavioral response to the situation, and the extent to which this phobia impairs everyday functioning. The avoidance or severe distress associated with SP needs to have a duration of at least 6 months. Specific phobia is considered one of the most prevalent types of anxiety disorders in childhood and adolescence. Based on Costello *et al.*'s meta-analysis (see Chapter 3, this volume), SP has an identical prevalence rate in

6–12- and 12–18-year-olds (6.7%); they also report an average age of onset of around 7–8 years old. There is considerable variety from one type of SP to another, but the most prevalent seem to be the animal and natural environmental phobias, followed by situational phobias, blood-injury, and other kinds of phobias.

Obsessive–compulsive disorder (OCD) is defined by two main features – *obsessions* and *compulsions* – which are both excessively time-consuming and cause a great deal of child or adolescent distress. Obsessions are recurrent, intrusive thoughts, images, or impulses (e.g., related to germs, harm, or contamination) that are disliked, inappropriate, and leave the individuals extremely impaired. Compulsions are repetitive behavioral or mental actions (e.g., touching, washing, checking, counting) aimed at reducing the anxiety or distress resulting from the obsessions, or at preventing the occurrence of feared events. Findings from recent studies suggest that OCD is not a common disorder among children; its prevalence rates usually range from 0.25% (Ford *et al.*, 2003) to 0. 6% (Bolton *et al.*, 2006). It is, however, possible that children and adolescents conceal symptoms of OCD or that their parents misinterpret the symptoms as "quirky," meaningless, or even oppositional behaviors, with the true prevalence being much higher than found in epidemiological studies. Age of onset of OCD is most common between 9 and 12 years, although in some cases it may occur earlier (see Albano, Chorpita, & Barlow, 2003).

Post-traumatic stress disorder (PTSD) is characterized by the experience of intense anxiety, horror, or helplessness following exposure to an event involving the threat (to self or to another) of death, injury, or loss of physical integrity. The main symptoms of PTSD consist of re-experiencing the traumatic event (e.g., nightmares, flashbacks, intrusive thoughts/images, or repetitive play), avoiding stimuli associated with the trauma, emotional numbing, and evidence of persistent autonomic arousal (e.g., sleep difficulties, irritability, and hypervigilance). When the symptoms resulting from the exposure to the traumatic event cause significant impairment, lasting for more than 2 days following that experience and persisting for less than 4 weeks, a diagnosis of *acute stress disorder* should be made (DSM-IV: APA, 2000). Bolton and collaborators (2006) reported prevalence rates of 0.3% a nationally representative sample of 6-year-old British twins; Ford *et al.* (2003) reported a prevalence of 0.14% in the British child and adolescent mental health survey; and Essau, Conradt, and Petermann (1999) a prevalence of 1.6% in a large sample of German adolescents.

In the DSM-IV, there is also a broad category of **anxiety disorder not otherwise specified** (ADNOS), an umbrella for symptoms that do not meet the criteria for any of the single disorders mentioned above (e.g., regarding duration or number of symptoms). Although research data on this condition are scarce, the findings of a British community study place its prevalence around 1% (Ford *et al.*, 2003). Two other categories included in the DSM-IV, that have been studied less and have uncertain validity, are anxiety disorder due to general medical condition or substance-induced anxiety disorder. Finally, anxiety appears as an important element of adjustment disorder with anxiety or with mixed anxiety and depressed mood.

In the ICD-10 (WHO, 1992), children's anxiety disorders are listed under a general category of "emotional disorders with onset specific to childhood," which also includes phobic anxiety disorder of childhood, social anxiety disorder of childhood, and sibling rivalry disorder. As in the DSM-IV, phobic anxiety disorder is characterized by excessive fear of specific stimuli (e.g., animals, heights) and social anxiety disorder by persistent fears of strangers or social situations to a degree that is outside the normal limits for the child. There is also a category of mixed disorders of conduct and emotions that involves a combination of antisocial behaviors and emotional difficulties (e.g., anxiety and depression). Similar to DSM-IV, the ICD-10 also allows anxiety disorders listed in the adult section of the manual to be applied to children and adolescent, when appropriate.

As mentioned above, both the DSM and ICD approaches to the diagnosis of anxiety disorders are categorical systems that afford certain advantages: they allow for reliable communication between clinicians and researchers; they facilitate the prediction of other symptoms when certain ones of the same syndrome are present; and they provide consistent criteria to compare results across studies. As Widiger and Samuel (2005) noted, it is simpler to inform a colleague that a youth has an anxiety disorder than to describe the patient in terms of several dimensions or facets of personality. Despite these advantages, the categorical systems also present with several limitations, notably when it comes to establishing clear boundaries among different diagnoses, or extending adult criteria downward to children and adolescents. These issues, which have been the focus of considerable debate among researchers and clinicians, are discussed next in more detail.

Validity issues

During the last two decades important advances were made to improve the reliability and validity of the classification of anxiety disorders in the main diagnostic systems (Saavedra & Silverman, 2002). The first step in improving those classification systems was to determine whether children and adolescents with anxiety conditions can be distinguished from their well-adjusted counterparts with regard to several criteria. In general, the evidence emerging from those studies, involving clinical and non-clinical samples, support the validity of a broad category of anxiety disorders, particularly if structured diagnostic interviews and standardized child self-rating scales are used (Dierker *et al.*, 2001; Saavedra & Silverman, 2002).

However, the evidence is less solid when it comes to separate anxiety disorders from other forms of psychopathology, as their boundaries are often blurred. One way of solving that problem was to introduce "mixed disorders" categories or "not otherwise classified" categories. The trouble with these new categories is that their validity is far from demonstrated. For example, in DSM-IV, people within the category of mixed mood and anxiety disorder cannot be distinctly diagnosed with either an anxiety or a mood disorder, even in cases where the specific symptoms of one or the other warrant clinical intervention. Moreover, as Widiger and Samuel (2005) pointed out, there is evidence that this mixed condition could be equally well classified as a personality disorder. Similarly, in a study of clinically referred children, Steinhausen and Reitzle (1996) found little evidence supporting the existence of a separate category of "mixed disorders of conduct and emotions" (including anxiety) as defined in ICD-10, because this category shares most of its characteristics with pure conduct disorder. Finally, as pointed out by Costello *et al.* (2004), there are instances where anxiety symptoms are associated with a high degree of disability even if they do not reach the threshold for a diagnosis.

The evidence is also scarce or inconsistent when it comes to internal validity (e.g., the existence of so many diagnostic categories of anxiety disorders rather than one single factor or dimension) of these diagnostic categories. For instance, a few studies based on factor analyses of questionnaires from large community samples found that DSM-IV anxiety disorders represent different problems dimensions in youths (Chorpita, Yim, Moffitt, Umemoto, & Francis, 2000; Spence, 1997; Spence, Barrett, & Tuner, 2003), while others using a similar approach claim there is only partial support (Lahey, Waldman, Hankin,

Applegate, Loft, & Rick, 2004) or no support to the distinctions between different anxiety constructs or diagnoses (Ferdinand, van Lang, Ormel, & Verhulst, 2006; Wardworth, Hudziak, Heath, & Achenbach, 2000). Furthermore, different disorders may share important features of anxiety, such as negative affect or worry (Brown & Barlow, 2002), and there is some evidence that interventions tailored to specific anxiety disorders (other than OCD and PTSD) do not clearly produce better outcomes (Dadds, James, Barrett, & Verhulst, 2004). Addressing these issues, Bodden *et al.* (2008), in their Christchurch longitudinal study, found that internalizing symptoms can be partitioned into components reflecting both a generalized tendency to internalizing and disorder-specific components. And they concluded that "at present time, there is no evidence to determine which of these interpretations is the more correct." The picture is not much different when the analysis is focused on the comorbidity rates of these disorders.

Comorbidity

One of the greatest challenges for the traditional diagnostic classification comes from the excessive overlap among diagnostic categories, usually referred to as comorbidity. In childhood and adolescence, this phenomenon is the rule rather than the exception (Curry, March, & Hervey, 2004). In decreasing order of frequency, the additional diagnoses are likely to be a second anxiety disorder (*homotypic comorbidity*), depressive disorder, disruptive behavior, or substance use disorders (*heterotypic comorbidity*). Interestingly, Costello *et al.* (Chapter 3, this volume) note several problems inherent in trying to establish comorbidity, but based on what evidence there is they concluded that (1) there were significant comorbidities among specific, social, and agoraphobia; (2) there was predictive comorbidity between overanxious disorder (OAD) and GAD; (3) controlling for other disorders, depression was significantly associated with anxiety disorders except OCD; and (4) in terms of heterotypic comorbidity, attention deficit hyperactivity disorder (ADHD) was comorbid with specific phobia, oppositional defiant disorder (ODD) with OCD, bipolar disorder with separation anxiety (in males), and alcohol abuse/dependence with OAD.

The frequent co-occurrence of other conditions with anxiety disorders and the special characteristics of comorbid cases raise important questions about the validity of the categories of the main diagnostic systems and highlights the need to consider new approaches to the conceptualization and classification of anxiety disorders (Weems & Stickle, 2005; Widiger & Samuel, 2005). The relevance of these issues is well documented in the scientific debate that is growing in psychology and related disciplines, on the eve of DSM-V, about the limitations of traditional diagnostic categories and possible ways of overcoming them (Tackett, Sellbom, Quilty, Rector, & Bagby, 2008). One of the suggestions that has been made is to integrate a dimensional approach in the new version of the DSM system.

Dimensional approach

In a dimensional approach, anxiety disorders are viewed as occurring along a continuum of severity, rather than falling above or below a "diagnostic threshold" or into discrete diagnostic categories. Further, the symptoms that constitute different anxiety disorders as well as the threshold between normal and abnormal anxiety are statistically derived from large samples, and are permitted to vary according to the individual's sex, age, or culture. As opposed to a committee of experts defining mental disease on the basis of clinical experience, the dimensional approach usually consists of asking parents, teachers, and children to answer questions about the child's behavior, and then factor-analysing the responses to derive severity levels and symptom clusters. The information is generally expressed on scales or questionnaires, which quantify the degree to which individuals manifest particular kinds of problems. Some of these instruments have been used already for many years whereas others are relatively recent (see Shear, Bjelland, Beesdo, Gloster, & Wittchen, 2007; Silverman & Ollendick, 2005).

By using instruments that measure symptoms on a continuum, it is possible to identify degrees and types of disturbance, as well as patterns of their manifestations, without the use of discrete categories and without presumptions regarding an underlying disease process. The level of impairment of the disorder is established according to statistical deviation from the norm of one's peers and may vary for different specific measures or research purposes. In support of the dimensional approach, Quay (1979) found a factor of anxiety-withdrawal, characterized by "feelings of tension, depression, inferiority and worthless, and behaviors of timidity, social withdrawal and hyper sensibility."

Similarly, Achenbach (1991a, 1991b, 1991c) identified an "anxious/depressed" factor derived from a variety of informants (e.g., parents, teachers, youths themselves) and across different settings (e.g., clinical or community samples), which includes symptoms such as "crying a lot, fear of doing or thinking bad things, the need to be perfect, to be nervous and fearful, guilty and self-conscious, worrying, feeling sad, or to feel lonely and worthless." Based on these items, several efforts have been made to generate constructs that reflect DSM disorders (Achenbach & Rescorla, 2001; Achenbach *et al.*, 2003; Connor-Smith & Compas, 2003). The items included in the Child Behavior Checklist/Youth Self-Report (CBCL/YSR) scale were supposed to reflect DSM-IV separation anxiety disorder, generalized anxiety disorder, and specific phobia. However, the existing empirical evidence provides little support for the concurrent validity of the DSM-IV anxiety problems scale (Ferdinand, 2006, 2008; van Lang, Ferdinand, Oldehinkel, Ormel, & Verhulst, 2005). A probable reason is that the number of items is small; and it does not assess symptom duration or level of associated impairment. Further research is needed before using this instrument as a screening instrument for anxiety disorders in research or clinical practice.

Other recent dimensional approaches have distinguished between higher-order features which reflect important processes common to most anxiety disorders, and lower-order features which refer to the contextual factors that differentiate the various disorders. Good illustrations of such new developments can be found in the tripartite model (Clark & Watson, 1991; Clark, Watson, & Reynolds, 1995) introduced to account for the co-occurrence between anxiety and depression, and in the transdiagnostic approach, aimed to develop a better treatment of these disorders (Mansell, Harvey, Watkins, & Shafran, 2009).

The approach of Clark, Watson, and colleagues cited above posits that anxiety and depression share a common component of negative affectivity (NA) and can be differentiated by low positive affect (PA) more commonly found in depressed individuals, and by the high physiological hyperarousal (PH) found in those with anxiety disorders. Further developments have led researchers to collapse anxiety and mood disorder into a higher-order construct of emotional disorder that will be organized in three subclasses: bipolar disorders, distress disorders, and fear disorders (Watson, 2005). Although originally tested in adult samples, the tripartite model has been extended recently to the study of anxiety disorders in childhood and adolescence. The results generally confirm the existence of three higher-order factors, which are independent but moderate to highly correlated (Chorpita, 2002; Joiner & Lonigan, 2000; Yang, Hong, Joung, & Kim, 2006). This led to the development of new scales to evaluate the tripartite model, for example the Positive Affect and Negative Affect Schedule for Children and Affect and Arousal Scale (Chorpita & Daleiden, 2002). However, the findings from these studies, both with clinical and non-clinical samples, have often been inconsistent. Based on their review of the literature, Anderson and Hope (2008) concluded that "more research in youth is needed in order to determine whether it is appropriate to extrapolate the functioning of the tripartite constructs across anxiety disorders from adult research" (p. 285).

The second approach, also known as a transdiagnostic or transprocess perspective, proposes that all anxiety disorders share similar maintaining psychological processes (e.g., interpretational biases, selective attention, problems of memory encoding or retrieval, cognitive avoidance, meta-cognitive and meta-emotional beliefs, and avoidance escape behaviors) (Barlow, Allen, & Choate, 2004; Mansell *et al.*, 2009). The differences among disorders relate to the contents rather than the processes. Accordingly, a person with combat-related PTSD would selectively attend to traumatic-event-related cues whereas a person with a blood phobia would primarily attend to the blood-related cues (Clark & Taylor, 2009). In other words, such an approach emphasizes empirically supported common dimensions of emotional disorders over disorder-specific criteria sets favored by the dominant diagnostic systems. Naturally it may have important implications for the development of new and broader treatment protocols that can be efficaciously applied to a variety of disorders (e.g., anxiety and depression) by targeting their shared features.

The growing recognition of (and importance attached to) symptomatic overlap among the anxiety disorders, the negative affect shared between anxiety and depression, and the transdiagnostic processes that appear to operate across all emotional disorders is likely to reinvigorate debate over dimensional versus categorical approaches to anxiety. Questionnaires that tap the overlapping features of anxiety disorders (e.g., frequency of avoidance, worry, hyperarousal) could be enhanced by inclusion of items reflecting negative and positive affectivity, to the extent possible – transdiagnostic fators (e.g., anxiety sensitivity, meta-beliefs about worry), and functional impairment (e.g., school, peers, family, chores, fun, etc.). Such a questionnaire could be administered to children and adolescents with known (identified) DSM anxiety disorders, those with other disorders, and those with no disorders, and across a wide demographic rage (e.g., age, gender, culture/race, income, treatment-seeking/general population) to establish norms and clinical cut-offs for anxiety. In addition, the data from surveys using such a questionnaire could help identify important developmental changes in the trajectory of proposed maintaining factors for anxiety. Also, as the questionnaire taps process variables linked to current evidenced-based treatments for anxiety, it might be more useful as a measure of treatment outcome than existing dimensional (trait) measures. Additional benefits include the relatively lower cost of using questionnaires versus psychiatric interviews to screen the population and a diminished emphasis on (or concern about) the frequent comorbidity that occurs among the anxiety disorders and which (arguably) does not change the primary components of effective treatment (e.g., exposure, cognitive restructuring, coping skills training, contingent reinforcement and parent training).

Despite these potential advantages, the dimensional will continue to face stiff opposition from those who favour the categorical (diagnostic) approach. Questionnaires tapping broad anxiety constructs are not particularly adept at detecting specific or uncommon symptom clusters (e.g., OCD and PD) or symptoms that young people are unlikely to acknowledge outside of an in-depth interview with an understanding and empathic therapist. Second, clinical cut-offs for "caseness" or treatment always reflect an imperfect trade-off between over-inclusiveness and thereby identifying too many "false positives" (and potentially wasting limited resources) and over-exclusiveness and thereby missing "true positives" who need treatment. Generally speaking, scores on questionnaires do not give a full picture of the person's actual situation (e.g., everyday functioning and meeting role demands) (Blanton & Jaccard, 2006). Third, it is unclear how a theory-driven, dimensional approach to the diagnosis of mental disorders might be implemented across large public health systems. The categorical approach to diagnoses has become dominant partly because it is atheoretical and because users of this information find it easy to understand, and useful in organizing treatment and support and in communicating with patients and their families. Movement away from the long-established categorical approach will require a solid conceptual basis for why such a change would be needed and a very large evidence base to support such a change, as well as recognition of the practical challenges (and cost) involved in any implementation (Barlow, 2002; Pilgrim, 2007).

Other approaches

In addition to dimensional and categorical approaches, other strategies have been used in the classification of anxious disorders. Two good examples are the classifications based on the nature of the eliciting stimuli and the functional analytic techniques. The first strategy, which consists of classifying the fear or anxiety according to the eliciting stimuli, was employed largely in early studies (Morris & Kratochwill, 1983), and may be useful for identifying treatment targets. However, it is limited by its use of seemingly endless lists of fears and anxieties (e.g., aquaphobia, mikrophobia, xenophobia), and its assumption of homogeneity within each particular category of fear when, in fact, there is considerable variety of symptom presentation. Moreover, the same treatment approach may be successful with several of those various conditions. This is one of the basic tenets of the recent transdiagnostic/transprocess approach already mentioned above.

The second strategy for classifying anxiety is the functional analytic approach, which also focuses on the eliciting stimuli but identifies specific target responses and their immediate consequences. Specifically, it assumes that the same fear or anxiety response may develop and be maintained in various ways, without resorting to pre-set diagnostic categories or dimensions. This is well illustrated in recent conceptualizations of school refusal behavior (Kearney, 2001, 2008). Accordingly, this behavior may have several different functions: avoiding anxiety and depression; escaping from aversive social or evaluative situations at school; attention-seeking, especially in cases of disruptive conduct; and providing access to positive tangible reinforcement, such as watching TV or staying longer in bed at home, instead of going to school. Thus, some children refuse attending classes for negative reinforcement whereas other children may refuse it for positive reinforcement. To test this model Kearney and Silverman (1990, 1996) developed the School Refusal Assessment Scale, which is now available in versions for children and for parents. Evidence supports this conceptualization of school refusal behavior, which paves the way to the development of new forms of interventions focused on the functions of school refusal that are more relevant in each case (Kearney, 2001, 2006).

In summary, all of the aforementioned classification systems have strengths and weaknesses and, thus, it may be difficult to decide upon which to use. The superiority of any one approach still requires a good deal of comparative research. In particular, it remains to be seen whether the dimensional or categorical approach is better at predicting external criteria for anxiety disorders, and which of these approaches is best at dealing with the considerable comorbidity found in anxious children. Also, as Kearney and Silverman (1996) pointed out, the validity of any classification system must, in the main, lead to reliable methods of assessment and effective treatments for the anxiety problem in question. When more treatment trials begin to appear for childhood anxiety disorders, derived from different classification systems, then the validity of the various classification schemes can be better evaluated. In particular it is necessary to know more about the development of anxiety and its associated problems before introducing changes to the current classification of youth anxiety disorders. Nevertheless, the classification systems described above clearly show that anxiety is not a unidimensional construct and, as such, a comprehensive assessment requires detailed knowledge of its diverse manifestations and associated features. Accordingly, this should lead to new measures capable of encompassing the different dimensions of anxiety and related disorders, and demonstrating greater sensitivity to their developmental changes.

Developmental considerations

As anxiety disorders are prevalent across the lifespan, it is important to consider whether childhood anxiety disorders persist in both form and function over time (i.e., homotypic continuity), remit (developmental discontinuity), or change into other disorders (i.e., heterotypic continuity). For example, is panic disorder in adulthood the outcome of childhood SAD? Are anxiety symptoms tied to sequential developmental tasks or challenges? Or do anxiety disorders usually precede depressive disorders? Such questions are relevant because if childhood anxiety disorders are unrelated to adolescent or adult anxiety disorders, or to other forms of psychopathology, then they may be of low priority when it comes to allocating resources to their prevention or treatment.

Costello *et al.* (Chapter 3, this volume) review the evidence and conclude that, for example, although there is evidence that childhood anxiety predicts adolescent depression, there is also evidence that early depression predicts anxiety. Similarly, they report that GAD, PD, and AG were the adult anxiety disorders most likely to have child and adolescent precursors, but there was little homotypic continuity within specific forms of anxiety. This finding could suggest that the categories are valid but that anxiety disorders are developmentally discontinuous. One could argue that the discontinuous hypothesis simply mirrors the developmental changes in anxiety seen in normal children (e.g., separation anxiety is replaced by more performance-related concerns during the school years). In other words, the disorders would reflect the developmental tasks and stresses children and adolescents are confronted with in specific periods of their lives (Warren & Sroufe, 2004).

Thus, it is not surprising that the prevalence of SAD decreases while OAD increases from childhood to adolescence (Costello *et al.*, 1988; Velez, Johnson, & Cohen, 1989) or that younger children often refuse to go to school to gain attention or proximity to caregivers while older children and adolescents may refuse school to avoid social evaluative situations (Kearney & Silverman, 1996). However, Costello *et al.* (Chapter 3, this volume) also concluded that there was relatively little heterotypic continuity for anxiety disorders, which implies that the diagnostic categories for the anxiety disorders across childhood and adolescence have some predictive validity. This conclusion is consistent with the findings from recent studies showing that anxiety symptoms in childhood moderately predict anxiety symptoms in adolescence or young adulthood (Bittner, Egger, Erkanli, Costello, Foley, & Angold, 2007; Ferdinand, Dieleman, Ormel, & Verhulst, 2007; Gregory & Eley, 2007; Pine, Cohen, Gurley, Brook, & Ma, 1998). Yet it must be also stressed that many anxious children and adolescents lose their anxiety disorders with age, whereas a large proportion of anxious-disordered adults had no anxiety disorder in childhood or adolescence.

Accordingly, it behoves the assessor to consider whether the anxiety symptoms are deviant for the child's age, and to assess comprehensively the fears and anxieties most relevant to each age level. One may even ask whether it is not justified to weight some symptoms differentially for specific developmental levels. In other words, the appropriate assessment and diagnosis of youths' anxiety disorders require an extended knowledge of their stability and changes over time and the utilization of measures that are sensitive to such changes. In this sense, age-downward extensions of instruments designed originally for adults may be misleading and, consequently, the utilization of adult criteria for anxiety disorders with children and adolescents may be of limited value. These issues are currently the focus of much research and debate concerning the next edition of DSM, which is due within 2 years (APA, 2009).

Current developments in the classification of anxiety disorders

Since the DSM-IV appeared in 1994, an impressive amount of new information about anxiety and its disorders has emerged and, as a result, several arguments have been put forward in support of changes in their assessment and diagnostic procedures. Some of the proposed alterations are rather broad in scope and apply to most of the anxiety disorders both in youths and in adults. They include renewed calls for incorporating a dimensional approach in the traditional classification system (Andrews, Anderson, Slade, & Sunderland, 2008), an increased attention to cultural factors in the definition of diagnostic criteria (Lewis-Fernández et al., 2010), a stronger emphasis in a developmental perspective that may lead to new subtypes of anxiety disorders based on the age of onset of their symptoms (Pine et al., 2002), or the introduction of higher-order structures to account for the strong association between anxiety and other internalizing problems (Andrews et al., 2008; Wittchen, Beesdo, & Gloster, 2009).

In addition to this, a considerable number of studies have focused on more specific issues, namely on how to organize the various anxiety disorders in relation to each other. The changes proposed aim at reclassifying in another diagnostic category some anxiety disorders such as OCD (Hollander, Braun, & Simeon, 2008; Stein et al., 2010) or PTSD (McNally, 2009); removing AG from DSM (Wittchen, Gloster, Beesdo-Baum, Fava, & Craske, 2010); or subsuming other anxiety disorders such as PD with and without AG under a single broader category (Craske et al., 2010). Moreover, it is believed that SAD would be reclassified from *Disorders Usually First Diagnosed in Infancy, Childhood, or Adolescence* to *Anxiety Disorders* (APA, 2010), while suggestions have been made to extend and adapt the criteria of PTSD to preschool children (Meiser-Stedman, Smith, Glucksman, Yule, & Dalgleish, 2008; Pynoos, Steinberg, Layne, Briggs, Ostrowski, & Fairbank, 2009). Finally, during the preparation of DSM-V, increased attention has also been paid to the question of how best to categorize GAD (Andrews et al., 2010), social phobia (Bögels et al., 2010), and SP (LeBeau et al., 2010).

However, despite the great deal of research going on into each of these issues, it is not clear which of the proposed changes will finally take place in the forthcoming revision of

DSM, let alone the implications that such revision will have for the development of new measures to assess and diagnose anxiety disorders in childhood and adolescence.

Assessment methods and instruments

Clinicians and researchers working in the field of youth's anxiety disorders can use a wide range of instruments and procedures, including diagnostic interviews, parent/teacher rating scales, children's self-reports, and direct observation or psychophysiological recordings (where possible). Twenty years ago, Barrios and Hartman (1988) described 100 instruments used in the assessment of childhood anxiety, with most of them focused on the motor or behavioral component. Since then, several other techniques have been developed, keyed to the most recent theoretical developments in the study of anxiety and the many revisions of the DSM and ICD. Some of them are multiple informant measures, in an attempt to overcome the low agreement among child and adults reports that has been observed in the study of anxiety disorders (Comer & Kendall, 2004). Furthermore, there has been an increasing effort to incorporate some measure of impairment in those instruments in order to facilitate diagnoses.

These advances are well documented in recent, extensive reviews of the literature (see American Academy of Child and Adolescent Psychiatry, 2007; Greco & Morris, 2004; Langley, Bergman, & Piacentini, 2002; Muris, 2007; Myers & Winters, 2002; Silverman & Ollendick, 2005). This chapter will focus only on those more psychometrically sound and most frequently used both for research and clinical purposes. Further, our review will be restricted to general self-report measures of anxiety and structured, semi-structured interviews or diagnostic interviews, and observational methods.

Interviews

An unstructured clinical interview with the parent(s) and the child is perhaps the most commonly used method for assessing anxiety disorders. Unstructured interviews have the advantage of great flexibility, permitting a relationship of trust to be developed with the child and parent, while at the same time allowing for a wide range of issues to be assessed. Moreover, unstructured interviews provide an excellent opportunity to observe family interactions and, in particular, how they influence the child's problems. However, because the interviewer may not ask the same questions of all family members, there are likely to be considerable differences in the information obtained from each informant. In addition, family members may disagree with one another regarding the occurrence, nature, and meaning of the same behavior or emotion. As a consequence, the rate of agreement between interviewers is generally low (McClelland & Werry, 2000).

To overcome these shortcomings, structured and semi-structured diagnostic interviews have been developed to increase the accuracy and reliability of diagnosis in children. As such, structured interviews consist of a long series of standardized questions covering a large range of problems which are asked in the same predetermined order and which yield DSM or, less often, ICD diagnoses. Most have parent and child forms, thus providing the interviewer with a more complex picture of the child's difficulties and allowing for the comparison of information from different informants. The parent and child forms are generally identical except for changes in the phrasing of questions. Additionally, some include visual prompts (e.g., fear thermometers, calendars, diaries) for use with younger children to elicit more accurate responses.

The most well researched and widely used structured and semi-structured interviews are the Schedule for Affective Disorders and Schizophrenia in School-Age Children (K-SADS) (Ambrosini, 2000), the Diagnostic Interview for Children and Adolescents (DICA) (Herjanic & Reich, 1982; Reich, 2000), the Child Assessment Schedule (CAS) (Hodges, McKnew, Cytryn, Stern, & Kline, 1982), the Diagnostic Interview Schedule for Children (DISC) (Costello, Edelbrock, Dulcan, Kalas, & Klaric, 1984), the Anxiety Disorders Interview Schedule for DSM-IV: Child and Parent Versions (ADIS-C/P) (Silverman & Albano, 1996; Silverman, Saavedra, & Pina, 2001), and the Child and Adolescent Psychiatric Assessment (CAPA) (Angold & Costello, 1995, 2000). Data on the validity and reliability of these instruments have been analyzed and discussed in several publications (e.g., Greco & Morris, 2004; Silverman, 1994; Silverman & Ollendick, 2005; Wood, Piacentini, Bergman, McCraken, & Barrios, 2002) and can be summarized as follows: they all use a structured or semi-structured format; have equivalent versions for parents and children; are able to generate diagnoses based on DSM criteria; allow for recording of the child's behavior during interview; can be used across a wide age range; and cover most childhood disorders. Generally, these interviews are diverse in their flexibility of presentation, the number of items included, the time required for administration, the rating format, the amount of training required, and the attention paid to anxiety and related disorders.

One of the few interviews specifically designed to assess anxiety disorders in children and adolescents, the ADIS-C/P (Silverman & Albano, 1996), is now one of the best known and most widely used. Like other semi-structured diagnostic interviews, it has parent and child versions. The interview, which follows a pre-set format, covers all of the anxiety disorders as defined in DSM-IV. The parent and child versions are administered separately, have slightly different coverage, and provide two independent scores which are then combined to arrive at a diagnosis. Each diagnosis is rated for severity and level of impairment, and detailed information can be collected on most of the other main child and adolescent DSM-IV disorders (e.g., depression, conduct disorder), precipitating events, and course of the disorder. Additionally, it includes questions that can help in a functional analysis of the child's anxiety symptoms.

The ADIS-C/P has been shown to have good inter-rater agreement for principal diagnosis as well as for the individual anxiety disorders, test–retest reliability, and sensitivity to treatment-produced change (Lyneham, Abbott, & Rapee, 2007; Silverman & Ollendick, 2005). In a study with a clinic sample, Silverman and Eisen (1992) calculated test–retest reliabilities over a period of 10–14 days. Overall Kappas for diagnoses were good for the child, parent, and combined diagnoses. Similarly a good inter-rater agreement was found in the assessment of preschool children (Rapee, Kennedy, Ingram, Edwards, & Sweeney, 2005), although the interview was designed to be used in children aged 6 years or older. Finally there are data showing concurrent validity between the diagnoses derived from the ADIS-C/P (i.e., separation anxiety, panic disorder, and social phobia), and the empirically derived factor scores on the Multidimensional Anxiety Scale for Children (Wood *et al.*, 2002).

To conclude, the ADIS-C/P provides coverage of all the anxiety disorders, seems to fare better than other existing interviews in differentiating among the different types of anxiety disorders, and is generally considered the gold standard interview for clinicians and researchers in this field. Of course, like most structured and semi-structured interviews it can take a long time to administer when the child meets criteria for multiple anxiety disorders. Some children may find it difficult to sit through the entire interview, necessitating breaks. Also, like most interviews, its diagnostic validity for younger children (e.g., those under 9–10 years) requires further investigation. Moreover, as noted earlier by Edelbrock, Greenbaum, and Conover (1985), structured clinical interviews with children below 8 years of age may be extremely unreliable and, consequently, data gathered by this method should be compared and complemented with those obtained through other procedures (see also Edwards, Rapee, Kennedy, & Spence, 2010).

Self-report measures

Because many symptoms of anxiety are internal to the child, they may pass undetected by other people. As such, the information provided by the child about their feelings, perceptions, or cognitions becomes of paramount importance in the assessment process. Some of the earliest studies on childhood anxiety relied exclusively on children's or adolescents' answers to a single question such as "What do you fear the most?" or "Which is the thing to be more afraid of?" The answers obtained by this procedure could be subsequently subjected to statistical analysis of variable complexity (e.g., frequency tallies, factor analysis, analysis of correspondence), leading to the classification of fears and anxieties in various categories.

It is currently most common to use standardized self-report measures such as rating scales or questionnaires in the assessment of childhood disorders, especially in research settings. These measures appear in a great variety of formats: behavior checklists, symptom checklists, personality questionnaires, and anxiety rating scales. One of the most widely used behavior checklists is the Youth Self-Report Questionnaire (Achenbach, 1991a), designed to assess child and adolescent (11–18 years) problems as well as adaptive behaviors. Social competencies are assessed through eight items, in a separate section at the beginning of the checklist, and in 16 items from a larger problem section. The main section of the checklist includes 102 items focusing on various behavior problems to which the child responds by circling *0* (not true), *1* (somewhat or sometimes true), and *2* (very true or often true). Principal component analyses of these items have consistently produced eight factors thought to reflect an equal number of statistically derived syndromes.

Of relevance here is the Anxious–Depressed subscale, which includes such symptoms as crying, a fear of doing things wrong, a need to be perfect, feeling nervous, worrying, and other related symptoms. A second subscale includes items relating to withdrawal. Through statistical analysis, it is possible to obtain one broad-band internalizing score that is derived from both the Anxious–Depressed and Withdrawn scales. This broad-band measure has been shown to successfully discriminate between referred and non-referred youngsters and has good test–retest reliability, although this varies according to age and gender. However, evidence supporting the validity of the anxiety measure remains scarce despite the widespread use of the Youth Self-Report (Aschenbrand, Angelosante, & Kendall, 2005; van Lang *et al.*, 2005).

Two other similar instruments are the Strengths and Difficulties Questionnaire (Goodman, 1997) and the Child Symptom Inventory-4 (Sprafkin, Gadow, Salisbury, Schneider, & Loney, 2002). They both include an anxiety scale and raise the same criticisms. In particular, the validity and clinical utility of that scale have not yet been fully demonstrated.

Contrasting with these general purpose questionnaires there are other self-report instruments specifically designed to assess children's fears and anxieties. Some of them provide global anxiety scores while others are aimed at evaluating specific anxiety disorder symptoms. One of the most researched and frequently used is the revised version of the Children's

Manifest Anxiety Scale (RCMAS: Reynolds & Richmond, 1978). The original CMAS was developed by Castaneda, McCandless, and Palermo (1956) and consisted of 53 items (42 Anxiety and 11 Lie scale items). In order to facilitate its administration, improve its psychometric properties and provide new normative data, the CMAS was revised to include 37 items (28 Anxiety and 9 Lie items) suitable for children 6–19 years of age (Reynolds & Richmond, 1978). Children respond to each item in a *yes/no* format. The authors found three statistically derived factors on this scale: Physiological, Worry/Oversensivity, and Concentration. Interestingly, some subsequent studies failed to replicate this factor structure but supported its use as a global measure of trait anxiety (Lee, Piersel, & Unruh, 1989). It has also been shown that the RCMAS possesses good test–retest reliability, across different time periods, and good convergent validity, as reflected in the high correlations between the RCMAS and the Trait Anxiety scale but not with the State Anxiety Scale of the State–Trait Anxiety Inventory for Children (STAIC) (Spielberger, 1973). Similarly, recent studies supported the factorial invariance as well as the construct validity of the RCMAS across White and Hispanic samples (Pina, Little, Knight, & Silverman, 2009), and showed its treatment sensitivity (Silverman & Ollendick, 2005). Data on its discriminant validity are generally mixed, as it has been shown to discriminate anxiety-disordered and normal controls but not anxiety-disordered from depressed children (Brady & Kendall, 1992) or children with attention deficit hyperactivity disorder (Perrin & Last, 1992). Further, the scores of younger children in this scale may be affected by social desirability (Pina, Silverman, Saavedra, & Weems, 2001).

Other self-report instruments traditionally used to assess youth's global level of anxiety-related stress or fears are the Revised Fear Survey Schedule for Children (FSSC-R: Ollendick, 1983) and the STAIC-T (State–Trait Anxiety Inventory for Children: Spielberger, 1973). However, they are less useful to assess symptoms clusters or anxiety disorders as described in the main diagnostic manuals (Langley *et al.*, 2002). Many of the limitations of these traditional measures have been overcome by the development of new ones based on DSM-IV criteria (see Brooks & Kutcher, 2003). One of them is the Multidimensional Anxiety Scale for Children (MASC: March, Parker, Sullivan, Stallings, & Conners, 1997), which can be completed by youth and their parents and yields a total anxiety disorder index as well as four main factor scores (i.e., physical symptoms, social anxiety, separation anxiety, and harm avoidance).

The MASC has good internal consistency, good test–retest reliability, satisfactory convergent validity both for the global index and for the subscales (Langley *et al.*, 2002; March, 1998; Wood *et al.*, 2002), as well as good discriminant validity (Rynn *et al.*, 2006). Another self-report measure is the Screen for Child Anxiety Related Emotional Disorders (SCARED: Birmaher *et al.*, 1997). The original SCARED consists of 38 items (both for children and parents) rated on a three-point scale. These items have been statistically grouped into five factors or subscales, including a general anxiety, separation anxiety, social phobia, somatic/panic, and school phobia scales. Data on the psychometric properties of this measure come from one large study of clinically referred children and adolescents (aged 9–18 years), and have shown its good test–retest reliability and internal consistency, as well as satisfactory validity. In particular, the SCARED succeeded in differentiating not only anxious from non-anxious children but also amongst various types of anxiety disorders (Birmaher, Brent, Chiappetta, Bridge, Monga, & Baugher, 1999). More recently, a revised version of the SCARED was developed (the SCARED-R) in order to provide a fuller account of children's and adolescents' anxiety disorders described in DSM-IV. This revised measure has

69 items, in versions for parents and children, and possesses good psychometric qualities (Muris, 2007).

Another DSM-based anxiety measure is the Spence Children's Anxiety Scale (SCAS: Spence, 1997). It consists of 45 items (38 anxiety items and 7 filler items) rated on a *0* (never) to *3* (always) scale. Factor analyses (exploratory and confirmatory) from a large community study with children (aged 8–12 years), revealed five interpretable factors across sex: panic–agoraphobia, social phobia, separation anxiety, obsessive–compulsive problems, generalized anxiety, and physical fears. It appeared to have good internal consistency, satisfactory test–retest reliability, and good convergent and discriminant validity. For example, strong significant correlations were found between this scale and the RCMAS or between its subscales and the SCARED-R. However, there were also several criticisms regarding the validity of some of its subscales, which led to its subsequent modification (Chorpita *et al.*, 2000). The new version – Revised Child Anxiety and Depression Scales – is considerably longer but continues to demonstrate good psychometric qualities (Chorpita, Moffitt, & Gray, 2005). There is also evidence that these qualities can be found in samples from different countries or cultures (Mellon & Moutavelis, 2007). However, its clinical utility still needs further investigation.

Taken together, self-report measures constitute a rapid, flexible, and cost-efficient means of assessing children's level of anxiety. In this sense, they are particularly useful as screening instruments at the beginning of the assessment process. Yet their clinical utility could be improved through the inclusion of items relating to the severity and associated impairment due to symptoms, or by reducing item overlap with measures of separate constructs (e.g., depression and behavior disorders). However, such instruments may be difficult for use with younger children whose reading abilities can vary greatly as well as their capacity to describe their anxiety. This could be partially compensated by the utilization of other sources of information.

Ratings by significant others

Questionnaires and checklists completed by parents, teachers, and other significant adults have often been used in the assessment of childhood anxiety disorders. The rationale behind using parent/teacher ratings of the child's anxiety is that those adults, who observe children over a long period of time, across numerous settings and stages of development, are in an excellent position to give an account of their problems. Further, they are also the persons who generally refer children for assessment and often become closely involved in treatment (Myers & Winters, 2002).

One of the most widely used checklists of this type is the Child Behavior Checklist (CBCL: Achenbach, 1991a, 1991b; Achenbach & Rescorla, 2001), available in separate forms for parents and teachers. It was designed to assess, in a standardized format, the social competencies and behavior problems of children and adolescents (4–18 years of age). As such, it includes questions about demographic characteristics, child competence in school and elsewhere, and a list of 118 specific problems, some of them related to anxiety.

Like the Youth Self-Report, discussed above, the CBCL version for parents and teachers provides a global score, separate scores for internalizing and externalizing problems, and eight narrow-band scales, including an Anxious–Depressed scale. Test–retest reliability coefficients are high for both girls and boys (Achenbach, 1991a). Main advantages of this checklist over similar measures are that it has a large normative database, can discriminate gender and age levels (increasing its sensitivity to developmental factors), and presents good psychometric properties demonstrated in large standardization samples. In particular, the existence of parallel forms for parents, teachers (Teacher Report Form – TRF), and adolescents allows for a comparative assessment by informant over a range of symptoms (Kendall, Puliafico, Barmish, Choudhury, Henin, & Treadwell, 2007). Moreover, the CBCL has been translated and standardized in several languages, which makes it especially useful for cross-cultural studies (Hartman *et al.*, 1999; Ivanova *et al.*, 2007a, 2007b; Rescorla *et al.*, 2007). As to its clinical utility, data are still scarce and often inconsistent. Thus, Gould, Bird, and Jaramillo (1993) found low but significant correlations between the CBCL internalizing scales and DSM-III-R diagnoses of anxiety and depression in an epidemiological sample, while Achenbach (1991a) reported high correlations between this scale and other measures of anxiety. Efforts to generate DSM-IV diagnoses based on CBCL/YSR scores produced no compelling data supporting the discriminant validity of these teachers' and parents' versions in the assessment of anxiety disorders (Ferdinand, 2008). Instead, the internalizing Cluster and the Anxiety–Depression scale appeared to measure a more global construct such as negative affect (Chorpita & Daleiden, 2002).

There are a number of other broadband measures of child psychopathology completed by parents and teachers that have been used to assess anxiety in clinical or research settings. These include the Conner's Rating Scales (Goyette, Conners, & Ulrich, 1978), the Revised Behavior Problems Checklist (Quay & Peterson, 1987), Rutter Scales (Rutter, 1967; Rutter, Tizard, & Whitemore, 1970), and the Strengths and Difficulties Questionnaire (Goodman, 1997). All have equivalent forms for parents and teachers, have been extensively used in community studies (Boyle & Jones, 1985; Weisz & Eastman, 1994), and display good psychometric properties. However, like the Achenbach checklist, their anxiety subscales generally encompass other symptoms and, therefore, lack specificity. Further, as they rely on adult ratings of the child's anxiety they are subject to certain biases (see McGee, Feehan, Williams, & Anderson, 1983; Turner, Beidel, & Costello, 1987). In particular, parents' perception of their children's difficulties can be influenced by their own depression or anxiety (McGee *et al.*, 1983; Moretti, Fine, Haley, & Marriage, 1985), which means that parent rating scales should only be used as part of a comprehensive package that also includes direct assessment of the child (Cole, Hoffman, Tram, & Maxwell, 2000). Similar comments can be made regarding other scales for clinicians working in pediatric settings such as the Pediatric Anxiety Rating Scale or PARS (Research Units on Pediatric Psychopharmacology Anxiety Study Group, 2002), aimed at assessing children's and adolescents' SAD, SOP, and GAD, as well as several other scales used to assess specific youths' anxiety disorders. However, the PARS' psychometric properties are not yet fully established (for a brief review of their strengths and weaknesses see Muris, 2007).

Direct observation methods

The central feature of direct observation methods is their focus on anxious behaviors as they actually occur in vivo or in situ, with particular emphasis on their antecedents and consequences. Assessment of this antecedent–behavior–consequence (A–B–C) relationship goes beyond the typical assessment of antecedent only (i.e., fear items on the Revised Fear Survey Schedule for Children [FSSC-R]), to provide a truly ideographic view of the anxious child. Also, direct observations are generally more useful in the development of treatment interventions than responses on most questionnaires. Indeed, direct observation of anxiety, by children themselves or another person, forms the backbone of most cognitive–behavioral treatments for anxious children.

There are two main categories of direct observations: those that occur in natural settings and those set up by the clinician such as Behavior Avoidance Tests (BATs). Under natural observation conditions, the clinician or the child monitors a target anxiety symptom for setting, frequency, duration, and intensity over well-defined periods. Naturalistic observation is useful, for example, in the assessment of fears of dental surgery, separation anxiety, test anxiety, public speaking anxiety, and many other situations. A variant typical example of this method is to have the child record his or her mood, thoughts, and behaviors during particular intervals throughout the day in a diary (self-monitoring). Glennon and Weisz (1978) developed an observation method for separation anxiety among preschool children that involves rating the occurrence of 30 behaviors (e.g., physical complaints, avoidance of eye contact, using words such as "afraid" and "scared") believed to reflect anxiety, while the child performs tasks in the presence and absence of the mother.

Another standardized measure is the Direct Observation Form (DOF) (see McConaughy, 1985) designed to monitor children's behavior in the classroom as well as in other group settings. It involves writing a narrative of the child's behavior as it occurs over 10-minute intervals at different times of the day. Drawing on this narrative, the observer rates the 96 behavior problems using a *0* (not observed) to *4* (definitely occurred) point scale. Although it is considered a general observation measure, some of its items are directly related to anxiety and fears. The DOF is typically administered by a trained observer (other than a teacher/parent) for use in the classroom with children of any age.

In contrast to the above, BATs use observational methods to directly assess the child's anxiety when confronted with the threat-related stimuli under controlled and standardized situations. For example, a BAT for a child with a specific spider phobia would consist of asking him or her to enter a room where a spider could be found in a cage, and register in detail their reactions. Several indices of anxiety can be derived with this strategy, including: response latency, distance from feared objects, number of tasks performed, number of approach responses, physiological reactions, and other reactions believed to reflect anxiety. This technique may be very helpful to evaluate the effects of treatment for specific phobias, but its usefulness is rather limited when the fear-eliciting stimuli cannot be clearly defined (e.g., in cases of generalized anxiety disorder).

There have been also some efforts to develop observational techniques that can account for the interactions of anxious children with other members of their family. Underlying this approach is the idea that parenting styles, family psychopathology, and family interactions generally play an important role in the etiology and maintenance of childhood anxiety. A good example of this approach is the Family Anxiety Coding Schedule developed by Dadds and colleagues (1994, 1996). This schedule was designed to register, in specified time periods, the anxious behaviors of the child and parents, as well as their mutual influences (defined in terms of antecedents and consequences). This should lead to the identification of family variables that may seem to maintain anxiety. One difference from other traditional methods of observation is that it focuses not only on the child's individual reactions but also on the interdependencies between several people's behavior (Hudson & Rapee, 2002).

Generally speaking, direct observation has several advantages over self- and parent-reports of childhood anxiety disorders: greater objectivity and flexibility, good inter-raters reliability (Ferrell, Beidel, & Turner, 2004; Moore, Whaley, & Sigman, 2004), and the focus on target behaviors for intervention. However, despite the increasing sophistication of direct observation methods (e.g., cameras, microphones, videotapes), many aspects of the child's anxiety remain inaccessible to the outside observer. Objective and detailed records of the frequency and duration of anxiety reactions do not necessarily provide relevant information on the child's subjective experience of feared events. Indeed, the same score on a given BAT may represent different levels of distress for different children (e.g., it is difficult to know if crying reflects anxiety, fear, aggressiveness, opposition, or other emotional states). Also, there is not as yet sufficient empirical evidence that observational methods are any better able to discriminate between anxious and non-anxious children, or between various forms of anxiety disorders than adult questionnaires or self-reports. In particular it is difficult to generalize these techniques across situations, given the lack of standardization of the tasks and coding procedures. Furthermore, observational methods are often costly, seem unlikely to provide any useful data about anxiety symptoms that are of very low frequency, and can be perceived as intrusive by the children or the family. Still, when the necessary precautions are taken, observational techniques become an important part of the assessment and treatment process of children's anxiety disorders.

Issues for further research

There is currently a number of excellent methods and instruments to choose from, when attempting to assess children's and adolescents' anxiety disorders, many of them developed over the last 30 years. Naturally, this has contributed to a more valid diagnosis of these disorders, a more accurate estimation of their prevalence rates, a better understanding of comorbidity in this field, and a higher consistency across studies and evaluations (Costello *et al.*, 2004). However, they often have important flaws and none of them fit in all situations. Thus, the selection of measures that best meet the needs and characteristics of a given child can be quite a challenging task. It depends not only on the purposes of the assessment and the qualities of the instruments, but also on the conceptualization of childhood anxiety disorders, the child's age, the symptoms profile, the sources of information available, the classification system of anxiety disorders selected, and the settings where the assessment is to be done. For instance, structured diagnostic interviews are better suited to categorical classification of anxiety disorders in clinical referred groups, while self-report or problems checklists are more suited to a dimensional approach classification or for screening purposes in general population. Therefore, a priority should be to determine which measures are useful for what purposes, and to think critically about which future developments are most needed in this domain. Among the issues deserving further research are improving the cross-cultural validity of anxiety measures, handling of discrepant information from multiple informants, improving the discriminant validity of existing measures, demonstrating their clinical relevance, and possibly developing new instruments that reflect the current conceptual and theoretical advances in the field of anxiety disorders as well as eventual changes suggested for the next edition of DSM (Beesdo *et al.*, 2009).

Conclusion

Data from epidemiological and longitudinal studies show that youth anxiety disorders are as prevalent and disturbing as any other form of child and adolescent psychopathology. In the first part of this chapter, we have provided an overview of the phenomenology and classification of those disorders. In this context, anxiety was presented as tripartite in nature (i.e., fear/worry, avoidance, and hyperarousal). Although this view is now being challenged in the literature, it remains the dominant influence on the characterization of anxiety disorders in the DSM. In addition, the limitations and strengths of the DSM and its "all-or-none" approach were contrasted with those that place anxiety on a continuum with no clear cut-offs to indicate where clinical significance begins.

In the second part, we discussed the various measures of anxiety (e.g., structured interviews, adult ratings, child self-reports, and direct observation), their psychometric properties, the diversity of symptoms that they are supposed to cover, the availability of adequate normative data, and their clinical utility. It is apparent from this review that, despite important advances registered in childhood assessment during the last 20 years, the psychometric properties of the widely used anxiety measures are uneven, their coverage is often rather limited, and their sensitivity to developmental aspects of anxiety often remains rather poor. In particular, no single measure has succeeded to account for all facets of anxiety, and no definitive rule has been provided to integrate the information from different sources and instruments.

It is crucial that mental health researchers and clinicians take notice of the progress already made (as well as of the challenges that lie ahead) in this field and, whenever possible, integrate such a knowledge in their professional practice, so that children and adolescents with anxiety disorders can be accurately diagnosed and successfully cared for in the community or in clinical settings.

Acknowledgments

Preparation of this chapter was supported by the Centro de Psicopedagogia da Universidade de Coimbra (FEDER/160–490: POCTI 2010) and the Grant PTDC/PSI-PED/104849/2008.

References

Achenbach, T. M. (1991a). *Manual for the Youth Self-Report and 1991 Profile*. Burlington, VT: University of Vermont Department of Psychiatry.

Achenbach, T. M. (1991b). *Manual for the Child Behaviour Checklist/4–18 and 1991 Profile*. Burlington, VT: University of Vermont Department of Psychiatry.

Achenbach, T. M. (1991c). *Manual for the Teachers Report Form and 1991 Profile*. Burlington, VT: University of Vermont Department of Psychiatry.

Achenbach, T. M. & Rescorla, L. A. (2001). *Manual for ASEBA School-Age Forms and Profiles*. Burlington, VT: Univerity of Vermont, Research Center for Children, Youth, and Families.

Achenbach, T. M., Dumenci, L., & Rescorla, L. (2003). Are American children's problems still getting worse? A 23-year comparison. *Journal of Abnormal Child Psychology*, **31**, 1–11.

Albano, A. M., Chorpita, B. F., & Barlow, D. H. (2003). Childhood anxiety disorders. In: E. J. Mash & R. A. Barkley (eds.) *Child Psychopathology*, pp. 279–329. New York: Guilford Press.

Ambrosini, P. J. (2000). Historical development and present status of the Schedule for Affective Disorders and Schizophrenia for School-Age Children (K-SADS). *Journal of the American Academy of Child and Adolescent Psychiatry*, **39**, 49–58.

American Academy of Child and Adolescent Psychiatry (2007). Practice parameter for the assessment and treatment of children and adolescents with anxiety disorders. *Journal of the American Academy of Child and Adolescent Psychiatry*, **46**, 267–283.

American Psychiatric Association (1994). *Diagnostic and Statistical Manual of Mental Disorders*, 4th edn. Washington, DC: American Psychiatric Association.

American Psychiatric Association (2000). *Diagnostic and Statistical Manual of Mental Disorders,* 4th edn, text revision. Washington, DC: American Psychiatric Association.

American Psychiatric Association (2009). *Report of the DSM-V Anxiety, Obsessive–Compulsive Spectrum, Posttraumatic, and Dissociative Disorders Work Group.* Arlington, VA: American Psychiatric Association. Available at www.psych.org/MainMenu/Research/DSMIV/DSMV/ DSMRevisionActivities/DSM-V-Work-Group-Reports/Anxiety-Obsessive-Compulsive-Spectrum-Posttraumatic-and-Dissociative-Disorders-Work-Group-Report.aspx.

American Psychiatric Association (2010). DSM-5 development. Available at www.dsm5.org/ Proposedrevisions/Pages/AnxietyDisorders.aspx.

Anderson, E. R. & **Hope, D. A.** (2008). A review of the tripartite model for understanding the link between anxiety and depression in youth. *Clinical Psychology Review,* **28**, 275–287.

Anderson, J. C., Williams, S. M., McGee, R., & **Silva, P.** (1987). DSM-III disorders in preadolescent children: prevalence in a large sample from the general population. *Archives of General Psychiatry,* **44**, 69–76.

Andrews, G., Anderson, T. M., Slade, T., & **Sunderland, M.** (2008). Classification of anxiety and depressive disorders: problems and solutions. *Depression and Anxiety,* **25**, 274–281.

Andrews, G., Hobbs, M. J., Borkovec, T. D., Beesdo, K., Craske, M. G., Heimberg, R. G., *et al.* (2010). Generalized worry disorder: a review of DSM-IV generalized anxiety disorder and options for DSM-V. *Depression and Anxiety,* **27**, 134–147.

Angold, A. & **Costello, E. J.** (1995). A test–retest reliability study of child-reported psychiatric symptoms and diagnoses using the Child and Adolescent Psychiatric Assessment (CAPA-C). *Psychological Medicine,* **25**, 755–762.

Angold, A. & **Costello, E. J.** (2000). The Child and Adolescent Psychiatric Assessment (CAPA). *Journal of the American Academy of Child and Adolescent Psychiatry,* **39**, 39–48.

Aschenbrand, S. G., Angelosante, A. G., & **Kendall, P. C.** (2005). Discriminant validity and clinical utility of the CBCL with anxiety disordered youth. *Journal of Clinical Child and Adolescent Psychology,* **34**, 735–746.

Austin, A. A. & **Chorpita, B. F.** (2004). Temperament, anxiety and depression: comparisons across five ethnic groups of children. *Journal of Clinical Child and Adolescent Psychology,* **33**, 216–226.

Barlow, D. H. (2002). *Anxiety and its Disorders: The Nature and Treatment of Anxiety and Panic,* 2nd edn. New York: Guilford Press.

Barlow, D. H., Allen, L. B., & **Choate, M. L.** (2004). Toward a unified treatment for emotional disorders. *Behaviour Therapy,* **35**, 205–230.

Barrios, B. A. & **Hartmann, D. P.** (1988). Fears and phobias. In: **E. J. Mash** & **L. G. Tardal** (eds.) *Behavioural Assessment of Childhood Disorders,* pp. 196–262. New York: Guilford Press.

Beesdo, K., Knappe, S., & **Pine, D. S.** (2009). Anxiety and anxiety disorders in children and adolescents: developmental issues and implications for DSM-V. *Psychiatric Clinics of North America,* **32**, 483–524.

Birmaher, B., Brent, D. A., Chiappetta, L., Bridge, J., Monga, S., & **Baugher, M.** (1999). Psychometric properties of the Screen for Child Anxiety Related Emotional Disorders (SCARED): a replication study. *Journal of the American Academy of Child and Adolescent Psychiatry,* **38**, 1230–1236.

Birmaher, B., Khertarpal, S., Brent, D., Cully, M., Balach, L., Kaufman, J., *et al.* (1997). The Screen for Child Anxiety Related Emotional Disorders (SCARED): scale construction and psychometric characteristics. *Journal of the American Academy of Child and Adolescent Psychiatry,* **36**, 545–553.

Bittner, A., Egger, H. L., Erkanli, A., Costello, E. J., Foley, D. L., & **Angold, A.** (2007). What do childhood anxiety disorders predict? *Journal of Child Psychology and Psychiatry,* **48**, 1174–1183.

Blanton, H. & **Jaccard, J.** (2006). Arbitrary metrics in psychology. *American Psychologist,* **61**, 27–41.

Bodden, D., Dirksen, C., & Bogels, M. (2008). Societal burden of clinically anxious youth referred for treatment: a cost-of-illness study. *Journal of Abnormal Child Psychology*, **36**, 487–497.

Bögels, S. M., Alden, L., Beidel, D. C., Clark, L. A., Pine, D. S., Murray, B. S., *et al.* (2010). Social anxiety disorder: questions and answers for the DSM-V. *Depression and Anxiety*, **27**, 168–189.

Bolton, D., Eley, T., O'Connor, T., Perrin, S., Rabe-Hesketh, S., Rijsdijk, F., *et al.* (2006). Prevalence and genetic and environmental influences on anxiety disorders in 6-year-old twins. *Psychological Medicine*, **36**, 335–344.

Boyle, M. H. & Jones, S. C. (1985). Selecting measures of emotional and behavioral disorders of childhood for use in general populations. *Journal of Child Psychology and Psychiatry*, **26**, 137–159.

Brady, E. U. & Kendall, P. C. (1992). Comorbidity of anxiety and depression in children and adolescents. *Psychological Bulletin*, **111**, 244–255.

Brooks, S. J. & Kutcher, S. (2003). Diagnosis and measurement of anxiety disorders in adolescents: a review of commonly used instruments. *Journal of Child and Adolescent Psychopharmacology*, **13**, 351–400.

Brown, T. A. & Barlow, D. H. (2002). Classification of anxiety and mood disorders. In: D. H. Barlow (ed.) *Anxiety and Its Disorders: The Nature and Treatment of Anxiety and Panic*, 2nd edn, pp. 292–327. New York: Guilford Press.

Campbell, J. M. (2006). Anxiety disorders. In: R. Kamphaus & J. Campbell (eds.) *Psychodiagnostic Assessment of Children: Dimensional and Categorical Approaches*, pp. 212–245. New York: Wiley & Sons.

Canino, G., Shrout, P., Rubio-Stipec, M., Bird, H., Bravo, M., Ramirez, R., *et al.* (2004). The DSM-IV rates of child and adolescent disorders in Puerto Rico. *Archives of General Psychiatry*, **61**, 85–93.

Cartwright-Hatton, C., McNicol, K., & Doubleday, E. (2006). Anxiety in a neglected population: prevalence of anxiety disorders in pre-adolescent children. *Clinical Psychology Review*, **26**, 817–833.

Castaneda, A., McCandless, B. R., & Palermo, D. S. (1956). The children's form of the Manifest Anxiety Scale. *Child Development*, **27**, 317–326.

Chorpita, B. F. (2002). The tripartite model and dimensions of anxiety and depression: an examination of structure in a large school sample. *Journal of Abnormal Child Psychology*, **30**, 177–190.

Chorpita, B. F. & Daleiden, E. L. (2002). Tripartite dimensions of emotion in a child clinical sample: measurement strategies and implications for clinical utility. *Journal of Consulting and Clinical Psychology*, **70**, 1150–1160.

Chorpita, B. F., Moffitt, C. E., & Gray, J. (2005). Psychometric properties of the Revised Child Anxiety and Depression Scale in a clinical sample. *Behaviour Research and Therapy*, **43**, 309–322.

Chorpita, B. F., Yim, L., Moffitt, C., Umemoto, L. A., & Francis, S. E. (2000). Assessment of symptoms of DSM-IV anxiety and depression in children: a revised child anxiety and depression scale. *Behaviour Research and Therapy*, **38**, 835–855.

Clark, D. A. & Taylor, S. (2009). The transdiagnostic perspective on cognitive-behavioral therapy for anxiety and depression: new wine for old wineskins? *Journal of Cognitive Psychotherapy*, **23**, 60–66.

Clark, L. A. & Watson, D. (1991). Tripartite model of anxiety and depression: psychometric evidence and taxonomic implications. *Journal of Abnormal Psychology*, **107**, 74–85.

Clark, L. A., Watson, D., & Reynolds, S. (1995). Diagnosis and classification of psychopathology: challenges to the current system and future directions. *Annual Review of Psychology*, **46**, 121–153.

Cole, D. A., Hoffman, K., Tram, J. M., & Maxwell, S. E. (2000). Structural differences in parent and child reports of children's symptoms of depression and anxiety. *Psychological Assessment*, **12**, 174–185.

Comer, J. S. & Kendall, P. C. (2004). A symptom-level examination of parent–child agreement in the diagnosis of anxious youth. *Journal of the American Academy of Child and Adolescent Psychiatry*, **43**, 878–886.

Cone, J. D. (1998). Hierarchical views of anxiety: what do they profit us? *Behavior Therapy*, **29**, 325–332.

Connor-Smith, J. K. & Compas, B. E. (2003). Analogue measures of DSM-IV mood and anxiety disorders based on behaviour check-lists. *Journal of Psychopathology and Behavioral Assessment*, **25**, 37–48.

Costello, E. J., Costello, A. J., Edelbrock, C. S., Burns, B. J., Dulcan, M. J., Brent, D., *et al.* (1988). DSM-III disorders in pediatric primary care: prevalence and risk factors. *Archives of General Psychiatry*, **45**, 1107–1116.

Costello, E. J., Edelbrock, C., Dulcan, M. K., Kalas, R., & Klaric, S. (1984). *Report on the NIMH Diagnostic Interview Schedule for Children (DISC)*. Washington, DC: National Institutes of Mental Health.

Costello, E. J., Egger, H. L., & Angold, A. (2004). Developmental epidemiology of anxiety disorders. In: J. March & T. Ollendick (eds.) *Phobic and Anxiety Disorders in Children and Adolescents: A Clinician's Guide to Effective Psychosocial and Pharmacological Interventions*, pp. 61–92. Oxford, UK: Oxford University Press.

Craske, M. G., Kircanski, K., Phil, M. A. C., Epstein, A., Wittchen, H., Pine, D. S., *et al.* (2010). Panic disorder: a review of DSM-IV panic disorder and proposals for DSM-V. *Depression and Anxiety*, **27**, 93–112.

Curry, J. F., March, J. S., & Hervey, A. S. (2004). Comorbidity of childhood and adolescence anxiety. In: J. March & T. Ollendick (eds.) *Phobic and Anxiety Disorders in Children and Adolescents: A Clinician's Guide to Effective Psychosocial and Pharmacological Interventions*, pp. 116–141. Oxford, UK: Oxford University Press.

Dadds, M. R., Barrett, P. M., Rapee, R. M., & Ryan, S. (1996). Family process and child anxiety and aggression: an observational analysis. *Journal of Abnormal Child Psychology*, **24**, 715–734.

Dadds, M. R., James, R. C., Barrett, P. M., & Verhulst, F. C. (2004). Diagnostic Issues. In: J. March & T. Ollendick (eds.) *Phobic and Anxiety Disorders in Children and Adolescents: A Clinician's Guide to Effective Psychosocial and Pharmacological Interventions*, pp. 3–33. Oxford, UK: Oxford University Press.

Dadds, M. R., Rapee, R. M., & Barrett, P. M. (1994). Behavioral observation. In: T. H. Ollendick, N. J. King, & W. Yule (eds.) *The International Handbook of Phobic and Anxiety Disorders in Children and Adolescents*, pp. 349–364. New York: Plenum Press.

Dierker, L., Albano, A. M., Clarke, G. N., Heimberg, R. G., Kendall, P. C., Merikangas, K. R., *et al.* (2001). Screening for anxiety and depression in early adolescence. *Journal of the American Academy of Child and Adolescent Psychiatry*, **40**, 929–936.

Edelbrock, C., Greenbaum, R., & Conover, N. C. (1985). Reliability and concurrent relations between the Teacher Version of the Child Behaviour Profile and the Conners Revised Teacher Rating Scale. *Journal of Abnormal Child Psychiatry*, **13**, 295–304.

Edwards, S. L., Rapee, R. M., Kennedy, S. J., & Spence, S. H. (2010). The assessment of anxiety symptoms in preschool-aged children: the Revised Preschool Anxiety Scale. *Journal of Clinical Child and Adolescent Psychology*, **39**, 400–409.

Essau, C., Conradt, J., & Petermann, F. (1999). Frequency and comorbidity of social phobia and social fears in adolescents. *Behaviour Research and Therapy*, **37**, 831–843.

Feng, X., Shaw, D. S., & Silk, J. S. (2008). Developmental trajectories of anxiety symptoms among boys across early and middle childhood. *Journal of Abnormal Psychology*, **117**, 32–47.

Ferdinand, R. F. (2006). Predicting anxiety diagnoses with the Youth Self-Report. *Depression and Anxiety*, **24**, 32–40.

Ferdinand, R. F. (2008). Validity of the CBCL/YSR DSM-IV scales Anxiety Problems and Affective Problems. *Journal of Anxiety Disorders*, **22**, 126–134.

Ferdinand, R. F., Dieleman, G., Ormel, J., & Verhulst, F. C. (2007). Homotypic versus heterotypic continuity of anxiety symptoms in young adolescents: evidence for distinctions between DSM-IV subtypes. *Journal of Abnormal Child Psychology*, **35**, 325–333.

Ferdinand, R. F., van Lang, N. D. J., Ormel, J., & Verhulst, F. C. (2006). No distinctions between different types of anxiety symptoms in pre-adolescents from the general population. *Journal of Anxiety Disorders*, **20**, 207–221.

Ferrell, C., Beidel, D., & Turner, S. (2004). Assessment and treatment of socially phobic children: a cross-cultural comparison. *Journal of Clinical Child and Adolescent Psychology*, **33**, 260–268.

Foley, D. L., Pickles, A., Maes, H. M., Silberg, J. L., & Eaves, L. J. (2004). Course and short-term outcomes of separation anxiety disorder in a community sample of twins. *Journal of the American Academy of Child and Adolescent Psychiatry*, **43**, 1107–1114.

Ford, T., Goodman, R., & Meltezer, H. (2003). The British Child and Adolescent Mental Health Survey 1999: the prevalence of DSM-IV disorders. *Journal of the American Academy of Child and Adolescent Psychiatry*, **40**, 1203–1211.

Glennon, B. & Weisz, J. R. (1978). An observational approach to the assessment of anxiety in young children. *Journal of Consulting and Clinical Psychology*, **46**, 1246–1257.

Goodman, R. (1997). The Strengths and Difficulties Questionnaire: a research note. *Journal of Child Psychology and Psychiatry*, **38**, 581–586.

Gould, M. S., Bird, H., & Jaramillo, B. S. (1993). Correspondence between statistically derived behaviour problem syndromes and child psychiatric diagnoses in a community sample. *Journal of Abnormal Child Psychology*, **21**, 287–313.

Goyette, C., Conners, C., & Ulrich, R. (1978). Normative data on Revised Conners Parent and Teachers Rating Scales. *Journal of Abnormal Child Psychology*, **6**, 221–236.

Greco, L. A. & Morris, T. L. (2004). Assessment. In: T. L. Morris & J. S. March (eds.) *Anxiety Disorders in Children and Adolescents*, pp. 98–121. New York: Guilford Press.

Gregory, A. M. & Eley, T. C. (2007). Genetic influences on anxiety in children: what we've learned and where we're heading. *Clinical Child and Family Psychology Review*, **10**, 199–212.

Grinde, B. (2005). An approach to the prevention of anxiety-related disorders based on evolutionary medicine. *Preventive Medicine*, **40**, 904–909.

Hartman, C. A., Hox, J., Auerbach, J., Erol, N., Fonseca, A. C., Nevik, T. S., *et al.* (1999). Syndrome dimensions of the Child Behavior Checklist and the Teacher Report Form: a critical empirical evaluation. *Journal of Child Psychology and Psychiatry*, **40**, 1095–1116.

Herjanic, B. & Reich, W. (1982). Development of a structured psychiatric interview: agreement between child and parent on individual symptoms. *Journal of Abnormal Child Psychology*, **10**, 307–324.

Hodges, K., McKnew, D., Cytryn, L., Stern, L., & Kline, J. (1982). The Child Assessment Schedule (CAS) Diagnostic Interview: a report on reliability and validity. *Journal of the American Academy of Child Psychiatry*, **21**, 468–473.

Hollander, E., Braun, A., & Simeon, D. (2008). Should OCD leave the anxiety disorders in DSM-V? The case for obsessive compulsive-related disorders. *Depression and Anxiety*, **25**, 317–329.

Hudson, J. L. & Rapee, R. M. (2002). Parent–child interactions in clinically anxious children and their siblings. *Journal of Clinical Child and Adolescent Psychology*, **31**, 548–555.

Ivanova, M. Y., Achenbach, T. M., Dumenci, L., Rescorla, L. A., Almqvist, F., Bilenberg, N., *et al.* (2007a). Testing the 8-Syndrome of the Child Behavior Checklist (CBCL) in 30 societies. *Journal of Clinical Child and Adolescent Psychology*, **36**, 405–417.

Ivanova, M. Y., Achenbach, T. M., Rescorla, L. A., Dumenci, L., Almqvist, F., Bathiche, M., *et al.* (2007b). The generalizability of Teacher's Report Form syndromes in 20 cultures. *School Psychology Review*, **36**, 468–483.

Joiner, T. E. & Lonigan, C. J. (2000). Tripartite model of depression and anxiety in youth psychiatric inpatients: relations with diagnostic status and future symptoms. *Journal of Clinical Child Psychology*, **29**, 372–382.

Kashdan, T. B. & Herbert, J. D. (2001). Social anxiety disorder in childhood and adolescence: current status and future directions. *Clinical Child and Family Psychology Review*, **1**, 37–61.

Kearney, C. A. (2001). *School Refusal Behavior in Youth: A Functional Approach and Treatment.* Washington, DC: American Psychological Association.

Kearney, C. A. (2006). Confirmatory factor analysis of the school refusal assessment scale revisited: child and parent versions. *Journal of Psychopathology and Behavioral Assessment*, **28**, 139–144.

Kearney, C. A. (2008). School absenteeism and school refusal behaviour in youth: a contemporary review. *Clinical Psychology Review*, **28**, 451–471.

Kearney, C. A. & Silverman, W. K. (1990). A preliminary analysis of a functional model of assessment and treatment for school refusal behaviour. *Behavioural Modification*, **14**, 344–360.

Kearney, C. A. & Silverman, W. K. (1996). The evolution and reconciliation of taxonomic strategies for school refusal behaviour. *Clinical Psychology Science and Practice*, **3**, 339–354.

Kendall, P. C., Puliafico, A. C., Barmish, A. J., Choudhury, M. S., Henin, A., & Treadwell, K. (2007). Assessing anxiety with the Child Behavior Checklist and the Teacher Report Form. *Journal of Anxiety Disorders*, **21**, 1004–1015.

Kessler, R. C., Berglund, P., Demler, O., Jin, R., Merikangas, K. R., & Walters, E. E. (2005). Lifetime prevalence and age-of-onset distributions of DSM-IV disorders in the national comorbidity survey replication. *Archives of General Psychiatry*, **62**, 593–602.

Kim-Cohen, J., Caspi, A., Moffit, T., Harrington, H., Milne, B., & Poulton, R. (2003). Prior juvenile diagnoses in adults with mental disorder. *Archives of General Psychiatry*, **60**, 709–717.

Lahey, B. B., Waldman, I. D., Hankin, B. L., Applegate, B., Loft, J. D., & Rick, J. (2004). The structure of child and adolescent psychopathology: generating new hypotheses. *Journal of Abnormal Psychology*, **113**, 358–385.

Lang, P. J. (1968). Fear reduction and fear behaviour. In: J. Schlein (ed.) *Research in Psychotherapy*, pp. 85–103. Washington, DC: American Psychological Association.

Langley, A. K., Bergman, L. R., & Piacentini, J. C. (2002). Assessment of childhood anxiety. *International Review of Psychiatry*, **14**, 102–113.

LeBeau, R. T., Glenn, D., Liao, B., Wittchen, H., Beesdo-Baum, K., Ollendick, T., *et al.* (2010). Specific phobia: a review of DSM-IV specific phobia and preliminary recommendations for DSM-V. *Depression and Anxiety*, **27**, 148–167.

Lee, S. W., Piersel, W. C., & Unruh, L. (1989). Concurrent validity of the physiological subscale of the Revised Children's Manifest Anxiety Scale: a multitrait–multimethod analysis. *Journal of Psychoeducational Assessment*, **7**, 246–254.

Lewis-Fernández, R., Hinton, D. E., Laria, A. J., Patterson, E. H., Hofmann, S. G., Craske, M. G., *et al.* (2010). Culture and the anxiety disorders: recommendations for DSM-V. *Depression and Anxiety*, **27**, 212–229.

Lyneham, H. J., Abbott, M. J., & Rapee, R. M. (2007). Inter-rater reliability of the Anxiety Disorders Interview Schedule for DSM-IV: child and parent version. *Journal of the American Academy of Child and Adolescent Psychiatry*, **46**, 731–737.

Mansell, W., Harvey, A., Watkins, E., & Shafran, R. (2009). Conceptual foundations of the transdiagnostic approach to CBT. *Journal of Cognitive Psychotherapy*, **23**, 6–19.

March, J. (1998). *Manual for the Multidimensional Anxiety Scale for Children (MASC)*. Toronto, ON: Multi-Health Systems.

March, J. S., Parker, J. D. A., Sullivan, K., Stallings, P., & Conners, K. (1997). The Multidimensional Anxiety Scale for Children (MASC): factor structure, reliability and validity. *Journal of the American Academy of Child and Adolescent Psychiatry*, **36**, 554–565.

McClellan, J. M. & Werry, J. S. (2000). Introduction (Special section: Research psychiatric diagnostic interviews for children and adolescents). *Journal of the American Academy of Child and Adolescent Psychiatry*, **39**, 19–27.

McConaughy, S. H. (1985). Using the Child Behaviour Checklist and related instruments in school-based assessment of children. *School Psychology Review*, **14**, 479–494.

McGee, R., Feehan, M., Williams, S., & Anderson, J. (1983). Prevalence of self-reported depressive symptoms and associated social factors in mothers in Dunedin. *British Journal of Psychiatry*, **143**, 473–479.

McNally, R. J. (2009). Can we fix PTSD in DSM-V? *Depression and Anxiety*, **26**, 597–600.

Meiser-Stedman, R., Smith, P., Glucksman, E., Yule, W., & Dalgleish, T. (2008). The posttraumatic stress disorder diagnosis in preschool- and elementary school-age children exposed to motor vehicle accidents. *American Journal of Psychiatry*, **165**, 1326–1337.

Mellon, R. & Moutavelis, A. G. (2007). Structure, developmental course, and correlates of children's anxiety-related behaviour in a Hellenic community sample. *Journal of Anxiety Disorders*, **21**, 1–21.

Moffitt, T., Caspi, A., Harrington, H., Milne, B., Melchior, M., Goldberg, D., *et al.* (2007). Generalized anxiety disorder and depression: childhood risk factors in a birth cohort followed to age 32. *Psychological Medicine*, **37**, 441–452.

Moore, P. S., Whaley, S. E., & Sigman, M. (2004). Interactions between mothers and children: impacts of maternal and child anxiety. *Journal of Abnormal Psychology*, **113**, 471–476.

Moretti, M. M., Fine, S., Haley, G., & Marriage, K. (1985). Childhood and adolescent depression: child-report versus parent-report information. *Journal of the American Academy of Child and Adolescent Psychiatry*, **24**, 298–302.

Morris, R. J. & Kratochwill, T. R. (1983). *Treating Children's Fears and Phobias: A Behavioral Approach*. New York: Pergamon Press.

Muris, P. (2007). *Normal and Abnormal Fear and Anxiety in Children and Adolescents*. New York: Elsevier.

Myers, K. & Winters, N. C. (2002). Ten-year review of rating scales. II. Scales for internalizing disorders. *Journal of the American Academy of Child and Adolescent Psychiatry*, **41**, 634–659.

Nelles, W. B. & Barlow, D. H. (1988). Do children panic? *Clinical Psychology Review*, **8**, 359–372.

Ollendick, T. H. (1983). Reliability and validity of the Revised Fear Survey Schedule for Children (FSSC-R). *Behaviour Research and Therapy*, **21**, 685–692.

Ollendick, T. H., Birmaher, B., & Mattis, S. G. (2004). In: **T. L. Morris & J. S. March** (eds.) *Anxiety Disorders in Children and Adolescents*, pp. 198–211. New York: Guilford Press.

Ollendick, T. H., Yang, B., King, N. J., Dong, Q., & Akande, A. (1996). Fears in American, Australian, Chinese, and Nigerian children and adolescents: a cross-cultural study. *Journal of Child Psychology and Psychiatry*, **37**, 213–220.

Perrin, S. G. & Last, C. G. (1992). Do childhood anxiety measures measure anxiety? *Journal of Abnormal Child Psychology*, **20**, 567–578.

Pilgrim, D. (2007). The survival of psychiatric diagnosis. *Social Science and Medicine*, **65**, 536–547.

Pina, A. A., Little, M., Knight, G. P., & Silverman, W. K. (2009). Cross-ethnic measurement equivalence of the RCMAS in Latino and Caucasian youth with anxiety disorders. *Journal of Personality Assessment*, **91**, 58–61.

Pina, A. A., Silverman, W. K., Saavedra, L. M., & Weems, C. F. (2001). An analysis of the RCMAS Lie scale in a clinic sample of anxious children. *Journal of Anxiety Disorders*, 15, 443–457.

Pine, D. S., Alegria, M., Cook, E. H. Jr., Costello, E. J., Dahl, R. E., Koretz, D., *et al.* (2002). Advance in Developmental Science and DSM-V. In: D. J. Kupfer, M. B. First, & D. A. Regier (eds.) *A Research Agenda for DSM-V*, pp. 85–122. Washington, DC: American Psychiatric Association.

Pine, D. S., Cohen, P., Gurley, D., Brook, J., & Ma, Y. (1998). The risk for early adulthood anxiety and depressive disorder in adolescents with anxiety and depressive disorders. *Archives of General Psychiatry*, 55, 56–64.

Pynoos, R. S., Steinberg, A. M., Layne, C. M., Briggs, E. C., Ostrowski, S. A., & Fairbank, J. A. (2009). DSM-V PTSD diagnostic criteria for children and adolescents: a developmental perspective and recommendations. *Journal of Traumatic Stress*, 22, 391–398.

Quay, H. C. (1979). Classification. In: H. C. Quay & J. S. Werry (eds.) *Psychopathological Disorders of Childhood*, pp. 1–42. New York: Wiley & Sons.

Quay, H. C. & Peterson D. R. (1987). *Manual for the Revised Behaviour Problem Checklist*. Coral Gables, FL: Quay & Peterson.

Rachman, S. J. (1978). Human fears: a three-systems analysis. *Scandinavian Journal of Behavior Therapy*, 7, 237–245.

Rachman, S. J. (1990). *Fear and Courage*, 2nd edn. New York: W.H. Freeman.

Rapee, R. M., Kennedy, S., Ingram, M., Edwards, S., & Sweeney, L. (2005). Prevention and early intervention of anxiety disorders in inhibited preschool children. *Journal of Consulting and Clinical Psychology*, 73, 488–497.

Rapee, R. M., Schniering, C. A., & Hudson, J. L. (2009). Anxiety disorders during childhood and adolescence: origins and treatment. *Annual Review of Clinical Psychology*, 5, 311–341.

Reich, W. (2000). Diagnostic Interview for Children and Adolescents (DICA). *Journal of the American Academy of Child and Adolescent Psychiatry*, 39, 59–66.

Rescorla, L., Achenbach, T. M., Ivanova, M., Dumenci, L., Bilenberg, N., Domuta, A., *et al.* (2007). Consistency of teacher reported problems for students in 21 countries. *School Psychology Review*, 36, 91–110.

Research Units on Pediatric Psychopharmacology Anxiety Study Group (2002). The Pediatric Anxiety Rating Scale (PARS): development and psychometric properties. *Journal of the American Academy of Child and Adolescent Psychiatry*, 41, 1061–1069.

Reynolds, C. R. & Richmond, B. O. (1978). "What I Think and Feel": a revised measure of children's manifest anxiety. *Journal of Abnormal Child Psychology*, 6, 271–280.

Roza, S. J., Hofstra, M.-B., van der Ende, J., & Verhulst, F. C. (2003). Stable prediction of mood and anxiety disorders based on behavioral and emotional problems in childhood: a 14-year follow-up during childhood, adolescence, and young adulthood. *American Journal of Psychiatry*, 160, 2116–2121.

Rutter, M. (1967). Children's behaviour questionnaire for completion by teachers. *Journal of Child Psychology and Psychiatry*, 8, 1–11.

Rutter, M., Tizard, J., & Whitemore, K. (1970). *Education, Health and Behaviour*. London: Longman.

Rynn, M. A., Barber, J. P., Khalid-Khan, S., Siqueland, L., Dembiski, M., McCarthy, K. S., *et al.* (2006). The psychometric properties of the MASC in a pediatric psychiatric sample. *Journal of Anxiety Disorders*, 20, 139–157.

Saavedra, L. & Silverman, W. (2002). Classification of anxiety disorders in children: what a difference two decades make. *International Review of Psychiatry*, 14, 87–101.

Schniering, C. A., Hudson, J. L., & Rapee, R. M. (2000). Issues in the diagnosis and assessment of anxiety disorders in children and adolescents. *Clinical Psychology Review*, 20, 453–478.

Shear, M. K., Bjelland, I., Beesdo, K., Gloster, A., & Wittchen, H. (2007). Supplementary dimensional assessment in anxiety disorders. *International Journal of Methods in Psychiatric Research*, **16**, 52–64.

Silverman, W. K. (1994). Structured diagnostic interviews. In: T. H. Ollendick, N. J. King, & W. Yule (eds.) *The International Handbook of Phobic and Anxiety Disorders in Children and Adolescents*, pp. 87–110. New York: Plenum Press.

Silverman, W. K. & Albano, A. M. (1996). *Anxiety Disorders Interview Schedule for DSM-IV: Child and Parent Versions*. San Antonio, TX: Psychological Corporation/Graywind.

Silverman, W. K. & Eisen, A. R. (1992). Age differences in the reliability of parental and child reports of child-anxious symptomatology using a structured interview. *Journal of the American Academy of Child and Adolescent Psychiatry*, **31**, 117–124.

Silverman, W. K. & Ollendick, T. H. (2005). Evidence-based assessment of anxiety and its disorders in children and adolescents. *Journal of Child and Adolescent Psychology*, **34**, 380–411.

Silverman, W. K., Saavedra, L. M., & Pina, A. A. (2001). Test–retest reliability of anxiety symptoms and diagnoses using the Anxiety Disorders Interview Schedule for DSM-IV: Child and Parent Versions (ADIS for DSM-IV: C/P). *Journal of the American Academy of Child and Adolescent Psychiatry*, **40**, 937–944.

Spence, S. H. (1997). Structure of anxiety symptoms among children: a confirmatory factor-analytic study. *Journal of Abnormal Child Psychology*, **22**, 280–297.

Spence, S. H., Barrett, P. M., & Tuner, C. M. (2003). Psychometric properties of the Spence Children's Anxiety Scale with young adolescents. *Journal of Anxiety Disorders*, **17**, 605–625.

Spielberger, C. D. (1973). *Manual for the State–Trait Anxiety Inventory for Children*. Palo Alto, CA: Consulting Psychologists Press.

Sprafkin, J., Gadow, K. J., Salisbury, H., Schneider, J., & Loney, J. (2002). Further evidence of reliability and validity of the Child Symptom Inventory-4: parent checklist in clinically referred boys. *Journal of Child and Adolescent Psychology*, **31**, 513–524.

Stein, D. J., Fineberg, N. A., Bienvenu, O. J., Denys, D., Lochner, C., Nestadt, G., et al. (2010). Should OCD be classified as an anxiety disorder in DSM-V? *Depression and Anxiety*, **27**, 495–506.

Steinhausen, H. C. & Reitzle, M. (1996). The validity of mixed disorders of conduct and emotions in children and adolescents: a research note. *Journal of Child Psychology and Psychiatry*, **37**, 339–343.

Sweeney, M. & Pine, D. (2004). Etiology of fear and anxiety. In: T. H. Ollendick & J. S. March (eds.) *Phobic and Anxiety Disorders in Children and Adolescents: A Clinician's Guide to Effective Psychosocial and Pharmacological Interventions*, pp. 34–60. Oxford, UK: Oxford University Press.

Tackett, J. L., Sellbom, M., Quilty, L. C., Rector, N. A., & Bagby, R. M. (2008). Additional evidence for a quantitative hierarchical model of mood and anxiety disorders for DSM–V: the context of personality structure. *Journal of Abnormal Psychology*, **117**, 812–825.

Turner, S. M., Beidel, D. C., & Costello, A. (1987). Psychopathology in the offspring of anxiety disorder patients. *Journal of Consulting and Clinical Psychology*, **55**, 229–235.

Twenge, J. M. (2000). The age of anxiety? Birth cohort change in anxiety and neuroticism, 1952–1993. *Journal of Personality and Social Psychology*, **79**, 1007–1021.

Twenge, J. M., Gentile, B., DeWall, C. N., Ma, D., Lacefield, K., & Schurtz, D. R. (2010). Birth cohort increases in psychopathology among young Americans, 1938–2007: a cross-temporal meta-analysis of the MMPI. *Clinical Psychology Review*, **30**, 145–154.

van Lang, N.D., Ferdinand, R.F., Oldehinkel, A. J., Ormel, J., & Verhulst, F. C. (2005). Concurrent validity of DSM-IV scales affective problems and anxiety problems of the Youth Self-Report. *Behaviour Research and Therapy*, **43**, 1485–1494.

Velez, C. N., Johnson, J., & Cohen, P. (1989). A longitudinal analysis of selected risk factors for childhood psychopathology. *Journal of the American Academy of Child and Adolescent Psychiatry*, **28**, 861–864.

Wakefield, J. C. (1992). The concept of mental disorder: on the boundary between biological facts and social values. *American Psychologist*, **47**, 373–388.

Wakefield, J. C., Horwitz, A. V., & Schmitz, M. (2004). Are we overpathologizing the socially anxious? Social phobia from a harmful dysfunction perspective. *Canadian Journal of Psychiatry*, **49**, 736–742.

Wakefield, J. C., Horwitz, A. V., & Schmitz, M. (2005). Social disadvantage is not mental disorder: response to Campbell-Sills and Stein. *Canadian Journal of Psychiatry*, **50**, 317–319.

Wardworth, M. E., Hudziak, J. J., Heath, A. C., & Achenbach, T. M. (2000). Latent class analysis of Child Behaviour Checklist anxiety/depression in children and adolescents. *Journal of the American Academy of Child and Adolescent Psychiatry*, **40**, 106–114.

Warren, S. L. & Sroufe, L. A. (2004). Developmental issues. In: T. H. Ollendick & J. S. March (eds.) *Phobic and Anxiety Disorders in Children and Adolescents: A Clinician's Guide to Effective Psychosocial and Pharmacological Interventions*, pp. 92–115. Oxford, UK: Oxford University Press.

Watson, D. (2005). Rethinking mood and anxiety disorders: a quantitative hierarchical model for DSM-V. *Journal of Abnormal Psychology*, **114**, 522–536.

Weems, C. & Stickle, T. (2005). Anxiety disorders in childhood: casting a nomological net. *Clinical Child and Family Psychology Review*, **8**, 107–134.

Weisz, J. R. & Eastman, K. L. (1994). Cross-natural research on child and adolescent psychology. In: F. C. Verhulst & H. M. Koot (eds.) *The Epidemiology of Child and Adolescent Psychopathology*, pp. 42–65. Oxford, UK: Oxford University Press.

Widiger, T. & Samuel, D. (2005). Diagnostic categories or dimensions? A question for the Diagnostic and Statistical Manual of Mental Disorders – fifth edition. *Journal of Abnormal Psychology*, **114**, 494–504.

Wilson, K. A. & Hayward, C. (2005). A prospective evaluation of agoraphobia and depression symptoms following panic attacks in a community sample of adolescents. *Journal of Anxiety Disorders*, **19**, 87–103.

Wittchen, H. U., Beesdo, K., & Gloster, A. T. (2009). The position of anxiety disorders in structural models of mental disorders. *Psychiatric Clinics of North America*, **32**, 465–481.

Wittchen, H., Gloster, A. T., Beesdo-Baum, K., Fava, G., & Craske, M. G. (2010). Agoraphobia: a review of the diagnostic classificatory position and criteria. *Depression and Anxiety*, **27**, 113–133.

Wood, J. J., Piacentini, J. C., Bergman, R. L., McCraken, J., & Barrios, V. (2002). Concurrent validity of anxiety disorders section of the Anxiety Disorders Interview Schedule for DSM-IV: child and parent versions. *Journal of Clinical Child and Adolescent Psychology*, **31**, 335–342.

World Health Organization (1992). *The International Classification of Mental and Behavioural Disorders: Clinical Descriptions and Diagnostic Guidelines*, 10th edn (ICD-10). Geneva, Switzerland: World Health Organization.

Yang, J. W., Hong, S. D., Joung, Y. S., & Kim, J. H. (2006). Validation study of tripartite model of anxiety and depression in children and adolescents: clinical sample in Korea. *Journal of Korean Medical Science*, **21**, 1098–1102.

Zinbarg, R. (1998). Concordance and synchrony in measures of anxiety and panic reconsidered: a hierarchical model of anxiety and panic. *Behavior Therapy*, **29**, 301–323.

3

The developmental epidemiology of anxiety disorders: phenomenology, prevalence, and comorbidity

E. Jane Costello, Helen L. Egger, William Copeland, Alaattin Erkanli, and Adrian Angold

In this chapter we review the prevalence and comorbidity of anxiety disorders in general, and where possible the specifics of separation anxiety disorder (SAD), generalized anxiety disorder (GAD), specific phobias, panic, social phobia, and panic disorder. There were too few reports of agoraphobia to make a reliable estimate. We have not included post-traumatic stress disorder (PTSD) and obsessive–compulsive disorder (OCD), because their status as anxiety disorders is a topic still being debated for the revision of the *Diagnostic and Statistical Manual of Mental Disorders* (American Psychiatric Association, 1994). Most recent studies have omitted overanxious disorder (OAD) after its omission from the latest edition of the *Diagnostic and Statistical Manual of Mental Disorders* (American Psychiatric Association, 1994), but we shall have something to say about OAD later on.

New studies of the prevalence of child and adolescent anxiety disorders in recent years have resolved several issues. First, longitudinal epidemiological as well as laboratory-based studies have made it clear that different types of anxiety have different correlates, predictors, and courses across childhood and adolescence (see elsewhere in this volume). Second, although there are still many problems with assessment, the situation is improving. Direct assessment of young children is always difficult, because they often lack the cognitive abilities needed to talk about worry, fear, and panic (Dadds, James, Barrett, & Verhulst, 2004). But parents have been shown to be reliable reporters about their young children's anxieties (Egger & Angold, 2006a). In addition, most current assessment instruments incorporate measures of functioning, so that researchers can decide what level of impairment they require to make a diagnosis. When functional impairment is included in the diagnosis, prevalence of some anxiety disorders, such as specific phobias, falls dramatically (Shaffer, Fisher, Dulcan, & Davies, 1996) and rates become much more consistent across studies (Costello, Egger, & Angold, 2004).

A third issue where some progress has been made is the overlap between depression and anxiety. The two types of disorder have been shown to predict one another developmentally (Costello, Mustillo, Keeler, & Angold, 2004; Keenan, Feng, Hipwell, & Klostermann, 2009;

Based in part on: (a) Costello, E. J., Egger, H. L., & Angold, A. (2005). Developmental epidemiology of anxiety disorders. In: S. Swedo & D. Pine (eds.) *Child and Adolescent Anxiety Disorders*, Child and Adolescent Psychiatry Clinics of North America No. 14, pp. 631–648. Amsterdam: Elsevier and (b) Costello, E. J., Egger, H. L., & Angold, A. (2004). The developmental epidemiology of anxiety disorders. In: T. Ollendick & J. March (eds.) *Phobic and Anxiety Disorders in Children and Adolescents*, pp. 61–91. New York: Oxford University Press.

Silberg, Rutter, & Eaves, 2001) and often respond to the same treatments (Ferdinand, Barrett, & Dadds, 2004). This has led some to treat them as part of the same syndrome (Achenbach, 1991). However, as we shall discuss later, recent evidence suggests that the overlap between anxiety and depression applies only to some anxiety disorders (Costello, Mustillo, *et al.*, 2004). Despite these advances, there is still much that is unresolved about the epidemiology of anxiety disorders.

Prevalence and comorbidity

We reviewed the epidemiologic literature for studies that could contribute to a meta-analysis of the prevalence of anxiety disorders. We searched the literature using Google Advanced Scholar Search, augmented by our own database of epidemiologic studies that we have compiled over the past 20 years. Studies were selected for the meta-analysis if they used a reasonably representative population sample, permitted individuals under 18 to be identified, and used a psychiatric assessment with known psychometric properties that permitted one or more anxiety diagnoses to be made. We present the available data from 55 data sets that report the prevalence of one or more DSM-III-R, DSM-IV, or ICD-10 anxiety disorders (table available from first author). Three of the studies are specific to children up to age 8, 13 studies cover ages 6 through 12, 26 studies cover ages 13 through 18, and a further 13 include ages 2 through 21, but do not provide separate analyses for children and adolescents. Table 3.1 presents data from the three preschool studies, and Tables 3.2 through 3.4 show the results of meta-analyses for ages 5–12, 13–18, and all studies. Figure 3.1 presents results for each diagnosis by age group.

Methods for the meta-analyses

For a sufficiently large sample size, the logit transform of the prevalence estimate p_i for the ith study is normally distributed with mean $\mu_i = \log[p_i/(1 - p_i)]$ and standard error $se_i = se(p_i)/[p_i(1 - p_i)]$, where $se(p_i)$ is the standard error of prevalence. We imputed $se(p_i)$ for studies that did not provide the value using a separate simulation model having a Gamma prior with unknown scale and shape parameters estimated from the data. We then used these estimates in the logit models. First, the baseline overall prevalence estimate was computed using a logit model with a random effect intercept having a non-informative multivariate normal prior fitted separately to younger, older, and combined cohorts, respectively. The combined logits from separate anxiety diagnoses were assumed to have a multivariate normal distribution with a diagonal variance–covariance matrix consisting of variances (se_i^2) some of which were imputed using the Gamma technique as described above. The random effect intercept vector accounted for both study-to-study heterogeneity and comorbidity among different diagnoses within a single study.

To estimate the effects of age at entrance to study, duration of the study, taxonomy, and time-frame, we added these as fixed effects to the above model. For the combined cohort, a cohort contrast variable was also added as an extra fixed effect. All the computations were implemented in WinBUGS using Gibbs sampling (Gilks *et al.*, 1993).

Anxiety in preschool children

Formal meta-analysis of anxiety in preschool children is not possible because there are too few published studies. Most of the research on anxiety and fear in young children has been conducted from the perspective of temperament and normal development, not psychopathology. In these approaches, anxiety/fear in young children is seen either as a normative phase of development or, in a subset of children, a risk factor for anxiety disorders. Between 7 and 12 months, most infants develop a fear of strangers and express distress when separated from their primary caregivers. These fears peak between 9 and 18 months of age and decrease for most children by age $2\frac{1}{2}$ (Warren & Sroufe, 2004). About 15% of young children display "behavioral inhibition": compared with other children, they show more intense and persistent fear, shyness, and social withdrawal in response to unfamiliar people, situations, or objects (Biederman *et al.*, 1990; Hirshfeld *et al.*, 1992; Kagan & Snidman, 1991).

Behaviorally inhibited young children display characteristic patterns of physiology such as high heart rate, low heart rate variability, high baseline morning cortisol, and elevated startle responses (Kagan, Reznick, & Snidman, 1987) and are more likely to develop an anxiety disorder later in childhood or adolescence or to have first-degree relatives with anxiety disorders (Biederman *et al.*, 1993; Hirshfeld *et al.*, 1992; Kagan & Snidman, 1999; Rosenbaum, Biederman, Bolduc, Hirshfeld, Faraone, & Kagan, 1992; Rosenbaum, Biederman, Hirshfeld, Bolduc, & Chaloff, 1991; Rosenbaum, Biederman, Hirshfeld, Bolduc, Faraone, *et al.*, 1991). Recent advances in the nosology and diagnosis of psychiatric symptoms and disorders in preschool children (Angold, Egger, & Carter, 2007; Sterba, Egger, & Angold, 2007) have made it possible to begin to define the boundaries between normative anxiety, temperamental variation, and clinically significant anxiety disorders in very young children. It is also clear from the literature that "Overall the DSM-IV provided as good a description of preschool psychopathology as it does for the mental health problems of older children" (Sterba *et al.*, 2007, p. 1011).

In recent years there have been several studies of psychiatric disorders in young children, using newly developed instruments. The Preschool Age Psychiatric Assessment (PAPA) (Angold *et al.*, 2007; Egger, Ascher, & Angold, 1999) was developed for use with parents of children aged 2 through 5 years old. The Dominic (Murphy, Cantwell, Jordan, Lee, Cooley-Quille, & Lahey, 2000; Valla, Bergeron, & Smolla, 2000) is a pictorial interview developed for children aged 6 through 11, and their parents. Third, the Development and Well-Being Assessment (DAWBA), an interview for children and parents that is now widely used around the world, is used with parents of children as young as 5 (Meltzer, Gatward, Goodman, & Ford, 1999). Other researchers have adapted instruments for older children for use with parents of preschool- and kindergarten-age children.

As Table 3.1 shows, data are now available from three studies of children aged between 2 and 8, most of them around age 6. The median estimate for any anxiety disorder in young children was 9.4%, with a range from 6.1% to 14.8% (Figure 3.1). The median estimate for young children is only slightly lower than the 10.1% estimate for the whole of Table 3.1.

The higher prevalence seen in the Twins Early Development Study (TEDS) (Caspi *et al.*, 2004) was largely attributable to the high rate of specific phobias. As we shall see, decisions made in a study about the measurement of impairment related to specific phobia have a dramatic effect on prevalence estimates for this disorder at every age.

Neither Egger and Angold (2006a) nor Briggs-Gowan *et al.* (Briggs-Gowan, Carter, Skuban, & Horwitz, 2001) reported any significant differences by child sex for anxiety disorders overall, or for specific anxiety disorders. In the Egger and Angold study, 4- and 5-year-olds were significantly more likely than 2- and 3-year-olds to have any anxiety disorder (11.9% vs. 7.7%) or PTSD (1.3% vs. 0.0%). African-American children were less likely to meet criteria for any anxiety disorder (6.4% vs. 14.0%) or social phobia (0.6%

Table 3.1 Prevalence estimates from three studies of young children (aged 2–8)

Study[a]	Nationality	Interview[b]	Time-frame	Taxonomy	Age range	Number of participants	Any anxiety	GAD	SAD	Social phobia	Specific phobia	Panic disorder
(1)	USA	DISC	6 mo.	DSM-IIIR	4–8	1886	6.1%		3.6%		2.8%	
(2)	USA	PAPA	3 mo.	DSM-IV	2–5	307	9.4%	6.5%	2.4%	2.1%	2.3%	
(3)	UK	ADIS	Current	DSM-IV	6–6.5	9324/1708[c]	14.8%	1.8%	2.8%	2.9%	10.8%	0.1%

[a] (1) Briggs-Gowan, Horwitz, Schwab-Stone, Leventhal, & Leaf (2000).
(2) Egger & Angold (2006b).
(3) Bolton et al. (2006).

[b] DISC, Diagnostic Interview Schedule for Children (Shaffer, Fisher, Dulcan, & Davies, 1996).
PAPA, Preschool-Age Psychiatric Assessment (Egger, Erkanli, Keeler, Potts, Walter, & Angold, 2006).
ADIS, Anxiety Disorders Interview Schedule for DSM-IV (Silverman, Saavedra, & Pina, 2001).

[c] Screened/interviewed.

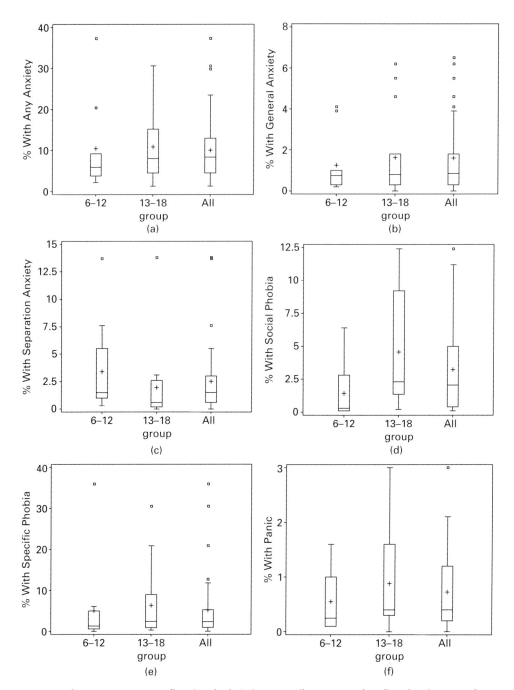

Figure 3.1 Mean, median (marked +), interquartile range, and outliers for six types of anxiety disorder. Data from 55 data sets (details from first author). (a) Any anxiety disorder; (b) generalized anxiety disorder; (c) separation anxiety disorder; (d) social phobia; (e) specific phobia; (f) panic disorder.

Table 3.2 Estimates of prevalence, standard error (SE), and 95% credible interval for any anxiety disorder, GAD, SAD, social phobia, specific phobia, and panic disorder, in children aged 6 through 12, from a meta-analysis of 13 data sets[a]

Disorder	Mean (%)	SE (%)	2.5%	97.5%
Any anxiety disorder	12.3	5.4	7.1	28.2
Generalized anxiety disorder	1.7	1.2	0.9	5.0
Separation anxiety disorder	3.9	1.5	2.6	8.5
Social phobia	2.2	2.2	1.0	8.8
Specific phobia	6.7	3.6	4.0	18.0
Panic disorder	1.5	3.2	0.2	8.9

[a] Bergeron, Valla, & Breton, (1992); Almqvist *et al.* (1999); McArdle, Prosser, & Kolvin (2004); Mullick & Goodman (2005); Green, Elvidge, Owen, & Craddock (2003); Green *et al.* (2003); Petersen, Bilenberg, Hoerder, & Gillberg (2006); Heiervang *et al.* (2007); Gau, Chong, Chen, & Cheng (2005); E. J. Costello, unpublished data; E. J. Costello, unpublished data; E. J. Costello, unpublished data; Costello *et al.* (2003).

vs. 4.3%) than non-African-American children. It is not clear whether the reported differences might be caused by cultural differences in reporting or expressing verbally the presence of anxiety problems. Comorbidity with other psychiatric disorders was common, ranging from 53% of cases of generalized anxiety disorder to 100% of cases of specific phobia. The most common type of comorbidity with non-anxiety disorders was with depression. Two of the studies came from the USA, and one from the UK, so it is not possible to say much about cultural variation in this age group.

Prevalence of anxiety disorders in elementary-school-age children

Table 3.2 summarizes information on prevalence from recent epidemiologic studies that permit us to look separately at children between 6 and 12 years of age.

From our meta-analysis, the mean estimate for any anxiety disorder is 12.3% (SE 5.4%); the 95% credible range (roughly comparable to a 95% confidence interval) is from 7.1% to 28.2%. The most common anxiety disorder is specific phobia (mean 6.7%, SE 3.6%), but as Figure 3.1 shows the range is very wide, especially above the mean. This diversity is because a few studies had very high rates, probably because they did not impose any impairment requirement before making the diagnosis. Separation anxiety was the next most prevalent anxiety disorder in this age range (3.9%, SE 1.5%), followed by social phobia (2.2%, SE 2.2%), and generalized anxiety disorder (1.7%, SE 1.2%). There were too few studies including panic disorder to make a reliable estimate.

Prevalence of anxiety disorders in children aged 13 through 18

Table 3.3 shows the results of the meta-analysis for adolescents. The standard errors are much smaller in this age range, partly because there are more studies. However, the mean estimates are similar: any anxiety disorder 11.0% (SE 0.5%), specific phobia 6.7% (SE 1.6%), social phobia 5.0% (SE 1.3%), SAD 2.3% (SE 0.9%), GAD 1.9% (SE 0.5%), and panic disorder 1.1% (SE 0.3%).

Table 3.3 Estimates of prevalence, standard error (SE), and 95% credible interval for any anxiety disorder, GAD, SAD, social phobia, specific phobia, and panic disorder in adolescents aged 13 through 18, from a meta-analysis of 26 data sets[a]

Disorder	Mean (%)	SE (%)	2.5%	97.5%
Any anxiety disorder	11.0	0.5	10.3	12.2
Generalized anxiety disorder	1.9	0.5	1.3	3.3
Separation anxiety disorder	2.3	0.9	1.4	4.8
Social phobia	5.0	1.3	3.5	8.4
Specific phobia	6.7	1.6	4.7	10.9
Panic disorder	1.1	0.3	0.7	1.8

[a] Costello *et al.* (2003); Verhulst, van der Ende, Ferdinand, & Kasius (1997); Beals *et al.* (1997); Canals, Domenech, Carbajo, & Blade (1997); Krueger, Caspi, Moffitt, & Silva (1998); Lewinsohn, Rohde, & Seeley (1998); Lewinsohn, Rohde *et al.* (1998b); Rueter, Scaramella, Wallace, & Conger (1999); Johnson, Cohen, Pine, Klein, Stephanie, & Brook (2000); Fergusson & Horwood (2001); Fergusson & Horwood (2001); Romano, Tremblay, Vitaro, Zoccolillo, & Pagani (2001); Gau *et al.* (2005); Gau *et al.* (2005); Gau *et al.* (2005); Gau *et al.* (2005); Green *et al.* (2003); Green *et al.* (2003); Lynch, Mills, Daly, & Fitzpatrick (2006); Ehringer, Rhee, Young, Corley, & Hewitt (2006); Shear, Jin, Ruscio, Walters, & Kessler (2006); Ehringer *et al.* (2006); E. J. Costello, unpublished data; E. J. Costello, unpublished data; E. J. Costello, unpublished data; Benjet, Borges, Medina-Mora, Zambrano, & Aguilar-Gaxiola (2009).

Table 3.4 Estimates of prevalence, standard error (SE), and 95% credible interval for any anxiety disorder, GAD, SAD, social phobia, specific phobia, and panic disorder in children and adolescents age 2 through 21, from a meta-analysis of 55 data sets[a]

Disorder	Mean (%)	SE (%)	2.5%	97.5%
Any anxiety disorder	10.2	0.5	9.3	11.3
Generalized anxiety disorder	1.6	0.2	1.2	2.3
Separation anxiety disorder	2.6	0.5	1.9	4.0
Social phobia	3.6	0.7	2.7	5.4
Specific phobia	5.4	0.8	4.2	7.6
Panic disorder	0.8	0.2	0.6	1.3

[a] Those listed in Tables 3.1 through 3.3, plus: Steinhausen (2006); Ravens-Sieberer, Wille, Bettge, & Erhart (2007); Srinath *et al.* (2005); Canino *et al.* (2004); Fleitlich-Bilyk & Goodman (2004); Shaffer *et al.* (1996); Kandel *et al.* (1997); Simonoff *et al.* (1997); Breton, Bergeron, Valla, Berthiaume, & Gaudet (1999); Johnson *et al.* (2000); Eapen, Al-Gazali, Bin-Othman, & Abou-Saleh (1998); Eapen, Jakka, & Abou-Saleh (2003); Angold *et al.* (2002); Perkonigg, Lieb, & Wittchen (1998).

All data sets

Including all the data sets, with the addition of those that did not permit age-specific estimates, did not change the picture much: any anxiety disorder 10.2% (SE 0.5%), specific phobia 5.4% (SE 0.8%), social phobia 3.6% (SE 0.7%), SAD 2.6% (SE 0.5%), panic disorder 0.8% (SE 0.2%).

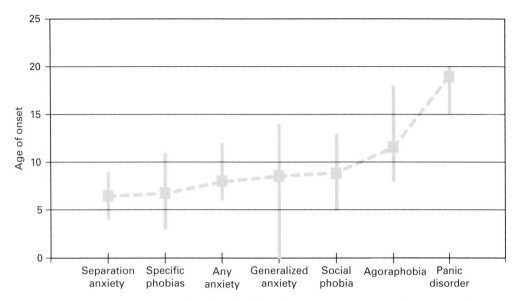

Figure 3.2 Age at onset of anxiety disorders through age 21: mean and interquartile range. Data from the Great Smoky Mountains Study.

Age differences in the prevalence of anxiety disorders

Figure 3.2 provides a summary of ages of onset of different anxiety disorders, through age 21, in the one study for which onset dates are available (the Great Smoky Mountains Study, GSMS). It shows that the mean (and median) age at onset of any anxiety disorder by age 21 was 8 years, with 50% of cases falling between 6 and 12 years of age. The earliest to begin was SAD, with a median age of 6 (mean 6.5), while panic disorders rarely began before mid-adolescence. It is important to note that the range is very wide for some anxiety disorders, especially GAD. It is also worth noting that in every diagnosis except SAD, new cases were still being reported at the latest interview (age 21); the latest case of separation anxiety disorder occurred at age 15.

It is difficult to draw conclusions about age trends in prevalence from a simple review of the studies in the meta-analysis, because in many cases age of participants is confounded with the time-frame of the interview. Thus, the 3-month studies tend to have both the lowest prevalence rates and the youngest participants, whereas the 12-month studies tend to have the highest prevalence as well as the oldest particpants.

Results from the meta-analysis that control for sample size, taxonomy, and time-frame of the interview showed only one significant age difference: panic disorders were more likely to occur in adolescents than in young children. Apart from this finding, there were no significant differences either within age group (children, adolescents) or in comparisons between the two age ranges.

Sex differences in the prevalence of anxiety disorders

It was not possible to use meta-analytic methods to look at sex differences, because too few studies reported rates separately by sex. The clinical data suggest that girls are somewhat more likely than boys to report an anxiety disorder of some sort. Lewinsohn (Lewinsohn, Gotlib, Seeley, & Allen, 1998), in one of the few studies to examine the effects of potentially confounding factors associated with both sex and anxiety, found that controlling for 15 such factors (for example, single-parent family or family poverty) did not eliminate the excess of anxiety disorders in girls. However, at the level of individual diagnoses very few of the sex differences are large, possibly because the number of cases for specific anxiety disorders is too small. In a comparison of three diagnostic interviews used with the same 1200 participants (E. J. Costello, unpublished data), all the differences were in the direction of more girls than boys with anxiety disorders. With the exception of specific phobia, however, few of the sex differences were statistically significant, and these differences varied across interviews. More work is needed to understand what aspects of different diagnostic interviews lead to these findings. Analysis of cumulative prevalence up to age 21 in the GSMS showed a slight but non-significant excess of female anxiety disorders by the beginning of adulthood. It is reasonable to conclude that where large sex differences are found in clinical studies, these may be the result of referral bias (Costello & Janiszewski, 1990).

Developmental changes in sex distribution

Lewinsohn identified a female preponderance in anxiety disorders that emerged by age 6 (Lewinsohn, Lewinsohn *et al.*, 1998). In the GSMS (unpublished data), the only anxiety disorder to be more common in pre-adolescent girls was separation anxiety. In adolescence the difference was significant only for social phobia and GAD. This difference continued into early adulthood, when young women also had significantly more cases of panic disorder.

Anxiety and disability

One of the most hotly debated areas in the past few years has been the relationship between psychiatric diagnosis and level of functioning. When the first versions of the Diagnostic Interview Schedule for Children (DISC) were introduced in the 1980s, they were found to generate extremely high prevalence rates for some disorders, among them some anxiety disorders (Costello, Edelbrock, Dulcan, Kalas, & Klaric, 1984; Shaffer *et al.*, 1996). For example, according to data from the four-site Methods for the Epidemiology of Child and Adolescent Mental Disorders (MECA) Study (Lahey *et al.*, 1994) 39.5% of the children had at least one anxiety diagnosis in the past 12 months (Shaffer *et al.*, 1996). At the same time, Health Maintenance Organizations (HMOs), insurance companies, and governmental agencies were concerned about whether all these children "really" needed treatment (Costello, Burns, Angold, & Leaf, 1993).

One solution to both problems was to require that, to receive a diagnosis, a child should show a significant degree of functional impairment or disability (to use the World Health Organization's preferred term). In 1993 the Federal Register (the official daily publication for rules, proposed rules, and notices of federal agencies and organizations) defined a new class of psychiatric disorders, called Serious Emotional Disturbance (SED), which required significantly impaired functioning or disability in addition to a diagnosis (Hodges, Doucette-Gates, & Liao, 1999). The SED classification was to be used as the criterion for assessing the prevalence of child psychiatric disorder in each American state, for the purpose of allocating federal block grants. Disability can be measured at several different levels. Each symptom can require impaired functioning, or disability can be evaluated at the level of the syndrome or diagnosis, or in the presence of any diagnosis, irrespective of which one causes impaired functioning. Alternatively, the interviewer could rate the child's level of functioning without making a diagnosis, using a separate measure (e.g., Hodges *et al.*, 1999; Shaffer, 1992), or, of course, more than one method can be used.

The effects on the prevalence of anxiety disorders of assessing disability in different ways can been seen in the four-site MECA study using the DISC 2.3. The study used two kinds of disability assessment. One was attached to each symptom cluster, such that the interviewer asked about disability if the child or parent endorsed "half plus one" symptoms (i.e., one more than half the symptoms needed for the diagnosis). The other required the interviewer to rate the child on a scale of 0–100 on level of functioning, using the Children's Global Assessment Scale (CGAS) (Shaffer, 1992) after the interview was ended. Adding *either* diagnosis-specific impairment *or* "mild impairment" (70 or less) on the CGAS halved the prevalence rate; adding both reduced it by two-thirds; requiring both diagnosis-specific impairment and "severe" (50 or below) impairment on the CGAS reduced it by almost 90% (Shaffer, Gould, *et al.*, 1996). Anxiety was of all diagnoses (including behavioral disorders), the area most severely affected by requiring impairment, and among the anxiety disorders, specific phobia was the most affected; the prevalence estimate fell from 21.6% (no impairment requirements) to 0.7% (diagnosis-specific plus CGAS <50).

Requiring disability as a criterion for making the diagnosis brings the rates down to levels that certainly make provider institutions more comfortable. However, there is growing evidence that disability can be associated with anxiety symptoms that do not reach the threshold for a diagnosis (Angold, Costello, Farmer, Burns, & Erkanli, 1999; Copeland, Shanahan, Costello, & Angold, 2009) and that even controlling for comorbidity with other psychiatric disorders anxiety disorders are associated with a high degree of disability (Ezpeleta, Keeler, Erkanli, Costello, & Angold, 2001). The true burden to children, families, and society associated with these conditions is still unclear and needs further longitudinal research.

Race, ethnic, and cultural differences in rates of anxiety disorders

The meta-analysis was based on data drawn from 19 different countries, and included a wide range of races, ethnicities, and cultures both among and within them. Of the studies with the highest rates of any anxiety disorder (over 20%) two were from Holland, one was from Mexico, and two from the USA, one with both White and African-American participants, and one with both Whites and American Indians. The only thing that can be said is that none of the studies with the highest rates came from Asian studies, but there may well be cultural reasons for this, such as a reluctance to report emotional problems (Tiwari & Wang, 2006).

The wide variability in prevalence rates among studies means that conclusions about race/ethnic/cultural differences can only safely be drawn when there is more than one group within the same study. The studies that permit comparison between White and African-American children (those of Egger, Costello, Angold) show a slight but generally non-significantly lower prevalence of anxiety disorders in African-American than in White youth (Angold *et al.*, 2002), and (in the case of the GSMS) a lower prevalence in the American Indian than the White participants. The Duke Validity study is interesting because each of 1200 youths aged 9 to 16 years, recruited from a primary care pediatric clinic, was given two psychiatric assessments about 1 week apart. They received two out of three interviews: the DISC, the Child and Adolescent Psychiatric Assessment (CAPA), and the DAWBA, in a counterbalanced design. Of this sample 41% was White, 47% African-American, and 12% Hispanic or "mixed." Despite the differences observed among the interviews, after correcting for multiple tests there were no significant differences by race/ethnicity whichever interview was used.

In summary, apart from a tendency for White youth to report more anxiety disorders than other race/ethnic groups within the USA, there is a lack of data from which to draw any conclusions about race/ethnic/cultural differences.

Comorbidity among anxiety disorders

Comorbidity among anxiety disorders has historically been a problem, not only for nosology and epidemiology, but also for diagnosis and treatment. This is an area where the high level of comorbidity found in clinical samples is mirrored in community samples. A review of published studies yields inconclusive results because: (1) not all diagnoses are included in every study, and the number of anxiety disorders included in the analyses of comorbidity varies from study to study; (2) there is a lack of consensus about whether to control for comorbidity with other anxiety disorders, or with other diagnoses, when examining the strength of a particular association; and (3) concurrent and sequential comorbidities are not always distinguished clearly. The two published papers to explore the issue of comorbidity among anxiety disorders (Lewinsohn, Zinbarg, Lewinsohn, & Sack, 1997; Simonoff *et al.*, 1997) used bivariate analyses (corrected for sex and age in the latter case), so it is hard to interpret the finding that the majority of comparisons yielded significant differences. We attempted to conduct a meta-analysis of the available data sets, along the lines of work on psychiatric comorbidity that we have previously published (Angold, Costello, & Erkanli, 1999). However, for many of the diagnostic comparisons there were too few data sets for such analyses to be feasible. Therefore we can only draw some very tentative conclusions, based mainly on studies for which we had direct access to the data (Angold *et al.*, 2002; Costello *et al.*, 1988; Costello, Mustillo, Erkanli, Keeler, & Angold, 2003; Egger *et al.*, 2006).

A question of nosologic interest is the extent to which the old overanxious disorder category overlaps with the DSM-IV generalized anxiety diagnosis. The intention was that children who would formerly have received a diagnosis of overanxious disorder of childhood would be subsumed into the new GAD category. The criteria for GAD were loosened for children, who could receive the diagnosis if they had only one of the six symptoms of Criterion C (*restlessness, fatigue, difficulty concentrating, irritability, muscle tension, sleep disturbance*).

However, with one exception these symptom classes are very different from those defined for overanxious disorder (*worries about the past or future, concerns about one's competence, need for reassurance, somatic symptoms, self-consciousness, muscle tension*). While mentioned briefly in the description of Criterion A (*excessive anxiety or worry*), the latter are not set out in the new formal diagnostic criteria. On the other hand, five of the six new Criterion C symptoms are very similar to symptoms of major depressive episode; it is difficult to write diagnostic questions that reliably capture the subtle differences between, for example, the fatigue associated with depression and that associated with GAD. Thus, any examination

Table 3.5 Prediction from disorder in any previous wave to current disorder, across age 9–21 in the Great Smoky Mountains Study ($n = 8806$ observations)

Outcome > Predictor V	Overanxious disorder	Generalized anxiety	OAD + GAD	Social phobia	MDD
Previous GAD					
Absent%	1.3	1.9	0.8	0.4	2.1
Present%	8.6	8.3	3.6	1.3	7.7
OR	7.2***	4.2***	4.5***	3.0*	3.9***
Previous OAD					
Absent%	1.4	1.9	0.8	0.4	2.2
Present%	11.6	13.6	7.9	1.8	8.2
OR	9.3***	8.2***	11.3***	4.2***	4.0***
OAD+GAD					
Absent%	1.5	2.0	0.8	0.4	2.3
Present%	11.5	14.1	6.6	2.3	6.5
OR	8.6***	8.2***	8.3***	5.4***	3.0***

OR, odds ratio; ***, $p < 0.001$; *, $p < 0.01$.

of the overlap between OAD and GAD should take into account the possibility of their overlap with depression.

We used GSMS data to examine *concurrent* comorbidity among OAD using DSM-III-R criteria, GAD using DSM-IV criteria, and DSM-IV depression. Over the course of the study 182 children and adolescents (11.6% of the sample) had one or more of the three diagnoses by the age of 16. Of those who were comorbid (5.4% of the sample, or 47% of those with any of the three diagnoses) more than half (52%) had all three disorders. Given that GAD was supposed to subsume OAD, one might expect this combination to be common. In fact, only 12 children (weighted 16% of those with either GAD or OAD) had both disorders *without depression* over the course of the study. Of the children with OAD without GAD, 36/88 (weighted 42%) also had a depressive disorder, not far from the 135/296 (weighted 34%) of children with GAD but not OAD.

Table 3.5 shows *predictive* comorbidity between GAD and OAD, also using data from the GSMS. It shows that prediction from GAD to OAD and vice versa is, if anything, higher than homotypic prediction (to the same disorder). As noted earlier, there is a great deal of similarity between many of the symptoms of depression and GAD in DSM-IV. So one might have expected more prediction from depression to GAD or vice versa than between depression and OAD, but this did not occur. In summary, although there is evidence for considerable concurrent and predictive comorbidity among GAD and OAD, tracing the extent to which this degree of comorbidity is real rather than methodological will require detailed longitudinal investigation. It is to be hoped that the DSM-V process will consider the pros and cons of reintroducing OAD, and possibly avoidant disorder, in its revision of the anxiety disorders.

Comorbidity among the phobias

Almost all the available studies confirmed significant comorbidities among the phobias: specific, social, and agoraphobia.

Comorbidity among separation anxiety and panic disorder

The concurrent association between panic disorder and separation anxiety was non-significant in three out of the four studies that measured it.

Absence of comorbidity

Evidence for lack of comorbidity among disorders generally lumped together under the label "anxiety" is as interesting as evidence for comorbidity. Little connection was found between separation anxiety and the group of phobias, or between separation anxiety and overanxious disorder. Both GAD and OAD were unrelated to simple/specific phobias. There was, however, a consistent pattern of significant association between OAD and social phobia. Interestingly, in light of the clinical data suggesting a *developmental* link, there was absolutely no evidence of a *cross-sectional* association between separation anxiety and panic disorder. However, it must be emphasized that the evidence is often patchy; some associations could only be examined in two or three studies. Also, most studies examined were cross-sectional and could not test for possible sequential or developmental relationships, in either children or adolescents.

Comorbidity with other disorders

A review of comorbidity with anxiety disorders, published in 1999 (Angold, Costello, & Erkanli, 1999) showed that controlling for other comorbid conditions, the highest level of anxious comorbidity was with depression, with a median odds ratio of 8.2 (95% CI 5.8–12.0). The odds ratio for comorbidity with conduct disorder and/or oppositional defiant disorder (CD/ODD) was 3.1 (95% CI 2.2–4.6), and that with attention deficit hyperactivity disorder (ADHD) was 3.0 (95% CI 2.1–4.3). These confidence intervals all exclude 1, indicating a statistically and substantively significant degree of comorbidity. In the case of substance use or abuse, although the bivariate odds ratios were significant in some studies, the association disappeared once comorbidity between anxiety and other psychiatric disorders was controlled (Armstrong & Costello, 2002).

There are very few published papers that permit a review of comorbidity between *specific* anxiety disorders and other psychiatric diagnoses. Comorbidity analyses of the Lewinsohn's Oregon Adolescent Depression Study (Lewinsohn *et al.*, 1997) looking at lifetime diagnoses, showed that depression was significantly associated with each of the anxiety disorders except OCD, controlling for other disorders. Other lifetime associations found were ADHD with specific phobia, ODD with OCD, bipolar disorder with separation anxiety (in males), and alcohol abuse/dependence with OAD. In preschool children, Sterba *et al.* (2007) used confirmatory factor analysis to show that the best-fitting model for the emotional disorders had three factors: social phobia, separation anxiety, and a factor that combined GAD and depression. The same analyses showed significant correlations of between 0.41 and 0.89 between these three factors and conduct disorder, oppositional disorder, and ADHD. The same strong association between GAD and depression was found by Moffitt *et al.* (2007) in the Dunedin, New Zealand longitudinal study, with GAD predicting depression and depression predicting GAD across the life course. Similar heterotypic prediction was seen in the GSMS (Costello *et al.*, 2003).

The importance of looking at anxiety disorders separately is shown by Kaplow's reanalysis of the data from the GSMS described above (Kaplow, Curran, Angold, & Costello, 2001). This reanalysis found that different anxiety disorders had different relationships to risk of beginning substance use. Children with separation anxiety symptoms were *less* likely than other children to begin drinking alcohol, and did so later than others, while those with generalized anxiety symptoms were *more* likely than other children to begin drinking, and did so earlier.

Homotypic and heterotypic continuity

An important question for clinicians is whether children with anxiety disorders can be expected to have further episodes of the same disorder (homotypic continuity), or to develop other psychiatric conditions (heterotypic continuity). There are few studies that deal with issues of concurrent versus sequential comorbidity (but see Orvaschel, Lewinsohn, & Seeley, 1995). Some studies have suggested that childhood anxiety predicts adolescent depression (Costello, Mustillo *et al.*, 2004) but there is also evidence that early depression predicts anxiety (Silberg *et al.*, 2001) The study of GSMS participants cited earlier (Kaplow *et al.*, 2001) demonstrated that the relationships among OAD, SAD, and alcohol use changed across development. The confused temporal relationship between anxiety and depression (see Table 3.5) may also need more fine-grained analysis before we understand it properly.

There are few epidemiologic studies that provide information about continuity *among* the anxiety disorders. The clinical literature suggests that separation anxiety is a predictor of later panic disorder (Black, 1994; Klein, 1995; Silove, Manicavasagar, Curtis, & Blaszczynski, 1996) for which there is some support in the GSMS (Bittner, Egger, Erkanli, Costello, Foley, & Angold, 2007). Controlling for concurrent comorbidity among the anxiety disorders, the GSMS showed a high degree of homotypic continuity of separation anxiety and social phobia from childhood to adolescence. Data from DSM-III-R OAD also showed significant continuity. There was relatively little heterotypic continuity, which suggests a level of predictive validity in the diagnostic categories for the anxiety disorders across childhood and adolescence.

Copeland *et al.* (2009) added to Bittner *et al.*'s (2007) review with analyses of prediction from childhood to young adulthood (age 19–21). After adjusting for other comorbidities, there was little prediction from childhood anxiety disorders to adolescence: in females only, childhood GAD predicted adolescent substance abuse. Predictions from childhood to adulthood were stronger: childhood OAD predicted adult panic, childhood separation anxiety and GAD predicted adult agoraphobia, and childhood depression predicted adult GAD and panic disorder. Occurrence of OAD in adolescence predicted young adult GAD, panic, and depression, GAD in adolescence predicted adult GAD (in girls) and depression, while adolescent depression predicted adult agoraphobia. Further understanding is needed of the role of puberty as, possibly, a time-limited perturbation in the genetic predisposition to anxiety disorders. In summary, GAD, panic disorder, and agoraphobia were the adult anxiety disorders most likely to be have child and adolescent precursors, but there was little homotypic continuity within specific forms of anxiety.

Conclusions

We argue in this chapter that as the quality (accuracy, reliability, validity) of measures used to assess anxiety disorders in the child and adolescent population have improved in the past few years, prevalence estimates are less erratic, our understanding of comorbidity is increasing, and the role of impairment as a criterion for "caseness" has been more carefully considered. Several of the instruments developed for epidemiologic research are now being used in clinical settings. Further integration of research methods can be expected in the next few years as, for example, laboratory methods for testing stress response become available for use in the field. The integration of laboratory, clinical, and epidemiologic ideas and methods can only benefit children with anxiety disorders and their families.

References

Achenbach, T. M. (1991). *Manual for the Child Behavior Checklist 4–18 and 1991 Profile.* Burlington, VT: University of Vermont Department of Psychiatry.

Almqvist, F., Puura, K., Kumpulainen, K., Tuompo-Johansson, E., Henttonen, I., Huikko, E., et al. (1999). Psychiatric disorders in 8–9-year-old children based on a diagnostic interview with the parents. *European Child and Adolescent Psychiatry*, **8**, IV/17–IV/28.

American Psychiatric Association (1994). *Diagnostic and Statistical Manual of Mental Disorders*, 4th edn. Washington, DC: American Psychiatric Association.

Angold, A., Costello, E. J., & Erkanli, A. (1999). Comorbidity. *Journal of Child Psychology and Psychiatry*, **40**, 57–87.

Angold, A., Costello, E. J., Farmer, E. M. Z., Burns, B. J., & Erkanli, A. (1999). Impaired but undiagnosed. *Journal of the American Academy of Child and Adolescent Psychiatry*, **38**, 129–137.

Angold, A., Egger, H., & Carter, A. (2007). The measurement of psychopathology in children under the age of six. In: **W. Narrow, M. First, P. Sirovatka, & D. Regier** (eds.) *Age and Gender Considerations in Psychiatric Diagnosis: A Research Agenda for DSM-V*, pp. 177–189. Arlington, VA: American Psychiatric Association.

Angold, A., Erkanli, A., Farmer, E. M. Z., Fairbank, J. A., Burns, B. J., Keeler, G., et al. (2002). Psychiatric disorder, impairment, and service use in rural African American and White youth. *Archives of General Psychiatry*, **59**, 893–901.

Armstrong, T. D. & Costello, E. J. (2002). Community studies on adolescent substance use, abuse, or dependence and psychiatric comorbidity. *Journal of Consulting and Clinical Psychology*, **70**, 1224–1239.

Beals, J., Piasecki, J., Nelson, S., Jones, M., Keane, E., Dauphinais, P., et al. (1997). Psychiatric disorder among American Indian adolescents: prevalence in northern plains youth. *Journal of the American Academy of Child and Adolescent Psychiatry*, **36**, 1252–1259.

Benjet, C., Borges, G., Medina-Mora, M. E., Zambrano, J., & Aguilar-Gaxiola, S. (2009). Youth mental health in a populous city of the developing world: results from the Mexican Adolescent Mental Health Survey. *Journal of Child Psychology and Psychiatry*, **50**, 386–395. doi: JCPP1962 [pii] 10.1111/j.1469–7610.2008.01962.x

Bergeron, L., Valla, J. P., & Breton, J. J. (1992). Pilot study for the Quebec Child Mental Health Survey. I. Measurement of prevalence estimates among 6 to 14 year olds. *Canadian Journal of Psychiatry*, **37**, 374–405.

Biederman, J., Rosenbaum, J. F., Bolduc-Murphy, E. A., Faraone, S. V., Chaloff, J., Hirshfeld, D. R., et al. (1993). A three-year follow-up of children with and without behavioural inhibition. *Journal of the American Academy of Child and Adolescent Psychiatry*, **32**, 814–821.

Biederman, J., Rosenbaum, J. F., Hirshfeld, D. R., Faraone, S. V., Bolduc, E. A., Gersten, M., et al. (1990). Psychiatric correlates of behavioural inhibition in young children of parents with and without psychiatric disorders. *Archives of General Psychiatry*, **47**, 21–26.

Bittner, A., Egger, H. L., Erkanli, A., Costello, E. J., Foley, D., & Angold, A. (2007). What do childhood anxiety disorders predict? *Journal of Child Psychology and Psychiatry*, **48**, 1174–1183.

Black, B. (1994). Separation anxiety disorder and panic disorder. In: **J. March** (ed.) *Anxiety Disorders in Children and Adolescents*, pp. 212–234. New York: Guilford Press.

Bolton, D., Eley, T. C., O'Connor, T. G., Perrin, S., Rabe-Hesketh, S., Rijsdijk, F., *et al.* (2006). Prevalence and genetic and environmental influences on anxiety disorders in 6-year-old twins. *Psychological Medicine*, **36**, 335–344.

Breton, J.-J., Bergeron, L., Valla, J.-P., Berthiaume, C., & **Gaudet, N.** (1999). Quebec child mental health survey: prevalence of DSM-III-R mental health disorders. *Journal of Child Psychology and Psychiatry*, **40**, 375–384.

Briggs-Gowan, M. J., Carter, A. S., Skuban, E. M., & **Horwitz, S. M.** (2001). Prevalence of social– emotional and behavioral problems in a community sample of 1- and 2-year old children. *Journal of the American Academy of Child and Adolescent Psychiatry*, **40**, 811–819.

Briggs-Gowan, M. J., Horwitz, S. M., Schwab-Stone, M. E., Leventhal, J. M., & **Leaf, P. J.** (2000). Mental health in pediatric settings: distribution of disorders and factors related to service use. *Journal of the American Academy of Child and Adolescent Psychiatry*, **39**, 841–849.

Canals, J., Domenech, E., Carbajo, G., & **Blade, J.** (1997). Prevalence of DSM-III-R and ICD-10 psychiatric disorders in a Spanish population of 18-year-olds. *Acta Psychiatrica Scandinavica*, **96**, 287–294.

Canino, G., Shrout, P. E., Rubio-Stipec, M., Bird, H. R., Bravo, M., Ramirez, R., *et al.* (2004). The DSM-IV rates of child and adolescent disorders in Puerto Rico: prevalence, correlates, service use, and the effects of impairment. *Archives of General Psychiatry*, **61**, 85–93.

Caspi, A., Moffitt, T. E., Morgan, J., Rutter, M., Taylor, A., Arseneault, L., *et al.* (2004). Maternal expressed emotion predicts children's antisocial behavior problems: using monozygotic-twin differences to identify environmental effects on behavioral development. *Developmental Psychology*, **40**, 149–161.

Copeland, W. E., Shanahan, L., Costello, E. J., & **Angold, A.** (2009). Childhood and adolescent psychiatric disorders as predictors of young adult disorders. *Archives of General Psychiatry*, **66**, 764–772.

Costello, E. J. & **Janiszewski, S.** (1990). Who gets treated? Factors associated with referral in children with psychiatric disorders. *Acta Psychiatrica Scandinavica*, **81**, 523–529.

Costello, E. J., Burns, B. J., Angold, A., & **Leaf, P. J.** (1993). How can epidemiology improve mental health services for children and adolescents? *Journal of the American Academy of Child and Adolescent Psychiatry*, **32**, 1106–1113.

Costello, E. J., Costello, A. J., Edelbrock, C., Burns, B. J., Dulcan, M. K., Brent, D., *et al.* (1988). Psychiatric disorders in pediatric primary care: prevalence and risk factors. *Archives of General Psychiatry*, **45**, 1107–1116.

Costello, A. J., Edelbrock, C. S., Dulcan, M. K., Kalas, R., & **Klaric, S. H.** (1984). *Development and Testing of the NIMH Diagnostic Interview Schedule for Children in a Clinic Population: Final Report (contract no. RFP-DB-81–0027)*. Rockville, MD: NIMH Center for Epidemiologic Studies.

Costello, E. J., Egger, H. L., & **Angold, A.** (2004). The developmental epidemiology of anxiety disorders. In: **T. Ollendick** & **J. March** (eds.) *Phobic and Anxiety Disorders in Children and Adolescents: A Clinician's Guide to Effective Psychosocial and Pharmacological Interventions*, pp. 61–91. Oxford, UK: Oxford University Press.

Costello, E. J., Mustillo, S., Erkanli, A., Keeler, G., & **Angold, A.** (2003). Prevalence and development of psychiatric disorders in childhood and adolescence. *Archives of General Psychiatry*, **60**, 837–844.

Costello, E. J., Mustillo, S., Keeler, G., & **Angold, A.** (2004). Prevalence of psychiatric disorders in childhood and adolescence. In: **B. Lubotsky, J. Petrila,** & **K. Hennessy** (eds.) *Mental Health Services: A Public Health Perspective*, pp. 111–128. Oxford, UK: Oxford University Press.

Dadds, M. R., James, R. C., Barrett, P. M., & Verhulst, F. C. (2004). Diagnostic issues. In: T. H. Ollendick & J. S. March (eds.) *Phobic and Anxiety Disorders in Children and Adolescents: A Clinician's Guide to Effective Psychosocial and Pharmacological Interventions*, pp. 3–33. Oxford, UK: Oxford University Press.

Eapen, V., Al-Gazali, L., Bin-Othman, S., & Abou-Saleh, M. (1998). Mental health problems among schoolchildren in United Arab Emirates: prevalence and risk factors. *Journal of the American Academy of Child and Adolescent Psychiatry*, **37**, 880–886.

Eapen, V., Jakka, M. E., & Abou-Saleh, M. T. (2003). Children with psychiatric disorders: the Al Ain Community Psychiatric Survey. *Canadian Journal of Psychiatry*, **48**, 402–407.

Egger, H. L. & Angold, A. (2006a). Anxiety disorders. In: J. Luby (ed.) *Handbook of Preschool Mental Health: Development, Disorders, and Treatment*, pp. 137–164. New York: Guilford Press.

Egger, H. L. & Angold, A. (2006b). Common emotional and behavioral disorders in preschool children: presentation, nosology, and epidemiology. *Journal of Child Psychology and Psychiatry*, **47**, 313–337.

Egger, H. L., Ascher, B. H., & Angold, A. (1999). *The Preschool Age Psychiatric Assessment*, Version 1.1. Durham, NC: Center for Developmental Epidemiology, Department of Psychiatry and Behavioural Sciences, Duke University Medical Center.

Egger, H. L., Erkanli, A., Keeler, G., Potts, E., Walter, B., & Angold, A. (2006). The test–retest reliability of the Preschool Age Psychiatric Assessment (PAPA). *Journal of the American Academy of Child and Adolescent Psychiatry*, **45**, 538–549.

Ehringer, M. A., Rhee, S. H., Young, S., Corley, R., & Hewitt, J. K. (2006). Genetic and environmental contributions to common psychopathologies of childhood and adolescence: a study of twins and their siblings. *Journal of Abnormal Child Psychology*, **34**, 1–17. doi: 10.1007/s10802–005-9000–0.

Ezpeleta, L., Keeler, G., Erkanli, A., Costello, E. J., & Angold, A. (2001). Epidemiology of psychiatric disability in childhood and adolescence. *Journal of Child Psychology and Psychiatry*, **42**, 901–914.

Ferdinand, R., Barrett, J., & Dadds, M. R. (2004). Anxiety and depression in childhood: prevention and intervention. In: T. H. Ollendick & J. S. March (eds.) *Phobic and Anxiety Disorders in Children and Adolescents: A Clinician's Guide to Effective Psychosocial and Pharmacological Interventions*, pp. 459–475. Oxford, UK: Oxford University Press.

Fergusson, D. & Horwood, L. (2001). The Christchurch health and development study: review of findings on child and adolescent mental health. *Australian and New Zealand Journal of Psychiatry*, **35**, 287–296.

Fleitlich-Bilyk, B. & Goodman, R. (2004). Prevalence of child and adolescent psychiatric disorders in southeast Brazil. *Journal of the American Academy of Child and Adolescent Psychiatry*, **43**, 727–734.

Gau, S., Chong, M., Chen, T., & Cheng, A. (2005). A three-year panel study of mental disorders among adolescents in Taiwan. *American Journal of Psychiatry*, **162**, 1344–1350.

Gilks, W. R., Clayton, D. G., Spiegelhalter, D. J., Best, N. G., McNeil, A. J., Sharples, L. D., *et al.* (1993). Modelling complexity: applications of Gibbs sampling in medicine. *Journal of the Royal Statistical Society*, **55**, 39–52.

Green, E. K., Elvidge, G. P., Owen, M. J., & Craddock, N. (2003). Mutational analysis of two positional candidate susceptibility genes for bipolar disorder on chromosome 12q23–q24: phenylalanine hydroxylase and human LIM-homeobox LHX5. *Psychiatric Genetics*, **13**, 97–101.

Heiervang, E. M., Stormark, K., Lundervold, A. J., Heimann, M., Goodman, R., Posserud, M., *et al.* (2007). Psychiatric disorders in Norwegian 8- to 10-year-olds: an epidemiological survey of prevalence, risk factors, and service use. *Journal of the American Academy of Child and Adolescent Psychiatry*, **46**, 438–447.

Hirshfeld, D. R., Rosenbaum, J. F., Biederman, J., Bolduc, E. A., Faraone, S. V., Snidman, N. S., *et al.* (1992). Stable behavioral inhibition and its association with anxiety disorder. *Journal of the American Academy of Child and Adolescent Psychiatry*, **31**, 103–111.

Hodges, K., Doucette-Gates, A., & Liao, Q. (1999). The relationship between the Child and Adolescent Functional Assessment Scale (CAFAS) and indicators of functioning. *Journal of Child and Family Studies*, **8**, 109–122.

Johnson, J. G., Cohen, P., Pine, D. S., Klein, D. F., Stephanie, K., & Brook, J. S. (2000). Association between cigarette smoking and anxiety disorders during adolescence and early adulthood. *Journal of the American Medical Association*, **284**, 2348–2351.

Kagan, J. & Snidman, N. (1991). Infant predictors of inhibited and uninhibited profiles. *Psychological Science*, **2**, 40–44.

Kagan, J. & Snidman, N. (1999). Early childhood predictors of adult anxiety disorders. *Biological Psychiatry*, **46**, 1536–1541.

Kagan, J., Reznick, S., & Snidman, N. (1987). The physiology and psychology of behavioral inhibition in children. *Child Development*, **58**, 1459–1473.

Kandel, D. B., Johnson, J. G., Bird, H. R., Canino, G., Goodman, S. H., Lahey, B. B., *et al.* (1997). Psychiatric disorders associated with substance use among children and adolescents: findings from the Methods for the Epidemiology of Child and Adolescent Mental Disorders (MECA) study. *Journal of Abnormal Child Psychology*, **25**, 121–132.

Kaplow, J. B., Curran, P. J., Angold, A., & Costello, E. J. (2001). The prospective relation between dimensions of anxiety and the initiation of adolescent alcohol use. *Journal of Clinical Child Psychology*, **30**, 316–326.

Keenan, K., Feng, X., Hipwell, A., & Klostermann, S. (2009). Depression begets depression: comparing the predictive utility of depression and anxiety symptoms to later depression. *Journal of Child Psychology and Psychiatry*, **50**, 1167–1175. doi: JCPP2080 [pii] 10.1111/j.1469–7610.2009.02080.x

Klein, R. G. (1995). Is panic disorder associated with childhood separation anxiety disorder? *Clinical Neuropharmacology*, **18**(Suppl. 2), S7–S14.

Krueger, R., Caspi, A., Moffitt, T., & Silva, P. (1998). The structure and stability of common mental disorders (DSM-III-R): a longitudinal–epidemiological study. *Journal of Abnormal Psychology*, **107**, 216–227.

Lahey, B. B., Flagg, E. W., Bird, H. R., Schwab-Stone, M., Canino, G., Dulcan, M. K., *et al.* (1994). The NIMH Methods for the Epidemiology of Child and Adolescent Mental Disorders (MECA) Study: background and methodology. *Journal of the American Academy of Child and Adolescent Psychiatry*, **35**, 855–864.

Lewinsohn, P. M., Lewinsohn, M., Gotlib, I. H., Seeley, J. R., & Allen, N. B. (1998). Gender differences in anxiety disorders and anxiety symptoms in adolescents. *Journal of Abnormal Psychology*, **107**, 109–117.

Lewinsohn, P. M., Rohde, P., & Seeley, J. R. (1998). Major depressive disorder in older adolescents: prevalence, risk factors, and clinical implications. *Clinical Psychology Review*, **18**, 765–794.

Lewinsohn, P., Zinbarg, J., Lewinsohn, M., & Sack, W. (1997). Lifetime comorbidity among anxiety disorders and between anxiety disorders and other mental disorders in adolescents. *Journal of Anxiety Disorders*, **11**, 377–394.

Lynch, F., Mills, C., Daly, I., & Fitzpatrick, C. (2006). Challenging times: prevalence of psychiatric disorders and suicidal behaviours in Irish adolescents. *Journal of Adolescence*, **29**, 555–573.

McArdle, P., Prosser, J., & Kolvin, I. (2004). Prevalence of psychiatric disorder: with and without psychosocial impairment. *European Child and Adolescent Psychiatry*, **13**, 347–353.

Meltzer, H., Gatward, R., Goodman, R., & Ford, T. (1999). *The Mental Health of Children and Adolescents in Great Britain*. London: Office for National Statistics.

Moffitt, T. E., Harrington, H., Caspi, A., Kim-Cohen, J., Goldberg, D., Gregory, A. M., *et al.* (2007). Depression and generalized anxiety disorder: cumulative and sequential comorbidity in a birth cohort followed prospectively to age 32 years. *Archives of General Psychiatry*, **64**, 651–660.

Mullick, M. S. I. & Goodman, R. (2005). The prevalence of psychiatric disorders among 5–10 year olds in rural, urban and slum areas in Bangladesh. *Social Psychiatry and Psychiatric Epidemiology*, **40**, 663–671.

Murphy, D. A., Cantwell, C., Jordan, D. D., Lee, M. B., Cooley-Quille, M. R., & Lahey, B. B. (2000). Test–retest reliability of Dominic anxiety and depression items among young children. *Journal of Psychopathology and Behavioral Assessment*, **22**, 257–270.

Orvaschel, H., Lewinsohn, P. M., & Seeley, J. R. (1995). Continuity of psychopathology in a community sample of adolescents. *Journal of the American Academy of Child and Adolescent Psychiatry*, **34**, 1525–1535.

Perkonigg, A., Lieb, R., & Wittchen, H.-U. (1998). Prevalence of use, abuse and dependence of illicit drugs among adolescents and young adults in a community sample. *European Addiction Research*, **4**, 58–66.

Petersen, D. J., Bilenberg, N., Hoerder, K., & Gillberg, C. (2006). The population prevalence of child psychiatric disorders in Danish 8- to 9-year-old children. *European Child and Adolescent Psychiatry*, **15**, 71–78.

Ravens-Sieberer, U., Wille, N., Bettge, S., & Erhart, M. (2007). Psychische Gesundheit von Kindern und Jugendlichen in Deutschland. *Bundesgesundheitsblatt–Gesundheitsforschung–Gesundheitsschutz*, **50**, 871–878.

Romano, E., Tremblay, R. E., Vitaro, F., Zoccolillo, M., & Pagani, L. (2001). Prevalence of psychiatric diagnoses and the role of perceived impairment: findings from an adolescent community sample. *Journal of Child Psychology and Psychiatry*, **42**, 451–461.

Rosenbaum, J. F., Biederman, J., Bolduc, E. A., Hirshfeld, D. R., Faraone, S. V., & Kagan, J. (1992). Comorbidity of parental anxiety disorders as risk for childhood-onset anxiety in inhibited children. *American Journal of Psychiatry*, **149**, 475–481.

Rosenbaum, J. F., Biederman, J., Hirshfeld, D. R., Bolduc, E. A., & Chaloff, J. (1991). Behavioral inhibition in children: a possible precursor to panic disorder or social phobia. *Journal of Clinical Psychiatry*, **52**, 5–9.

Rosenbaum, J. F., Biederman, J., Hirshfeld, D. R., Bolduc, E. A., Faraone, S. V., Kagan, J., *et al.* (1991). Further evidence of an association between behavioural inhibition and anxiety disorders: results from a family study of children from a non-clinical sample. *Journal of Psychiatric Research*, **25**, 49–65.

Rueter, M. A., Scaramella, L., Wallace, L. E., & Conger, R. D. (1999). First onset of depressive or anxiety disorders predicted by the longitudinal course of internalizing symptoms and parent–adolescent disagreements. *Archives of General Psychiatry*, **56**, 726–732.

Shaffer, D. (1992). *The Diagnostic Interview Schedule for Children*. New York: New York State Psychiatric Institute.

Shaffer, D., Fisher, P., Dulcan, M. K., & Davies, M. (1996). The NIMH Diagnostic Interview Schedule for Children, Version 2.3 (DISC 2.3): description, acceptability, prevalence rates, and performance in the MECA study. *Journal of the American Academy of Child and Adolescent Psychiatry*, **35**, 865–877.

Shaffer, D., Gould, A., Fisher, P., Trautman, P., Moreau, D., Kleinman, M., *et al.* (1996). Psychiatric diagnosis in child and adolescent suicide. *Archive of General Psychiatry*, **53**, 339–348.

Shear, K., Jin, R., Ruscio, A. M., Walters, E. E., & Kessler, R. C. (2006). Prevalence and correlates of estimated DSM-IV child and adult separation anxiety disorder in the national comorbidity survey. *American Journal of Psychiatry*, **163**, 1074–1083.

Silberg, J., Rutter, M., & Eaves, L. (2001). Genetic and environmental influences on the temporal association between earlier anxiety and later depression in girls. *Biological Psychiatry*, **49**, 1040–1049.

Silove, D., Manicavasagar, V., Curtis, J., & Blaszczynski, A. (1996). Is early separation anxiety a risk factor for adult panic disorder? A critical review. *Comprehensive Psychiatry*, **37**, 167–179.

Silverman, W., Saavedra, L. M., & Pina, A. A. (2001). Test–retest reliablity of anxiety symptoms and diagnoses with the anxiety disorders interview schedule for DSM-IV: Child and Parent Versions. *Journal of the American Academy of Child and Adolescent Psychiatry*, **40**, 937–944.

Simonoff, E., Pickles, A., Meyer, J. M., Silberg, J. L., Maes, H. H., Loeber, R., *et al.* (1997). The Virginia Twin Study of adolescent behavioral development: influences of age, sex and impairment on rates of disorder. *Archives of General Psychiatry*, **54**, 801–808.

Srinath, S., Girimaji, S., Gururaj, G., Seshadri, S., Subbakrishna, D., Bhola, P., *et al.* (2005). Epidemiological study of child and adolescent psychiatric disorders in urban and rural areas of Bangalore, India. *Indian Journal of Medical Research*, **122**, 67–79.

Steinhausen, H. C. (2006). Developmental psychopathology in adolescence: findings from a Swiss study: the NAPE Lecture 2005. *Acta Psychiatrica Scandinavica*, **113**, 6–12. doi: 10.1111/j.1600–0447.2005.00706.x

Sterba, S., Egger, H. L., & Angold, A. (2007). Diagnostic specificity and nonspecificity in the dimensions of preschool psychopathology. *Journal of Child Psychology and Psychiatry*, **48**, 1005–1013. doi: 10.1111/j.1469–7610.2007.01770.x

Tiwari, S. K. & Wang, J. (2006). The epidemiology of mental and substance use-related disorders among white, Chinese, and other Asian populations in Canada. *Canadian Journal of Psychiatry*, **51**, 904–912.

Valla, J.-P., Bergeron, L., & Smolla, N. (2000). The Dominic-R: a pictorial interview for 6- to 11-year-old children. *Journal of the American Academy of Child and Adolescent Psychiatry*, **39**, 85–93.

Verhulst, F. C., van der Ende, J., Ferdinand, R. F., & Kasius, M. C. (1997). The prevalence of DSM-III-R diagnoses in a national sample of Dutch adolescents. *Archives of General Psychiatry*, **54**, 329–336.

Warren, S. L. & Sroufe, L. A. (2004). Developmental issues. In: T. H. Ollendick & J. S. March (eds.) *Phobic and Anxiety Disorders in Children and Adolescents: A Clinician's Guide to Effective Psychosocial and Pharmacological Interventions*, pp. 92–115. Oxford, UK: Oxford University Press.

4

The "normal" development of fear

Peter Muris and Andy P. Field

Children seem to be particularly prone to experience anxiety phenomena. Research has shown that worry (Muris, Meesters, Merckelbach, Sermon, & Zwakhalen, 1998; Silverman, La Greca, & Wasserstein, 1995), night-time anxiety (Gordon, King, Gullone, Muris, & Ollendick, 2007; King, Ollendick, & Tonge, 1997; Muris, Merckelbach, Ollendick, King, & Bogie, 2001), scary dreams and nightmares (Mindell & Barrett, 2002), anxiety-related physiological symptoms (Weems, Zakem, Costa, Cannon, & Watts, 2005), panic attacks (Hayward, Killen, & Taylor, 1989; King, Gullone, Tonge, & Ollendick, 1993), and obsessive–compulsive disorder related rituals (Leonard, Goldberger, Rapoport, Cheslow, & Swedo, 1990) are commonly observed in non-clinical youths.

Quite a number of studies have focused on childhood fear (Gullone, 2000). Findings of this research generally indicate that fear is in essence benign and non-pathological by nature (e.g., Craske, 1997). Children experience relatively mild fears that appear and disappear spontaneously and follow a predictable course. These developmentally appropriate or "normal" fears should be distinguished from phobias and anxiety disorders, which are out of proportion to the demands of the situation that evokes it, cannot be rationalized, are involuntary, lead to avoidance of the situation, and interfere with daily functioning (American Psychiatric Association, 2000). Although for most children normal fears naturally wax and wane, as this chapter shows, it is likely that childhood fears may be the seeds for more pervasive and severe anxiety symptoms or disorders (in the sense that a normal fear may, for whatever reason, increase in magnitude and persist beyond its natural course: Muris, 2006, 2007).

This chapter examines the developmental pathway of normal fears and their link to clinical anxiety. We begin by investigating how normal fears are measured before describing their developmental pattern and moderating influences such as gender. We then discuss some possible explanations for these developmental patterns before concluding by bridging the gap between normal fear and clinical anxiety.

What do children fear?

Over the past 100 years, researchers have used a variety of methods to try to measure common fear and anxiety in childhood. Although there is no space to review every study in the literature (for an excellent review see Gullone, 2000), in this section we summarize some of the key approaches and the findings from them before drawing the main conclusions.

Anxiety Disorders in Children and Adolescents, 2nd edn, ed. W. K. Silverman and A. P. Field. Published by Cambridge University Press. © Cambridge University Press 2011.

Child report

Many early studies into children's fears simply asked children about their fears within an interview. Jersild and Holmes (1935), for example, report data from interviews with 398 5–12-year-old children. The most commonly reported fears were animals (17.4%), injury or pain (15.3%), imaginary creatures and ghosts (10%), and robbers, burglars, kidnappers etc. (9.5%). In a later study by Bauer (1976), 4–12-year-old children were interviewed by asking them "What are you afraid of most?" Responses to this question were coded into categories of fear. Results showed that the most highly cited sources of fears were similar to those found by Jersild and Holmes, although the percentage of children reporting these fears had increased dramatically: 39% of children reported fears of bodily injury or physical danger, 43% reported fears of monsters and ghosts, and 30% reported fears of animals. In addition, 50% had night-time fears and 65% had frightening dreams (compared to only 5.6% in Jersild and Holmes's study). Gullone (2000) reviewed many other interview-based studies using youths aged from 4 to 19. This author concluded that the average number of fears is typically between two and five per child, but that there is also considerable variation across studies (with one study even reporting an average of 9.3 fears per child). However, these interviews did seem to elicit general themes such as animals, death/injury, the unknown (strange sounds or situations), and social concerns (e.g., being teased).

However, interview methods are problematic because interviews have to be coded by the experimenter who may interpret responses in a way that fits the experimenter's pre-existing expectancies about what children fear. This problem can be overcome through standardized coding schemes, and multiple coders whose responses are checked for agreement. However, these checks have seldom been done in this research field (Gullone, 2000), although Bauer (1976) did report an inter-rater agreement of 0.94.

Another way to solicit information from children is through questionnaires. Gullone (2000) reports that around 20 different questionnaires have been used to measure children's fears. The most widely used is the Fear Survey Schedule for Children (FSSC: Scherer & Nakamura, 1968) and in particular its revision, the FSSC-R (Ollendick, 1983). The FSSC-R is a standardized 80-item measure, which asks children to rate how much fear they experience in response to a wide range of specific stimuli and situations, using a three-point response scale ("none," "some," or "a lot"). In this way, information can be obtained on the number, severity, and types of fears that children experience.

Factor analysis has consistently demonstrated that the FSSC-R contains five factors: fear of danger and death (e.g., "Being hit by a car or truck"), fear of failure and criticism (e.g., "Looking foolish"), fear of the unknown (e.g., "Going to bed in the dark"), fear of small animals (e.g., "Snakes"), and medical fears (e.g., "Getting an injection from the doctor") (see Ollendick, 1983). The psychometric properties of the FSSC-R are generally satisfactory, and hence this instrument seems to reflect a suitable method to investigate normal fears in children.

Surveys based on FSSC-R have generally indicated that non-clinical children report a surprisingly large number of fears. For example, Ollendick, King, and Frary (1989) found an average of 14 fears reported by American and Australian youths aged 7 to 17 years, and comparable high numbers have been reported for children and adolescents in other countries (e.g., Ollendick, Yang, King, Dong, & Akande, 1996). Most of the common fears as obtained with the FSSC-R pertain to dangerous situations and physical harm. Thus, fear items such as "Not being able to breathe," "Bombing attacks or being invaded," "Being hit by a car or truck," "Fire or getting burned," and "Falling from high places" typically feature high in FSSC-R-based fear rank orders (e.g., King, Hamilton, & Ollendick, 1988).

Since the development of the FSSC-R in the early 1980s, society has changed and youths are increasingly confronted with "new" threatening stimuli and situations: school violence, sexual assaults, domestic violence, parental divorce, abuse, and neglect are real-life threats for a growing number of children and adolescents (e.g., Fishkin, Rohrbach, & Anderson-Johnson, 1997). In addition, television makes youths increasingly aware of new diseases (e.g., AIDS), disasters (e.g., floods), and other threatening events (e.g., drugs, terrorist attacks) that may occur (e.g., Lengua, Long, Smith, & Meltzoff, 2005). Research with updated versions of the FSSC-R, which include more of these contemporary fear stimuli and situations, has indicated that a number of the new fear items list high in the top 10 of most common fears, although most prevalent fears are still concerned with the theme of danger and harm (e.g., Burnham & Gullone, 1997; Muris & Ollendick, 2002; Shore & Rapport, 1998).

Although questionnaires like the FSSC-R may yield valuable information on children's fears in a standardized fashion (e.g., Weems, Silverman, Saavedra, Pina, & Lumpkin, 1999), it is also good to keep in mind that this method is also prone to a number of shortcomings. To begin with, it is clear that this type of assessment is determined by the items that are included in the scale. This point was nicely illustrated by Muris and colleagues (Muris, Merckelbach, & Collaris, 1997; Muris, Merckelbach, Meesters, & Van Lier, 1997) who examined the prevalence of common childhood fears by employing the FSSC-R, but also by asking children what they feared most without specifying items a priori (i.e., "free option" method). Results indicated that the top 10 fears generated using the FSSC-R were remarkably similar to those obtained in the studies performed by Ollendick and colleagues almost a decade or more earlier. Using the free option method many items were spontaneously generated that matched items from the FSSC-R (e.g., burglary, being hit by a car), but there were other prevalent fears not tapped by the FSSC-R (e.g., being kidnapped, parents dying).

In addition, it has been noted that by prompting children to think about potential threats, questionnaires like the FSSC-R may not tap what children actually fear but how aversive they find the thought of the threat happening. For example, children may not actually experience a fear of their parents arguing because this idea has never occurred to them, but when prompted, the thought of their parents arguing is something that they find fearful. As such, some FSSC-R items might not index the *actual* frequency of fears, but rather reflect negative affective responding to the thought of the actual occurrence of these specific events were they to occur (McCathie & Spence, 1991). Additional support for this notion was provided by a diary study (Muris, Merckelbach, Ollendick, King, Meesters, & Van Kessel, 2002), which indicated that frequent FSSC-R danger and death fears have a low prevalence rate in children's daily life.

Parent report

Although most studies on childhood fears have relied on youths' self-report, there is a small body of research using other informants such as parents. In an older study, Hagman (1932) interviewed 70 mothers about the fears of their children who were aged between 23 months and 6 years. The most frequently mentioned fears pertained to dogs, doctors, storms, deep water, and darkness. Parents reported an average of 2.7 fears per child, which is at the low end of the range of fears reported by children themselves in the studies mentioned in the previous section. Jersild and Holmes (1935) collected questionnaires over a 21-day period from 153 parents of children from birth to 8 years old. Each child had, on average, 4.64 fears; the most frequently reported fears were noises, animals, physical harm or danger, strange persons, and pain. These studies illustrate several problems with the parent report of childhood fear (see Silverman & Ollendick, 2005). First, parent and child reports of fears typically differ – especially in younger children. Jersild and Holmes directly compared parent and child report in their study; adults underestimated fears of animals, criminal characters, imaginary creatures, and bodily injury compared to reports of 5–12-year-old children, but overestimated fears of pain, noise, and strange objects. Second, a parent's ability to report on fear will vary as a function of their experiences of seeing the child in situations in which it is scared or the extent to which the child is willing to communicate about fear. In other words, parents and teachers can only report fears of situations that they have actually experienced with their child.

Regardless of the differences resulting from methodology, the data seem to indicate that children typically yield a range of fears that bear some intuitive relation to the phobic conditions that can readily be observed in adults, such as animal phobia ("Spiders"), height phobia ("Falling from a high place"), claustrophobia ("Not being able to breathe"), and blood–injection–illness phobia ("Getting a serious disease"). Although the studies described in this section focused on childhood fears, there is also a body of research examining the prevalence of other anxiety symptoms among youths. An example is a study by Bell-Dolan, Last, and Strauss (1990), who examined the prevalence of symptoms of DSM-defined anxiety disorders in a sample of 62 non-clinical children and adolescents. These children and adolescents had never displayed any serious psychiatric problems, but child- and parent-based semi-structured interviews revealed that subclinical anxiety disorders symptoms were fairly common among these youths. Not only phobic symptoms were highly prevalent, but also symptoms of generalized anxiety disorder, separation anxiety disorder, and social phobia. In other words, just like fears, other anxiety symptoms are quite common among non-clinical children.

Altogether, the data show that children have a realistic sense of the global threats in the world, even though these global threats manifest themselves in idiosyncratic fears within a given child. The fact that normative fear and anxiety of children seem to reflect the content of phobias and other anxiety disorders provides a strong basis for assuming that the seeds of clinical anxiety are sown in childhood (Muris, 2007). This does not mean, however, that all fears that become manifest during childhood are pathological in nature. Fears wax and wane as children grow older, and even follow a predictable course. We now turn our attention to how these fears change over age and what variables may mediate and moderate the content and intensity of normal fears.

Developmental patterns

Research has shown that normal anxiety phenomena in youths follow a predictable developmental pattern. One of the first studies that addressed this issue was that of Jersild and Holmes (1935) who, based on parent report, concluded that between birth and 6 years reports of fears of noise, pain, falling, and strange events declined; whereas reports of fears of imaginary creatures, physical harm, and nightmares increased. Bauer (1976) found, based on child report, that 74% of the 4–6-year-olds, 53% of the 6–8-year-olds, but only 5% of the 10–12-year-olds reported fear of ghosts and monsters. In contrast, only 11% of the 4–6-year-olds, but 53% of the 6–8-year-olds and 55% of the 10–12-year-olds reported fear of bodily injury and physical danger. Muris, Merckelbach, Gadet, and Moulaert (2000) investigated the prevalence of fears, worries, and scary dreams among 4–12-year-old children by means of a semi-structured interview, which included pictures to explain these anxiety phenomena to the (younger) children. Inspection of the developmental pattern of these phenomena revealed that fears and scary dreams were common among 4–6-year-olds, became even more prevalent in 7–9-year-olds, and then decreased in frequency in 10–12-year-olds. Worry showed the opposite developmental pattern: it was more prevalent in older children (i.e., 7–12-year-olds) than in younger children. As to the frequency of specific types of fears, some developmental patterns emerged that were similar to those obtained by Bauer (1976). For example, the prevalence of fears and scary dreams pertaining to imaginary creatures decreased with age, whereas worry about performance at school increased as children became older.

A further investigation by Westenberg, Drewes, Goedhart, Siebelink, and Treffers (2004) also performed a developmental analysis of fears in 8–18-year-old youths. Based on the observation that childhood fears can be divided in two broad categories of physical harm and social problems, these researchers focused their analysis on the developmental pattern of fears concerning physical danger and fears concerning social evaluation. For this purpose, children in three age groups (i.e., 8–11-year-olds, 12–14-year-olds, and 15–18-year-olds) completed the FSSC-R. Results indicated that scores on FSSC-R subscales pertaining to physical fears substantially decreased across the three age groups. A differential pattern was observed within the category of social fears. That is, whereas fears of social evaluation (e.g., "Being criticized by others") and achievement evaluation (e.g., "Failing a test") clearly increased when children were older, fear of punishment (e.g., "Getting punished by mother") significantly decreased with age.

Altogether, although it should be noted that most of the abovementioned studies have relied on cross-sectional designs, findings suggest that fears and other anxiety phenomena follow a predictable course during childhood. In the next section, we discuss how this developmental pattern can be explained.

Explanations of normal fears

Evolution

One possible explanation for the developmental pattern in children's normal fear and anxiety is that evolutionary pressures have selected for a fear system that naturally focuses on certain environmental threats at ages at which these threats would have been pertinent to our pre-technological ancestors. For example, Öhman, Dimberg, and Öst (1985) argued that in infancy, evolution should have selected for fear and avoidance of all potentially dangerous things because at this age children are defenseless and this innate fear will keep infants within protective distance of their parents. As children grow emotionally and physically (4 to 8 years) they will begin to explore their environment alone. At this age, encounters with predators are more likely to be fatal than for adolescents and adults because, despite their new autonomy, children are still small and relatively powerless against an attack. As such, it will be extremely important for them to learn about threat efficiently at this age to avoid potentially catastrophic encounters with predators. Evolution should, therefore, select for a system that allows rapid learning about threat from animals.

As children move towards the teenage years they become physically stronger and more cognitively developed and are better able to defend themselves or outwit predators. Natural wariness of predators should therefore wane. However, during the teenage years children's social position within the group becomes more vital: assuming a prominent position in the hierarchy could mean the difference between survival or not. Again, therefore, evolution might select for a system that shifts the focus of threat into the social world. All in all, it can be argued that normative fears seem to mirror plausible evolutionary concerns across children's development.

Cognitive development

Another explanation for the developmental pattern of childhood fear and anxiety is concerned with the progress in children's cognitive capacities. The basic idea is that fear and anxiety originate from threat, and threat has to be conceptualized. Conceptualization, in turn, critically depends on cognitive abilities (Vasey, 1993). Thus, at a very young age, fear and anxiety are primarily directed at immediate, concrete threats (loud noises, loss of physical support). As cognitive abilities reach a certain maturational stage, fear and anxiety become more sophisticated. For example, at about 9 months, children learn to differentiate between familiar and unfamiliar faces, and consequently separation anxiety and fear of strangers become manifest. Following this, fears of imaginary creatures occur, and it is believed that these are closely linked to the magical thinking of toddlers (Bauer, 1976). Fears of small animals and unknown stimuli in the environment also develop during this phase, and are believed to be functionally related to the increased mobility of children and their exploration and awareness of the external world. From 7 years onwards, children are increasingly able to infer physical cause–effect relationships and to anticipate potential negative consequences. These cognitive changes are thought to broaden the range of fear-provoking stimuli and enhance the more cognitive features of anxiety (e.g., worry).

Whereas the evolutionary-based explanation for the developmental pattern in childhood fear is difficult to demonstrate empirically (Muris, Merckelbach, de Jong, & Ollendick, 2002), there is evidence that cognitive development mediates manifestations of fear and anxiety in youths. For example, the study by Westenberg *et al.* (2004) also examined whether developmental patterns in fears were predicted by youths' level of cognitive maturation. As discussed earlier, the researchers found that children's fears of physical danger decreased with age, whereas fears concerning social evaluation increased as children got older. Most importantly, however, the results indicated that the age effect in social–evaluative fears was fully explained by developmental trends in cognitive maturity. This led the authors to the conclusion that social fear and anxiety, which frequently arise during adolescence, are a corollary of cognitive development.

Another investigation by Muris, Merckelbach, Meesters, and Van den Brand (2002) explored the connection between cognitive development and worry. Children were interviewed about the presence and content of their main worry. Furthermore, the ability to catastrophize was assessed by asking children to think up as many potential negative outcomes associated with a series of worry topics as possible. A number of Piaget's conservation tasks also was administered to assess children's level of cognitive maturation. Results revealed a mediation model in which increased age and, in its wake, cognitive development lead to enhanced ability to catastrophize, which in turn increases the possibility of a personal worry to emerge. On the basis of these results, Muris *et al.* (2002) concluded that worry becomes increasingly manifest in middle childhood when children reach a certain level of cognitive maturation.

The cross-sectional studies described above clearly suggest that fears and anxiety-related phenomena are to some extent mediated by the progress in children's cognitive development. It seems plausible that cognition is involved in developmental issues such as biological regulation in infants, magical thinking in toddlers, school adjustment in middle childhood, and formation of friendship during puberty, which according to some authors also determine the content of youths' fear and anxiety (Warren & Sroufe, 2004). As mentioned earlier, there are currently no long-term prospective studies investigating the developmental course of childhood fear and anxiety, and so this type of research would be welcome to prove the notion that at least the content of such phenomena are guided by age and cognitive maturation.

Moderators of normal fears

Gender

It is well established that girls report higher levels of fear than boys (e.g., Ollendick, King, & Muris, 2002). For example, on a standardized fear rating scale like the FSSC-R, girls consistently display higher scores as compared to boys (e.g., Muris & Ollendick, 2002). One explanation for the finding that girls are more fearful and anxious than boys has to do with individual differences in gender role orientation (Ollendick, Yang, Dong, Xia, & Lin, 1995). Briefly, this explanation implies that girls and boys are socialized to develop gender-linked feminine and masculine behaviors, traits, and skills. According to theories on the development of gender roles (e.g., Bem, 1981), the expression of fear and anxiety is in agreement with the feminine gender role, which is generally acquired by girls and which tolerates the expression of negative emotions and related behaviors (e.g., avoidance behavior). Conversely, fearfulness and anxiety are inconsistent with the masculine gender role. Such emotions are less accepted in boys who are expected to behave bravely and to display active and purposeful coping behavior (see Ginsburg & Silverman, 2000).

Several studies have examined the link between gender role orientation and fear and anxiety in children. Brody, Hay, and Vandewater (1990) investigated relations between gender and gender role orientation and children's feelings towards peers as indexed by an Emotional Story Task in 120 non-clinical youths aged 6 to 12 years. Results showed that girls reported higher levels of fear towards peers than boys. Most importantly, gender role orientation accounted for more of the variance in predicting fear than did the child's sex. That is, biological gender was no longer associated with fear towards peers, after the influence of gender role orientation was partialled out. In general, boys and girls who scored higher on feminine gender role traits were more prone to report higher levels of fears towards peers.

There are also survey studies indicating that gender role orientation, and a related phenomenon like toy and activity preferences, are associated with children's scores on fear and anxiety questionnaires (Ginsburg & Silverman, 2000; Muris, Meesters, & Knoops, 2005; Palapattu, Newman Kingery, & Ginsburg, 2006). Results generally indicate that femininity and a preference for girls' toys and activities were positively associated with fear and anxiety, whereas masculinity and a preference for boys' toys and activities were negatively related to these emotions. Overall, although there is some support for the notion that gender role orientation is involved in the gender differences of fear and anxiety in youths, more research on this issue is certainly required.

Culture and socioeconomic status

Researchers have observed that fear levels in children and adolescents may vary as a function of cultural group membership. Most studies have been carried out in the United States and have generally found that children and adolescents from ethnic minorities (e.g., African American, Hispanic American) display higher levels of fear and anxiety than White children (e.g., Glover, Pumariega, Holzer, Wise, & Rodriguez, 1999; Last & Perrin, 1993; Neal, Lilly, & Zakis, 1993; Pina & Silverman, 2004; Varela, Vernberg, Sanchez-Sosa, Riveros, Mitchell, & Mashunkashey, 2004).

Similar results have been obtained in the Netherlands. In a recent study, Hale, Raaijmakers, Muris, and Meeus (2005) collected anxiety disorders symptoms scores of White Dutch children and adolescents and youths from various ethnic minorities (e.g., Moroccan, Turkish, Surinam). Results demonstrated that ethnic minority youths consistently exhibited higher anxiety scores than the White Dutch youths.

Several investigations have made an attempt to compare the fear and anxiety levels of youths across Western and non-Western countries. Ollendick *et al.* (1996) assessed fears in a sample of 1200 American, Australian, Chinese, and Nigerian children and adolescents. Nigerian children and adolescents reported higher levels of fears than American and Australian youths, whereas the fear levels of Chinese children and adolescents were in between. Furthermore, cultural differences emerged with respect to the content of fears. Although some fears were highly prevalent in all countries, there were fears that appeared to be highly specific and idiosyncratic to each of the nations (e.g., looking foolish in America, snakes in Africa, ghosts in China).

Another study by Elbedour, Shulman, and Kedem (1997) compared self-reported fears of Jewish and Bedouin children in Israel. Results revealed quantitative and qualitative differences between the two groups, with the Bedouin children reporting higher levels of fear and a greater variety of fear-provoking stimuli and situations than the Jewish children. Altogether, the results of these and other studies (e.g., Essau, Sakano, Ishikawa, & Sasagawa, 2004; Maduewesi, 1982; Opolot, 1976) suggest that manifestations of fear and anxiety are at least to some extent culturally determined.

This point is further illustrated by a series of studies that have been carried out in South Africa (Burkhardt, Loxton, & Muris, 2003; Muris, Loxton, Neumann, DuPlessis, King, & Ollendick, 2006; Muris, Schmidt, Engelbrecht, & Perold, 2002). Children and adolescents from various cultural backgrounds completed fear and anxiety questionnaires. Results consistently demonstrated that youths from the Black and Colored communities displayed higher fear and anxiety scores as compared to South African youths from the White community. Interestingly, the latter group showed similar fear and anxiety levels as those observed for children and adolescents in Western countries (Muris *et al.*, 2002).

Thus, there seem to be variations in the content and intensity of fear and anxiety in children and adolescents with different cultural backgrounds. As noted by Weisz, Sigman, Weiss, and Mosk (1993), differences in socialization practices across the various cultures may account for these findings. Compared to Western cultures, Asian and African societies more strongly emphasize self-control, social inhibition, and compliance with social norms, which in turn may foster the development of fear and anxiety. There is some evidence to support this hypothesis: Muris *et al.* (2006) found that differences in parental rearing behaviors (i.e., higher levels of anxious rearing, overprotection, and rejection) accounted for a significant proportion of the differences in anxiety symptoms among White, Black, and Colored South-African youths. However, an important part of the cultural variations in childhood fear and anxiety seemed to be explained by children's socioeconomic status. That is, compared to White South African youths, Black and Colored children tend to live in neighborhoods characterized by deprivation, violence, and poverty. This not only means that children are exposed to certain threat stimuli, which may instill specific fears. It is also likely that the environment in which these children are raised is more stressful, and that this enhances general feelings of fear and anxiety.

The bridge between normal and abnormal fear and anxiety

In conclusion, fear and anxiety are common during childhood. In most youths, fear and anxiety represent relatively mild and transitory phenomena that seem to be guided by children's (cognitive) developmental level. As this chapter has shown, at a group level, gender, culture, and socioeconomic status moderate the content and intensity of children's fears and anxiety. Still, an important question remains how serious childhood fears and anxiety are, and whether they may represent clinically relevant phenomena. In other words, to what extent do children and adolescents engage in worry about feared stimuli and situations at a frequent or regular basis? Do they engage in avoidance behavior to prevent their occurrence? Do these fear and anxiety symptoms interfere with youths' daily functioning? (Ollendick & King, 1994).

To obtain a better picture of the clinical significance of "normal" fear and anxiety symptoms among youths, their connection to DSM-defined phobias and anxiety disorders should be considered. A study by Muris, Merckelbach, Mayer, and Prins (2000) explored this issue. In that study, fears of 290 children aged 8 to 13 years were assessed and then their severity was evaluated by means of a structured diagnostic interview measuring anxiety disorders in terms of DSM criteria. Results showed that in a sizeable minority of the children (22.8%), fears reflected significant anxiety disorders, notably specific phobias.

Similar findings were reported in a follow-up study that investigated the connection between childhood fears and specific phobias by interviewing children's parents (Muris & Merckelbach, 2000). Other studies that examined the severity of normal children's night-time fears and worries through their links with DSM classifications (Muris et al., 1998, 2001) also revealed that such fear and anxiety phenomena reflect serious problems in a fair proportion of the youths. Thus, while there has been a strong tendency in the literature to portray childhood fear and anxiety as mild and non-pathological, there seems to be at least a subgroup of children displaying significant phobias and anxiety disorders, which not only hinder current functioning but also may have a negative impact on their future life (see also Weems, Silverman, & La Greca, 2000; Weems et al., 1999).

Current etiological models adopt a developmental psychopathology perspective, which proposes that childhood phobias and anxiety disorders are in fact radicalizations of normative fear and anxiety (Craske, 1997; Muris, 2006, 2007; Vasey & Dadds, 2001). During the past decades, knowledge of the factors that are involved in the exacerbation of fear and anxiety in youths has increased (Muris & Broeren, 2009; Murray, Creswell, & Cooper, 2009; Rapee, Schniering, & Hudson, 2009). A large number of vulnerability factors have been identified, including (1) child-related vulnerability such as biological sensitivity and genetically based individual difference variables (i.e., neuroticism, negative affectivity: Lonigan, Phillips, Wilson, & Allan, Chapter 10, this volume), (2) environmental risk factors, which pertain to negative life events, specific learning experiences (i.e., conditioning, modeling, and negative information transmission) (Field & Purkis, Chapter 11), and family-based vulnerability Creswell, Murray, Stacey, & Cooper, Chapter 14, this volume), and (3) maintaining factors, which are concerned with avoidance and cognitive distortions (Field, Hadwin, & Lester, Chapter 6, this volume).

In addition, there is recent research emphasizing the role of protective factors that incorporate regulatory processes, positive cognition, and coping mechanisms, which may all shield youths against the development of high fear and anxiety (Chorpita, 2001; Thompson, 2001). The basic idea is that various vulnerability and protective factors interact with each other to produce an adaptive or a maladaptive outcome.

There seems to be a clear bridge between normal and abnormal fear and anxiety in youths. As this volume is on anxiety disorders in children and adolescents, it will certainly tell us more about factors that push children and adolescents towards the "abnormal" side of the bridge and the variables that (fail to) pull youths back to the "normal" (non-pathological) side.

References

American Psychiatric Association (2000). *Diagnostic and Statistical Manual of Mental Disorders*, 4th edn, text revision *(DSM-IV-TR)*. Washington, DC: American Psychiatric Association.

Bauer, D. H. (1976). An exploratory study of developmental changes in children's fears. *Journal of Child Psychology and Psychiatry*, **17**, 69–74.

Bell-Dolan, D. J., Last, C. G., & **Strauss, C. C.** (1990). Symptoms of anxiety disorders in normal children. *Journal of the American Academy of Child and Adolescent Psychiatry*, **25**, 759–765.

Bem, S. L. (1981). Gender schema theory: a cognitive account of sex typing. *Psychological Review*, **88**, 354–364.

Brody, L. R., Hay, D. H., & **Vandewater, E.** (1990). Gender, gender role identity, and children's reported feelings toward the same and opposite sex. *Sex Roles*, **23**, 363–387.

Burkhardt, K., Loxton, H., & **Muris, P.** (2003). Fears and fearfulness in South-African children. *Behaviour Change*, **20**, 94–102.

Burnham, J. J. & **Gullone, E.** (1997). The fear survey schedule for children. II. A psychometric investigation with American data. *Behaviour Research and Therapy*, **35**, 165–173.

Chorpita, B. F. (2001). Control and the development of negative emotion. In: **M. W. Vasey** & **M. R. Dadds** (eds.) *The Developmental Psychopathology of Anxiety*, pp. 112–142. New York: Oxford University Press.

Craske, M. G. (1997). Fear and anxiety in children and adolecents. *Bulletin of the Menninger Clinic*, **61** (Suppl. A), A4–A36.

Elbedour, S., Shulman, S., & **Kedem, P.** (1997). Children's fears: cultural and developmental perspectives. *Behaviour Research and Therapy*, **35**, 491–496.

Essau, C. A., Sakano, Y., Ishikawa, S., & **Sasagawa, S.** (2004). Anxiety symptoms in Japanese and in German children. *Behaviour Research and Therapy*, **42**, 601–612.

Fishkin, S. A., Rohrbach, L. A., & **Anderson-Johnson, C.** (1997). Correlates of youths' fears of victimization. *Journal of Applied Social Psychology*, **27**, 1601–1616.

Ginsburg, G. S. & **Silverman, W. K.** (2000). Gender role orientation and fearfulness in children with anxiety disorders. *Journal of Anxiety Disorders*, **14**, 57–67.

Glover, S. H., Pumariega, A. J., Holzer, C. E., Wise, B. K., & **Rodriguez, M.** (1999). Anxiety symptomatology in Mexican–American adolescents. *Journal of Child and Family Studies*, **8**, 47–57.

Gordon, J., King, N. J., Gullone, E., Muris, P., & **Ollendick, T. H.** (2007). Nighttime fears of children and adolescents: frequency, content, severity, harm expectations, disclosure, and coping behaviours. *Behaviour Research and Therapy*, **45**, 2464–2472.

Gullone, E. (2000). The development of normal fear: a century of research. *Clinical Psychology Review*, **20**, 429–451.

Hagman, E. R. (1932). A study of fears of children of pre-school age. *Journal of Experimental Education*, **1**, 110–130.

Hale, W. W., Raaijmakers, Q., Muris, P., & **Meeus, W.** (2005). Psychometric properties of the Screen for Child Anxiety Related Emotional Disorders (SCARED) in the general adolescent population. *Journal of the American Academy of Child and Adolescent Psychiatry*, **44**, 283–290.

Hayward, C., Killen, J. D., & **Taylor, C. B.** (1989). Panic attacks in young adolescents. *American Journal of Psychiatry*, **146**, 1061–1062.

Jersild, A. T. & **Holmes, F. B.** (1935). *Children's Fears*, Child Development Monographs No. 20. New York: Columbia University Press.

King, N. J., Gullone, E., Tonge, B. J., & **Ollendick, T. H.** (1993). Self-reports of panic attacks and manifest anxiety in adolescents. *Behaviour Research and Therapy*, **31**, 111–116.

King, N. J., Hamilton, D. I., & **Ollendick, T. H.** (1988). *Children's Phobias: A Behavioral Perspective*. New York: Wiley & Sons.

King, N. J., Ollendick, T. H., & **Tonge, B. J.** (1997). Children's nighttime fears. *Clinical Psychology Review*, **17**, 431–443.

Last, C. G. & **Perrin, S.** (1993). Anxiety disorders in African-American and white children. *Journal of Abnormal Child Psychology*, **21**, 153–164.

Lengua, L. J., Long, A. C., Smith, K. I., & **Meltzoff, A. N.** (2005). Pre-attack symptomatology and temperament as predictors of children's responses to the September 11 terrorist attacks. *Journal of Child Psychology and Psychiatry*, **46**, 631–645.

Leonard, H. L., Goldberger, E. L., Rapoport, J. L., Cheslow, D. L., & **Swedo, S. E.** (1990). Childhood rituals: normal development or obsessive–compulsive symptoms? *Journal of the American Academy of Child and Adolescent Psychiatry*, **29**, 17–23.

Maduewesi, E. (1982). Nigerian elementary children's interests and concerns. *Alberta Journal of Educational Research*, **28**, 204–211.

McCathie, H. & **Spence, S. H.** (1991). What is the Revised Fear Survey Schedule for Children measuring? *Behaviour Research and Therapy*, **29**, 495–502.

Mindell, J. A. & **Barrett, K. M.** (2002). Nightmares and anxiety in elementary-aged children: is there a relationship? *Child Care and Development*, **28**, 317–322.

Muris, P. (2006). The pathogenesis of childhood anxiety disorders: considerations from a developmental psychopathology perspective. *International Journal of Behavioral Development*, **31**, 4–10.

Muris, P. (2007). *Normal and Abnormal Fear and Anxiety in Children and Adolescents*. Oxford, UK: Elsevier.

Muris, P. & **Broeren, S.** (2009). Twenty-five years of research on childhood anxiety disorders: publication trends between 1982 and 2006 and a selective review of the literature. *Journal of Child and Family Studies*, **18**, 388–395.

Muris, P. & **Merckelbach, H.** (2000). How serious are common childhood fears? II. The parent's point of view. *Behaviour Research and Therapy*, **38**, 813–818.

Muris, P. & **Ollendick, T. H.** (2002). The assessment of contemporary fears in adolescents using a modified version of the Fear Survey Schedule for Children – Revised. *Journal of Anxiety Disorders*, **16**, 567–584.

Muris, P., Loxton, H., Neumann, A., DuPlessis, M., King, N. J., & Ollendick, T. H. (2006). DSM-defined anxiety disorders symptoms in South African youths: their assessment and relationship with perceived parental rearing behaviors. *Behaviour Research and Therapy*, **44**, 897–910.

Muris, P., Meesters, C., & Knoops, M. (2005). The relation between gender role orientation and fear and anxiety in non-clinic referred children. *Journal of Clinical Child and Adolescent Psychology*, **34**, 326–332.

Muris, P., Meesters, C., Merckelbach, H., Sermon, A., & Zwakhalen, S. (1998). Worry in normal children. *Journal of the American Academy of Child and Adolescent Psychiatry*, **37**, 703–710.

Muris, P., Merckelbach, H., & Collaris, R. (1997). Common childhood fears and their origins. *Behaviour Research and Therapy*, **35**, 929–937.

Muris, P., Merckelbach, H., Gadet, B., & Moulaert, V. (2000). Fears, worries, and scary dreams in 4- to 12-year-old children: their content, developmental pattern, and origins. *Journal of Clinical Child Psychology*, **29**, 43–52.

Muris, P., Merckelbach, H., de Jong, P. J., & Ollendick, T. H. (2002). The aetiology of specific fears and phobias in children: a critique of the non-associative account. *Behaviour Research and Therapy*, **40**, 185–195.

Muris, P., Merckelbach, H., Mayer, B., & Prins, E. (2000). How serious are common childhood fears? *Behaviour Research and Therapy*, **38**, 217–228.

Muris, P., Merckelbach, H., Meesters, C., & Van den Brand, K. (2002). Cognitive development and worry in normal children. *Cognitive Therapy and Research*, **26**, 775–785.

Muris, P., Merckelbach, H., Meesters, C., & Van Lier, P. (1997). What do children fear most often? *Journal of Behavior Therapy and Experimental Psychiatry*, **28**, 263–267.

Muris, P., Merckelbach, H., Ollendick, T. H., King, N. J., & Bogie, N. (2001). Children's night-time fears: parent–child ratings of frequency, content, origins, coping behaviours, and severity. *Behaviour Research and Therapy*, **39**, 13–28.

Muris, P., Merckelbach, H., Ollendick, T. H., King, N. J., Meesters, C., & Van Kessel, C. (2002). What is the Revised Fear Survey Schedule for Children measuring? *Behaviour Research and Therapy*, **40**, 1317–1326.

Muris, P., Schmidt, H., Engelbrecht, P., & Perold, M. (2002). DSM-IV defined anxiety disorder symptoms in South-African children. *Journal of the American Academy of Child and Adolescent Psychiatry*, **41**, 1360–1368.

Murray, L., Creswell, C., & Cooper, P. J. (2009). The development of anxiety disorders in childhood: an integrative review. *Psychological Medicine*, **39**, 1413–1423.

Neal, A. M., Lilly, R. S., & Zakis, S. (1993). What are African American children afraid of? A preliminary study. *Journal of Anxiety Disorders*, **7**, 129–139.

Öhman, A., Dimberg, U., & Öst, L. G. (1985). Animal and social phobias: biological constraints on learned fear responses. In: S. Reiss & R. R. Bootzin (eds.) *Theoretical Issues in Behavior Therapy*, pp. 107–133. Orlando, FL: Academic Press.

Ollendick, T. H. (1983). Reliability and validity of the Revised Fear Survey Schedule for Children (FSSC-R). *Behaviour Research and Therapy*, **21**, 685–692.

Ollendick, T. H. & King, N. J. (1994). Fears and their level of interference in adolescents. *Behaviour Research and Therapy*, **32**, 635–638.

Ollendick, T. H., King, N. J., & Frary, R. B. (1989). Fears in children and adolescents: reliability and generalizability across gender, age and nationality. *Behaviour Research and Therapy*, **27**, 19–26.

Ollendick, T. H., King, N. J., & Muris, P. (2002). Fears and phobias in children: phenomenology, epidemiology, and aetiology. *Child and Adolescent Mental Health*, **7**, 98–106.

Ollendick, T. H., Yang, B., Dong, Q., Xia, Y., & Lin, L. (1995). Perceptions of fear in other children and adolescents: the role of gender and friendship status. *Journal of Abnormal Child Psychology*, **23**, 439–452.

Ollendick, T. H., Yang, B., King, N. J., Dong, Q., & Akande, A. (1996). Fears in American, Australian, Chinese, and Nigerian children and adolescents: a cross-cultural study. *Journal of Child Psychology and Psychiatry*, **37**, 213–220.

Opolot, J. A. (1976). Normative data on the Children's Manifest Anxiety Scale in a developing country. *Psychological Reports*, **39**, 587–590.

Palapattu, A. G., Newman Kingery, J., & Ginsburg, G. S. (2006). Gender role orientation and anxiety symptoms among African American adolescents. *Journal of Abnormal Child Psychology*, **34**, 441–449.

Pina, A. A. & Silverman, W. K. (2004). Clinical phenomenology, somatic symptoms, and distress in Hispanic/Latino and European American youths with anxiety disorders. *Journal of Clinical Child and Adolescent Psychology*, **33**, 227–236.

Rapee, R. M., Schniering, C. A., & Hudson, J. L. (2009). Anxiety disorders during childhood and adolescence: origins and treatment. *Annual Review of Clinical Psychology*, **5**, 311–341.

Scherer, M. W. & Nakamura, C. Y. (1968). A fear survey schedule for children (FSS-FC): a factor analytic comparison with manifest anxiety (CMAS). *Behaviour Research and Therapy*, **6**, 173–182.

Shore, G. N. & Rapport, M. D. (1998). The Fear Survey Schedule for Children-Revised (FSSC-HI): ethnocultural variations in children's fearfulness. *Journal of Anxiety Disorders*, **12**, 437–461.

Silverman, W. K. & Ollendick, T. H. (2005). Evidence-based assessment of anxiety and its disorders in children and adolescents. *Journal of Clinical Child and Adolescent Psychology*, **34**, 380–411.

Silverman, W. K., La Greca, A. M., & Wasserstein, S. (1995). What do children worry about? Worries and their relationship to anxiety. *Child Development*, **66**, 671–686.

Thompson, R. A. (2001). Childhood anxiety disorders from the perspective of emotion regulation and attachment. In: M. W. Vasey & M. R. Dadds (eds.) *The Developmental Psychopathology of Anxiety*, pp. 160–182. New York: Oxford University Press.

Varela, R. E., Vernberg, E. M., Sanchez-Soza, J. J., Riveros, A., Mitchell, M., & Mashunkashey, J. (2004). Anxiety reporting and culturally associated interpretation biases and cognitive schemas: a comparison of Mexican, Mexican American, and European American families. *Journal of Clinical Child and Adolescent Psychology*, **33**, 237–247.

Vasey, M. W. (1993). Development and cognition in childhood anxiety: the example of worry. *Advances in Clinical Child Psychology*, **15**, 1–39.

Vasey, M. W. & Dadds, M. R. (eds.) (2001). *The Developmental Psychopathology of Anxiety*. New York: Oxford University Press.

Warren, S. L. & Sroufe, L. A. (2004). Developmental issues. In: T. H. Ollendick & J. S. March (eds.) *Phobic and Anxiety Disorders in Children and Adolescents: A Clinician's Guide to Effective Psychosocial and Pharmacological Interventions*, pp. 92–115. Oxford, UK: Oxford University Press.

Weems, C. F., Silverman, W. K., & La Greca, A. M. (2000). What do youth referred for anxiety problems worry about? Worry and its relationship to anxiety and anxiety disorders in children and adolescents. *Journal of Abnormal Child Psychology*, **28**, 63–72.

Weems, C. F., Silverman, W. K., Saavedra, L. M., Pina, A. A., & Lumpkin, P. W. (1999). The discrimination of children's phobias using the Revised Fear Survey Schedule for Children. *Journal of Child Psychology and Psychiatry*, **40**, 941–952.

Weems, C. F., Zakem, A. H., Costa, N. M., Cannon, M. F., & Watts, S. E. (2005). Physiological response and childhood anxiety: association with symptoms of anxiety disorders and cognitive bias. *Journal of Clinical Child and Adolescent Psychology*, **34**, 712–723.

Weisz, J. R., Sigman, M., Weiss, B., & Mosk, J. (1993). Parent reports of behavioral and emotional problems among children in Kenya, Thailand, and the United States. *Child Development*, **64**, 98–109.

Westenberg, P. M., Drewes, M. J., Goedhart, A. W., Siebelink, B. M., & Treffers, P. D. A. (2004). A developmental analysis of self-reported fears in late childhood through mid-adolescence: social-evaluative fears on the rise? *Journal of Child Psychology and Psychiatry*, **45**, 481–495.

5

Social anxiety disorder: a normal fear gone awry?

Caroline L. Bokhorst and P. Michiel Westenberg

Introduction

As described by Muris and Field in Chapter 4, the age-related developmental trend in non-clinical fears mirrors that of the age of onset of clinical fears and therefore, the various phobias may have their origin in these "normal" fears. For example, the early onset and high prevalence of specific phobia in childhood is mirrored by the waxing and waning of similar fears in children and adolescents from community samples: fears of animals, the dark, and fantasized objects occur most frequently in children under 10 years of age, and fears of natural phenomena and other concrete situations (e.g., transportation devices) are reported most frequently in late childhood and early adolescence (see Gullone, 2000; Wenar, 1994). Given the substantive and developmental parallels between normal and deviant anxiety it has been suggested that an anxiety disorder is a normal fear development gone awry (see Muris & Field, Chapter 4 this volume; Westenberg, Siebelink, & Treffers, 2001).

Social anxiety may however be the exception to this rule. Contrary to the well-established link between specific phobia and childhood fears of animals, accidents, and natural disasters there is little evidence to support the link between social anxiety disorder and non-clinical social anxiety or social fears.[1] On the one hand, a clear developmental trend has been observed for social anxiety disorder: it is relatively rare in children under 10 years of age, its prevalence increases sharply during middle to late adolescence, and retrospective studies with socially phobic adults indicate an average age of onset in the mid-teenage years (Kashdan & Herbert, 2001; Lecrubier, Wittchen, Faravelli, Bobes, Patel, & Knapp, 2000; Ollendick, King, & Yule, 1994; Öst, 1987; Strauss, & Last, 1993; Westenberg, Siebelink, Warmerhoven, & Treffers, 1999). Several authors concluded that these age differences for social anxiety disorder would be connected to age differences for non-clinical social fear (Kashdan & Herbert, 2001; Ollendick & Hirshfeld-Becker, 2002). However, only piecemeal evidence has been provided for the idea that non-clinical social fear increases during adolescence. Most research with the Fear Survey Schedule for Children (FSSC) shows that the level of social fear is stable or even declines between late childhood and adolescence (e.g., Gullone & Lane, 2002; Muris & Ollendick, 2002; see Gullone, 2000, for a review). Likewise, research using other measures of social anxiety failed to demonstrate an increase of social

---

[1] In this chapter, social anxiety disorder refers to clinical levels of social anxiety, whereas the terms social anxiety and social fears are used to refer to non-clinical or normal levels of fear.

Anxiety Disorders in Children and Adolescents, 2nd edn, ed. W. K. Silverman and A. P. Field. Published by Cambridge University Press. © Cambridge University Press 2011.

anxiety during adolescence: the level of social anxiety either was stable or decreased with age (Garcia-Lopez, Olivares, Hidalgo, Beidel, & Turner, 2001; Gullone, King, & Ollendick, 2001; Hale, Meeus, Raaijmakers, Van Hoof, & Muris, 2008; Inderbitzen-Nolan & Walters, 2000).

In their literature review on the etiology of social anxiety disorder, Rapee and Spence (2004, p. 741) thus concluded that it is mere "folklore" to believe that the teenage-bound increase of social anxiety disorder is related to a normative intensification of social fearfulness during adolescence. In the present chapter we instead argue that the failure to detect developmental trends in non-clinical social fear may be due to a number of theoretical and methodological issues. To observe developmental trends in non-clinical social fear it may be crucial: (a) to study developmental maturity in addition to age, (b) to distinguish among social fear subtypes, (c) to study the level of avoidance in addition to level of distress, and (d) to investigate relative levels of social anxiety in addition to absolute levels. We also argue that in making the connection between clinical and non-clinical forms of social anxiety it is important to distinguish among social anxiety subtypes.

How to observe normal developmental trends?

Development versus age

Warren and Sroufe (2004) argue that it is important to take the developmental level of an individual into account, regardless of their chronological age, when evaluating children for anxiety disorders. To use the developmental level of an individual successfully for clinical purposes, knowledge about the relation between different factors and social anxiety is a prerequisite. Most research on the development of social anxiety is restricted to age differences and is not directly aimed at developmental level. Age, however, is an "empty," non-explanatory construct (Kazdin, 1989). Age alone does not provide us with explanations as to why a specific fear would be more salient at a particular age period. Furthermore, age is only a rough estimate of the developmental stage of an individual; the relation between age and development is far from perfect (e.g., Galambos, Barker, & Tilton-Weaver, 2003). Individuals differ in the pace of development and hence developmental variability is present *within* each age cohort and this might obscure developmental differences *between* age cohorts. The problem of differential development seems particularly relevant for the adolescent period, given individual differences in the timing and speed of physical and psychological maturation. To detect a developmental trend for social anxiety, it may therefore be important to focus on developmental level, rather than age.

Investigators have suggested that several maturational factors contribute to an increase in social anxiety, such as pubertal, cognitive, and psychosocial development.

Pubertal development

It has been suggested that the dramatic bodily changes during puberty yield a heightened awareness of oneself in social interactions and transient fears of negative social evaluation (Buss, 1980). Deardorff, Hayward, Wilson, Bryson, Hammer, and Agras (2007) is the only study to investigate directly the relation between puberty and self-reported social anxiety. In a non-clinical sample of 106 children, ages 9.5 to 11 years, pubertal development was measured by child self-reported Tanner staging. Children's social anxiety was assessed using the Social Anxiety subscale of the Multidimensional Anxiety Scale for Children (MASC: March, Parker, Sullivan, Stallings, & Conners, 1997). Three developmental groups were created: (1) a group of children who were pre-pubertal at ages 9.5 and 11, (2) a transition group of children who were pre-pubertal at age 9.5, but pubertal at age 11, and (3) a group of children who were pubertal at ages 9.5 and 11; because the ages were equal in each developmental group, the effect of puberty could be studied regardless of age. A main effect for developmental group emerged for girls only. The more developed girls reported higher levels of social anxiety at age 11. The analyses were also conducted with other subscales of the MASC (Harm Avoidance, Physical Symptoms, and Separation/Panic) as dependent variables. No significant effects were found for the other subscales, indicating that pubertal development was specifically related to social anxiety, at least for girls.

Recently, it has been proposed that puberty-related changes in the brain might create greater stress sensitivity and consequently a greater vulnerability to negative social evaluation (Dahl, 2004; Dahl & Gunnar, 2009; Nelson, Leibenluft, McClure, & Pine, 2005; Spear, 2009). The connection between puberty and biological reactivity to a social-evaluative task was evaluated in two studies. Gunnar, Wewerka, Frenn, Long, and Griggs (2009) used the child version of the Trier Social Stress Task (TSST-C: Buske-Kirschbaum *et al.*, 1997) in a non-referred sample of 9–15-year-olds ($n = 82$). The TSST-C is known to stimulate the HPA-axis reactivity leading to increases in cortisol levels. Increases in cortisol levels are indicative of social stress rather than general stress (Dickerson & Kemeny, 2004). The TSST-C involves an impromptu speech followed by an arithmetic task in front of an unfamiliar adult audience. Pubertal development was assessed with the Pubertal Development Scale (Peterson, Crockett, Richards, & Boxer, 1988). Gunnar *et al.* (2009) found evidence for a significant positive relation between puberty and biological reactivity. The correlation between puberty and cortisol reactivity *within* the cohort of 13-year-olds was close to statistical significance. This finding indicates a positive relation between pubertal maturity and cortisol reactivity regardless of age. It should however be noted that gender differences were present in this particular age group with girls demonstrating a stronger cortisol response. The girls were also more advanced in puberty. Therefore, gender and puberty effects might be confounded in this study.

The second study investigated the relation between age, pubertal development, and stress reactivity in 295 non-referred 9–17-year-olds (Sumter, Bokhorst, Miers, Van Pelt, & Westenberg, 2010). Pubertal development was measured with the Pubertal Development Scale (Peterson *et al.*, 1988). Stress reactivity was measured by cortisol and alpha-amylase (AA) during the Leiden Public Speaking Task (Leiden-PST: Westenberg *et al.*, 2009). Cortisol can be seen as a measure for prolonged stress, whereas AA is a measure of the acute stress response (Granger, Kivlighan, Sheikh, Gordis, & Stroud, 2008; Nicolson, 2008). In the Leiden-PST, participants give a prepared speech in front of a prerecorded neutral audience of eight age peers and a teacher. Four puberty groups were created, that is, pre-pubertal ($n = 46$), beginning-pubertal ($n = 50$), mid-pubertal ($n = 76$), and advanced/post-pubertal ($n = 112$). Participants at the advanced/post-pubertal stage had higher cortisol levels *before* the task than the three least-developed groups, suggesting that more mature participants were more stressed by the upcoming task before it took place. For AA levels a linear upward trend was observed during the task with stronger reactivity for the more mature participants, indicating that the stress system of the more mature group is more reactive during a social-evaluative situation. Similar findings were obtained if age groups were used as the independent variable.

In sum, these studies provide preliminary evidence for the connection between puberty and social fear. However, age and gender are highly correlated with puberty and thus it remains difficult to disentangle the unique contribution of puberty. Another caveat concerns the usage of subjective measures of pubertal development. Different effects may be obtained with more objective assessments.

Cognitive development

Elkind and Bowen (1979) argue that the advent of abstract thinking leads to a period of "adolescent egocentrism," characterized by the belief that one is the continual object of everyone's attention. Gullone and King (1997) speculate that this belief may be responsible for the presumed increase of social-evaluative anxiety during adolescence. To date, only one study investigated the relationship empirically. Rosso, Young, Femia, and Yurgelun-Todd (2004) provide preliminary evidence on a small sample size for a link between cognitive development and social anxiety. In their study on 20 non-referred children and adolescents, aged 9 to 18 years, abstract reasoning ability was measured with a subtest of the Wechsler Adult Intelligence Scale, Version-III, i.e., Matrix Reasoning. The level of social anxiety was assessed with the MASC. The results demonstrated a positive signifi-cant relation between abstract reasoning and social anxiety. This relationship was hardly affected if age was controlled for. Therefore, the authors conclude that "the maturation of abstract reasoning may be an enabling factor in the increased vulnerability to social anxiety disorder during adolescence" (p. 361). The findings of this study should be inter-preted with caution, given the small sample and specific operationalization of cognitive development.

Psychosocial development

Kashdan and Herbert (2001) note that "adolescence is widely agreed to be a critical develop-mental stage of identity formation and social skill development, in which concerns about peer acceptance and body image become paramount" (p. 39). Westenberg *et al.* (2001) selected Loevinger's (1976, 1993) model of ego development to conceptualize the possible link between social fears and psychosocial maturation. The proposed model was tested in a study of 882 non-referred children and adolescents (aged 8 to 18 years: Westenberg, Drewes, Goedhart, Siebelink, & Treffers, 2004). The findings indicated a positive significant correlation between psychosocial maturation and social anxiety (with gender and verbal ability controlled for). The connection between ego level and social anxiety remained after age had been controlled for. This means that relatively mature teenagers (be they age 12, 15, or 18) were more likely to express fears about social evaluation than their less mature age peers.

Overall, these studies provide preliminary support for the contribution of maturational factors in the development of social fearfulness in non-referred youth. However, a number of limitations should be noted. First, despite the long history of speculations regarding the developmental underpinnings of social anxiety in youth, we found only five studies that investigated these suggestions empirically. Second, small samples were employed in three of these studies and four studies were cross-sectional rather than longitudinal. Finally, to dissect development from age, it is imperative to recruit samples containing sufficient developmental variation within age groups.

Social fear factors

Research on clinical forms of social anxiety refers to different subtypes: a generalized subtype is differentiated from a non-generalized, specific subtype (e.g., fear of public speaking; see Blöte, Kint, Miers, & Westenberg, 2009). A clear developmental trend may be present for non-clinical forms of specific social anxiety and might not be present for generalized social anxiety, or vice versa.

Most research on the normal development of social fear makes use of one global social fear factor, for example the Fear of Failure and Criticism factor in the Fear Survey Schedule or the Social Phobia subscale in the Screen for Child Anxiety Related Emotional Disorders (SCARED). These global factors can be viewed as the non-clinical representation of generalized social anxiety. As was mentioned earlier, studies using these global measures of social fear do not report clear and consistent age differences. Most studies report no effect of age and a few studies unexpectedly observed an age-related decrease of social anxiety.

In contrast, research on specific types of social fear has revealed differential age patterns that are consistent with the hypothesis that fear of negative evaluation increases during adolescence. Westenberg *et al.* (2004) analyzed young people's responses to the Failure and Criticism scale of the Fear Survey Schedule for Children – Revised (FSSC-R) using a factor analysis which separated out the various types of social fears: fear of social evaluation, fear of achievement evaluation, and fear of punishment. Their study of 882 non-referred children and adolescents (aged 8 to 18 years) confirmed that social fearfulness as assessed by the one Failure and Criticism scale does not increase with age, and revealed that subsets of items included in this scale display opposite age patterns. Fear of punishment (e.g., being sent to the principal) decreased between middle childhood and early adolescence, whereas fears associated with social evaluation and achievement (e.g., giving an oral report or being criticized) increased between early and mid adolescence. This differential age pattern was replicated in a cross-sectional sample of 910 7–18-year-olds (Westenberg, Gullone, Bokhorst, Heyne, & King, 2007).

Research findings indicate that the increase with age is strongest for fear of situations in which the evaluative component is most explicit, such as public speaking. Sumter, Bokhorst, and Westenberg (2009) investigated age-related differences in distress for various social situations. A group of 260 non-referred 9–17-year-old adolescents was presented with 20 situations taken from the Anxiety Disorder Interview Schedule for Children (ADIS-C: Silverman & Albano, 1996) and were asked whether they would feel distressed in each situation. Analyses yielded no significant age differences for general distress in social situations. However, analyses on different social domains revealed diverging patterns: whereas no age differences were found for situations of "informal speaking and interaction" and only weak differences for "observation by others," distress in "formal speaking and interaction" situations clearly increased with age.

One study compared the age patterns for public-speaking anxiety specifically and social anxiety more generally (C. L. Bokhorst *et al.*, unpublished data). A large sample of 1031 adolescents aged 9 to 18 years completed the Social Anxiety Scale for Adolescents (La Greca & Lopez, 1998) and the adjusted version of the Personal Rating of Public Speaking Anxiety (McCroskey, 1970). Divergent age differences emerged: general social anxiety was unrelated to age, but public-speaking anxiety was positively related to age.

The importance to differentiate across different sources of social anxiety is supported by results from factor-analytic and cluster-analytic studies. The aforementioned study of 882 non-referred children and adolescents (aged 8 to 18 years: Westenberg *et al.*, 2004) demonstrated the existence of three clusters of fears within the Fear of Failure and Criticism factor: (1) social evaluation fears, (2) achievement evaluation fears, and (3) punishment fears. In a study of social fears in 3803 non-referred children and adolescents aged 6 to

18 years confirmatory factor analysis was used to test which factor solution (one general Failure and Criticism subscale or three separate clusters of social fears) provided the best fit across several age groups (Bokhorst, Westenberg, Oosterlaan, & Heyne, 2008). Results showed that one global social fear scale was sufficient to describe the data in children aged 6–9 years, and that from the age of 10 years onwards the social fears became more differentiated. In the adolescent period, the three separate clusters of social fears were necessary for a sufficient fit.

In sum, these studies demonstrate the importance of distinguishing among different aspects of social anxiety when investigating normal developmental patterns, particularly during the adolescent period. It appears that adolescents become more sensitive to explicitly evaluative situations whereas fear of other social situations is less affected by age.

Level of avoidance versus distress

For a diagnosis of social anxiety disorder not only the level of social anxiety is important, but also the level of interference in daily life. Only if the anxiety is accompanied by substantial interference a diagnosis is given. Although the level of social anxiety and the amount of interference are expected to be highly correlated, it is possible that both aspects follow different developmental patterns. Rapee and Spence (2004) argue that "the apparent onset of social phobia [social anxiety disorder] in early adolescence may perhaps have more to do with the increases in life interference caused by social anxiety at this developmental stage than with increases in actual levels of social distress" (p. 741). Social anxiety might become increasingly impairing during social interactions with age peers. Whereas in childhood particular levels of social anxiety are not yet a hindrance, the same levels of social anxiety can become a problem due to the changing challenges of the adolescent period and may lead to avoidance of social situations.

Some evidence for this idea is provided by two recent studies, in which both the level of distress and the level of avoidance were measured. Rao, Beidel, Turner, Ammerman, Crosby, and Sallee (2007) investigated the level of distress and avoidance for several social situations in a sample of children and adolescents diagnosed with social anxiety disorder. The results showed that the level of avoidance of social situations increased from childhood to adolescence. However, the level of distress increased as well. It should be noted that they studied a clinical sample where the level of distress and avoidance might be more severe (and more strongly related) than in community samples.

Sumter *et al.* (2009) investigated distress and avoidance towards 20 social situations (see above) in 260 non-referred 9–17-year-old adolescents. Results showed that no significant age differences were present for general level of distress, whereas the level of avoidance had a positive significant relation to age.

In sum, the level of avoidance increased more than the level of distress in a non-referred adolescent sample. Hence, these results emphasize the importance in distinguishing between distress and avoidance of social situations. It should however be noted that the level of avoidance, as measured in the two described studies, may not capture the whole construct of interferences in daily life. More research assessing the broader construct of life interference is necessary.

Relative levels versus absolute levels of social anxiety

Most research on the developmental underpinnings of social fear is based on the comparison of average fear scores across age cohorts. Weems and Costa (2005) argue that the developmental trend for general fear level needs to be taken into account. General fear-fulness – thus not restricted to social anxiety – has been studied extensively and it is a consistent finding that it steadily declines between late childhood and middle adolescence (Gullone, 2000; Gullone *et al.*, 2001, Westenberg *et al.*, 2004, 2007). Weems and Costa (2005) pointed out that the developmental course of social anxiety should be viewed in light of this overall decrease. Social anxiety levels, in absolute terms, might remain stable but become more salient in comparison to general fears. This differential expression of fears is important for clinical practice as it shows which fears are most prominent during a specific period of time.

Two studies indicate that relative social fear scores (i.e., relative to general fear score) consistently increase with age. Weems and Costa (2005) investigated age differences in the expression of fears and anxiety in a sample of 145 non-referred children and adolescents aged 6 to 17 years. They assessed fears with the FSSC-R and anxiety with the Revised Child Anxiety and Depression Scales (RCADS). To test the differential expression of specific fears, mixed-design repeated-measures ANCOVAs were carried out, with age and sex as between-subject variables and the specific fears as within-subject variables. Total fear was used as the covariate and was thus controlled to account for differences in general fearfulness. The results demonstrated that fear of failure and criticism and characteristics of social anxiety became more salient from childhood to adolescence. In the ages 14 to 17 years, social fears became most predominant, relative to total fear. Westenberg *et al.* (2007) replicated these findings in a cross-sectional sample of 7–18-year-olds ($n = 910$) as well as in the longitudinal analyses on a subsample ($n = 261$): social fears increased with age when total fear scores were taken into account.

In sum, these studies demonstrate the importance of taking general fear level into account when looking for developmental patterns in social fearfulness.

Conclusion

Overall, the reviewed studies indicate that fear and avoidance of social situations, particu-larly social-*evaluative* situations, is part and parcel of normal adolescent development. At the same time, the findings should be interpreted with some caution.

First, most studies were cross-sectional whereas longitudinal designs are needed to confirm the developmental nature of social fearfulness. Longitudinal designs are required to investigate the developmental pattern itself (e.g., by estimation of growth curves) and to fully understand the relationship with pubertal, cognitive, and psychosocial development.

Second, most research appears to be based on the assumption of measurement invariance across different age cohorts, that is, measures are assumed to have equivalent meaning for participants from different age cohorts. However, measurement equivalence has not always been well tested for the social anxiety instruments that were used in the reviewed studies. We need to establish measurement invariance across age in order to properly interpret age differences, or similarities, in social anxiety scores.

Third, an important issue in research regarding age and social anxiety is the manner in which age is treated statistically in each study. Although age is a continuous variable, it is almost never treated that way in empirical studies. In contrast, most researchers have divided their sample into different age groups and have compared these groups on the dependent variables of interest. According to MacCallum, Zhang, Preacher, and Rucker (2002), however, splitting a continuous variable into groups (e.g., by dichotomizing it on the basis of the median) is rarely justified from a conceptual or statistical perspective. In their paper, they illustrate the negative consequences of dichotomization of individual differences measures by comparing the results of analyses based on the original continuous scores and after dichotomization. The comparison of both procedures shows that dichotomization generally leads to the loss of information, the loss of effect size, and the loss of statistical significance. Furthermore, it increases the risk of overlooking non-linear effects. The authors state that these problems "can be easily avoided by application of standard methods of regression and correlational analysis to original (undichotomized) measures" (MacCallum *et al.*, 2002, p. 38). Up to now, most studies on the developmental pattern of social anxiety have relied on the comparison of age groups. For future research, it is recommended to treat age as a continuous variable to avoid the abovementioned problems.

Social anxiety disorder: a normal fear gone awry

The reviewed findings suggest that normal adolescent development plays a role in the development of social anxiety disorder. Investigations into the "how" and "why" normal development escalates into a social anxiety disorder have not yet been carried out. Theoretical models regarding the etiology of social anxiety disorder do not include normal adolescent development as a key factor. In Rapee and Spence's model (2004), for example, several factors are mentioned, including intrapersonal ones (genetics, temperament, cognitive factors, and social skill deficits) and interpersonal or environmental ones (parent–child interaction, aversive social experiences, and negative life events). These factors all describe individual differences, whereas no attention is paid to the contribution of normal development. Furthermore, etiological models generally do not distinguish explicitly between different types of social anxiety disorder, but describe social anxiety subtypes as lying on a continuum of severity of social anxiety (e.g., Rapee & Spence, 2004; see also Kimbrel, 2008). However, the present review lends additional support for the idea that social anxiety subtypes are qualitatively different and may therefore require a different explanatory model (Blöte *et al.*, 2009; Kimbrel, 2008).

As was mentioned earlier, two types of social anxiety disorder are described in the DSM-IV-TR: (a) the generalized type in which individuals are "anxious in virtually any situation that involves social interaction," and (b) the non-generalized or "circumscribed type of social phobia in which the focus of worry is on the embarrassment that might arise when performing a particular activity in public". The latter type is also referred to as "performance anxiety" (First, Frances, & Pincus, 2004, p. 240). Non-generalized social anxiety disorder occurs particularly in situations where one might be observed or scrutinized by others and therefore fear of social evaluation plays a central role in this subtype. Generalized social anxiety disorder is more related to interpersonal interactions (i.e., interaction anxiety), although the majority of individuals with generalized social anxiety disorder also fears performance situations, such as public speaking (see Summerfeldt, Kloosterman, Antony, & Parker, 2006).

Research has shown that generalized and non-generalized social anxiety disorder follow distinct developmental pathways (see for an overview Wittchen & Fehm, 2003). Whereas the generalized form often is already present by late childhood, the onset of non-generalized social anxiety disorder seems to be more adolescent bound. The findings of the current review on non-clinical forms of social anxiety reveal the same age pattern: general social anxiety is fairly stable between late childhood and adolescence, whereas social-evaluation fear more specifically increases in prominence during adolescence.

The distinct developmental course for non-clinical social anxiety and the specific social-evaluative fear factor is mirrored by findings concerning the heritability and continuity of both types of social anxiety disorder. Findings from family and twin studies indicate a heritable component for social anxiety (disorder) (see for an overview Stein & Chavira, 1998), but the estimates differ according to anxiety subtype. Mannuzza, Schneier, Chapman, Liebowitz, Klein, and Fyer (1995) found that generalized social anxiety disorder is familial, whereas non-generalized social anxiety disorder is not familial. Furthermore, generalized social anxiety disorder appears related to (innate) temperamental factors, such as shyness and behavioral inhibition, whereas non-generalized social anxiety disorder is less related to these factors (Chavira, Stein, & Malcarne, 2002; Hofmann, Heinrichs, & Moscovitch, 2004; Stemberger, Turner, Beidel, & Calhoun, 1995).

The heritability differences are reflected in differences for the continuity of both subtypes. A higher level of continuity between childhood and adolescence is observed for generalized social anxiety than for social-evaluative anxiety more specifically. Studies on generalized social anxiety (disorder) report a moderate to high level of continuity between early childhood and adolescence (see Rapee & Spence, 2004). In contrast, lower continuity has been observed for social-evaluation fear more specifically; this fear does not seem to stabilize until mid or late adolescence. In their longitudinal study of social-evaluation fear in a non-referred sample, Westenberg *et al.* (2007) demonstrated that continuity of individual differences increases with age: no continuity was observed for the youngest age group (7–8-year-olds at Time 1), low continuity for the 9–12-year-olds (across time $r = 0.33$), and moderate continuity for the 13–16-year-olds ($r = 0.53$). The study also showed that the continuity of the highest levels of social evaluation fear was very low. These results suggest that levels of social evaluation fear can easily change in childhood and that individual differences are not stabilized until mid to late adolescence.

Hence, it seems plausible that a vulnerability to develop generalized social anxiety disorder is already present in infancy or early childhood, whereas a vulnerability to develop non-generalized social anxiety disorder emerges during adolescence. In the absence of empirical research we may speculate about the role of normal development in the etiology of clinical forms of social anxiety. Normal development may interact differently with environmental factors in the etiology of both anxiety disorder subtypes. It is plausible that the parent–child relationship during (early) childhood plays a key role in the emergence of generalized social anxiety, whereas peer relations may play a key role in the emergence of the non-generalized type. Early experiences with parents (e.g., insecure attachment, overprotection) in combination with specific characteristics of the child (e.g., shy or inhibited temperament) might contribute to generalized social anxiety disorder. In contrast, the advent of non-generalized social anxiety disorder during adolescence might be more influenced by adverse interactions with peers. In the adolescent period peer relations become increasingly important, and it is conceivable that the normal increase in social evaluation anxiety makes adolescents specifically sensitive to negative evaluation by peers. If an adolescent is sensitive to social evaluation, negative feedback from peers could tip the balance, particularly if other risk factors are present (e.g., shyness). At the same time, positive peer evaluation and low levels of peer exclusion may decrease the risk of a social anxiety disorder (see Oh, Rubin, Bowker, Booth-LaForce, Rose-Krasnor, & Laursen, 2008, for a related study on social withdrawal).

Overall conclusion

The present review suggests that maturational factors are related to non-clinical forms of social anxiety which play a key role in the etiology of social anxiety disorder. Research directly looking into this relationship is lacking. Longitudinal studies are needed to investigate the complex and reciprocal relations between normal development and the various risk factors in the etiology of social anxiety disorder. To investigate the specific contribution of normal development future research should incorporate various maturational factors (pubertal, cognitive, and psychosocial), in addition to individual and interpersonal factors. Only by studying these constructs together, it is possible to understand better the interplay between maturational factors and individual differences in the emergence of generalized and non-generalized social anxiety disorders.

References

Blöte, A. W., Kint, M. J. W., Miers, A. C., & Westenberg, P. M. (2009). The relation between public speaking anxiety and social anxiety: a review. *Journal of Anxiety Disorders*, **23**, 305–313.

Bokhorst, C. L., Westenberg, P. M., Oosterlaan, J., & Heyne, D. A. (2008). The changing structure of social fears during childhood and adolescence: from 5 to 7 factors in the Fear Survey Schedule for Children-Revised. *Journal of Anxiety Disorders*, **22**, 135–142.

Buske-Kirschbaum, A., Jobst, S., Psych, D., Wustmans, A., Kirschbaum, C., Rauh, W., *et al.* (1997). Attenuated free cortisol response to psychosocial stress in children with atopic dermatitis. *Psychosomatic Medicine*, **59**, 419–426.

Buss, A. H. (1980). *Self-Consciousness and Social Anxiety*. San Francisco, CA: W.H. Freeman.

Chavira, D. A., Stein, M. B., & Malcarne, V. L. (2002). Scrutinizing the relationship between shyness and social phobia. *Journal of Anxiety Disorders*, **16**, 585–598.

Dahl, R. E. (2004). Adolescent brain development: a period of vulnerabilities and opportunities. *Annals of the New York Academy of Sciences*, **1021**, 1–22.

Dahl, R. E. & Gunnar, M. R. (2009). Heightened stress responsiveness and emotional reactivity during pubertal maturation: implications for psychopathology. *Development and Psychopathology*, **21**, 1–6.

Deardorff, J., Hayward, C., Wilson, K. A., Bryson, S., Hammer, L. D., & Agras, S. (2007). Puberty and gender interact to predict social anxiety symptoms in early adolescence. *Journal of Adolescent Health*, **41**, 102–104.

Dickerson, S. S. & Kemeny, M. E. (2004). Acute stressors and cortisol responses: a theoretical integration and synthesis of laboratory research. *Psychological Bulletin*, **130**, 355–391.

Elkind, D. & Bowen, R. (1979). Imaginary audience behavior in children and adolescents. *Developmental Psychology*, **15**, 33–44.

First, M. B., Frances, A., & Pincus, H. A. (2004). *DSM-IV-TR Guidebook: The Essential Companion to the Diagnostic and Statistical Manual of Mental Disorders*, 4th edn, text revision. Washington, DC: American Psychiatric Association.

Galambos, N. L., Barker, E. T., & Tilton-Weaver, L. C. (2003). Who gets caught at maturity gap? A study of pseudomature, immature, and mature adolescents. *International Journal of Behavioral Development*, **27**, 253–263.

Garcia-Lopez, L. J., Olivares, J., Hidalgo, M. D., Beidel, D. C., & Turner, S. M. (2001). Psychometric properties of the Social Phobia and Anxiety Inventory, the Social Anxiety Scale for Adolescents, the Fear of Negative Evaluation Scale, and the Social Avoidance and Distress Scale in an adolescent Spanish-Speaking sample. *Journal of Psychopathology and Behavioral Assessment*, **23**, 51–59.

Granger, D. A., Kivlighan, K. T., El-Sheikh, M., Gordis, E. B., & Stroud, L. R. (2008). Measurement of cortisol. In: **L. J. Luecken** & **L. C. Gallo** (eds.) *Handbook of Physiological Research Methods in Health Psychology*, pp. 37–74. Los Angeles, CA: Sage.

Gullone, E. (2000). The development of normal fear: a century of research. *Clinical Psychology Review*, **20**, 429–451.

Gullone, E. & King, N. J. (1997). Three-year follow-up of normal fear in children and adolescents aged 7 to 18 years. *British Journal of Developmental Psychology*, **15**, 97–111.

Gullone, E. & Lane, B. (2002). The Fear Survey Schedule for Children. II. A validity examination across response format and instruction type. *Clinical Psychology and Psychotherapy*, **9**, 55–67.

Gullone, E., King, N. J., & Ollendick, T. H. (2001). Self-reported anxiety in children and adolescents: a three-year follow-up study. *Journal of Genetic Psychology*, **162**, 5–19.

Gunnar, M. R., Wewerka, S., Frenn, K., Long, J. D., & Griggs, C. (2009). Developmental changes in hypothalamus–pituitary–adrenal activity over the transition to adolescence: normative changes and associations with puberty. *Development and Psychopathology*, **21**, 69–85.

Hale, W., Meeus, W., Raaijmakers, Q., Van Hoof, A., & Muris, P. (2008). Developmental trajectories of adolescent anxiety disorder symptoms: a five-year prospective community study. *Journal of the American Academy of Child and Adolescent Psychiatry*, **47**, 556–564.

Hofmann, S. G., Heinrichs, N., & Moscovitch, D. A. (2004). The nature and expression of social phobia: toward a new classification. *Clinical Psychology Review*, **24**, 769–797.

Inderbitzen-Nolan, H. M. & Walters, K. S. (2000). Social Anxiety Scale for Adolescents: normative data and further evidence of construct validity. *Journal of Clinical Child Psychology*, **29**, 360–371.

Kashdan, T. B. & Herbert, J. D. (2001). Social anxiety disorder in childhood and adolescence: current status and future directions. *Clinical Child and Family Psychology Review*, **4**, 37–61.

Kazdin, A. E. (1989). Developmental psychopathology: current research, issues, and directions. *American Psychologist*, **44**, 180–187.

Kimbrel, N. A. (2008). A model of the development and maintenance of generalized social phobia. *Clinical Psychology Review*, **28**, 592–612.

La Greca, A. M. & Lopez, N. (1998). Social anxiety among adolescents: linkages with peer relations and friendships. *Journal of Abnormal Child Psychology*, **26**, 83–94.

Lecrubier, Y., Wittchen, H. U., Faravelli, C., Bobes, J., Patel, A., & Knapp, M. (2000). A European perspective on social anxiety disorder. *European Psychiatry*, **15**, 5–16.

Loevinger, J. (1976). *Ego Development: Conceptions and Theories*. San Francisco, CA: Jossey-Bass.

Loevinger, J. (1993). Measurement of personality: true or false. *Psychological Inquiry*, **4**, 1–16.

MacCallum, R. C., Zhang, S., Preacher, K. J., & Rucker, D. D. (2002). On the practice of dichotomization of quantitative variables. *Psychological Methods*, **7**, 19–40.

Mannuzza, S., Schneier, F. R., Chapman, T. F., Liebowitz, M. R., Klein, D. F., & Fyer, A. J. (1995). Reliability and validity. *Archives of General Psychiatry*, **52**, 230–237.

March, J. S., Parker, J. D., Sullivan, K., Stallings, P., & Conners, C. K. (1997). The Multidimensional Anxiety Scale for Children (MASC): factor structure, reliability, and validity. *Journal of the American Academy of Child and Adolescent Psychiatry*, **36**, 554–565.

McCroskey, J. C. (1970). Measures of communication-bound anxiety. *Speech Monographs*, **37**, 269–277.

Muris, P. & Ollendick, T. H. (2002). The assessment of contemporary fears in adolescents using a modified version of the Fear Survey Schedule for Children – Revised. *Journal of Anxiety Disorders*, **16**, 567–584.

Nelson, E. E., Leibenluft, E., McClure, E., & Pine, D. S. (2005). The social re-orientation of adolescence: a neuroscience perspective on the process and its relation to psychopathology. *Psychological Medicine*, **35**, 163–174.

Nicolson, N. A. (2008). Measurement of cortisol. In: **L. J. Luecken** & **L. C. Gallo** (eds.) *Handbook of Physiological Research Methods in Health Psychology*, pp. 37–74. Los Angeles, CA: Sage.

Oh, W., Rubin, K. H., Bowker, J. C., Booth-LaForce, C., Rose-Krasnor, L., & **Laursen, B.** (2008). Trajectories of social withdrawal from middle childhood to early adolescence. *Journal of Abnormal Child Psychology*, **36**, 553–566.

Ollendick, T. H. & **Hirshfeld-Becker, D. R.** (2002). The developmental psychopathology of social anxiety disorder. *Biological Psychiatry*, **51**, 44–58.

Ollendick, T. H., King, N. J., & **Yule, W.** (1994). *International Handbook of Phobic and Anxiety Disorders in Children and Adolescents*. New York: Plenum Press.

Öst, L. G. (1987). Age of onset in different phobias. *Journal of Abnormal Psychology*, **96**, 223–229.

Peterson, A. C., Crockett, L., Richards, M., & **Boxer, A.** (1988). A self-report measure of pubertal status: reliability, validity, and initial norms. *Journal of Youth and Adolescence*, **17**, 117–133.

Rao, P. R., Beidel, D. C., Turner, S. M., Ammerman, R. T., Crosby, L. E., & **Sallee, F. R.** (2007). Social anxiety disorder in childhood and adolescence: descriptive psychopathology: *Behaviour Research and Therapy*, **45**, 1181–1191.

Rapee, R. M. & **Spence, S. H.** (2004). The etiology of social phobia: empirical evidence and an initial model. *Clinical Psychology Review*, **24**, 737–767.

Rosso, I. M., Young, A. D., Femia, L. A., & **Yurgelun-Todd, D. A.** (2004). Cognitive and emotional components of frontal lobe functioning in childhood and adolescence. *Annals of the New York Academy of Sciences*, **1021**, 355–362.

Silverman, W. K. & **Albano, A. M.** (1996). *Anxiety Disorders Interview Schedule for DSM-IV – Child Version*. San Antonio, TX: Graywind.

Spear, L. P. (2009). Heightened stress responsivity and emotional reactivity during pubertal maturation: implications for psychopathology. *Development and Psychopathology*, **21**, 87–97.

Stein, M. B. & **Chavira, D. A.** (1998). Subtypes of social phobia and comorbidity with depression and other anxiety disorders. *Journal of Affective Disorders*, **50**, S11–S16.

Stemberger, R. T., Turner, S. M., Beidel, D. C., & **Calhoun, K. S.** (1995). Social phobia: an analysis of possible developmental factors. *Journal of Abnormal Psychology*, **104**, 526–531.

Strauss, C. C. & **Last, C. G.** (1993). Social and simple phobias in children. *Journal of Anxiety Disorders*, **7**, 141–152.

Summerfeldt, L. J., Kloosterman, P. H., Antony, M. M., & **Parker, J. D. A.** (2006). Social anxiety, emotional intelligence, and interpersonal adjustment. *Journal of Psychopathology and Behavioral Assessment*, **28**, 57–68.

Sumter, S. R., Bokhorst, C. L., Miers, A. C., Van Pelt, J., & **Westenberg, P. M.** (2010). Age and puberty differences in stress responses during a public speaking task: Do adolescents grow more sensitive to social evaluation? *Psychoneuroendocrinology*, **35**, 1510–1516. doi: 10.1016/j.psyneuen.2010.05.004.

Sumter, S. R., Bokhorst, C. L., & **Westenberg, P. M.** (2009). Social fears during adolescence: is there an increase in distress and avoidance? *Journal of Anxiety Disorders*, **23**, 897–903.

Warren, S. L. & **Sroufe, L. A.** (2004). Developmental issues. In: **T. H. Ollendick** & **J. S. March** (eds.) *Phobic and Anxiety Disorders in Children and Adolescents: A Clinician's Guide to Effective Psychosocial and Pharmacological Interventions*, pp. 92–115. Oxford, UK: Oxford University Press.

Weems, C. F. & **Costa, N.** (2005). Developmental differences in the expression of childhood anxiety symptoms and fears. *Journal of the American Academy of Child and Adolescent Psychiatry*, **44**, 656–663.

Wenar, C. (1994). *Developmental Psychology: From Infancy through Adolescence*, 3rd edn. New York: McGraw-Hill.

Westenberg, P. M., Bokhorst, C. L., Miers, A. C., Sumter, S. R., Kallen, V. L., Van Pelt, J., *et al.* (2009). A prepared speech in front of a pre-recorded audience: subjective, physiological, and neuroendocrine responses to the Leiden Public Speaking Task. *Biological Psychology*, **82**, 116–124.

Westenberg, P. M., Drewes, M. J., Goedhart, A. W., Siebelink, B. M., & Treffers, P. D. A. (2004). A developmental analysis of self-reported fears in late childhood through mid-adolescence: social evaluative fears on the rise? *Journal of Child Psychology and Psychiatry*, **45**, 481–495.

Westenberg, P. M., Gullone, E., Bokhorst, C. L., Heyne, D. A., & King, N. J. (2007). Social evaluation fear in childhood and adolescence: normative developmental course and continuity of individual differences. *British Journal of Developmental Psychology*, **25**, 471–483.

Westenberg, P. M., Siebelink, B. M., & Treffers, P. D. A. (2001). Psychosocial developmental theory in relation to anxiety and its disorders. In: W. K. Silverman & P. D. A. Treffers (eds.) *Anxiety Disorders in Children: Research, Assessment, and Intervention*, pp. 72–89. Cambridge, UK: Cambridge University Press.

Westenberg, P. M., Siebelink, B. M., Warmenhoven, N. J. C., & Treffers, P. D. A. (1999). Separation anxiety and overanxious disorders: relations to age and level of psychosocial maturity. *Journal of the American Academy of Child and Adolescent Psychiatry*, **38**, 1000–1007.

Wittchen, H. U. & Fehm, L. (2003). Epidemiology and natural course of social fears and social phobia. *Acta Psychiatrica Scandinavica*, **108**, 4–18.

6

Information processing biases in child and adolescent anxiety: a developmental perspective

Andy P. Field, Julie A. Hadwin, and Kathryn J. Lester

Epidemiological studies consistently highlight the presence of anxiety as one of the most prevalent disorders in childhood and adolescence (see Costello, Egger, Copeland, Erkanli, & Angold, Chapter 3, this volume). Symptoms of childhood anxiety often persist beyond childhood, through adolescence and into adulthood (see Weems, 2008, for a review), and childhood anxiety is associated with academic difficulties and underachievement (Ashcraft, 2002; Crozier & Hostettler, 2003; Owens, Stevenson, Norgate, & Hadwin, 2008), impaired social functioning and peer difficulties (Asendorpf, Denissen, & van Aken, 2008; Erath, Flanagan, & Bierman, 2007) and is a major risk factor for subsequent psychological (Kim-Cohen, Caspi, Moffitt, Harrington, Milne, & Poulton, 2003; Lewinsohn, Holm-Denoma, Small, Seeley, & Joiner, 2008; Roza, Hofstra, van der Ende, & Verhulst, 2003) and physical health problems (Beesdo, Hoyer, Jacobi, Low, Höfler, & Wittchen, 2009). Given the prevalence and impact of anxiety on development, it is important to understand the causes of childhood anxiety to inform prevention and intervention methods (e.g., Cowart & Ollendick, 2010).

Clinical and experimental theories of anxiety include processing biases in attention and interpretation as a causal factor that mediates anxiety vulnerability by directly influencing cognitive representations (Beck & Clark, 1997; Williams, MacLeod, Watts, & Mathews, 1997). Distinctive patterns of information processing biases characterize anxiety (see Hadwin & Field, 2010, for a review): anxious individuals have a tendency to selectively attend to threat in the environment (attentional bias), and to make disproportionately threatening interpretations of ambiguous stimuli (interpretation bias). As in anxious adults, there is prima facie evidence that children and adolescents with anxiety demonstrate both attentional (see Field & Lester, 2010b; Garner, 2010; Heim-Dreger, Kohlmann, Eschenbeck, & Burkhardt, 2006; Nightingale, Field, & Kindt, 2010, for reviews) and interpretation biases (see Field & Lester, 2010b; Muris, 2010; Muris & Field, 2008, for reviews). Information processing biases have been found to play a causal role in the development of anxiety (Mathews & MacLeod, 2002). For example, in adult samples, if biases are trained in non-anxious individuals, then anxiety symptoms increase (e.g., Mathews & Mackintosh, 2000; Salemink, van den Hout, & Kindt, 2010; Wilson, MacLeod, Mathews, & Rutherford, 2006; Yiend, Mackintosh, & Mathews, 2005). Similarly, clinically anxious individuals become less anxious if biases are untrained (e.g., Amir, Beard, Burns, & Bomyea, 2009; Schmidt, Richey, Buckner, & Timpano, 2009; see MacLeod, & Bridle, 2009).

Anxiety Disorders in Children and Adolescents, 2nd edn, ed. W. K. Silverman and A. P. Field. Published by Cambridge University Press. © Cambridge University Press 2011.

This chapter explores the empirical evidence across diverse paradigms that supports the proposition that anxious children and young people demonstrate information processing biases similar to those found in anxious adults. It goes on to present and evaluate three different explanations or conceptual frameworks in which information processing biases develop in pre-adolescent children. The final part of the chapter reviews these different frameworks in the context of genetic and environmental influences in anxiety. The summary section presents a précis of theories of the mechanisms that underlie the acquisition of information processing biases.

Evidence for information processing biases in anxious children and young people

There have been several recent reviews of the literature on information processing biases and anxiety in children and young people (Hadwin & Field, 2010; Muris & Field, 2008). Rather than provide a detailed review of the literature; we aim to highlight some of the key studies and core theoretical issues in this area of research. Our overall aim is to give the reader a feel for the overall picture that emerges for the role of information processing biases in child and adolescent anxiety, the mechanisms that underlie these biases, and how they might be acquired.

Attentional biases in anxious children and adolescents

Inhibitory processes to threat and anxiety

Experimental studies have used an emotional Stroop task to explore the proposition that elevated trait or state anxiety is associated with poorer inhibitory processes (or selective attention) to threat versus neutral stimuli. This task requires participants to name the color of a word or picture and to ignore its meaning; if the meaning of the word interferes with color-naming, then the response time to that word will be slower. Individuals with anxiety are typically found to respond more slowly to color-name anxiety-related words (e.g., "web" or "fangs" for a spider phobic). This interference is argued to reflect an individual's inability to utilize top–down processing to inhibit attention to negative or threat meanings in order to complete the task efficiently (Eysenck, Derakshan, Santos, & Calvo, 2007). In the emotional Stroop task, stimuli can be presented either sequentially (single-trial-based Stroop), or concurrently (card-based Stroop format). Research with children and adolescents has found that color-naming is typically associated with both longer (though some studies have found shorter) latencies to color-name threat stimuli for specific anxieties, generalized anxiety, and state anxiety and in both analog and clinical samples (see Nightingale *et al.*, 2010, for a review).

In non-clinical populations, research has looked at both general (high vs. low trait anxiety) and specific anxiety (e.g., high vs. low spider fearful). In terms of specific anxiety, early research has shown that spider-fearful (compared with non-fearful) children (aged 6–13 years old), showed greater latencies to color-name spider-related words (e.g., "creepy," "hairy"), but not neutral words (e.g., "table," "cars"); and this finding was replicated in a slightly younger sample (4–5 years, 6–7 years, and 8–9 years) by the same researchers (M. Martin, Horder, & Jones, 1992; M. Martin & Jones, 1995). Similar results were found for 8–12-year-olds with social concerns when naming the color of words related to acceptance (e.g., "popular") and rejection (e.g., "hated") (J. M. Martin & Cole,

2000). Similarly, 6–12-year-old children with elevated social concerns were less able to inhibit attention to angry schematic faces (relative to neutral) when color-matching face outlines to the relevant color buttons (Hadwin, Donnelly, Richards, French, & Patel, 2009). With respect to general anxiety, youths aged 16–18 years (Richards, Richards, & McGeeney, 2000) and 10–11 years (Richards, French, Nash, Hadwin, & Donnelly, 2007), with high trait anxiety showed greater color-naming interference for anxiety-related words than low trait-anxious controls. Stroop interference was significantly correlated with both trait, $r = 0.40$, and state anxiety, $r = 0.42$ (Richards *et al.*, 2007). Although the Stroop paradigm is typically associated with low error rates, related work has found that children aged 6–10 years had increased color-naming errors on negative versus positive faces with elevated state or trait anxiety (Eschenbeck, Kohlmann, Heim-Dreger, Koller, & Leser, 2004).

In clinical samples, emotional Stroop interference effects have been found in children and adolescents (9–17 years) with post-traumatic stress disorder (PTSD) (Moradi, Taghavi, Neshat-Doost, Yule, & Dalgleish, 1999). Dubner and Motta (1999) studied foster-care children and adolescents who had developed PTSD after being either physically or sexually abused. The sample included 40 pre-adolescents (8–12 years of age), 72 early adolescents (13–15 years of age), and 38 late adolescents (16–19 years of age). This study found that children and adolescents who had been sexually abused had significantly longer color-naming latencies for sexual-abuse-related words (e.g., "naughty" and "sex") than non-abused controls. In addition, youths who had experienced sexual abuse and who had a diagnosis of PTSD showed significantly more interference for sexual-abuse-related words (compared with those without PTSD) and they were slower to color-name sexual abuse words compared to other anxiety, neutral, and positive words. Also, adolescents (13–14 years old) with a diagnosis of generalized anxiety disorder (GAD) demonstrated significantly greater color-naming latencies when asked to color-name emotionally aversive words (depression-related and trauma-related) compared with positive and neutral words relative to controls (Taghavi, Dalgleish, Moradi, Neshat-Doost, & Yule, 2003).

In summary, a small literature has replicated the basic emotional Stroop interference effect in child and adolescent samples who experience elevated anxiety or who have been diagnosed with an anxiety disorder. Although this body of research is growing, several studies using this paradigm have been unable to demonstrate the basic Stroop effect in anxiety in both non-clinical and clinical samples of children and young people.

Kindt, Brosschot, and Everaerd (1997), for example, used a Stroop paradigm to explore attention in typically developing children aged 8 to 9 years who were classified as high or low anxious in both a neutral situation and a stressful vaccination situation. The results showed that both anxiety groups demonstrated cognitive interference specific to information related to physical harm in both the stressful and neutral context. In addition, when the vaccination stressor was absent both high and low trait-anxious girls – but not boys – showed a processing bias for generally threatening information. Other studies have also shown an attentional bias in all children (regardless of their anxiety levels) for threat material (Eschenbeck *et al.*, 2004; Kindt & Brosschot, 1999). A further series of studies suggests that attentional biases have different developmental trajectories in anxious and non-anxious children. For example, in 8–12-year-olds, spider Stroop interference decreased with age for children who reported low spider fearfulness; but it increased with age in children who reported fear of spiders (Kindt, Bierman, & Brosschot, 1997). This developmental finding was replicated in a study in which spider-fearful and non-spider-fearful girls (8–11 years) were falsely informed that they might have to approach a real spider (Kindt, van den Hout, de Jong, & Hoekzema, 2000). The results showed no significant interference effect for spider-threat words or pictures; but the interference effect became greater with age in the spider-fearful girls and decreased with age in the non-spider-fearing girls.

Further studies have found Stoop interference effects in the opposite direction. For example, Morren, Kindt, van den Hout, and van Kasteren (2003) found *faster* responses to spider-related words relative to control words in a large sample of high ($n = 170$) and low spider-fearful children ($n = 215$) aged 7–11 years. Similarly, in two experiments Heim-Dreger *et al.*, (2006) demonstrated *avoidance* of drawings of faces depicting either friendly or threatening expressions in an emotional Stroop task. In both experiments trait anxiety did not significantly predict interference effects: it was best predicted by the absolute values of interference scores (i.e., when you ignore whether the effect shows vigilance or avoidance).

Evidence from "at-risk" and clinically diagnosed children and adolescents also suggests that the emotional Stroop does not always produce an interference effect. For example, young people "at risk" because of being classified as behaviorally inhibited at 2 years of age should exhibit greater threat-related interference in the Stroop task compared with those who are uninhibited. However, in a study of 12–13-year-olds, all participants (regardless of their earlier temperament classification) showed faster color-naming latencies for threat and positive words relative to neutral words (Schwartz, Snidman, & Kagan, 1996). Similarly, children and adolescents (aged 8–15 years) whose parent was diagnosed with panic disorder showed similar interference scores for panic-related words compared to those whose parent was diagnosed with animal phobia and those of healthy controls (Schneider, Unnewehr, In-Albon, & Margraf, 2008).

Failures to replicate the predicted Stroop interference effect have also been found in clinical samples diagnosed with PTSD and GAD (Dalgleish, Taghavi, Neshat-Doost, Moradi, Canterbury, & Yule, 2003), and using trauma-related stimuli in sexually abused adolescent girls (11–13 years old) with PTSD (Freeman & Beck, 2000), and in children and adolescents (7–18 years old) diagnosed with separation anxiety disorder (SAD), social phobia (SP), and/or GAD compared with typical controls (Kindt, Bögels, & Morren, 2003). Finally, children (7–12 years) and adolescents (13–17 years) with a range of clinically diagnosed anxiety disorders were slower to color-name images of adults and children depicting either neutral or emotional expressions (anger, disgust, or happiness) in general compared to controls (Benoit, McNally, Rapee, Gamble, & Wiseman, 2007).

Further research has used an emotional Go/NoGo task to explore inhibition to threat in anxiety (e.g., Hare, Tottenham, Davidson, Glover, & Casey, 2005; Ladouceur *et al.*, 2006; Waters & Valvoi, 2009). In this task, participants are asked to respond to a particular emotional face on some trials (Go trials) and avoid responding to any other face on other trials (NoGo trials). This task measures both inhibition (using the proportion of presses that they accidentally make on NoGo trials) and attentional control (using response times on Go trials when NoGo trials are relatively sparse). Waters and Valvoi (2009) found that girls diagnosed with clinical anxiety aged 8–12 years (compared with typically developing controls) were slower to respond to neutral face Go trials in the context of angry (versus happy) face NoGo trials. There was no corresponding significant effect of anxiety in boys.

Selective attention to threat

In the emotional Stroop task the word/picture and color appear at the same time and in the same physical location; hence, the emotional cue and the probe (i.e., the color of the word/picture) are spatially and temporally integrated. As such, the emotional Stroop task is a measure of emotional interference (van Strien & Valstar, 2004) because attention is distributed cognitively but not physically (i.e., in the visuo-spatial field). Other tasks, like the dot-probe paradigm, require a physical and temporal distribution of attention. In this task, a threatening and a neutral cue (e.g., a word or face) are presented simultaneously on a screen. These cues disappear and a probe appears either in the location of the threatening or the neutral cue. In this task, individuals with elevated or clinical levels of anxiety (relative to non-anxious controls) respond faster to probes appearing in the location of threatening rather than neutral cues and slower to probes following neutral cues. This finding is interpreted as showing that anxiety is associated with an attentional orientation towards threatening cues and that anxiety is linked to increased difficulty disengaging from these cues (e.g., Field, 2006b; Heim-Dreger *et al.*, 2006; Lipp & Derakshan, 2005).

Several studies have used the dot-probe paradigm for assessing attention bias to threat words in childhood and adolescent anxiety. For example, in an early paper Vasey, Daleiden, Williams, and Brown (1995) administered the dot-probe task to a group of 9–14-year-old children and adolescents diagnosed with anxiety disorders and a group of age-matched typically developing controls. The results showed that children and adolescents in the anxiety group had faster responses to probes preceded by a threatening rather than a neutral word. Similar findings have been shown in clinically referred adolescents diagnosed with GAD and PTSD (Dalgleish, Moradi, Taghavi, Neshat-Doost, & Yule, 2001; Dalgleish *et al.*, 2003; Taghavi, Neshat-Doost, Moradi, Yule, & Dalgleish, 1999), in children with elevated anxiety sensitivity (Hunt, Keogh, & French, 2007), and in non-clinical children and adolescents who experience high anxiety levels (Vasey, El Hag, & Daleiden, 1996). At least one study using word stimuli suggests that these biases might be relatively specific: adolescents (aged 10 to 13 years) reporting high levels of social stress showed vigilance to social threat words, but not physical threat words. In contrast, adolescents who reported low social stress showed no bias at all (Helzer, Connor-Smith, & Reed, 2009).

Consistent with the proposition that both clinical and non-clinical children demonstrate information processing biases for threat (see for example Kindt *et al.*, 2000), Waters and colleagues found that both non-selected and clinically anxious children between the ages of 9 and 12 years showed an attentional bias for emotionally valenced images (Waters, Lipp, & Spence, 2004). Similarly, clinically anxious and non-anxious control children (aged 7 to 12) showed a vigilance for happy faces compared to neutral, but only clinically anxious children (with GAD) showed a vigilance for angry faces compared to neutral (Waters, Henry, Mogg, Bradley, & Pine, 2010; Waters, Mogg, Bradley, & Pine, 2008).[1] Finally, pre-therapy attentional bias for threat pictures in clinically anxious 8–12-year-old children remained after 10 sessions of cognitive behavior therapy (CBT) (Waters, Wharton, Zimmer-Gembeck, & Craske, 2008).

---

[1] Figure 1 of Waters *et al.* (2010) seems to suggest that the bias for angry faces in clinically anxious children was as large as the bias for happy faces, suggesting that these children might have a bias for emotional faces in general, whereas low-anxious children have a bias only for happy faces.

The aforementioned work suggests that clinically anxious children show *vigilance* for angry faces; however, other research muddies the Waters findings. On the one hand, some research supports Waters's work: vigilance for angry facial expressions has been observed in children and adolescents (ages 7 to 18 years) with GAD, SP, and/or SAD, and did not differ significantly across these disorders (Roy *et al.*, 2008); trait anxiety has been positively associated with vigilance to angry faces in 11–18-year-old unselected adolescents and corresponds with activation in the right dorsolateral prefrontal cortex (Telzer *et al.*, 2008); and adolescents (with a mean age of 14) with a current diagnosis of bipolar disorder show vigilance for threat faces but only when they also have a lifetime history of anxiety (Brotman *et al.*, 2007).

On the other hand, there is evidence of *avoidance* of threat faces too. Avoidance of angry faces has been observed compared to controls in 7–13-year-old children and adolescents with PTSD (Pine *et al.*, 2005) and adolescents (mean age of 13–14) with a diagnosis of GAD (Monk, Telzer, *et al.*, 2008). This bias was evidenced using brain indices; there were no significant group differences using reaction times – both groups showed a bias towards angry faces. Avoidance of negative facial expressions has also been shown to correlate with social anxiety symptoms in a non-clinical sample of 8–11-year-olds (Stirling, Eley, & Clark, 2006). Finally, 8–16-year-old children and adolescents with anxiety disorders (GAD, SAD, SP, and specific phobia) showed avoidance of mildly threatening pictures, but an inability to disengage from severely threatening pictures (Legerstee *et al.*, 2009). In this study, children and adolescents who responded to CBT showed a tendency to avoid severely threatening pictures whereas non-responders tended to have difficulties in disengaging from severe threat before therapy. This finding is interesting because it implies qualitative differences in attentional allocation to threat within groups of anxiety-disordered children and adolescents.

Visual search and anxiety

Several studies within child and adolescent research have used a visual search task to explore attention in anxiety. In this task, participants are asked to make a decision about the presence or absence of a pre-specified target set amongst distractors (top–down search) or to decide whether all stimuli within a visual array are the same or different (bottom–up search). Searching for targets can be made easy or more difficult by increasing the similarity of targets and distracters or the number of targets or distractors in a set size (i.e., the number of stimuli within a visual array). Typically, absent (or same) trials take twice as long as present (or different) trials because participants search each location whereas in present (or different trials) they search on average about half of the locations before they find the target. Search efficiency in this task is usually reflected in increased reaction times to find target faces as the set size or number of distractors increases (i.e., the gradient of the search slope): flatter slopes reflect more efficient searches. Further research has also considered search intercepts, which reflect the difficulty of the search and can include, for example, cognitive or perceptual factors that influence response generation and that are unaffected by set size. Some have argued (Donnelly, Hadwin, Manneer, & Richards, 2010) that visual search paradigms have been used effectively to explore engagement or disengagement to threat in anxiety, and to demonstrate the moderating effect of anxiety on individuals' decisions about when to terminate search.

In relation to engagement with threat stimuli, research with adults has found that a clinical diagnosis of anxiety was associated with flatter search slopes for negative facial stimuli (Eastwood *et al.*, 2005). Similarly, feared objects (spiders and snakes) were found faster by adult participants with higher levels of related fearfulness (Soares, Esteves, & Flykt, 2009). Research in adults has also found that elevated trait anxiety is associated with slowed reaction times to find positive stimuli in the context of threatening distractors, indicating links between anxiety and difficulties with attentional disengagement from threat (Byrne & Eysenck, 1995; Rinck, Reinecke, Ellwart, Heuer, & Becker, 2005).

A growing body of work has utilized visual search paradigms to explore attention in anxiety in children and adolescents. In the context of searching for threat (angry faces), early research found that self-report trait anxiety (and not depression) in children aged 7–10 years was associated with increased search efficiency (flatter search slopes or lower intercepts) when making decisions about when to terminate absent search trials (Hadwin, Donnelly, French, Richards, Watts, & Daley, 2003). The authors argued that childhood anxiety is associated with a lowered decision threshold related to establishing the absence of threat in search. Recent work from the same laboratory also showed an association between anxiety and increased search efficiency (flatter search slopes) when detecting angry faces, where this effect was moderated by age (Perez-Olivas, Stevenson, & Hadwin, 2008). Consistent with Kindt and van den Hout's (2001) developmental account of the emergence of information processing biases in anxiety, the results showed that self-report separation anxiety was negatively correlated with angry search slopes, but only for those aged 10 years and above.

Most important, Perez-Olivas *et al.* (2008) were able to demonstrate the utility of visual search tasks in understanding the relationship between parenting factors and childhood anxiety (Hudson & Rapee, 2004; Rapee, 2001). Specifically, this study found that the vigilance for angry faces in older children was associated with maternal overprotection and acted as a potential mediator between this parenting factor and separation anxiety in the child. This study is significant in starting to delineate potential cognitive mechanisms that underpin the relationship between parenting and childhood anxiety.

The link between childhood anxiety and detection of threat has also been shown in further studies using visual search of emotional faces (Waters & Lipp, 2008b) or fear-related stimuli (Waters, Lipp, & Spence, 2008). Waters & Lipp (2008b), Experiment 2, used a visual search design to ask children aged 8–11 years to make decisions about the presence or absence of angry, happy, or sad faces (with neutral distractors; there was no manipulation of set size in this study so no slope or intercept statistics could be calculated). The authors used the 75th and 25th centiles of children's self-report anxiety scores to create a low and high anxiety group. The results were presented as intra-group differences in search rather than inter-group differences (see Bar-Haim, Lamy, Pergamin, Bakermans-Kranenburg, & van IJzendoorn, 2007). They showed that children in both anxiety groups were faster to find angry compared with happy faces; while only the children in the high anxiety group were faster to find sad compared with happy faces. Group differences were not supported in a correlational analysis, although self-report depression was negatively correlated with reaction times to find happy faces. The authors argued for a general vigilance for negative emotional faces in children with elevated anxiety.

Waters, Lipp, *et al.* (2008), Experiment 3, extended their findings with emotional faces to explore search for snakes and spiders in children aged 10 to 12 years. To explore the effect of fearfulness in search, the authors used a similar group split using spider and snake phobia questionnaires to create high and low spider- and snake-fearful groups. The results highlighted that children in the low fearful group were faster to make absent decisions if the stimulus array was made up of fearful (snakes or spiders) compared with neutral (flowers or mushroom) stimuli; this effect was not present in the high fearful group indicating that these children had more difficulty disengaging from these fearful stimuli.

The results of studies using visual search paradigms with children and adolescents are broadly consistent with research using other paradigms such as the dot-probe task, and adult research generally. Some studies have shown that elevated anxiety in childhood is associated with increased engagement and greater difficulty in disengagement from threat or fearful stimuli. Further research has indicated that decision-making in threat search is moderated by anxiety.

Interpretation and anxiety

A variety of tasks have been used to demonstrate that clinically anxious children and adolescents disproportionately interpret ambiguous situations in a threatening way. For example, children and adolescents can be asked to interpret homophones that have either a neutral or a threatening interpretation (e.g., dye versus die) or they can provide or choose endings for ambiguous sentences or stories. Trait anxiety levels in 7–9-year-old school children have been found to be positively correlated with choosing threat interpretations of these homophones (Hadwin, Frost, French, & Richards, 1997). Similarly, youths (aged 8–17) diagnosed with GAD made more threat interpretations than controls (Taghavi, Moradi, Neshat-Doost, Yule, & Dalgleish, 2000). Further research has shown that threat interpretation biases measured using homophone tasks reduce in clinically anxious children (aged 8 to 12) after CBT (Waters, Wharton, *et al.*, 2008).

Using a story-based methodology, youths with anxiety disorders and oppositional defiant disorder (aged between 7 and 14 years) more frequently interpreted ambiguous situations as threatening than controls (Barrett, Rapee, Dadds, & Ryan, 1996). In two similar studies, anxiety-disordered youths (SAD, GAD, and SP in both studies) interpreted ambiguous stories significantly more negatively than controls and youths (aged 9 to 18) with externalizing disorders (Bögels & Zigterman, 2000), and children (7 to 12) at risk of anxiety because of having parents with an anxiety diagnosis (Waters, Craske, Bergman, & Treanor, 2008). Several studies have also shown that the extent of this interpretation bias varies as a function of anxiety (Chorpita, Albano, & Barlow, 1996; Creswell & O'Connor, 2006, 2011; Creswell, O'Connor, & Brewin, 2006; Creswell, Shildrick, & Field, 2010) and worry (Suarez & Bell-Dolan, 2001) in non-clinical samples aged 5 to 13. Dineen and Hadwin (2004), for example, asked non-selected school children (6 to 10 years old) to judge how a protagonist and they themselves would interpret the ambiguous intention of a second character. Parent report was associated with increased negative attributions children made about the story protagonists, but not with attributions to themselves.

Considering the broader relationships between interpretation biases within families, further research has found positive associations between children's and mothers' interpretation biases (Creswell & O'Connor, 2006; Creswell *et al.*, 2006), as well as between children's interpretations and mothers' expectations about how their child would respond to ambiguity (Creswell & O'Connor, 2006). In addition, children's interpretations were also linked to their own beliefs about how their mothers behave towards them when faced with ambiguity (Lester, Seal, Nightingale, & Field, 2010). Interpretation biases are stable over time and have a reciprocal relationship with mothers' expectations about children's anxious cognitions: for example, children's interpretation biases create negative maternal expectancies that then magnify these interpretation biases in the future (Creswell & O'Connor, 2011; Creswell, Shildrick, *et al.*, 2010).

Muris and colleagues have also explored a related cognitive distortion, the Reduced Evidence for Danger (RED) bias, which measures how *quickly* youths make threatening interpretations when confronted with ambiguity. In the paradigm they developed, children and adolescents are given ambiguous vignettes but are told that some have scary or bad endings. Each vignette is read to the child a sentence at a time and each time the child has to decide whether they believe the vignette will have a bad ending (Muris, Rapee, Meesters, Schouten, & Geers, 2003). When non-clinical children and adolescents (8–13 years), high and low on social anxiety, were given vignettes describing social situations, those high on social anxiety needed to hear fewer sentences to decide that a story would have a bad outcome (Muris, Merckelbach, & Damsma, 2000). This bias has been replicated in several other studies and has been found to persist over time (Muris, Kindt, Bögels, Merckelbach, Gadet, & Moulaert, 2000; Muris, Luermans, Merckelbach, & Mayer, 2000; Muris, Rapee, *et al.*, 2003).

Interpretation biases have been causally linked to anxiety disorders: when biases are trained in non-anxious adults, their anxiety increases; treatment typically reduces interpretational biases; and training benign biases reduces anxiety (see Field & Lester, 2010a, for a review). In support of these findings, further studies have used an innovative analog (the "space odyssey" paradigm) of the adult bias modification studies to train interpretation biases in children (Muris, Huijding, Mayer, & Hameetman, 2008; Muris, Huijding, Mayer, Remmerswaal, & Vreden, 2009). Children imagine taking a journey to an unknown planet and are presented with ambiguous scenarios (e.g., "On the street, you encounter a spaceman. He has a sort of toy handgun and he fires at you … ") and select either a positive ("You are laughing: it is a water pistol and the weather is fine anyway") or a negative ("Oops, this hurts! The pistol produces a red beam which burns your skin!") outcome. They are told whether their decision is correct or wrong. The child is "trained" to interpret ambiguous situations positively or negatively by consistently reinforcing either the positive or negative outcome for each scenario. Following the modification phase, children rate the level of threat associated with various ambiguous scenarios describing everyday situations that could occur on Earth (e.g., going to school).

Interpretation bias scores were affected by the bias modification procedure in non-clinical children aged 8–12 years: they reported higher threat interpretations after negative modification compared with children who had received positive modification. Negative modification was particularly pronounced in children with pre-existing high levels of anxiety symptoms (Muris, Huijding, *et al.*, 2008). These results were broadly replicated in a second study (Muris, Huijding, *et al.*, 2009); however, they did not replicate the finding that trait anxiety moderated this effect. They also found a non-significant association between the induced bias and avoidance tendencies, which casts doubt on the causal effect of induced bias on anxiety, because if an interpretation bias created anxiety you would expect children to have become avoidant after the training procedure.

Emotional reasoning

Covariation bias is the tendency to overestimate the association between feared stimuli and negative outcomes. In adults, this phenomenon is demonstrated by showing participants slides consisting of fear-relevant (e.g., spiders) and neutral (e.g., flowers) pictures that are followed by an electric shock (or other aversive outcome), a tone, or nothing. Participants subsequently estimate the contingencies between the slides and the various outcomes. People with phobias typically overestimate the contingency between phobic stimuli and negative outcomes (Tomarken, Cook, & Mineka, 1989). Muris and colleagues have used thought experiments to assess covariation biases in adolescents; they are asked to imagine that they are in a covariation bias experiment as just described, or one involving a computer game in which participants won or lost candy while looking at various slides. High fearful non-clinical children and adolescents (8–16 years) estimated more negative and fewer positive outcomes in relation to spider pictures than low fearful youths (Muris, Huijding, Mayer, den Breejen, & Makkelie, 2007). However, an earlier study based on a card game failed to find a covariation bias in non-clinical children and adolescents aged 8 to 13 (Muris, de Jong, Meesters, Waterreus, & van Lubeck, 2005).

There is further evidence that verbal information can be used to induce covariation biases. Field and Lawson (2008) found that threat information about a novel animal led non-clinical 7–9-year-old children to more accurately estimate the contingency between that animal and negative outcomes (in the absence of verbal information children tended to overestimate the number of positive outcomes). A similar study extended these findings showing that covariation and other reasoning biases about novel animals could be induced using verbal information (Muris, Rassin, *et al.*, 2009).

A series of studies have explored how children reason about anxiety-related information. Children and adolescents were given vignettes describing anxiety-related (e.g., giving a talk, getting a report card from a teacher) or everyday (e.g., playing with a ball, drawing, watching TV) situations. The vignettes were manipulated to contain either danger or safety information; for example, believing a party to be "fancy dress" you turn up dressed as a clown but arrive to discover everyone else is dressed normally (danger) or they too are in costume (safety). In addition, some children and adolescents were given anxiety response information (e.g., you begin to sweat, or tremble). Participants rated how dangerous they found the vignette. Non-clinical children and adolescents' (7 to 13 years) danger ratings were affected by whether the vignette contained danger information; even in the safe vignettes danger ratings were higher when anxiety response information was given (Morren, Muris, & Kindt, 2004; Muris, Merckelbach, & van Spauwen, 2003; Muris, Vermeer, & Horselenberg, 2008). The tendency to use anxiety response information as a heuristic for evaluating the dangerousness of the safe stories was increased by trait anxiety and anxiety sensitivity (Muris, Merckelbach, *et al.*, 2003). In addition, age, cognitive development, and anxiety sensitivity were positively related to 4–13-year-old children and adolescents' ability to perceive physical symptoms as a signal of anxiety (Muris, Mayer, Freher, Duncan, & van den Hout, 2010). Finally, when 9–13-year-old non-clinical children and adolescents took part in a bogus pipeline experiment in which they believed they were hearing their heartbeat but were actually given false feedback, they gave higher threat ratings to ambiguous situations than children who listened to recordings of an African drum (Muris, Mayer, & Bervoets, 2010).

Interim summary

In this section we reviewed the evidence that anxiety is related to systematic biases in information processing. This review highlights the critical mass of evidence to suggest that anxious children and adolescents show attentional and interpretational biases to threat and emotional reasoning biases. Some of these biases can be improved by treatment (interpretational biases) but others appear resistant (attentional bias). Further evidence suggests that information processing biases play a causal role in anxiety (although the evidence is less comprehensive than adult research). We now turn our attention to the origins of these biases and the role of development in their genesis.

Theories of information processing biases

Adult models

Field and Lester (2010b) noted that developmental processes are overlooked in many of the theoretical frameworks related to information processing biases to threat. These theories typically emphasize innate brain circuitry dedicated to evaluating threat in the environment. One example of these systems is an evolved fear module with dedicated neural circuitry that responds automatically to threat stimuli and is impervious to cognitive control (Öhman & Mineka, 2001). Another is the behavioral inhibition system (BIS), an evolved system in the septo-hippocampal area of the brain that inhibits ongoing behavior and directs attentional resources to threats in the environment (Gray & McNaughton, 2003). These models are based on systems that are assumed to act automatically. It is likely that development reflects the interplay between automatic and controlled processing. It is acknowledged, for example, that the "automatic" BIS "tags" automatic motor processes as "needing to be checked" by controlled processes (Zinbarg & Mohlman, 1998), and that the conscious appraisal of the personal meaning of threat stimuli is necessary meaning that automatic processes would pass these stimuli onto a "conscious perception system."

Information processing *biases* to threat (rather than threat processing more generally) are probably best explained by Mathews and Mackintosh's (1998) model. This model explains attentional bias in terms of sensory input from threatening and benign stimuli activating threat and benign representations that compete for attention/cognitive resources. Interpretation biases are explained by ambiguous sensory input activating both threat and benign interpretations that compete for attention via inhibitory links. In both cases, the dominant representation enters awareness once it reaches a threshold activation level (and by inhibiting the weaker representation). Here, the strength of the representations/interpretations are proposed to be determined by two systems: an automatic threat evaluation system (TES), which processes the sensory input and evaluates its threat potential; and a positive emotional evaluative system (PES), which assesses cues relevant to attaining rewards. Controlled processing is suggested to gate these two systems: the attention allocated to and interpretation placed upon stimuli and events depends not just on the outputs of the TES and PES but also on an individual's cognitive effort.

Developmental models

Field and Lester (2010b) note that the adult models do not explicitly include a role for cognitive, social, and emotional development. They describe three broad conceptualizations of how child development might influence information processing biases. Field and Lester acknowledge that these three models are not an exhaustive list of possibilities, but merely the three most convenient ways to examine the extant literature. First, they describe an *integral bias model*, in which information processing biases are present during early childhood and do not change with development; they are innate constituents of emotion (M. Martin & Jones, 1995; M. Martin *et al.*, 1992). This model assumes that information processing biases should not differ across children and adolescents at different stages of development.

Second, Field and Lester (2010b) propose a *moderation model*, which assumes that information processing biases towards threat are present in all young children, but diminish over time as a function of individual factors (e.g., anxiety or the development of inhibitory processes). This assumption implies that the interaction between individual differences (e.g., temperament) and cognitive, social, and emotional development leads processing biases to follow different developmental trajectories in different children (or adolescents). A good example of a moderation model is Kindt and van den Hout's inhibition hypothesis (Kindt & van den Hout, 2001), which was based on Kindt's work with the emotional Stroop task (see earlier). They proposed that links between anxiety and cognitive processing biases for threat were dependent on the development of inhibitory skills. They suggested that in typical development children up to the age of 10 years had not developed a capacity to inhibit their attention to threat; and this ability developed after that time. The significant risk factor in this model was the absence of the development of relevant inhibitory skills in those children who experienced elevated levels of anxiety, which placed children at risk for processing biases to threat. This model can be summed up in terms of developmental trajectories, whereby processing biases decrease with age in some children (e.g., non-anxious) and are maintained or increase with age in others (e.g., anxious children).

The final model that Field and Lester (2010b) discuss is the *acquisition model*, in which the emergence of information processing biases towards threat is assumed to be linked to the development of the cognitive, social, and emotional skills necessary to sustain them (see Alfano, Beidel, & Turner, 2002; Manassis & Bradley, 1994; Muris, 2007). In contrast to the moderation model, an acquisition model assumes that processing biases towards threat are not present (or are present but not fully formed) in young children, but emerge with development. Here, individual differences will again interact with child development, but the moderation and acquisition models differ in the role that they place on anxiety. In the moderation model, trait anxiety is assumed to feed into child development to change the developmental course of the processing bias; this could also be the case in acquisition models but trait anxiety might also emerge (or worsen) as a *consequence* of acquiring a processing bias.

According to Field and Lester (2010b), these models can be distinguished empirically by establishing three things: (1) integral bias and moderation models can be distinguished from the acquisition model by establishing whether processing biases for threat exist from very early in a child's development; (2) if processing biases do exist from an early developmental stage then the integral bias and moderation models can be dissociated by establishing whether *at this early stage of development* they are present in all people (moderation model) or in only a subset of people (integral bias); and (3) the integral bias model can be differentiated from the moderation and acquisition models by establishing whether processing biases to threat have a developmental trajectory.

Field and Lester (2010b) review the existing evidence for each of the three propositions, and conclude that, notwithstanding a certain amount of inconsistency in the evidence, attentional and interpretational biases are best conceptualized by different models: attentional biases are probably best conceptualized by a moderation model, whereas interpretational biases develop in line with an acquisition model. We will briefly sum up the evidence on which Field and Lester (2010b) base their conclusions, but for more detail see their review.

In terms of attentional biases, first, attentional biases to threat have been demonstrated from very early in development: infants as young as 5 months (LoBue & DeLoache, 2010; Rakison & Derringer, 2008; Thrasher, LoBue, Coan, & DeLoache, 2009) and pre-school age children (LoBue & DeLoache, 2008) show attentional biases to fear-relevant stimuli such as snakes, spiders, and threatening faces. This research probably rules out the acquisition model. In these studies all infants and children showed an attentional bias to threat (i.e., there was no evidence that the effects were unique to children with specific temperaments or high anxiety). In addition, we have already reviewed evidence from samples in older childhood that show an attentional bias to threat in all children using the Stroop (Eschenbeck et al., 2004; Kindt & Brosschot, 1999; Kindt, Brosschot, et al., 1997) and dot-probe tasks (Waters & Lipp, 2008a, 2008b; Waters et al., 2004). We have also seen evidence of attentional biases to threat that are specific to anxiety disordered children, and these have often (but not always) used slightly older samples implying a developmental change at some point between infancy and adolescence (e.g., Brotman et al., 2007; Dalgleish et al., 2001, 2003; Legerstee et al., 2009; Monk, Klein, et al., 2008; Moradi et al., 1999; Taghavi et al. 1999, 2003; Vasey et al., 1995).

A developmental trajectory for attentional bias is also supported by Kindt and van den Hout's inhibition hypothesis (2001), which is based on evidence that Stroop interference decreased with age in low spider-fearful children, but increased with age in high fearful children (Kindt, Bierman, et al., 1997; Kindt et al., 2000). Kindt suggests that age 10 might be a critical period at which the trajectory of attentional biases changes in high and low anxious children, although the change is more likely to be dependent on cognitive, social, and emotional development than age per se (Field & Lester, 2010b). Field and Lester (2010b) concluded that, on balance, there is probably the best evidence that attentional biases follow a moderation model.

The evidence for interpretation biases to threat is far less clear. As we have already reviewed, studies have shown that childhood anxiety is associated with a bias towards making threat interpretations of ambiguous scenarios (e.g., Barrett et al., 1996; Bögels & Zigterman, 2000; Creswell & O'Connor, 2006), selecting the threat interpretation of ambiguous homophones (e.g., Hadwin et al., 1997; Taghavi et al., 2000) and being faster and requiring less information to conclude that ambiguous vignettes will have a threatening conclusion (e.g., Muris, Merckelbach, et al., 2000). There is also a small body of work showing that cognitive development is linked to interpretation biases: older non-clinical children are increasingly able to link physical symptoms with fear and anxiety (Muris, Merckelbach, & Luijten, 2002), especially from the age of 7 (Muris, Hoeve, Meesters, & Mayer, 2004); age and performance on Piagetian conservation tasks independently predict children's ability to relate physical symptoms to anxiety (Muris, Vermeer, et al., 2008); and performance on Piagetian conservation tasks and especially Theory of Mind (ToM) tests predict anxious interpretations and emotional reasoning scores (Muris, Mayer, Vermeulen, & Hiemstra, 2007). Finally, we have seen that interpretation biases can be 'trained' in non-anxious children (Muris, Huijding, et al., 2008, 2009), suggesting that they can be learned.

Field and Lester (2010b) concluded based on their review of this evidence that inter-pretation biases vary as a function of anxiety and child development, which rules out only the integral bias model. They suggest that there is no evidence of interpretation biases in infancy, which would distinguish moderation from acquisition models, and that there is a methodological Gordian knot for researchers to sever: how to demonstrate an interpretation bias in infants, who have yet to develop language ability.

The origins of information processing biases

In their review paper, Field and Lester (2010b) argued that the evidence for a role of developmental change in information processing biases is more compelling than that for an integral bias model. If we trust their assertion then the obvious question is through what mechanisms do these developmental changes take place?

Genetic and environmental influences on the development of information processing biases

It is generally accepted that the development of anxiety is associated with both genetic and environmental risks (Silberg, Rutter, Neale, & Eaves, 2001). From a genetic perspective, family members often share symptoms of anxiety: children whose parents are diagnosed with an anxiety disorder are more likely to develop anxiety compared with children whose parents do not have a disorder (see Creswell, Murray, Stacey, & Cooper, Chapter 14, this volume for a review). Similarly, twin studies indicate that genes can account for around 53% of the variance in anxious symptoms in childhood and adolescence (see Gregory & Eley, Chapter 8, this volume). With respect to the specific risk for information processing biases, Eley and colleagues used the scenario and homophone tasks described earlier in this chapter in a sample of 8-year-old twins and showed that just under one-third of the variance in interpretational biases (30% for the scenarios and 24% for the homophone task) was attributable to genes with non-shared environment explaining the remaining variance (Eley, Gregory, Clark, & Ehlers, 2007). In terms of attentional bias, in a study of 10-year-old twins no significant genetic influence was found on anxious children's avoidance of angry faces (Lau *et al.*, 2009). In this study, a common genetic factor explained 75% of the variance in the ability to identify *all* of the emotional facial expressions used (angry, fearful, sad, disgusted, and happy), leading the authors to speculate that environmental influences would contribute to the ability to identify specific emotional facial expressions.

This later finding highlights the fact that risk genes are likely to be shaped or influenced by feedback from the environment (Leonardo & Hen, 2008). Understanding the interaction of genes and environment in the development of anxiety becomes more difficult in a developing population. Leonardo and Hen (2008), for example, proposed that "gene by environment interaction is perhaps more appropriately conceived of as a gene by environment by time interaction, with some time periods being more susceptible to environmental manipulation than others" (p. 135). In other words, genetically determined developmental stages (i.e., critical or sensitive periods) are proposed to make individuals more or less susceptible to the influence of environment and the development of anxiety, where a sensitive period can be defined as "developmental phases at which the individual is more likely to acquire a new behavior pattern than at other times" (Schaffer, 2006).

Theoretical models of childhood anxiety and information processing biases typically recognize the interplay between genes and the environment, noting that genetically vulnerable children are more susceptible to the development of anxiety in the context of environmental risk (Field & Lester, 2010a; Rapee, 2001). Environmental risk has typically included some consideration of a child's own direct fearful experiences, as well as their experiences through observations or instruction from others (see Field and Purkis, Chapter 11, this volume and Hadwin, Garner, & Perez-Olivas, 2006, for a review of these pathways); because these different learning pathways are reviewed elsewhere in this book the next section focuses on the mechanisms that underlie the development of information processing biases.

Mechanisms of the development of information processing biases

Very little has been written on the mechanisms through which information processing to threat might be learnt. Hadwin *et al.* (2006) argued that information processing biases might be learnt through family processes. Essentially, they suggested that through giving children threat information (verbally or vicariously) in the course of family interactions will serve to reinforce avoidant behaviors. Field and Lester (2010a) put forward a slightly more specific take on this general idea: they suggest that biases develop early in life through reinforcement for paying attention to threat or making threat interpretations in the face of ambiguity. Parents and family members will, of course, be the primary source of this "reinforcement" but not the exclusive source (see Hudson & Rapee, 2004, who highlight a peer role in the emergence of information processing biases). Field and Lester (2010a) noted that if information processing biases are trained in non-anxious adults, children, and adolescents their anxiety increases (e.g., Mathews & Mackintosh, 2000; Muris, Huijding, *et al.*, 2008; Salemink *et al.*, 2010; Wilson *et al.*, 2006; Yiend *et al.*, 2005) and that these training paradigms mirror how information processing biases develop in the real world.

Field and Lester (2010a) suggested that children experience an ongoing stream of novel, often ambiguous situations and stimuli and that they may seek to resolve this ambiguity and uncertainty through significant others in their environment (parents, teachers, siblings, etc.). In doing so, they learn appropriate emotional and behavioral responses to novel stimuli and situations. The parent (or significant other) could resolve each ambiguous or novel event for their child in either a benign or a threatening manner. Across events the child is provided with an array of anxiogenic learning experiences, each of which is like a "trial" in a bias modification procedure. For each "trial/event" a benign or threat response is reinforced by the parent/significant other through verbal information (e.g., Field, Lawson, & Banerjee, 2008), gestures such as pointing, or subtle behavioral reactions (e.g., Murray, Cooper, Creswell, Schofield, & Sack, 2007). The intergenerational transmission of processing biases to threat (e.g., Creswell, Cooper, & Murray, 2010; Creswell & O'Connor, 2006; Creswell *et al.*, 2006; Creswell, Shildrick, *et al.*, 2010) is, therefore, explained by anxious parents, because of their own bias towards threat, consistently drawing the child's attention to threat or resolving ambiguity in a threatening way. As such, they "train" their children to have their own bias. As we noted earlier, there will be a gene by environment interaction such that the power of threat or positive "training" will depend upon genes (Belsky & Pluess, 2009): this differential susceptibility is illustrated by the finding that the s/s genotype of 5-HTTLPR is associated with elevated depressive symptoms or risk among adolescent women in high-stress environments but in low-stress environments the s/s genotype is associated with reduced depressive symptom levels or risk (Eley *et al.*, 2004).

Field and Lester (2010a) assume, therefore, that a parent's own cognitive biases towards threat extend to influence how they process aspects of their child's world; put another way, they view their child's world, as well as their own, as being threatening. This assumption appears to be true: as trait anxiety increased in mothers so did their tendency to interpret ambiguous child-related situations as threatening (Lester, Field, Oliver, & Cartwright-Hatton, 2009). In Lester *et al.*'s study, mediation analyses revealed that parental trait anxiety drives a self-referent interpretation bias in the mother, which in turn drives a bias for interpreting ambiguous situations involving their child in a threatening way. Field and Lester's (2010a) hypothesis also requires evidence that when faced with novelty and/or ambiguity anxious parents guide their child towards threat/a threat interpretation. There is some tentative evidence of this behavior. Using a task similar to the ambiguous scenarios task already described in this chapter, 6–11-year-old non-anxious children were asked how they thought their mother and father would react in a series of ambiguous situations in an open-ended way. This measure was intended as a proxy of the child's past experiences of ambiguity with their parents. There was a significant relationship between what children reported their mothers would do and the children's interpretation of a different set of ambiguous situations (Lester *et al.*, 2010). Of course it is possible that the children's existing interpretation biases drove their responses about how their mothers would react to ambiguous situations, but notwithstanding this criticism, the results support the idea interpretation biases develop through parents disambiguating situations for their children in a threatening way.

Assuming that processing biases are learnt through a real-world version of cognitive bias modification training, it is important to know the mechanism underlying this learning to inform treatment practices that target these biases (Cowart & Ollendick, 2010). Field and Lester (2010a) try to explain the learning process in terms of conditioning (see Field and Purkis, Chapter 11, this volume for a review of the role of conditioning in anxiety generally). In the case of attentional biases, there is evidence that biases can be trained to neutral stimuli through fear conditioning (Koster, Crombez, Verschuere, & De Houwer, 2006; Purkis & Lipp, 2009). Field and Lester (2010a) adopt Dickinson's distinction between goal-directed and habitual instrumental learning: the habitual learning system is used for stimulus–response learning and does not encode details of the outcome, whereas a separate system for learning goal-directed action does encode information about the outcome (Dickinson, Balleine, Watt, Gonzalez, & Boakes, 1995). Based on evidence that goal-directed instrumental learning becomes easier in humans aged over 2 years old (Klossek, Russell, & Dickinson, 2008), Field and Lester (2010a) argue that attentional biases to threat are acquired through the habitual system because they have been shown much earlier than 2 years old (e.g., Rakison & Derringer, 2008). They also point out that it is reasonable to assume that a stimulus–outcome association is learned through Pavlovian associative learning because in the real world there isn't a "correct" response so children are probably not reinforced for directing attention to threat. Instead, when faced with potential threat they pick up on other people's attention (through social referencing) or the consequences of being in the presence of the stimulus (e.g., their parent removes them from the situation).

In contrast, Field and Lester (2010a) argued that interpretational biases will take advantage of the more complex goal-oriented learning system because these biases require an understanding of the implicational meaning of responses. Theoretically interpretation biases *could* be learnt over successive trials through the habitual learning system with an association formed between an ambiguous cue and a threat response (the interpretation); however, Field and Lester (2010a) argue that it is more likely that children learn a simple stimulus–outcome association. In simple terms, they learn "when faced with ambiguity the outcome will be bad."

As such, Field and Lester's (2010a) theory suggests that attentional bias and interpretational biases are underpinned by different learning systems. Attentional biases are learnt through a habitual learning system that is present early in development, whereas interpretational biases are learnt through a more complex goal-oriented learning system that is in evidence more after the age of 2 years. One obvious prediction from this theory is that attentional biases should be present in infancy, whereas interpretational biases should not. As we have seen in this chapter the available evidence backs up this prediction (although there are good methodological reasons why to date interpretational biases have not been demonstrated in infants).

A final point that Field and Lester (2010a) make is that the "outcomes" to which we have referred need not be real because imagined outcomes are sufficient to sustain the formation of associative connections (see Field, 2006a, for a review). This implies that a parent/external agent's response to a stimulus/situation does not in itself need to be traumatic or negative, it needs only to trigger imagery or cognitions that are traumatic in the child; these mental representations alone can be a sufficiently negative outcome. Also, if attentional and interpretational biases develop through operant (stimulus–response) or classical (stimulus–stimulus) associations, the underlying mechanism driving them is an association in memory. Therefore, models of associative learning (see Field & Purkis, Chapter 11, this volume for a review) are a useful framework for predicting and correcting information processing biases. For example, these biases could be weakened through variations on extinction procedures.

Summary

In this chapter we have tried to present an overview of both the evidence for information processing biases in anxious children and adolescents, and the causal role that these biases play. In addition, we have focused on the existing theoretical frameworks that have been put forward for looking at how these biases interact with child development and the mechanisms that might underpin them. We have seen that the evidence base in child and adolescent samples is somewhat more variable than in adult samples; there are also relatively few theories that look specifically at developmental issues when trying to explain how these processing biases are acquired. In many ways this is a disappointing state of affairs, but it also leaves room for innovative and exciting research in the future. There are many questions to be answered, and many of them will involve creative methodological thinking. For example, distinguishing moderation from acquisition models of interpretation biases will require some serious thought about age-appropriate methods for testing interpretation biases in pre-linguistic children. Also, there is, as yet, very little direct evidence to support learning-based theories of processing biases and the role that the family plays in this learning. Researchers have a very challenging and thrilling journey ahead; we would not want it any other way.

Acknowledgment

Andy Field wrote this chapter while funded by Economic and Social Research Council grant number RES-062–23-0406.

References

Alfano, C. A., Beidel, D. C., & Turner, S. M. (2002). Cognition in childhood anxiety: conceptual, methodological, and developmental issues. *Clinical Psychology Review*, **22**, 1209–1238.

Amir, N., Beard, C., Burns, M., & Bomyea, J. (2009). Attention modification program in individuals with generalized anxiety disorder. *Journal of Abnormal Psychology*, **118**, 28–33. doi: 10.1037/a0012589

Asendorpf, J. B., Denissen, J. J. A., & van Aken, M. A. G. (2008). Inhibited and aggressive preschool children at 23 years of age: personality and social transitions into adulthood. *Developmental Psychology*, **44**, 997–1011. doi: 10.1037/0012–1649.44.4.997

Ashcraft, M. H. (2002). Math anxiety: personal, educational, and cognitive consequences. *Current Directions in Psychological Science*, **11**, 181–185.

Bar-Haim, Y., Lamy, D., Pergamin, L., Bakermans-Kranenburg, M. J., & van IJzendoorn, M. H. (2007). Threat-related attentional bias in anxious and nonanxious individuals: a meta-analytic study. *Psychological Bulletin*, **133**, 1–24.

Barrett, P. M., Rapee, R. M., Dadds, M. M., & Ryan, S. M. (1996). Family enhancement of cognitive style in anxious and aggressive children. *Journal of Abnormal Child Psychology*, **24**, 187–203.

Beck, A. T. & Clark, D. A. (1997). An information processing model of anxiety: automatic and strategic processes. *Behaviour Research and Therapy*, **35**, 49–58.

Beesdo, K., Hoyer, J., Jacobi, F., Low, N. C. P., Höfler, M., & Wittchen, H. U. (2009). Association between generalized anxiety levels and pain in a community sample: evidence for diagnostic specificity. *Journal of Anxiety Disorders*, **23**, 684–693. doi: 10.1016/j.janxdis.2009.02.007

Belsky, J. & Pluess, M. (2009). Beyond diathesis stress: differential susceptibility to environmental influences. *Psychological Bulletin*, **135**, 885–908. doi: 10.1037/a0017376

Benoit, K. E., McNally, R. J., Rapee, R. M., Gamble, A. L., & Wiseman, A. L. (2007). Processing of emotional faces in children and adolescents with anxiety disorders. *Behavior Change*, **24**, 183–194.

Bögels, S. M. & Zigterman, D. (2000). Dysfunctional cognitions in children with social phobia, separation anxiety disorder, and generalized anxiety disorder. *Journal of Abnormal Child Psychology*, **28**, 205–211.

Brotman, M. A., Rich, B. A., Schmajuk, M., Reising, M., Monk, C. S., Dickstein, D. P., *et al.* (2007). Attention bias to threat faces in children with bipolar disorder and comorbid lifetime anxiety disorders. *Biological Psychiatry*, **61**, 819–821. doi: 10.1016/j.biopsych.2006.08.021

Byrne, A. & Eysenck, M. W. (1995). Trait anxiety, anxious mood, and threat detection. *Cognition and Emotion*, **9**, 549–562.

Chorpita, B. F., Albano, A. M., & Barlow, D. H. (1996). Cognitive processing in children: relation to anxiety and family influences. *Journal of Clinical Child Psychology*, **25**, 170–176.

Cowart, M. J. W. & Ollendick, T. H. (2010). Attentional biases in children: implications for treatment. In: J. A. Hadwin & A. P. Field (eds.) *Information Processing Biases and Anxiety: A Developmental Perspective*, pp. 297–319. Chichester, UK: Wiley-Blackwell.

Creswell, C. & O'Connor, T. G. (2006). "Anxious cognitions" in children: an exploration of associations and mediators. *British Journal of Developmental Psychology*, **24**, 761–766.

Creswell, C. & O'Connor, T. G. (2011). Interpretation bias and anxiety in childhood: stability, specificity and longitudinal associations. *Behavioural and Cognitive Psychotherapy*, **39**, 191–204.

Creswell, C., Cooper, P., & Murray, L. (2010). Intergenerational transmission of anxious information processing biases. In: J. A. Hadwin & A. P. Field (eds.) *Information Processing Biases and Anxiety: A Developmental Perspective*, pp. 279–295. Chichester, UK: Wiley-Blackwell.

Creswell, C., O'Connor, T. G., & Brewin, C. R. (2006). A longitudinal investigation of maternal and child "anxious cognitions." *Cognitive Therapy and Research*, **30**, 135–147.

Creswell, C., Shildrick, S., & Field, A. P. (2010). Interpretation of ambiguity in children: a prospective study of associations with anxiety and parental interpretations. *Journal of Child and Family Studies*. doi: 10.1007/s10826–010–9390–7

Crozier, W. R. & Hostettler, K. (2003). The influence of shyness on children's test performance. *British Journal of Educational Psychology*, **73**, 317–328.

Dalgleish, T., Moradi, A., Taghavi, M., Neshat-Doost, H. T., & Yule, W. (2001). An experimental investigation of hypervigilance for threat in children and adolescents with post-traumatic stress disorder. *Psychological Medicine*, **31**, 541–547.

Dalgleish, T., Taghavi, R., Neshat-Doost, H., Moradi, A. R., Canterbury, R., & Yule, W. (2003). Patterns of processing bias for emotional information across clinical disorders: a comparison of attention, memory, and prospective cognition in children and adolescents with depression, generalized anxiety, and posttraumatic stress disorder. *Journal of Clinical Child and Adolescent Psychology*, **32**, 10–21.

Dickinson, A., Balleine, B., Watt, A., Gonzalez, F., & Boakes, R. A. (1995). Motivational control after extended instrumental training. *Animal Learning and Behavior*, **23**, 197–206.

Dineen, K. A. & Hadwin, J. A. (2004). Anxious and depressive symptoms and children's judgements of their own and others' interpretation of ambiguous social scenarios. *Journal of Anxiety Disorders*, **18**, 499–513. doi: 10.1016/s0887–6185(03)00030–6

Donnelly, N., Hadwin, J. A., Manneer, T., & Richards, H. (2010). The use of visual search paradigms to understand attentional biases in childhood anxiety. In: J. A. Hadwin & A. P. Field (eds.) *Information Processing Biases and Anxiety: A Developmental Perspective*, pp. 109–127. Chichester, UK: Wiley-Blackwell.

Dubner, A. E. & Motta, R. W. (1999). Sexually and physically abused foster care children and posttraumatic stress disorder. *Journal of Consulting and Clinical Psychology*, **67**, 367–373.

Eastwood, J. D., Smilek, D., Oakman, J. M., Farvolden, P., van Ameringen, M., Mancini, C., et al. (2005). Individuals with social phobia are biased to become aware of negative faces. *Visual Cognition*, **12**, 159–179. doi: 10.1080/13506280444000175

Eley, T. C., Gregory, A. M., Clark, D. M., & Ehlers, A. (2007). Feeling anxious: a twin study of panic/somatic ratings, anxiety sensitivity and heartbeat perception in children. *Journal of Child Psychology and Psychiatry*, **48**, 1184–1191. doi: 10.1111/j.1469–7610.2007.01838.x

Eley, T. C., Sugden, K., Corsico, A., Gregory, A. M., Sham, P., McGuffin, P., et al. (2004). Gene–environment interaction analysis of serotonin system markers with adolescent depression. *Molecular Psychiatry*, **9**, 908–915. doi: 10.1038/sj.mp.4001546

Erath, S. A., Flanagan, K. S., & Bierman, K. L. (2007). Social anxiety and peer relations in early adolescence: behavioral and cognitive factors. *Journal of Abnormal Child Psychology*, **35**, 405–416. doi: 10.1007/s10802–007–9099–2

Eschenbeck, H., Kohlmann, C. W., Heim-Dreger, U., Koller, D., & Leser, M. (2004). Processing bias and anxiety in primary school children: a modified emotional Stroop colour-naming task using pictorial facial expressions. *Psychology Science*, **46**, 451–465.

Eysenck, M. W., Derakshan, N., Santos, R., & Calvo, M. G. (2007). Anxiety and cognitive performance: attentional control theory. *Emotion*, **7**, 336–353. doi: 10.1037/1528–3542.7.2.336

Field, A. P. (2006a). Is conditioning a useful framework for understanding the development and treatment of phobias? *Clinical Psychology Review*, **26**, 857–875. doi: 10.1016/j.cpr.2005.05.010

Field, A. P. (2006b). Watch out for the beast: fear information and attentional bias in children. *Journal of Clinical Child and Adolescent Psychology*, **35**, 431–439.

Field, A. P. & Lawson, J. (2008). The verbal information pathway to fear and subsequent causal learning in children. *Cognition and Emotion*, **22**, 459–479. doi: 10.1080/02699930801886532

Field, A. P. & Lester, K. J. (2010a). Learning of information processing biases in anxious children and adolescents. In: J. A. Hadwin & A. P. Field (eds.) *Information Processing Biases and Anxiety: A Developmental Perspective*, pp. 253–278. Chichester, UK: Wiley-Blackwell.

Field, A. P. & Lester, K. J. (2010b). Is there room for 'development' in developmental models of information processing biases to threat in children and adolescents? *Clinical Child and Family Psychology Review*, **13**, 315–332. doi: 10.1007/s10567–010–0078–8

Field, A. P., Lawson, J., & Banerjee, R. (2008). The verbal information pathway to fear in children: the longitudinal effects on fear cognitions and the immediate effects on avoidance behavior. *Journal of Abnormal Psychology*, **117**, 214–224.

Freeman, J. B. & Beck, J. G. (2000). Cognitive interference for trauma cues in sexually abused adolescent girls with posttraumatic stress disorder. *Journal of Clinical Child Psychology*, **29**, 245–256.

Garner, M. (2010). Assessment of attentional bias using the dot-probe task in anxious children and adolescents. In: J. Hadwin & A. P. Field (eds.) *Information Processing Biases and Anxiety: A Developmental Perspective*, pp. 77–109. Chichester, UK: Wiley-Blackwell.

Gray, J. A. & McNaughton, N. (2003). *The Neuropsychology of Anxiety: An Enquiry into the Functions of the Septo-Hippocampal System*, 2nd edn. New York: Oxford University Press.

Hadwin, J. A. & Field, A. P. (eds.) (2010). *Information Processing Biases and Anxiety: A Developmental Perspective*. Chichester, UK: Wiley-Blackwell.

Hadwin, J. A., Donnelly, N., French, C. C., Richards, A., Watts, A., & Daley, D. (2003). The influence of children's self-report trait anxiety and depression on visual search for emotional faces. *Journal of Child Psychology and Psychiatry and Allied Disciplines*, **44**, 432–444.

Hadwin, J. A., Donnelly, N., Richards, A., French, C. C., & Patel, U. (2009). Childhood anxiety and attention to emotion faces in a modified Stroop task. *British Journal of Developmental Psychology*, **27**, 487–494.

Hadwin, J. A., Frost, S., French, C. C., & Richards, A. (1997). Cognitive processing and trait anxiety in typically developing children: evidence for an interpretation bias. *Journal of Abnormal Psychology*, **106**, 486–490.

Hadwin, J. A., Garner, M., & Perez-Olivas, G. (2006). The development of information processing biases in childhood anxiety: a review and exploration of its origins in parenting. *Clinical Psychology Review*, **26**, 876–894. doi: 10.1016/j.cpr.2005.09.004

Hare, T. A., Tottenham, N., Davidson, M. C., Glover, G. H., & Casey, B. J. (2005). Contributions of amygdala and striatal activity in emotion regulation. *Biological Psychiatry*, **57**, 624–632. doi: 10.1016/j.biopsych.2004.12.038

Heim-Dreger, U., Kohlmann, C. W., Eschenbeck, H., & Burkhardt, U. (2006). Attentional biases for threatening faces in children: vigilant and avoidant processes. *Emotion*, **6**, 320–325.

Helzer, E. G., Connor-Smith, J. K., & Reed, M. A. (2009). Traits, states, and attentional gates: temperament and threat relevance as predictors of attentional bias to social threat. *Anxiety Stress and Coping*, **22**, 57–76. doi: 10.1080/10615800802272244

Hudson, J. L. & Rapee, R. (2004). From anxious temperament to disorder: an etiological model of generalized anxiety disorder. In: R. G. Heimberg, C. L. Turk, & D. S. Mennin (eds.) *Generalized Anxiety Disorder: Advances in Research and Practice*, pp. 51–74. New York: Guilford Press.

Hunt, C., Keogh, E., & French, C. C. (2007). Anxiety sensitivity, conscious awareness and selective attentional biases in children. *Behaviour Research and Therapy*, **45**, 497–509. doi: 10.1016/j.brat.2006.04.001

Kim-Cohen, J., Caspi, A., Moffitt, T. E., Harrington, H., Milne, B. J., & Poulton, R. (2003). Prior juvenile diagnoses in adults with mental disorder: developmental follow-back of a prospective-longitudinal cohort. *Archives of General Psychiatry*, **60**, 709–717.

Kindt, M. & Brosschot, J. F. (1999). Cognitive bias in spider-phobic children: comparison of a pictorial and a linguistic spider Stroop. *Journal of Psychopathology and Behavioral Assessment*, **21**, 207–220.

Kindt, M. & **van den Hout, M.** (2001). Selective attention and anxiety: a perspective on developmental issues and the causal status. *Journal of Psychopathology and Behavioral Assessment*, **23**, 193–202.

Kindt, M., Bierman, D., & **Brosschot, J. F.** (1997). Cognitive bias in spider fear and control children: assessment of emotional interference by a card format and a single-trial format of the Stroop task. *Journal of Experimental Child Psychology*, **66**, 163–179.

Kindt, M., Bögels, S., & **Morren, M.** (2003). Processing bias in children with separation anxiety disorder, social phobia and generalised anxiety disorder. *Behaviour Change*, **20**, 143–150.

Kindt, M., Brosschot, J. F., & **Everaerd, W.** (1997). Cognitive processing bias of children in a real life stress situation and a neutral situation. *Journal of Experimental Child Psychology*, **64**, 79–97.

Kindt, M., van den Hout, M., de Jong, P., & **Hoekzema, B.** (2000). Cognitive bias for pictorial and linguistic threat cues in children. *Journal of Psychopathology and Behavioral Assessment*, **22**, 201–219.

Klossek, U. M. H., Russell, J., & **Dickinson, A.** (2008). The control of instrumental action following outcome devaluation in young children aged between 1 and 4 years. *Journal of Experimental Psychology – General*, **137**, 39–51. doi: 10.1037/0096–3445.137.1.39

Koster, E. H. W., Crombez, G., Verschuere, B., & **De Houwer, J.** (2006). Attention to threat in anxiety-prone individuals: mechanisms underlying attentional bias. *Cognitive Therapy and Research*, **30**, 635–643. doi: 10.1007/s10608–006-9042–9

Ladouceur, C. D., Dahl, R. E., Williamson, D. E., Birmaher, B., Axelson, D. A., Ryan, N. D., *et al.* (2006). Processing emotional facial expressions influences performance on a Go/NoGo task in pediatric anxiety and depression. *Journal of Child Psychology and Psychiatry*, **47**, 1107–1115. doi: 10.1111/j.1469–7610.2006.01640.x

Lau, J. Y. F., Burt, M., Leibenluft, E., Pine, D. S., Rijsdijk, F., Shiffrin, N., *et al.* (2009). Individual differences in children's facial expression recognition ability: the role of nature and nurture. *Developmental Neuropsychology*, **34**, 37–51. doi: 10.1080/87565640802564424

Legerstee, J. S., Tulen, J. H. M., Kallen, V. L., Dieleman, G. C., Treffers, P. D. A., Verhulst, F. C., *et al.* (2009). Threat-related selective attention predicts treatment success in childhood anxiety disorders. *Journal of the American Academy of Child and Adolescent Psychiatry*, **48**, 196–205. doi: 10.1097/CHI.0b013e31819176e4

Leonardo, E. D. & **Hen, R.** (2008). Anxiety as a developmental disorder. *Neuropsychopharmacology*, **33**, 134–140. doi: 10.1038/sj.npp.1301569

Lester, K. J., Field, A. P., Oliver, S., & **Cartwright-Hatton, S.** (2009). Do anxious parents interpretive biases towards threat extend into their child's environment? *Behaviour Research and Therapy*, **47**, 170–174. doi: 10.1016/j.brat.2008.11.005

Lester, K. J., Seal, K., Nightingale, Z. C., & **Field, A. P.** (2010). Are children's own interpretations of ambiguous situations based on how they perceive their mothers have interpreted ambiguous situations for them in the past? *Journal of Anxiety Disorders*, **24**, 102–108. doi: 10.1016/j.janxdis.2009.09.004

Lewinsohn, P. M., Holm-Denoma, J. M., Small, J. W., Seeley, J. R., & **Joiner, T. E.** (2008). Separation anxiety disorder in childhood as a risk factor for future mental illness. *Journal of the American Academy of Child and Adolescent Psychiatry*, **47**, 548–555. doi: 10.1097/CHI.0b013e31816765e7

Lipp, O. V. & **Derakshan, N.** (2005). Attentional bias to pictures of fear-relevant animals in a dot probe task. *Emotion*, **5**, 365–369.

LoBue, V. & **DeLoache, J. S.** (2008). Detecting the snake in the grass: attention to fear-relevant stimuli by adults and young children. *Psychological Science*, **19**, 284–289.

LoBue, V. & **DeLoache, J. S.** (2010). Superior detection of threat-relevant stimuli in infancy. *Developmental Science*, **13**, 221–228. doi: 10.1111/j.1467–7687.2009.00872.x

Manassis, K. & Bradley, S. J. (1994). The development of childhood anxiety disorders: toward an integrated model. *Journal of Applied Developmental Psychology*, **15**, 345–366. doi: 10.1016/0193–3973(94)90037-X

Martin, J. M. & Cole, D. A. (2000). Using the personal Stroop to detect children's awareness of social rejection by peers. *Cognition and Emotion*, **14**, 241–260.

Martin, M. & Jones, G. V. (1995). Integral bias in the cognitive processing of emotionally linked pictures. *British Journal of Psychology*, **86**, 419–435.

Martin, M., Horder, P., & Jones, G. V. (1992). Integral bias in naming of phobia-related words. *Cognition and Emotion*, **6**, 479–486.

Mathews, A. & Mackintosh, B. (1998). A cognitive model of selective processing in anxiety. *Cognitive Therapy and Research*, **22**, 539–560.

Mathews, A. & Mackintosh, B. (2000). Induced emotional interpretation bias and anxiety. *Journal of Abnormal Psychology*, **109**, 602–615.

Mathews, A. & MacLeod, C. (2002). Induced processing biases have causal effects on anxiety. *Cognition and Emotion*, **16**, 331–354.

Monk, C. S., Klein, R. G., Telzer, E. H., Schroth, E. A., Mannuzza, S., Moulton, J. L., et al. (2008). Amygdala and nucleus accumbens activation to emotional facial expressions in children and adolescents at risk for major depression. *American Journal of Psychiatry*, **165**, 90–98.

Monk, C. S., Telzer, E. H., Mogg, K., Bradley, B. P., Mai, X. Q., Louro, H. M. C., et al. (2008). Amygdala and ventrolateral prefrontal cortex activation to masked angry faces in children and adolescents with generalized anxiety disorder. *Archives of General Psychiatry*, **65**, 568–576.

Moradi, A. R., Taghavi, M. R., Neshat-Doost, H. T., Yule, W., & Dalgleish, T. (1999). Performance of children and adolescents with PTSD on the Stroop colour-naming task. *Psychological Medicine*, **29**, 415–419.

Morren, M., Kindt, M., van den Hout, M., & van Kasteren, H. (2003). Anxiety and the processing of threat in children: further examination of the cognitive inhibition hypothesis. *Behaviour Change*, **20**, 131–142.

Morren, M., Muris, P., & Kindt, M. (2004). Emotional reasoning and parent-based reasoning in normal children. *Child Psychiatry and Human Development*, **35**, 3–20.

Muris, P. (2007). *Normal and Abnormal Fear and Anxiety in Children and Adolescents*. Oxford, UK: Elsevier Science.

Muris, P. (2010). Anxiety-related reasoning biases in children and adolescents. In: J. Hadwin & A. P. Field (eds.) *Information Processing Biases and Anxiety: A Developmental Perspective*, pp. 21–45. Chichester, UK: Wiley-Blackwell.

Muris, P. & Field, A. P. (2008). Distorted cognition and pathological anxiety in children and adolescents. *Cognition and Emotion*, **22**, 395–421. doi: 10.1080/02699930701843450

Muris, P., de Jong, P. J., Meesters, C., Waterreus, B., & van Lubeck, J. (2005). An experimental study of spider-related covariation bias in 8- to 13-year-old children. *Child Psychiatry and Human Development*, **35**, 185–201.

Muris, P., Hoeve, I., Meesters, C., & Mayer, B. (2004). Children's conception and interpretation of anxiety-related physical symptoms. *Journal of Behavior Therapy and Experimental Psychiatry*, **35**, 233–244.

Muris, P., Huijding, J., Mayer, B., den Breejen, E., & Makkelie, M. (2007). Spider fear and covariation bias in children and adolescents. *Behaviour Research and Therapy*, **45**, 2604–2615. doi: 10.1016/j.brat.2007.06.002

Muris, P., Huijding, J., Mayer, B., & Hameetman, M. (2008). A space odyssey: experimental manipulation of threat perception and anxiety-related interpretation bias in children. *Child Psychiatry and Human Development*, **39**, 469–480.

Muris, P., Huijding, J., Mayer, B., Remmerswaal, D., & Vreden, S. (2009). Ground control to Major Tom: experimental manipulation of anxiety-related interpretation bias by means of the "space odyssey" paradigm and effects on avoidance tendencies in children. *Journal of Anxiety Disorders*, **23**, 333–340. doi: 10.1016/j.janxdis.2009.01.004

Muris, P., Kindt, M., Bögels, S., Merckelbach, H., Gadet, B., & Moulaert, V. (2000). Anxiety and threat perception abnormalities in normal children. *Journal of Psychopathology and Behavioral Assessment*, **22**, 183–199.

Muris, P., Luermans, J., Merckelbach, H., & Mayer, B. (2000). "Danger is lurking everywhere": the relation between anxiety and threat perception abnormalities in normal children. *Journal of Behavior Therapy and Experimental Psychiatry*, **31**, 123–136.

Muris, P., Mayer, B., & Bervoets, S. (2010). Listen to your heart beat and shiver! An experimental study of anxiety-related emotional reasoning in children. *Journal of Anxiety Disorders*, **24**, 612–617. doi: 10.1016/j.janxdis.2010.04.002

Muris, P., Mayer, B., Freher, N. K., Duncan, S., & van den Hout, A. (2010). Children's internal attributions of anxiety-related physical symptoms: age-related patterns and the role of cognitive development and anxiety sensitivity. *Child Psychiatry and Human Development*, **41**, 535–548. doi: 10.1007/s10578–010-0186–1

Muris, P., Mayer, B., Vermeulen, L., & Hiemstra, H. (2007). Theory-of-mind, cognitive development, and children's interpretation of anxiety-related physical symptoms. *Behaviour Research and Therapy*, **45**, 2121–2132. doi: 10.1016/j.brat.2007.02.014

Muris, P., Merckelbach, H., & Damsma, E. (2000). Threat perception bias in non-referred, socially anxious children. *Journal of Clinical Child Psychology*, **29**, 348–359.

Muris, P., Merckelbach, H., & Luijten, M. (2002). The connection between cognitive development and specific fears and worries in normal children and children with below-average intellectual abilities: a preliminary study. *Behaviour Research and Therapy*, **40**, 37–56.

Muris, P., Merckelbach, H., & van Spauwen, I. (2003). The emotional reasoning heuristic in children. *Behaviour Research and Therapy*, **41**, 261–272.

Muris, P., Rapee, R., Meesters, C., Schouten, E., & Geers, M. (2003). Threat perception abnormalities in children: the role of anxiety disorders symptoms, chronic anxiety, and state anxiety. *Journal of Anxiety Disorders*, **17**, 271–287.

Muris, P., Rassin, E., Mayer, B., Smeets, G., Huijding, J., Remmerswaal, D., *et al.* (2009). Effects of verbal information on fear-related reasoning biases in children. *Behaviour Research and Therapy*, **47**, 206–214. doi: 10.1016/j.brat.2008.12.002

Muris, P., Vermeer, E., & Horselenberg, R. (2008). Cognitive development and the interpretation of anxiety-related physical symptoms in 4- to 12-year-old non-clinical children. *Journal of Behavior Therapy and Experimental Psychiatry*, **39**, 73–86.

Murray, L., Cooper, P., Creswell, C., Schofield, E., & Sack, C. (2007). The effects of maternal social phobia on mother–infant interactions and infant social responsiveness. *Journal of Child Psychology and Psychiatry*, **48**, 45–52. doi: 10.1111/j.1469–7610.2006.01657.x

Nightingale, Z. C., Field, A. P., & Kindt, M. (2010). The emotional Stroop task in anxious children. In: J. A. Hadwin & A. P. Field (eds.) *Information Processing Biases and Anxiety: A Developmental Perspective*, pp. 47–75. Chichester, UK: Wiley-Blackwell.

Öhman, A. (1993). Fear and anxiety as emotional phenomena. In: M. Lewis & J. Haviland (eds.) *Handbook of Emotions*, pp. 511–536. New York: Guilford Press.

Öhman, A. & Mineka, S. (2001). Fears, phobias, and preparedness: toward an evolved module of fear and fear learning. *Psychological Review*, **108**, 483–522.

Owens, M., Stevenson, J., Norgate, R., & Hadwin, J. A. (2008). Processing efficiency theory in children: working memory as a mediator between trait anxiety and academic performance. *Anxiety Stress and Coping*, **21**, 417–430. doi: 10.1080/10615800701847823

Perez-Olivas, G., Stevenson, J., & Hadwin, J. A. (2008). Do anxiety-related attentional biases mediate the link between maternal over involvement and separation anxiety in children? *Cognition and Emotion*, **22**, 509–521. doi: 10.1080/02699930801886656

Pine, D. S., Mogg, K., Bradley, B. P., Montgomery, L., Monk, C. S., McClure, E., *et al.* (2005). Attention bias to threat in maltreated children: implications for vulnerability to stress-related psychopathology. *American Journal of Psychiatry*, **162**, 291–296.

Purkis, H. M. & Lipp, O. V. (2009). Are snakes and spiders special? Acquisition of negative valence and modified attentional processing by non-fear-relevant animal stimuli. *Cognition and Emotion*, **23**, 430–452. doi: 10.1080/02699930801993973

Rakison, D. H. & Derringer, J. L. (2008). Do infants possess an evolved spider-detection mechanism? *Cognition and Emotion*, **107**, 381–393.

Rapee, R. M. (2001). The development of generalized anxiety. In: M. W. Vasey & M. R. Dadds (eds.) *The Developmental Psychopathology of Anxiety*, pp. 481–503. Oxford, UK: Oxford University Press.

Richards, A., French, C. C., Nash, G., Hadwin, J. A., & Donnelly, N. (2007). A comparison of selective attention and facial processing biases in typically developing children who are high and low in self-reported trait anxiety. *Development and Psychopathology*, **19**, 481–495.

Richards, A., Richards, L. C., & McGeeney, A. (2000). Anxiety-related Stroop interference in adolescents. *Journal of General Psychology*, **127**, 327–333.

Rinck, M., Reinecke, A., Ellwart, T., Heuer, K., & Becker, E. S. (2005). Speeded detection and increased distraction in fear of spiders: evidence from eye movements. *Journal of Abnormal Psychology*, **114**, 235–248. doi: 10.1037/0021–843x.114.2.235

Roy, A. K., Vasa, R. A., Bruck, M., Mogg, K., Bradley, B. P., Sweeney, M., *et al.* (2008). Attention bias toward threat in pediatric anxiety disorders. *Journal of the American Academy of Child and Adolescent Psychiatry*, **47**, 1189–1196. doi: 10.1097/CHI.0b013e3181825ace

Roza, S. J., Hofstra, M. B., van der Ende, J., & Verhulst, F. C. (2003). Stable prediction of mood and anxiety disorders based on behavioral and emotional problems in childhood: a 14-year follow-up during childhood, adolescence, and young adulthood. *American Journal of Psychiatry*, **160**, 2116–2121.

Salemink, E., van den Hout, M., & Kindt, M. (2010). How does cognitive bias modification affect anxiety? Mediation analyses and experimental data. *Behavioural and Cognitive Psychotherapy*, **38**, 59–66. doi: 10.1017/s1352465809990543

Schaffer, H. R. (2006). *Key Concepts in Developmental Psychology*. London: Sage.

Schmidt, N. B., Richey, J. A., Buckner, J. D., & Timpano, K. R. (2009). Attention training for generalized social anxiety disorder. *Journal of Abnormal Psychology*, **118**, 5–14. doi: 10.1037/a0013643

Schneider, S., Unnewehr, S., In-Albon, T., & Margraf, J. (2008). Attention bias in children of patients with panic disorder. *Psychopathology*, **41**, 179–186.

Schwartz, C. E., Snidman, N., & Kagan, J. (1996). Early temperamental predictors to Stroop interference to threatening information at adolescence. *Journal of Anxiety Disorders*, **10**, 89–96.

See, J., MacLeod, C., & Bridle, R. (2009). The reduction of anxiety vulnerability through the modification of attentional bias: a real-world study using a home-based cognitive bias modification procedure. *Journal of Abnormal Psychology*, **118**, 65–75. doi: 10.1037/a0014377

Silberg, J., Rutter, M., Neale, M., & Eaves, L. (2001). Genetic moderation of environmental risk for depression and anxiety in adolescent girls. *British Journal of Psychiatry*, **179**, 116–121.

Soares, S. C., Esteves, F., & Flykt, A. (2009). Fear, but not fear-relevance, modulates reaction times in visual search with animal distractors. *Journal of Anxiety Disorders*, **23**, 136–144. doi: 10.1016/j.janxdis.2008.05.002

Stirling, L. J., Eley, T. C., & Clark, D. M. (2006). Preliminary evidence for an association between social anxiety symptoms and avoidance of negative faces in school-age children. *Journal of Clinical Child and Adolescent Psychology*, **35**, 440–445.

Suarez, L. & Bell-Dolan, D. (2001). The relationship of child worry to cognitive biases: threat interpretation and likelihood of event occurrence. *Behavior Therapy*, **32**, 425–442.

Taghavi, M. R., Dalgleish, T., Moradi, A. R., Neshat-Doost, H. T., & Yule, W. (2003). Selective processing of negative emotional information in children and adolescents with Generalized Anxiety Disorder. *British Journal of Clinical Psychology*, **42**, 221–230.

Taghavi, M. R., Moradi, A. R., Neshat-Doost, H. T., Yule, W., & Dalgleish, T. (2000). Interpretation of ambiguous emotional information in clinically anxious children and adolescents. *Cognition and Emotion*, **14**, 809–822.

Taghavi, M. R., Neshat-Doost, H. T., Moradi, A. R., Yule, W., & Dalgleish, T. (1999). Biases in visual attention in children and adolescents with clinical anxiety and mixed anxiety–depression. *Journal of Abnormal Child Psychology*, **27**, 215–223.

Telzer, E. H., Mogg, K., Bradley, B. P., Mai, X. Q., Ernst, M., Pine, D. S., *et al.* (2008). Relationship between trait anxiety, prefrontal cortex, and attention bias to angry faces in children and adolescents. *Biological Psychology*, **79**, 216–222. doi: 10.1016/j.biopsycho.2008.05.004

Thrasher, C., LoBue, V., Coan, J. A., & DeLoache, J. S. (2009). Infants orient more quickly to threatening voices. *Psychophysiology*, **46**, S138–S139.

Tomarken, A. J., Cook, M., & Mineka, S. (1989). Fear-relevant selective associations and covariation bias. *Journal of Abnormal Psychology*, **98**, 381–394.

van Strien, J. W. & Valstar, L. H. (2004). The lateralized emotional Stroop task: left visual-field interference in women. *Emotion*, **4**, 403–409.

Vasey, M. W., Daleiden, E. L., Williams, L. L., & Brown, L. M. (1995). Biased attention in childhood anxiety disorders: a preliminary study. *Journal of Abnormal Child Psychology*, **23**, 267–279.

Vasey, M. W., El Hag, N., & Daleiden, E. L. (1996). Anxiety and the processing of emotionally threatening stimuli: distinctive patterns of selective attention among high- and low-test-anxious children. *Child Development*, **67**, 1173–1185.

Waters, A. M. & Lipp, O. V. (2008a). The influence of animal fear on attentional capture by fear-relevant animal stimuli in children. *Behaviour Research and Therapy*, **46**, 114–121. doi: 10.1016/j.brat.2007.11.002

Waters, A. M. & Lipp, O. V. (2008b). Visual search for emotional faces in children. *Cognition and Emotion*, **22**, 1306–1326. doi: 10.1080/02699930701755530

Waters, A. M. & Valvoi, J. S. (2009). Attentional bias for emotional faces in pediatric anxiety disorders: an investigation using the emotional go/no go task. *Journal of Behavior Therapy and Experimental Psychiatry*, **40**, 306–316.

Waters, A. M., Craske, M. G., Bergman, R. L., & Treanor, M. (2008). Threat interpretation bias as a vulnerability factor in childhood anxiety disorders. *Behaviour Research and Therapy*, **46**, 39–47. doi: 10.1016/j.brat.2007.10.002

Waters, A. M., Henry, J., Mogg, K., Bradley, B. P., & Pine, D. S. (2010). Attentional bias towards angry faces in childhood anxiety disorders. *Journal of Behavior Therapy and Experimental Psychiatry*, **41**, 158–164. doi: 10.1016/j.jbtep.2009.12.001

Waters, A. M., Lipp, O. V., & Spence, S. H. (2004). Attentional bias toward fear-related stimuli: an investigation with non-selected children and adults and children with anxiety disorders. *Journal of Experimental Child Psychology*, **89**, 320–337. doi: 10.1016/j.jecp.2004.06.003

Waters, A. M., Lipp, O., & Spence, S. H. (2008). Visual search for animal fear-relevant stimuli in children. *Australian Journal of Psychology*, **60**, 112–125. doi: 10.1080/00049530701549346

Waters, A. M., Mogg, K., Bradley, B. P., & Pine, D. S. (2008). Attentional bias for emotional faces in children with generalized anxiety disorder. *Journal of the American Academy of Child and Adolescent Psychiatry*, **47**, 435–442. doi: 10.1097/CHI.0b013e3181642992

Waters, A. M., Wharton, T. A., Zimmer-Gembeck, M. J., & Craske, M. G. (2008). Threat-based cognitive biases in anxious children: comparison with non-anxious children before and after cognitive behavioral treatment. *Behaviour Research and Therapy*, **46**, 358–374. doi: 10.1016/j.brat.2008.01.002

Weems, C. F. (2008). Developmental trajectories of childhood anxiety: identifying continuity and change in anxious emotion. *Developmental Review*, **28**, 488–502. doi: 10.1016/j.dr.2008.01.001

Williams, J. M. G., MacLeod, C., Watts, F., & Mathews, A. (1997). *Cognitive Psychology and Emotional Disorders*, 2nd edn. Chichester, UK: Wiley & Sons.

Wilson, E. J., MacLeod, C., Mathews, A., & Rutherford, E. M. (2006). The causal role of interpretive bias in anxiety reactivity. *Journal of Abnormal Psychology*, **115**, 103–111.

Yiend, J., Mackintosh, B., & Mathews, A. (2005). Enduring consequences of experimentally induced biases in interpretation. *Behaviour Research and Therapy*, **43**, 779–797. doi: 10.1016/j.brat.2004.06.007

Zinbarg, R. E. & Mohlman, J. (1998). Individual differences in the acquisition of affectively valenced associations. *Journal of Personality and Social Psychology*, **74**, 1024–1040.

7

Adult models of anxiety and their application to children and adolescents

Sam Cartwright-Hatton, Shirley Reynolds, and Charlotte Wilson

In recent years, a number of sophisticated cognitive models of anxiety disorders have emerged in the adult literature, for example Clark and Wells's model of social anxiety disorder (Clark & Wells, 1995), Wells's model of generalized anxiety disorder (GAD) (Wells, 1999) and Salkovskis' model of obsessive–compulsive disorder (OCD) (Salkovskis, 1985). These developments have allowed refinements in treatment of anxiety disorders for adults (Clark *et al.*, 2006; Wells, 1999; Whittal, Thordarson, & McLean, 2005).

In comparison, childhood anxiety disorders are usually treated using generic cognitive–behavioral approaches (e.g., Kendall, Gosch, Furr, & Sood, 2008), as few disorder-specific cognitive models have been developed for these younger populations. Therefore, investigators have begun to examine whether specific cognitive models that have been developed for adults can also be used to explain and treat anxiety disorders in children and adolescents. The previous chapter (Field, Hadwin, & Lester, Chapter 6, this volume) highlighted the importance of considering developmental models of information processing biases when thinking about anxiety in children and adolescents. That chapter looked at the role of child development in anxiogenic cognitive processing that span multiple anxiety disorders, whereas this chapter focuses on the applicability of theories and treatments of particular anxiety disorders to child and adolescent samples. As such, whereas the previous chapter looked at the role of child development in transprocess models of anxiety, we will focus on models that relate to the etiology and treatment of three anxiety disorders: social anxiety disorder, OCD, and GAD. These disorders have been selected because they are amongst the most common anxiety diagnoses in children and adolescents, and are the disorders for which adult models are best explored in a younger population (see Costello, Egger, Copeland, Erkanli, & Angold, Chapter 3, this volume).

We will show that, at least for older children and adolescents, adult models of disorder do appear to be largely applicable. Although there is currently less evidence that these processes can be manipulated in youth through treatment, we will argue that the evidence suggests that disorder-specific models of anxiety should be adapted for use with older children and subjected to careful evaluation of their efficacy.

Cognitive development and child and adolescent anxiety

As will become clear, the majority of the research that has explored adult models in young populations has done so in late childhood or adolescence. There is very little research into

Anxiety Disorders in Children and Adolescents, 2nd edn, ed. W. K. Silverman and A. P. Field. Published by Cambridge University Press. © Cambridge University Press 2011.

these questions in young children. Similarly, researchers have generally taken a pragmatic approach: "does this technique/theoretical construct hold with the age group with which I am working?" Most researchers have been applied psychologists, rather than developmental psychologists, and this is apparent in the research that has been conducted. Little of the work that is described below uses constructs from the developmental psychology literature to inform their hypotheses or design. Thus, for example, there is little consideration of children's cognitive development, either in general or in relation to specific disorders and related theories. At a general level a key element of cognitive development, and a key requirement of cognitive behavior therapy, is the ability of children to reflect on their own thinking and experiences and to examine the relationships between their thoughts and feelings, and thoughts and behaviors (Quakley, Reynolds, & Coker, 2004). Reflecting and thinking over the past and the future is a core aspect of GAD and requires a high level of self-reflection, the creation of hypothetical scenarios, and engaging in " . . . if, then . . . ", thinking all of which involve complex cognitive processes. Similarly, the ability to take the perspective of another person and to imagine oneself "in another person's shoes" as well as to compare the self to others, are key features of social anxiety disorder. In OCD, a key theoretical model, thought–action fusion (TAF) (Rachman, 1997), suggests that people with OCD tend to make the assumption that thinking about doing a bad thing is equivalent to actually doing that bad thing, and that thinking about a bad thing happening makes that bad thing more likely to happen. Bolton (1996) suggested that TAF corresponds closely to "magical thinking" which is often observed as a normal developmental phase in children, but this association is little understood.

In developmental terms, we can easily identify cornerstones of cognitive development that map onto these clinical constructs: the ability to reflect on multiple aspects of a situation equates to Piaget's (Piaget, 1936/1953; Piaget & Inhelder, 1956) notion of *centration*, the ability to see situations from other's perspectives relates to Piagetian *egocentrism*, and magical thinking pertains to a child's understanding of the fantasy–reality distinction. Before the age of about 6 years, children tend to focus on single aspects of a situation (*centration*), cannot view situations from multiple perspectives (*egocentrism*), and engage more in magical and fantasy-based thought (Harris, Brown, Marriott, Whittall, & Harmer, 1991). Although children younger than 6 years can understand some aspects of the fantasy–reality distinction above this age they better understand fantasy material and tend to use evidence-based approaches to determine whether entities are real or fantasy (Boerger, Tullos, & Woolley, 2009; Tullos & Woolley, 2009). As such, many of the cognitive processes that underpin anxiety disorders are still developing in children under 10; therefore, attempts to explain the origins of anxiety disorders and the information processing patterns that underlie them need to consider these developmental stepping stones (Alfano, Beidel, & Turner, 2002; Field & Lester, 2001b; Muris, 2007). Similarly, treatment packages need also to be mindful of the cognitive capabilities of the child especially given that targeting cognition is not always necessary nor sufficient for positive treatment outcome in childhood anxiety disorders (Alfano *et al.*, 2002).

Although age is often measured and analyzed in the research literature, specific markers of development are not and although age correlates with development it is something of an "empty variable" that adds little or no specific information about cognitive mediators of anxiety (Field & Lester, 2010b). There are two issues here. First, children develop at different speeds and an able 10-year-old might achieve levels of performance that are not present in the average 12-year-old. Likewise, although a study shows that an average 12-year-old can demonstrate a particular cognitive process, this does not mean that this process should be assumed in all 12-year-olds. Second, age-related effects tell us little about the mechanisms underlying those effects. For example, in a study by Muris, Hoeve, Meesters, and Mayer (2004) 4–12-year-old children had to decide whether a character in a story was happy, sad, angry, anxious, or in pain based on brief scenarios in which the character experienced an anxiety-related physical symptom (e.g., heart beating very fast). From the age of 7, children were increasingly able to link physical symptoms to anxiety, suggesting a cognitive shift occurring at this age. However, much as this age-related change is interesting, it tells us little about the specific cognitive building blocks that bring about this change.

Some researchers have, however, tried to look at how cognitive development, rather than age, affects anxiety responses. In a community sample of 6–11-year-olds, Banerjee and Henderson (2001), for example, measured social anxiety using the Social Phobia and Anxiety Inventory for Children (SPAI-C) (Beidel, Turner, & Morris, 1995), Theory of Mind using a standard second-order false-belief task, children's understanding of scenarios involving a faux pas, and children's understanding of deceptive presentational displays (such as not crying when hurt because the person does not want to be perceived as a wimp). Unexpectedly, Theory of Mind did not significantly correlate with social anxiety. In highly shy children, social anxiety was not linked to general deficiencies in mental state understanding; but it was associated with a relatively poor insight into how self-presentational motives can create effective emotional displays and a poorer appreciation of the unintentional emotional consequences of faux pas.

Attempts have also been made to link cognitive development to anxiogenic information processing in community samples. For example, cognitive development has been measured using Piagetian conservation tasks (Muris, Mayer, Vermeulen, & Hiemstra, 2007; Muris, Vermeer, & Horselenberg, 2008). In one study, 4–13-year-old children were interviewed after listening to vignettes across which the presence of anxiety-related physical symptoms was systematically varied. Supporting his previous finding, Muris' data showed that from 7 years, children were increasingly able to relate physical symptoms to the anxiety emotion and that cognitive development (broadly measured) enhanced this understanding of anxiety-related physical symptoms (Muris et al., 2008). Another study showed that 4–12-year-old children's performance on conservation tasks and on a Theory of Mind test both predicted anxious interpretations and emotional reasoning scores (Muris et al., 2007).

Although these studies are very useful in starting to dissociate the effects of age from the effects of cognitive development, they have tended to (quite understandably) measure very global markers of development such as conservation and mental state understanding. However, as Banerjee and Henderson's study (2001) shows it is not necessarily global cognitive skills (e.g. mental state understanding) that predict anxious responses but rather more specific ones (e.g., understanding of faux pas and self-presentation strategies). Field and Lester (2010a, 2010b) have, therefore, argued that researchers studying child and adolescent anxiety need to think carefully about the specific cognitive (and social) skills that might mediate the development and treatment of anxiety responses.

Field and Lester (2010b) note that studying cognitive development as a mediator of anxiety also brings with it inherent methodological problems. For example, although a study might demonstrate that one age group (most often individuals in late childhood or early adolescence) show the outcomes predicted by adult models, another set of children, even just slightly less cognitively developed, might not have done. Likewise, the same set of children, if the question were posed slightly differently, and the experiment constructed a little more sensitively, to take advantage of better-developed cognitive processes, might have produced quite different results (Hadwin & Field, 2010b). Grave and Blissett (2004) cite a range of studies of cognitive development in which young participants' abilities were underestimated by the way that they were tested. In these studies, younger children were initially unable to complete a task in the way expected of older children, but with sensitive cueing, appropriate training, and use of familiar and concrete aids and language, were able to perform at a much higher level. (Similar findings have famously been shown for many Piagetian skills – see Donaldson [1984] for a review.) Similarly, Quakley *et al.* (2004) demonstrated that the use of concrete visual cues with children aged 4 to 7 significantly improved their ability to discriminate amongst thoughts, feelings, and behaviors.

  To sum up, the relative absence of developmental psychology in research into child and adolescent anxiety should be borne in mind when considering the findings of the studies reported here. We have raised several issues that are not currently addressed adequately in the literature and which limit what we can say about the developmental appropriateness of adult models at different ages, and more importantly, different levels of cognitive development.

General processes in social anxiety

Adult models of social anxiety disorder (Clark & Wells, 1995; Rapee & Heimberg, 1997) have shown that people with social anxiety (or in many studies, individuals with high levels of social anxiety symptoms) have unusual patterns of cognition and behavior in several realms. The key findings in the adult social anxiety area are:

- Socially anxious individuals have attentional biases toward social threat in their environment: e.g., for threat words (Becker, Rinck, Margraf, & Roth, 2001) and emotional faces (Gilboa-Schechtman, Foa, & Amir, 1999).
- Once threatening social cues (e.g., emotional faces) are detected, socially anxious people turn their attention away from these cues (Amir, Foa, & Coles, 1998; Mansell & Clark, 1999). Instead, it appears that they turn their attention to internal stimuli (e.g., Clark & Wells, 1995). Thus, these individuals are more likely to notice noxious physical sensations, such as increased heart rate and sweating, which exacerbates their social anxiety further.
- During social situations (and afterwards when recalling them), socially anxious individuals are prone to viewing social situations from an "observer perspective" (Coles, Turk, & Heimberg, 2002; Spurr & Stopa, 2003; Wells, Clark, & Ahmad, 1998). This means that they view the situation as if they were watching it from outside of their own body. This observer perspective often generates an unflattering image of their social performance because they are paying attention to their current aroused physical state (and the physical symptoms that they feel, such as sweating and hyperventilating). The observer perspective contrasts with the "field perspective" (Wells *et al.*, 1998), which is usually adopted by less anxious individuals. When using the field perspective, individuals view the situation through their own eyes, thus allowing them to gather more accurate information on the success of the social interaction in which they are engaged. For example, when giving a public speech, a socially anxious person adopting the observer perspective will gather information about their subjective appearance, which could include images of the self sweating, stumbling over words, blushing, and so on. However, the same individual

adopting the field perspective would gather information about the audience's reaction to their performance, which would, in most cases, be positive (e.g., members of the audience smiling, appearing interested) or at worst neutral.

- When presented with ambiguous social information, socially anxious people will often interpret this in an anxiety-provoking fashion (Amir *et al.*, 1998; Harvey, Richards, Dziadosz, & Swindell, 1993). For example, a socially anxious adult who sees a companion yawn is likely to interpret this yawn as a reaction to his/her boring conversational style, compared to a less anxious person who might interpret it as showing that his/her companion is tired.
- Adults who suffer from social anxiety have a tendency to overestimate the likelihood of negative outcomes to social events (Gilboa-Schechtman *et al.*, 1999).
- Socially anxious adults are likely to engage in "safety behaviors," such as planning sentences before they speak, in an attempt to improve their social performance (or avoid social catastrophe). However, there is evidence that such safety behaviors often have a negative impact on the outcome of the social situation (Alden & Bieling, 1998).
- After a stressful social encounter, socially anxious adults are likely to engage in a period of rumination or post-event processing, which has been termed the "post-mortem" (e.g., Clark & Wells, 1995; Mellings & Alden, 2000). This has the effect of increasing the individual's propensity to predict a poor outcome for future social encounters.
- There is evidence that socially anxious adults experience distressing negative imagery during, before, and after social encounters. This imagery both increases their anxiety and increases use of safety behaviors (Hackmann, Surawy, & Clark, 1998; Hirsch, Mathews, Clark, Williams, & Morrison, 2006).

The impact of these cognitive and behavioral features serves to maintain symptoms of social anxiety in adults and thus they have become key targets of cognitive behavioral treatment (e.g., Clark *et al.*, 2006). If such treatment is to be adapted for use with children and adolescents then it is important to demonstrate that similar processes operate to maintain their social anxiety. In recent years, some of these features of the social anxiety model have been tested in children and/or adolescents. Is there evidence that similar processes are at play when children and adolescents experience social anxiety?

Do socially anxious children have attentional biases towards social threat in their environment?

Field, Hadwin, and Lester (this volume) reviewed the evidence for attentional biases to threat in anxious children and adolescents and concluded that there is evidence for these biases in general (see Hadwin & Field, 2010a; Hadwin, Garner, & Perez-Olivas, 2006, for reviews). In terms of social anxiety disorder specifically, Roy *et al.* (2008) used a dot-probe attentional bias paradigm to examine attentional bias to emotional (happy, angry) and neutral faces in a large sample of children and adolescents (aged 7 to 18 years). Although children who were diagnosed with an anxiety disorder showed an increased attentional bias to threatening faces compared to "non-anxious" youths, this effect did not seem to depend on their primary anxiety disorder, with those having diagnoses of GAD and separation anxiety disorder performing equivalently to socially anxious participants. Although the high levels of comorbidity in anxiety disorders that often clouds this issue may have played a part in the result, it does suggest that attentional biases towards social threat might be present across anxiety disorders in this age group. Another issue here is that this study employed a very wide age range (participants were aged from 7 to 18 years). Hadwin *et al.*'s (2006) review of the area concludes that before about 10 years of age, most typically developing children have an attentional bias towards threat information, regardless of their level of anxiety, and that this may be adaptive. If this is the case, it is not clear to what extent attempting to modify attentional biases in this age group would be beneficial, and it could, in fact, be harmful.

Once threatening social cues (e.g., emotional faces) are detected, do socially anxious children turn their attention away from these and towards internal stimuli?

This question has been little explored in youth populations. However, Hodson, McManus, Clark, and Doll (2008) conducted a questionnaire-based study, in which they asked a large sample of non-referred 11–14-year-olds to complete self-report measures of social anxiety symptoms and also self-report measures of several processes that have been identified in socially phobic adults, including measures relating to self-focused attention. As has been found in adult populations, levels of self-reported self-focused attention were significantly and positively associated with self-reported levels of social anxiety symptoms. Unfortunately, this study cannot tell us whether these young people deflect their attention inwardly in direct response to detection of threatening social cues. Also, because this was a non-referred sample, it is not clear whether these processes are active in children with diagnosable social anxiety or merely those with some symptoms.

During social situations (and afterwards when recalling them), do socially anxious children view social situations from an "observer perspective"?

There is evidence that when anxious in a social situation, some adolescents adopt the observer perspective, as has been shown for socially anxious adults. Hignett and Cartwright-Hatton (2008) asked non-referred adolescents aged 12 to 18 years, with a range of self-reported levels of social anxiety symptoms, to give an unprepared speech to a video camera. Afterwards, they were asked to "try to get a picture in your mind about what you felt you were like whilst you were in front of the camera," and to report whether this image was viewed from an observer or a field perspective. Even the youngest participants were able to report on whether they had an observer or field perspective, and there was a small but significant correlation with levels of self-reported social anxiety symptoms, with the more anxious participants reporting a more "observer" perspective and the less anxious participants reporting a more "field" perspective. This research, however, included only non-referred adolescents. To our knowledge, only one paper has examined perspective-taking in a clinically anxious child: Ahrens-Eipper and Hoyer (2006) report a case study of an 11-year-old boy, who appeared to generate a spontaneous image of how he appeared to others (thus suggesting an observer perspective), when engaged in situations (class dictation) that triggered social anxiety.

Developmentally, it is reasonable to predict that taking an observer perspective depends upon having mental state understanding (or at least an ability to understand how others might perceive you). Such abilities are reflected in measures of self-presentation, in which a child's behavior is influenced by their beliefs about how others will perceive them (to use an earlier example, not crying to avoid looking like a wimp). These cognitive skills and the motives for using them are developing even by the ages of 4 to 6 (Banerjee & Yuill, 1999); therefore, it is not surprising (developmentally) that children in the aforementioned studies could take an observer perspective. Also, of course, this observation implies that an observer perspective could develop at a relatively young age (i.e., developmentally, there is nothing to suggest that by the age of 4–6 a child cannot at least be aware of how others might view their behavior).

When presented with ambiguous social information, do socially anxious children and adolescents interpret this information in an anxiety-provoking fashion?

Little research has examined this process in children and adolescents, although some research does indirectly imply that it happens when youth are socially anxious. For example, Simonian, Beidel, Turner, Berkes, and Long (2001) demonstrated that clinically diagnosed socially anxious children and adolescents aged between 9 and 15 showed poor recognition of facial emotion compared to non-referred controls. Although the authors did not specifically examine negatively biased errors, it appears likely that a bias towards negative interpretation of ambiguous facial emotion was at least partially responsible for this result.

Do children and adolescents who experience social anxiety have a tendency to overestimate the likelihood of negative social events?

Magnúsdóttir and Smári (1999) asked non-referred 14-year-olds to complete measures of social anxiety symptoms and to report how they would feel in response to a list of hypothetical, mildly negative, social and non-social situations. They were then asked to rate the same scenarios based on their view of how another person would feel. The results showed that the more socially anxious adolescents rated social events as more threatening than less socially anxious adolescents, and that this discrepancy arose *only* for social events, and was stronger when reporting for the self than for another. Similarly, Vassilopoulos and Banerjee (2008) found that in non-referred 11–13-year-olds, high levels of social anxiety symptoms were associated with more catastrophic interpretations of hypothetical, mildly negative, social encounters, and also with a tendency to discount positive encounters. These relationships remained strong even when symptoms of depression were statistically controlled.

Finally, in the only study in this area that employed a clinical population, Rheingold, Herbert, and Franklin (2003) compared 37 adolescents with diagnoses of social anxiety disorder with 29 non-clinical controls. The socially anxious adolescents rated hypothetical negative events as more costly and as more likely than the control participants. These results were confirmed when symptoms of depression were statistically controlled.

Are socially anxious children more likely to engage in "safety behaviors"?

In the Hodson *et al.* (2008) self-report survey of non-referred 11–14-year-olds, safety behaviors (such as "rehearsing what to say," "checking that you are coming across well") were widely reported, and were correlated with self-reported symptoms of social anxiety. Similarly, in the Ahrens-Eipper and Hoyer (2006) case study of an 11-year-old boy with a dictation phobia, several safety behaviors were reported, including gripping the pen tightly and repeating the word "concentrate" to himself.

After a stressful social encounter, are socially anxious children likely to engage in a post-mortem?

To our knowledge only one study has examined the post-mortem in children. Hodson *et al.* (2008) as part of their self-report survey of non-referred 11–14-year-olds asked participants whether they engaged in post-mortem-type activity after social encounters (for example whether they found themselves thinking about the event after it was over, or found it difficult to forget about), and found that many (especially those with high levels of social anxiety symptoms) reported doing so.

Do socially anxious children experience negative imagery?

Although imagery in social phobia of childhood and adolescence has been little studied, Alfano, Beidel, and Turner (2008) found that manipulating negative imagery in "non-phobic" 12–16-year-olds did not result in worse performance or substantially increased anxiety during several social tasks, and that their social performances were still rated as significantly better than that of a group of matched socially anxious youth. This finding suggests that even if youth in this age group do experience negative mental imagery when socially anxious, this may not have the same negative consequences as have been shown in adults.

Treatment

There is evidence that the procedures used to treat social anxiety disorders in adult clients also have utility with younger clients. General cognitive behavior therapy has been shown to be effective in the treatment of social anxiety (e.g., Spence, Donovan, & Brechman-Toussaint, 2000). Moreover, specific, model-led techniques that have been developed for adults based on observed cognitive and behavioral distortions show signs of being effective with children.

Video feedback is a technique that has been used with adult clients to directly challenge their negatively distorted perceptions of their social performance. It is highly effective at modifying beliefs about social skills, and increasing confidence in social situations (e.g., Harvey, Clark, Ehlers, & Rapee, 2000). Morgan and Banerjee (2006) attempted this technique with non-referred 11–13-year-olds with high levels of social anxiety symptoms, and reported good results, but notably only for those participants who had reasonably good social skills. For those children who did have social skill deficits, there was a suggestion that use of the technique may exacerbate their anxiety. Similarly, an unmodified version of video feedback was tested with a sample of non-referred adolescents who displayed high levels of social anxiety symptoms (aged 13 to 17 years). This intervention was tested in isolation, without any other procedures, but produced positive results from just one session (Parr & Cartwright-Hatton, 2009).

In summary, most aspects of the adult models of social anxiety that have been tested have yielded similar results for youth populations as they have done in their original adult populations. The one exception (that has been published) is that Alfano *et al.* (2008) failed to show any impact of negative imagery in social anxiety in a group of adolescents, suggesting that this may not be so important for this age group as adults. However, to our knowledge, no other studies have examined imagery in social anxiety in youth, so conclusions must be drawn with care.

General processes in obsessive–compulsive disorder

There are compelling reasons to develop and deliver effective treatments for obsessive–compulsive disorder in children and young people. Presentation of OCD in children and young people is similar to presentation of OCD in adults (March & Leonard, 1996) and is associated with severe impairment and disruption in children's academic, social, and family functioning (Piacentini, Bergman, Keller, & McCracken, 2003). Between 50% and

80% of adults with OCD identify their onset of symptoms before the age of 18 years (Pauls, Alsobrook, Goodman, Rasmussen, & Leckman, 1995). However, there are some developmental differences in the expression of OCD. For example, Ivarrson and Valderhaug (2006) examined the factor structure of OCD symptoms reported by 251 clinically referred children and adolescents (mean age = 12.8 years). They found five distinct sub types of OCD, which overlapped with subtypes identified amongst adults. However, they also noted that reassurance seeking was greater overall in children and young people than in adults. In addition, some elements of obsessive–compulsive behaviors, for example rituals and elements of "magical thinking," are common in early childhood (Evans, Milanak, Medieros & Ross, 2002; Mancini, Gragnani, Orazi & Pietrangeli, 1999), although normal childhood rituals are not distressing (Pollock & Carter, 1999).

Because of the general similarities in presentation across adults and younger people and the need for effective interventions there is much interest in adapting treatments developed originally for adults. The development of cognitive behavior therapy for OCD is based on the theory that, in adults, OCD is maintained both by specific behaviors (compulsions) and by beliefs and cognitive processes. The basic premise is that intrusive negative thoughts and images are common in the general population (Corcoran & Woody, 2008; Rachman, 1997) and that they are discounted or ignored by most individuals. Cognitive behavioral models propose that adults with OCD interpret their negative thoughts and images as meaningful, and that this increases their distress and leads them to adapt maladaptive strategies to manage or reduce this distress (e.g., rituals and compulsions). In turn, the rituals and compulsions interfere with normal functioning, maintain distress, and do not reduce the emotional impact of the negative thoughts or images.

Three key cognitive models have been the focus of research in adults and have contributed to the development of treatment. These are (1) the inflated responsibility model (Salkovskis, 1985), (2) the meta-cognitive model (Wells, 1999), and (3) the thought–action fusion model (Rachman, 1997).

In the inflated responsibility model Salkovskis (1985) proposed that people with OCD interpret their intrusive thoughts as meaning that they are responsible for harm to self or others, unless they take action to avoid that harm. Therefore, people with OCD try to reduce or neutralize their intrusions through repetitive and compulsive behaviors and try to avoid harm coming to others (Salkovskis, Richards, & Forrester, 1995). Salkovskis, Shafran, Rachman, and Freeston (1999) identified a number of pathways through which inflated responsibility may develop, including early experiences of having excessive amounts of responsibility, or in contrast, through being sheltered from age-appropriate responsibility for the self.

In adults, inflated responsibility is associated with OCD symptoms in non-clinical samples (e.g. Freeston, Ladouceur, Gagnon, & Thibodeau, 1993; Menzies, Harris, Cumming, & Epstein, 2000) and in individuals with OCD (Salkovskis et al., 2000) In addition, experimental work suggests that increasing perceived responsibility in non-clinical participants leads to them exhibiting OCD-type behaviors. For example, Ladouceur, Rhéaume, Freeston, Aublet, Jean, and Lachance (1995) manipulated responsibility by asking participants to sort medications. Those given high responsibility hesitated and checked more, were more preoccupied with errors, and were more anxious than those with lower responsibility.

Thought–action fusion (TAF) (Rachman, 1997; Rachman & Shafran, 1999) is a cognitive process where a person interprets their own thoughts and their actions as equivalent. Rachman identified two types of TAF: TAF-Morality is the belief that having an intrusive thought about an unacceptable behavior is morally equivalent to carrying out that behavior (e.g., thinking about sex with someone unacceptable would be morally equivalent to having sex with them); TAF-Likelihood is the belief that thinking about a bad situation will increase the probability of the situation actually occurring (e.g., thinking about family members having an accident would make it more likely they would have an accident).

Support for the TAF model in adults is supported by self-report questionnaire studies (Gwilliam, Wells, & Cartwright-Hatton, 2004; Smári & Hólmsteinsson, 2001) and experimental research (Rassin, Merkelbach, Muris, & Spann, 1999; Zucker, Craske, Barrios & Holguin, 2002). It appears that TAF is not OCD specific; for example, Rassin, Diepstraten, Merckelbach, and Muris (2000), found that levels of thought–action fusion were similar across a range of anxiety disorders, and were not significantly higher in persons with OCD.

In children the phenomenon of "magical thinking" is sometimes seen as parallel to TAF in adults (Bolton, Dearsley, Madronal-Luque, & Baron-Cohen, 2002). "Magical thinking" is seen as part of normal development in children and is believed to diminish as children begin to develop more greater understanding about their own thinking. Bolton (1996) hypothesized that thinking patterns in early-onset OCD can in part be explained by magical thinking failing to be appropriately redirected into normal cognitive development. In line with the idea that obsessive–compulsive characteristics lie on the normal developmental spectrum, it would seem that most children have sufficient protective factors to prevent exacerbation into adolescence and adulthood.

The meta-cognitive beliefs model of OCD (Wells & Papageorgiou, 1998) proposes that obsessional thoughts are negatively appraised because of the person's meta-cognitive beliefs about the meaning and/or dangerous consequences of having the thought. The model emphasizes two broad domains of belief: (1) beliefs about the importance, meaning, and power of thoughts; and (2) beliefs about the need to control thoughts and/or perform rituals. According to the meta-cognitive model, neutralizing and avoidance behaviors increase awareness of intrusions and prevent the testing of dysfunctional beliefs.

Empirical support for the meta-cognitive approach comes from evidence that meta-cognitive beliefs predict obsessional thoughts (Wells & Papageorgiou, 1998), and that meta-cognitive beliefs are positively associated with cognitive and behavioral symptoms of OCD (Janeck, Calamari, Riemann, & Heffelfinger, 2003). In addition, Fisher and Wells (2008) reported outcomes from a newly developed meta-cognitive therapy for OCD. They reported case series data from four adults who made statistically and clinically significant improvement at 3-month follow-up which was maintained at 6-month follow-up for three participants.

The promise of new and more effective treatment for OCD is a strong reason to establish if these models can be used to explain OCD symptoms in children and young people. Thus, the following section reviews the literature in relation to the three models outlined above: inflated responsibility, TAF, and meta-cognitive beliefs.

Is inflated responsibility associated with obsessive–compulsive symptoms in children and adolescents?

Several studies have examined the relationship between inflated responsibility and OCD symptoms in non-clinical children and adolescents. For example, Magnúsdóttir and Smári (2004) found that in 202 children aged 10 to 14 years, responsibility attitudes added significantly to the prediction of obsessive symptoms, when age, gender, and depression were controlled. Similarly, Matthews, Reynolds, and Derisley (2007) examined inflated responsibility and OCD symptoms in 223 adolescents aged 13 to 16 years and found that inflated responsibility was a better predictor of OCD symptoms than TAF or meta-cognitive beliefs. In addition, TAF did not independently predict OCD symptoms, but was linked to OCD through inflated responsibility.

Barrett and Healy-Farrell (2003) found that children (7 to 13 years) with OCD had higher responsibility scores than non-clinical controls, but that they did not significantly differ from children who had other anxiety disorders (but not OCD). In a slightly older group, aged 11 to 18 years, Libby, Reynolds, Derisley, and Clark (2004) found that young people with OCD reported significantly higher levels of responsibility than anxious children and non-clinical controls.

In correlational or observational studies it is not possible to determine if variables are causally related, and thus if inflated responsibility is the cause or consequence of obsessions or compulsions. Reeves, Reynolds, Coker, and Wilson (2010) reported an experimental study with 81 non-clinically referred children aged 9 to 12. Based on Ladouceur *et al.* (1995), children were randomized to three levels of responsibility. Their task was to sort sweets into those with and without nuts, for later distribution to a class of children one of whom had a nut allergy. Behaviors typical of OCD (checking, hesitating, time taken) were associated with the children's level of responsibility: children in the inflated responsibility group were slower and checked and hesitated more often and children in the moderate responsibility group fell between those with inflated and those with reduced responsibility. However, there was no effect of responsibility on anxiety, perhaps because the children were allowed to check their work as often as they liked and perhaps because the presence of an adult experimenter provided unintended reassurance.

Is thought–action fusion associated with obsessive–compulsive symptoms?

Thought–action fusion is of particular interest in children because of the related concept of magical thinking, which is common amongst younger children. Evans *et al.* (2002) found that in young children aged 3 to 8 years, there was a moderate relationship between magical thinking and rituals and compulsions. Bolton *et al.* (2002) recruited children of a wide age range (5 to 17 years) and also found significant associations between TAF and obsessive–compulsive thoughts, and obsessive–compulsive behaviors.

Thought-action fusion may be a general marker of psychopathology and negative affect rather than a specific indicator or maintaining factor of OCD. Muris, Meesters, Rassin, Merckelbach, and Campbell (2001) found that TAF was significantly associated with symptoms of OCD, anxiety, and depression in 427 Dutch adolescents aged 13 to 16 years. In two studies that used clinical samples, the results are equivocal. In children aged 7 to 13 years, Barrett and Healy-Farrell (2003) found that TAF was higher in children with OCD and children with anxiety than in non-clinical controls, suggesting that TAF is a general marker of negative affect or distress rather than specific to OCD. In contrast, in adolescents aged 11 to 18 (mean age 14.08), Libby *et al.* (2004) found that TAF-Likelihood was significantly higher in the OCD group than in the group with other anxiety disorders and those with no anxiety disorder.

Are meta-cognitive beliefs associated with obsessive–compulsive symptoms?

Research on meta-cognitive beliefs and obsessive–compulsive symptoms has so far focused exclusively on non-clinical samples of adolescents. Cartwright-Hatton, Mather, Illingworth,

Brocki, Harrington, and Wells (2004) found that in young people aged 13 to 17 years meta-cognitions, measured by questionnaire, were significantly associated with obsessive–compulsive symptoms. There were also significant associations between meta-cognition and symptoms of depression and anxiety, suggesting that, like TAF, meta-cognition may be a general indicator of negative affect or psychopathology. Subsequently, Mather and Cartwright-Hatton (2004) reported that after controlling for age, sex, and depressive symptoms, meta-cognition but not responsibility was a significant predictor of obsessive–compulsive symptoms. This is in contrast with the study of Matthews *et al.* (2007) which, as described above, found that inflated responsibility and meta-cognitions independently predicted OCD symptoms. The relationship between these constructs thus requires further clarification in future research and with younger children.

Do cognitions differ in children, adolescents, and adults who have OCD?

Generally the literature cited above suggests that cognitive processes that are related to OCD in adults can be detected in children and adolescents, are associated with OCD symptoms in non-clinical samples, and are elevated in those with OCD. Most research has relied on self-report and questionnaire methods and thus has has focused on older children and teenagers. Very little is known about how cognitive processes emerge, change, or develop during childhood and adolescence, let alone how, or if, they become dysfunctional.

Some studies have targeted a relatively narrow range of adolescents; others have targeted pre-pubescent children; and still others have recruited both children and adolescents. Such varied recruitment strategies make it difficult to disentangle changes in cognition, which unfold as part of the developmental process. This is particularly relevant in studies that examine TAF, because of the clear conceptual overlap between TAF and magical thinking, which appears to be developmentally normal in young children. The natural trajectory of magical thinking in children has not been systematically followed and thus it is not known how, or indeed if, this normal phenomenon transforms into a cognitive risk factor. Inflated responsibility has received the greatest attention from researchers, perhaps because it is a more discrete construct which can be more readily manipulated and measured.

We identified only one study which compared OCD-related cognitions across development. Farrell and Barrett (2006) compared children (aged 6–11 years), adolescents (12–17 years), and adults, all of whom met diagnostic criteria for OCD. They found that adolescents and adults were broadly similar in their cognitions but that children reported fewer intrusions than adults and adolescents. Children reported that their intrusive thoughts were less distressing and less uncontrollable than adolescents and adults. They also reported lower responsibility than the adolescents and adults. In contrast, there was no difference between the cohorts in reported frequency of TAF – reflecting perhaps the clear conceptual overlap between magical thinking and TAF. This study suggests that across childhood and adolescence there are interesting shifts in OCD-related cognitions which might reflect the changing cognitive capacities associated with development.

Treatment

Cognitive behavior therapy (CBT) is considered to be the treatment of choice for adults with OCD (e.g., Barrett & Piacentini, 2008; NICE, 2005). Evidence for CBT with children and young people has emerged fairly recently. In a recent meta-analysis, using fairly liberal inclusion criteria, Watson and Rees (2008) identified five randomized controlled trials of

CBT with children or young people with OCD, all of which were published since 2003. Effect sizes for CBT treatment were large (mean $d = 1.45$) and somewhat larger than effect sizes for pharmacological treatments (mean $d = 0.48$). Both active treatments were significantly superior to control conditions. However, follow-up data were not generally available so the meta-analysis could not determine whether treatment gains are well maintained. In addition, the CBT treatments were defined broadly – they included group interventions, individual treatment, and family-based treatments – and sample sizes were generally modest. Not surprisingly, effect sizes across CBT were varied and had wide confidence intervals; effect sizes for pharmacological treatment were much more consistent and had narrower confidence intervals, making those data somewhat more reliable.

Thus the emerging evidence for using CBT to treat children and young people who have OCD is promising but requires replication in more robustly designed randomized trials in which more focused modes of delivering treatment can be evaluated. Research reviewed in this section has focused specifically on the cognitive processes of children and young people but in the development and maintenance of OCD, thinking (cognition) takes place in a social context, often the family. In order to adapt CBT for OCD in children and young people, the delivery of CBT will often need to change. For example, younger children may prefer to have their parents present during treatment sessions and this may be helpful in many cases. In contract, with adolescents, issues around parental involvement in treatment need to be clarified as there is a potential conflict between older teenagers' entitlement to privacy, confidentiality, and autonomy, and the practical and emotional support that their parents may be able to provide though joint therapy sessions. Thus although we need more data from randomized controlled trials, this needs to be based in and on theory which is informed by other types of studies in which the role of family members, especially parents, is examined more closely.

General processes in generalized anxiety disorder

Generalized anxiety disorder (GAD) is characterized by excessive anxiety and worry that feels uncontrollable and is associated with somatic symptoms. Many adults with GAD report having had their symptoms since childhood, and although it is difficult to determine the mean age of onset of GAD due to problems with retrospective reports, it appears to be one of the earlier emotional disorders to emerge, prior to OCD, panic disorder, and depression (Costello, Egger, & Angold, 2004). DSM-IV (American Psychiatric Association, 1994) saw a change in the diagnostic criteria for GAD in children, which essentially made the diagnosis in children and adolescents continuous with the diagnosis in adults. Tracey, Chorpita, Douban, and Barlow (1997) examined the criteria for diagnosis of GAD in children and concluded that it was both reliable and valid, and that different criteria were not required for children and adults. Furthermore they concluded that different criteria were not required for different ages of children.

In both children and adults, the key feature of GAD is excessive worry about a variety of events or situations. Although worry can be reliably observed in children as young as 4 years old (Morris, Brown, & Halbert, 1977), it is by 7 or 8 years old that children can elaborate a number of future possibilities (Vasey, 1993) and therefore report more worries (Muris, Merckelbach, Gadet, & Moulaert, 2000). However, studies have shown that having a variety of worries (Weems, Silverman, & La Greca, 2000) and having excessive worry (Bell-Dolan, Last, & Strauss, 1990) can be found in children aged 5 upwards. Therefore excessive worry about a variety of events or situations can be seen from early childhood. For a diagnosis of GAD, the worry should feel difficult to control, impact significantly on the child's life, and be associated with at least one frequent somatic symptom of anxiety, such as feeling tense, being irritable, or having problems sleeping or concentrating. These three factors were found to differentiate children with GAD and non-referred children aged 8–13 (Muris, Meesters, Merckelbach, Sermon, & Zwakhalen, 1998), but have not been studied in younger children.

In terms of cognitive development, Vasey, Crnic, and Carter (1994) found that with increasing age, children are better able to envisage and elaborate on a greater variety of threatening outcomes, which increases the number of worries. These findings and others suggest that advances in cognitive development at around 7–8 years enhance the complexity of worry; it becomes more elaborate and abstract (Vasey, 1993; Vasey & Daleiden, 1994; Vasey *et al.*, 1994). Other studies have shown that an ability to elaborate is a mediator between age/cognitive development and the presence of personal worry (Muris, Merckelbach, Meesters, & van den Brand, 2002). The implication is that as cognitive development increases, so does the ability to elaborate on potential negative outcomes, subsequently increasing the probability of having a personal worry.

In general, the normal development of worry seems to follow a developmental trajectory consistent with Piaget's (1936/1953): children in the pre-operational stage (under 7 years old) appear restricted in their ability to consider multiple possible negative outcomes and report few worries and a low ability to elaborate on them. As children begin the concrete operational stage, bringing the ability of decentration and the increasing capacity to contemplate multiple possibilities, worry is more frequent and elaborate.

However, we reiterate our earlier point that age and general markers of cognitive development can only tell us so much about the developmental foundations upon which psychopathological processes rest. Based on the working definition of worry (Vasey, 1993; Vasey *et al.*, 1994), Grist and Field among others (e.g., Lagattuta, Muris, and Vasey) have argued that the specific cognitive competencies necessary to worry include the ability to anticipate threatening future events, which in turn requires the ability to think beyond what is observable and to consider what is possible, and the reasoning skills to elaborate on catastrophic possibilities (R. M. Grist & A. P. Field, unpublished data).

Grist and Field go on to argue that the capacity to mentally represent the future is an essential first step for the worry process and that these representations require the ability to think about possibilities beyond what we know about reality. In the developmental literature, these abilities are reflected in *counterfactual thinking*, in which one speculates about the possible outcome of an event, and *future hypothetical thinking*, in which alternatives that may have occurred can be considered when the reality of the situation is already known. Grist and Field found that this ability to consider multiple possible outcomes significantly mediated the relationship between age and the ability to elaborate on worry. These results highlight the importance of studying specific developmental abilities that explain cognitive processes in psychopathology rather than focusing on age as a proxy of these abilities.

However, it is clear that from early childhood children should be able to fulfill criteria for GAD, although it is likely that it becomes more prevalent in children aged 7 upwards. Given the continuity between the adult and child diagnoses, there is an important theoretical question about the key factors that maintain GAD in children and young people and the extent to which these resemble or replicate the factors that have been hypothesized to maintain GAD in adults. In comparison to social anxiety, where different models postulate rather similar processes, three rather different but overlapping models of GAD have emerged in relation to adults: the cognitive avoidance theory of GAD (Borkovec, Alcaine, & Behar, 2004); the intolerance of uncertainty model (Dugas, Gagnon, Ladouceur, & Freeston, 1998); and the meta-cognitive model (Wells, 1995). For excellent reviews of these models see Davey and Wells (2006) and Heimberg, Turk, and Mennin (2004).

Understanding the role of worry in GAD is key in all three models, but each model has postulated slightly different roles for worry. Each model requires slightly different cognitive and emotional abilities and therefore may apply differently to children of different ages. However, there are some common features. In each model the individual is required to recognize worry and anxiety, be able to reflect on them, and be able to systematically pursue strategies to deal with them. For example, in order for children to use worry to avoid imagery or somatic reactions or thinking about something highly emotional, the child has to be able to worry, to be aware of their imagery, bodily sensations of anxiety or thought processes, and would have to be able to deliberately employ strategies to avoid these things. Many of these processes start in early childhood, when children are as young as 2 to 3 years old (Dunn, 1988; Lagattuta, 2007; Piaget, 1951), but being able to deliberately employ a strategy to avoid or manage thoughts or feelings may not be possible until the child is 5 or older (Cole, Michel, & Teti, 1994). Being able to show intolerance for uncertainty requires the child to have greater understanding of emotions than needed to show simpler emotions such as anxiety, but even children's ability to report on complex and mixed emotions appears to be well developed by the age of 3 years (Harris, 1989). Indeed, perhaps the most complex ability required, the ability to reflect and report on beliefs about worry, can be seen in children as young as 6 years of age (Flavell, 1999).

Although all these abilities do appear in the early years, each ability develops significantly with age, with some abilities significantly improving into adulthood (Saarni, 1999; Schraw & Moshman, 1995). Furthermore, there is evidence that children can reflect on hypothetically experiencing and managing emotions before they can reflect on experiencing and managing their own emotions, and the ability to reflect on managing their own emotions may develop before the ability to manage emotions whilst they are occurring (Daleiden & Vasey, 1997). Thus, although the research suggests that by the time children are reporting a variety of worries and are able to elaborate a number of different negative outcomes, they also have the capacity to reflect on these worries and to use strategies to avoid them, we know very little about whether these processes are occurring in worried children.

Adult theories of generalized anxiety disorder

The cognitive avoidance theory of GAD (Borkovec *et al.*, 2004) proposes that worry, the central feature of GAD, plays several different avoidance functions. It hypothesizes that worry has a primary avoidance function, whereby it reduces and shortens distressing thoughts and images (Borkovec & Inz, 1990). In addition the theory proposes that worry has secondary avoidance functions including avoidance of somatic reactions (Borkovec & Hu, 1990; Vrana, Cuthbert, & Lang, 1986), avoidance of emotional reactions during subsequent difficult experiences, and avoidance of thinking about more emotional topics (Borkovec & Roemer, 1995). Significant differences have been found indicating different autonomic nervous system activity in adults with GAD than in non-referred adults (Thayer, Friedman, & Borkovec, 1996), but other researchers have failed to find the predicted reduced physiological reactivity associated with high levels of worry (Laguna, Ham, Hope, & Bell,

2004). Little research has been carried out on the specific avoidance functions in individuals with diagnosed GAD. This research has instead recruited students who met criteria for GAD (Borkovec & Roemer, 1995) or were reported to be speech phobic (Borkovec & Hu, 1990), or adults who report high levels of worry (Laguna *et al.*, 2004). Thus, although there is evidence for the model in general, the evidence that it is specifically relevant to individuals with GAD is limited.

In a complementary model of GAD, Dugas, Gosselin, and Ladouceur (2001) proposed that people with GAD have increased intolerance of uncertainty (IU). They have recently suggested that four cognitive variables are associated with the development and maintenance of pathological worry (Dugas, Buhr, & Ladouceur, 2004). These are: (1) intolerance of uncertainty, (2) positive beliefs about worry, (3) negative problem orientation defined as "a set of dysfunctional attitudes and perceptions related to the problem-solving process" (Koerner & Dugas, 2006, p. 207), and (4) cognitive avoidance, which consists of avoidance of distressing images and use of deliberate and effortful strategies to suppress unwanted thoughts and worries.

There is support for all four of these variables being associated with worry and GAD in adults. For intolerance of uncertainty, several cross-sectional, experimental and treatment studies have found that intolerance of uncertainty is specifically related to worry, as opposed to anxiety or depression. For example, in non-referred adults, intolerance of uncertainty has been found to be more highly related to worry than to obsessive–compulsive symptoms (Dugas *et al.*, 2001) or to depressive symptoms and depressive cognitions (Dugas, Schwartz, & Francis, 2004). Ladouceur, Gosselin, and Dugas (2000) found that manipulating intolerance of uncertainty led to increases in worry in a non-referred sample of adults, although it has been questioned whether the manipulation was changing intolerance of uncertainty. Studies of adults with GAD also support the theory. Adults with GAD report higher levels of intolerance of uncertainty than adults with other anxiety disorders (Dugas, Marchand, & Ladouceur, 2005; Ladouceur *et al.*, 1999) or no disorders (Dugas *et al.*, 1998), and in cognitive–behavioral treatment for GAD, changes in intolerance of uncertainty appear to precede changes in worry (Dugas & Ladouceur, 2000).

Positive beliefs about worry, the second proposed variable, have been found in adults with GAD. Borkovec and Roemer (1995) recruited students who met criteria for GAD, students who reported anxiety symptoms with no excessive worry, and students who weren't anxious or worried. Only higher ratings on beliefs in worry as a distraction from more emotional topics distinguished adults with GAD from the non-worried, anxious adults. In contrast Davis and Valentiner (2000) found that positive beliefs about worry did not distinguish students who met criteria for GAD from non-worried anxious students. However, they did find that positive beliefs about worry distinguished students who met criteria for GAD from students with no anxiety disorders. It is, however, unclear whether positive beliefs about worry distinguish adults referred to services with GAD from non-referred adults (Cartwright-Hatton & Wells, 1997; Wells & Carter, 2001).

Third, a negative problem orientation has been shown to be associated with high levels of worry (Dugas, Freeston, & Ladouceur, 1997; Dugas, Letarte, Rhéaume, Freeston, & Ladouceur, 1995) and is more evident in adults with GAD compared to adults with other anxiety disorders and non-clinical controls (Ladouceur *et al.*, 1999). There is less research on the final variable, cognitive avoidance, but Dugas *et al.* (1998) found that adults with GAD can be distinguished from non-referred adults by their endorsement of thought suppression as a control strategy. However, it is unclear that the strategy is specifically aimed at avoiding distressing images, as opposed to distressing thoughts in general, or avoiding thinking at all. There is little evidence that thought suppression is a strategy specific to GAD; indeed research would suggest that it is also endorsed by individuals with OCD and other emotional disorders (Purdon, 1999).

All four proposed variables are therefore associated with GAD, but they may not be specific to GAD, and it is still unclear whether these variables contribute to the development and/or maintenance of the disorder and therefore what role they may play in the treatment of it.

The meta-cognitive model of GAD (Wells, 1995) proposes that adults' appraisals of their worries cause worry to become pathological. Thus, Wells (1995) proposed that positive beliefs about worry prompt the use of worry as a strategy, but negative beliefs about worry lead to worry about worry, or "type 2" worry, which is the key feature that distinguishes between adults with GAD and non-anxious adults. He proposes that negative beliefs about worry are important in both the development of pathological worry and the maintenance of it. As reported above, although some researchers have found that positive beliefs in worry occur in adults who meet criteria for GAD, and distinguish between students who meet criteria for GAD from students with no anxiety disorders, Cartwright-Hatton and Wells (1997) and Wells and Carter (2001) have not found significant differences in positive beliefs when comparing adults referred to mental health services with GAD and adults without GAD. Not only were there no differences in positive beliefs about worry between participants with GAD and participants with other anxiety disorders, there were no differences between participants with GAD and non-referred participants with no emotional disorders. In contrast, some studies have found significant differences in adults' negative beliefs about worry, particularly beliefs about the dangerousness and uncontrollability of worry, and in type 2 worry when comparing adults with GAD and non-referred adults (Cartwright-Hatton & Wells, 1997; Davis & Valentiner, 2000; Nassif, 1999; Wells & Carter, 2001). Whilst a strength of the evidence lies in its use of clinically referred samples of adults with GAD, there is still minimal experimental evidence that positive and negative beliefs about worry play a causal role in the development and maintenance of GAD.

Overall, few longitudinal and experimental studies have tested the cognitive avoidance model, the intolerance of uncertainty model, and the meta-cognitive model of GAD, and many studies have used non-referred samples, or adults who report high levels of worry, rather than adults with diagnosed GAD. However, evidence exists for each of these three models in adults. The evidence for each of the models in children and adolescents is reviewed below.

Does worry play an avoidance function in children?

Much of the research on childhood worry has focused on what children worry about and whether there are gender, age, and ethnicity differences (Cartwright-Hatton, 2006). It is difficult, therefore, to conclude much about the functions of worry in children, especially whether there is an avoidance function. Vasey and Daleiden's (1994) definition of worry in children does state that worry is primarily verbal, and so could fulfill the function of distracting from images, and children do report that worry is helpful (see below), but we know little about whether worry in children does reduce and shorten distressing thoughts and images. Gosselin, Langlois, Freeston, Ladouceur, Laberge, and Lemay (2007) found that non-referred adolescents who reported high levels of worries endorsed the use of worry to transform negative images more than adolescents who reported low levels of worries, suggesting that they were keen to avoid the negative images. However, this strategy did not independently predict worry over and above other cognitive avoidance strategies. Furthermore, to the authors' knowledge, no studies have examined the impact of worry on somatic reactions and on emotional reactions during subsequent difficult experiences in children or adolescents. Children do report that worrying can help them not to think about more emotional topics, but these studies are only preliminary and these functions have not been examined in children or adolescents with GAD.

Is the intolerance of uncertainty model relevant to children?

One study has examined all four factors of the intolerance of uncertainty model in a non-referred sample of adolescents aged 14–18 years (Laugesen, Dugas, & Bukowski, 2003). Intolerance of uncertainty, positive beliefs about worry, negative problem orientation, and cognitive avoidance (thought suppression) were all correlated with increased tendency to worry as measured by the Penn State Worry Questionnaire for Children (PSWQ-C), with all but thought suppression contributing independent variance. Intolerance of uncertainty and negative problem orientation were the most effective at distinguishing adolescents reporting moderate levels of worry from adolescents reporting high levels of worry. In younger non-referred children (8–12 years), intolerance of uncertainty, cognitive avoidance, and negative problem orientation were all associated with worry and GAD symptoms (positive beliefs were not studied) and intolerance of uncertainty was the strongest predictor of these symptoms (P. Gosselin & A. Martin, unpublished data).

In further studies of cognitive avoidance strategies in non-referred adolescents, Gosselin, Langlois, Freeston, Ladouceur, Dugas, and Pelletier (2002) found that five different types of cognitive avoidance strategies (avoidance of triggers; thought substitution; distraction; thought suppression; and transformation of images) were significantly associated with worry and beliefs about worry. Furthermore, all five types of cognitive avoidance were elevated in adolescents reporting high levels of worry when compared to adolescents reporting moderate levels of worry (Gosselin et al., 2007). In a further regression analysis, all cognitive avoidance strategies except transformation of images contributed significant independent variance to the prediction of worry. Although adolescents who report high levels of worry are therefore reporting using a variety of cognitive avoidance strategies more than adolescents who report low levels of worry, we do not yet know whether adolescents with GAD report using the same strategies but to a greater extent, or whether there may be certain strategies that are implicated in worry that is part of a psychological disorder. Furthermore, we know little about the strategies children report using and whether they use worry to avoid unwanted thoughts and feelings.

Along with these two direct tests of the model, other studies provide support for aspects of the model. For positive beliefs about worry, significant associations between positive beliefs and worry have been found in adolescents aged 12–17 years recruited from the community (Wilson, 2008) and in children and adolescents aged 7–17 years with anxiety disorders (Bacow, Pincus, Ehrenreich, & Brody, 2009). However, in the clinical sample this relationship was no longer significant when worry excessiveness was controlled for, whereas in the non-referred sample worry and positive beliefs about worry continued to be significantly associated when trait anxiety was controlled for. Two studies of problem-solving in non-referred children aged 6–11 years have shown that it is children's poor confidence in their own problem-solving ability rather than lack of problem-solving skills that is associated with worry (Parkinson & Creswell, 2008; Wilson & Hughes, 2006) and in terms of cognitive avoidance, there are mixed findings. In an experimental study of thought suppression in a non-referred sample of children aged 7–11 years, Gaskell, Wells, and Calam (2001) found no significant immediate or delayed enhancement of thoughts. However, thought suppression has been linked with post-traumatic stress disorder symptoms in children following physical injury (Aaron, Zaglul, & Emery, 1999) and a variety of thought control strategies appear to be associated with OCD symptoms in non-referred adolescents (Hall & Wilson, 2008). There is therefore very little research on the strategies children and adolescents use to control their unwanted thoughts and feelings and whether any of these are specific to children and adolescents with high levels of worry or GAD.

Are negative and positive beliefs about worry associated with worry and generalized anxiety disorder?

To date, no studies have reported meta-cognitive beliefs about worry in children with GAD only. Instead studies have explored meta-cognitive beliefs in children and adolescents with emotional and anxiety disorders and in non-referred samples. In the validation study for a child version of the Meta-Cognitions Questionnaire (MCQ-C), Bacow et al. (2009) found that although a variety of negative beliefs about worry were significantly associated with worry in a sample of children aged 7–17 years with anxiety disorders, the only factor that distinguished children with and without anxiety disorders was cognitive monitoring, and contrary to the prediction the children without anxiety disorders scored higher on the cognitive monitoring scale. In the validation study for the adolescent version of the Meta-Cognitions Questionnaire (MCQ-A), Cartwright-Hatton et al. (2004) found that a small sample of 11 adolescents with any emotional disorder reported more beliefs about uncontrollability and dangerousness of worry, and about superstition, punishment, and responsibility, than a matched non-referred sample. As predicted, no significant differences were found in positive beliefs about worry.

In studies using non-referred samples of children and adolescents, a range of meta-cognitive beliefs, including positive and negative beliefs, have been found to be associated with anxiety symptoms (Cartwright-Hatton et al., 2004) and with worry (Laugesen et al., 2003; Patzelt, Gerlach, Adam, Marschke, & Melfsen, 2008; Wilson, 2008). Furthermore, Gosselin et al. (2007) found that negative beliefs about worry, such as "worry helps to solve problems" and "worry helps to avoid the worst," distinguished between adolescents reporting high levels of worry and those reporting moderate levels of worry in a large community sample ($n = 777$). Just as for cognitive avoidance, it is unclear whether children and adolescents with GAD report the same meta-cognitive beliefs about worry but to a greater extent than non-referred children and adolescents, or whether there may be certain meta-cognitive beliefs that are implicated in worry that is part of a psychological disorder

For both children and adults there is a dearth of longitudinal and experimental studies of these models of GAD. Furthermore very few studies have examined the proposed processes and mechanisms within these models in children or adolescents with diagnosed GAD. This may be especially significant when testing adult models in children and adolescents as the processes and mechanisms that maintain the disorder may be the same in children and adults, but the factors that lead to referral may be different, with many children and adolescents being referred because of parental concerns. It is likely that methodology of testing these models of GAD will be different but complementary when testing the models in children and adolescents, for example, using a greater focus on children who fulfill criteria for GAD who haven't been referred and comparing children who fulfill criteria for GAD who have and haven't been referred.

Treatment

At present there are, to the authors' knowledge, no interventions that have been specifically designed for childhood GAD. Instead, children with this diagnosis are usually treated with a more generic CBT package. These interventions are effective for many children (Kendall, Flannery-Schroeder, Panichelli-Mindel, Southam-Gerow, Henin, & Warman, 1997; Silverman, Kurtines, Ginsburg, Weems, Lumpkin, & Carmichael, 1999), including those with GAD (Eisen & Silverman, 1998), but there may be advantages in developing specific treatments based on specific models of GAD. One advantage of developing specific models of GAD is to determine whether specific or general models are more relevant in childhood and therefore whether specific or general treatments might be more effective or efficient. Understanding specific cognitive and behavioral factors may also lead for more specific searches for family origins of these factors and therefore lead to better understanding on when and how to involve parents in the treatment of childhood GAD. Finally, different models may propose contradictory strategies for treating GAD and therefore testing which factors are most relevant for children help to avoid doing harm within therapy. For example if worry is used as an avoidance strategy then the treatment may be to reduce worry and deal with the things the individual is avoiding. However, if worry about worry is key to understanding GAD, then exposure and perhaps increases in worry are required to test negative beliefs about worry.

Conclusions and implications

The research reviewed in this chapter gives some indication that the models of social phobia, GAD, and OCD that were developed for adults also have applicability for younger populations. In writing this chapter we found only a small number of studies that had *failed* to report applicability of an adult model for children or adolescents.

However, several considerations should be made before we can assume that adult models are applicable, in their entirety, to children and adolescents. First, publication bias is a well-known phenomenon. Studies that do not produce "interesting" results struggle to get published, for several reasons. It is highly likely that a paper purporting to show that children or adolescents did *not* show an effect that had been well established in the adult literature would not be published easily. Add to this the fact that many studies in this area are small and underpowered (for a myriad of reasons) and the probability of getting a "failure to replicate" study published grows further.

Even if we are to assume that the results described here are reliable and representative, many questions remain to be answered. As a cursory glance at the reference list to this chapter will indicate, this research is in its earliest stages. Thus far, much of the research has taken the form of small, unfunded studies. As a result, many of the studies reported here have made use of convenience (rather than clinical) samples, and have relied on inexpensive, self-report methodologies. These methods, whilst useful for preliminary marking out of the field, bring with them several limitations: First, whilst it is often assumed that the anxiety disorders are not discrete disorders, but exist on a continuum of symptoms throughout the population, there is less evidence of this for child and adolescent populations. Therefore, it may not be safe to assume that an effect present (or not present) for children with low to moderate symptom levels will also be present (or not present) for those with more severe symptoms. More research employing populations of children and adolescents with diagnosable disorders is now required. Second, much of the research reported here has relied on self-report of symptoms and of the psychological processes under investigation. Self-report studies, particularly where the reporting all comes from one source (usually the child), are prone to a number of biases. Furthermore, it is not possible, using this design, to determine anything about the *causal* nature of the processes in question. Further research employing experimental designs and more objective measures of the symptoms and processes under investigation will be needed if our understanding is to move forward.

The issue of developmental processes was raised at the beginning of this chapter. Childhood and adolescence spans a wide range of ages, within which an enormous amount of development takes place. It is likely that the same effects will not be associated with symptoms in the same way for young children as they are for older adolescents. Unfortunately, as yet, no systematic approach to this difficulty has been taken. Most of the processes under scrutiny in this chapter have just been studied in one narrow age group, and the results cannot reliably be generalized to other ages. As discussed earlier, very little research has focused on younger children. Most research has examined children who are in late childhood or adolescence; therefore we know extremely little about how these models apply to children in early or middle childhood. In some respects, therefore, it is unsurprising that the research reported here has been so positive in concluding that adult models are applicable to younger people – much of the research has taken place using participants who were in what Piaget termed the "formal operations" stage, in which he expected most cognitive functioning to take place at an adult level.

Clearly, therefore, more research is needed. Ideally, this research would be developmentally informed, and would examine key processes across a seamless range of ages. Moreover, if possible, the research would group children by developmental age, rather than chronological age, and would make use of sensitive tools to measure this.

If, however, we accept the conclusion that it is generally appropriate to apply the adult cognitive models to older children and adolescents, what implications does this have? It suggests that treatment of childhood anxiety might, in line with adult treatments, become more disorder-specific. As outlined above, we already have some specific treatments for children with OCD. Might we now develop specialized treatment approaches for childhood social phobia and GAD, which focus on manipulating the specific cognitive and behavioral processes that have been identified as important? The research reviewed here suggests that a range of sophisticated cognitive processes are at play in youth anxiety disorders. The extant treatment approaches are, in general, quite behaviorally focused, unlike modern cognitive–behavioral treatments for adult anxiety. This research suggests that some of the cognitions that are tackled as routine when treating adults are also deserving of attention when treating children and adolescents. For instance, in both children with GAD and OCD, meta-cognitive beliefs have been shown to be at play. If children and adolescents are able to report beliefs such as these, one might argue that these make a sensible target for treatment.

However, despite having evidence that adolescents, and in some cases children, do report sophisticated, disorder-specific, cognitive beliefs and processes, there remains little evidence that standard CBT techniques are effective in *modifying* these in youth. Although a limited amount of research has attempted such modification (as described above), this has largely been done for adolescents only. We know very little about the lower end of the age range, and, in particular, what age is too young for tackling this type of complex cognition. As outlined above, there is evidence from the developmental literature that when assessed carefully and sensitively, and when playing to children's developmental strengths rather than their weaknesses, even quite young children can achieve skill levels that had previously not been thought possible until they were older. Few applied psychologists have tested this hypothesis, particularly in the context of CBT. However, Reynolds and colleagues have demonstrated that children's understanding of their thoughts, feelings, and behaviors, and the relationships amongst these, develops rapidly at around the age of 6 or 7 years (Quakley, Coker, Palmer, & Reynolds, 2003). In addition, Quakley *et al.* (2004) found that using concrete cues (e.g., puppets and picture cues) can aid children's understanding. Importantly, children who have anxiety-related problems do not appear to differ from non-anxious children in their understanding of thoughts, feelings, and behaviors (Reynolds, Girling, Coker, & Eastwood, 2006; Quakley *et al.*, 2003). Similarly, Harter (1988, cited in Grave & Blissett, 2004) reports research showing that when considering strategies that they could use to manage unpleasant emotion, pre-adolescent children preferred active strategies, rather than thinking-based strategies. The authors concluded, therefore, that therapy employing more "active" techniques might be preferable to therapy using more abstract ones. Many proponents of CBT for children and younger adolescents do indeed now take this approach. For example, the widely used *Think Good – Feel Good* CBT-based workbook for children and young people (Stallard, 2003) uses lots of concrete metaphors, such as the "worry safe" and "anger volcano" to explain abstract concepts to young clients, and employs characters with whom the young client can relate. Also, rather than challenging beliefs and behaviors just by talking about them, it employs fun games and exercises to ensure that the young person is actively engaged with the process. Finally, clinicians would benefit from having a range of assessment tools that would facilitate their decision-making when evaluating an individual child's readiness for CBT.

In summary, although it seems likely that adolescents and older children experience some of the same processes as adults when they are anxious, we know little about individuals in early or middle childhood. We also know little about whether modifying these processes can be done, and if it can, whether this reduces anxiety.

References

Aaron, J., Zaglul, H., & Emery, R. E. (1999). Posttraumatic stress in children following acute physical injury. *Journal of Pediatric Psychiatry*, **24**, 335–343.

Ahrens-Eipper, S. & Hoyer, J. (2006). Applying the Clark–Wells model of social phobia to children: the case of a "dictation phobia." *Behavioural and Cognitive Psychotherapy*, **34**, 103–106.

Alden, L. E. & Bieling, P. (1998). Interpersonal consequences of the pursuit of safety. *Behaviour Research and Therapy*, **36**, 53–64.

Alfano, C. A., Beidel, D. C., & Turner, S. M. (2002). Cognition in childhood anxiety: conceptual, methodological, and developmental issues. *Clinical Psychology Review*, **22**, 1209–1238.

Alfano, C. A., Beidel, D. C., & Turner, S. M. (2008). Negative self-imagery among adolescents with social phobia: a test of an adult model of the disorder. *Journal of Clinical Child and Adolescent Psychology*, **37**, 327–336.

American Psychiatric Association (1994). *Diagnostic and Statistical Manual of Mental Disorders*, 4th edn. Washington, DC: American Psychiatric Association.

Amir, N., Foa, E. B., & Coles, M. E. (1998). Automatic activation and strategic avoidance of threat-relevant information in social phobia. *Journal of Abnormal Psychology*, **107**, 285–290.

Bacow, T. L., Pincus, D. B., Ehrenreich, J. T., & Brody, L. R. (2009). The metacognitions questionnaire for children: development and validation in a clinical sample of children and adolescents with anxiety disorders. *Journal of Anxiety Disorders*, **23**, 727–736.

Banerjee, R. & Henderson, L. (2001). Social–cognitive factors in childhood social anxiety: a preliminary investigation. *Social Development*, **10**, 558–572.

Banerjee, R. & Yuill, N. (1999). Children's understanding of self-presentational display rules: associations with mental-state understanding. *British Journal of Developmental Psychology*, **17**, 111–124.

Barrett, P. & Healy-Farrell, L. (2003). Perceived responsibility in juvenile obsessive–compulsive disorder: an experimental manipulation. *Journal of Clinical Child and Adolescent Psychology*, **32**, 430–441.

Barrett, P. & Piacentini, J. (2008). Evidence-based treatments for children and adolescent obsessive compulsive disorder. *Journal of Clinical Child and Adolescent Psychology*, **37**, 131–155.

Becker, E. S., Rinck, M., Margraf, J., & Roth, W. T. (2001). The emotional Stroop effect in anxiety disorders: general emotionality or disorder specificity? *Journal of Anxiety Disorders*, **15**, 147–159.

Beidel, D. C., Turner, S. M., & Morris, T. L. (1995). A new inventory to assess childhood social anxiety and phobia: the Social Phobia and Anxiety Inventory for Children. *Psychological Assessment*, **7**, 73–79.

Bell-Dolan, D. G., Last, C. G., & Strauss, C. C. (1990). Symptoms of anxiety disorders in normal children. *Journal of the American Academy of Child and Adolescent Psychiatry*, **29**, 759–765.

Boerger, E. A., Tullos, A., & Woolley, J. D. (2009). Return of the Candy Witch: individual differences in acceptance and stability of belief in a novel fantastical being. *British Journal of Developmental Psychology*, **27**, 953–970. doi: 10.1348/026151008x398557

Bolton, D. (1996). Developmental issues in obsessive–compulsive disorder. *Journal of Child Psychology and Psychiatry and Allied Disciplines*, **37**, 131–137.

Bolton, D., Dearsley, P., Madronal-Luque, R., & Baron-Cohen, S. (2002). Magical thinking in childhood and adolescence: development and relation to obsessive compulsion. *British Journal of Developmental Psychology*, **20**, 479–494.

Borkovec, T. D. & Hu, S. (1990). The effect of worry on cardiovascular response to phobic imagery. *Behaviour Research and Therapy*, **28**, 69–73.

Borkovec, T. D. & Inz, J. (1990). The nature of worry in generalized anxiety disorder: a predominance of thought activity. *Behaviour Research and Therapy*, **28**, 153–158.

Borkovec, T. D. & Roemer, L. (1995). Perceived functions of worry among generalised anxiety subjects: distraction from more emotionally distressing topics? *Journal of Behavior Therapy and Experimental Psychiatry*, **26**, 25–30.

Borkovec, T. D., Alcaine, O., & Behar, E. (2004). Avoidance theory of worry and generalized anxiety disorder. In: R. G. Heimberg, C. L. Turk, & D. S. Mennin (eds.) *Generalized Anxiety Disorder: Advances in Research and Practice*, pp. 77–108. New York: Guilford Press.

Cartwright-Hatton, S. (2006). Worry in childhood and adolescence. In: G. C. L. Davey & A. Wells (eds.) *Worry and Its Psychological Disorders: Theory, Assessment and Treatment*, pp. 81–97. Chichester, UK: Wiley.

Cartwright-Hatton, S. & Wells, A. (1997). Beliefs about worry and intrusions: the meta-cognitions questionnaire. *Journal of Anxiety Disorders*, **11**, 279–296.

Cartwright-Hatton, S., Mather, A., Illingworth, V., Brocki, J., Harrington, R., & Wells, A. (2004). Development and preliminary validation of the meta-cognitions questionnaire-adolescent version. *Journal of Anxiety Disorders*, **18**, 411–422.

Clark, D. M. & Wells, A. (1995). A cognitive model of social phobia. In: R. Heimberg, M. Liebowitz, D. A. Hope, & F. R. Schneier (eds.) *Social Phobia: Diagnosis, Assessment and Treatment*, pp. 69–93. New York: Guilford Press.

Clark, D. M., Ehlers, A., Hackmann, A., McManus, F., Fennell, M., Grey, N., *et al.* (2006). Cognitive therapy versus exposure and applied relaxation in social phobia: a randomized controlled trial. *Journal of Consulting and Clinical Psychology*, **74**, 568–578. doi: 10.1037/0022–006x.74.3.568

Cole, P. M., Michel, M. K., & Teti, L. (1994). The development of emotion regulation and dysregulation: a clinical perspective. *Monographs of the Society for Research in Child Development*, **59**, 73–100.

Coles, M. E., Turk, C. L., & Heimberg, R. G. (2002). The role of memory perspective in social phobia: immediate and delayed memories for role-played situations. *Behavioural and Cognitive Psychotherapy*, **30**, 415–425.

Corcoran, K. M. & Woody, S. R. (2008). Appraisals of obsessional thoughts in normal samples. *Behaviour Research and Therapy*, **46**, 71–83.

Costello, E. J., Egger, H. L., & Angold, A. (2004). Developmental epidemiology of anxiety disorders. In: T. H. Ollendick & J. S. March (eds.) *Phobic and Anxiety Disorders in Children and Adolescents*, pp. 61–91. Oxford, UK: Oxford University Press.

Daleiden, E. L. & Vasey, M. W. (1997). An information-processing perspective on childhood anxiety. *Clinical Psychology Review*, **17**, 407–429.

Davey, G. C. L. & Wells, A. (eds.) (2006). *Worry and Its Psychological Disorders: Theory, Assessment and Treatment*. Chichester, UK: Wiley.

Davis, R. N. & Valentiner, D. P. (2000). Does meta-cognitive theory enhance our understanding of pathological worry and anxiety? *Personality and Individual Differences*, **29**, 513–526.

Donaldson, M. (1984). *Children's Minds*. London: Fontana.

Dugas, M. J. & Ladouceur, R. (2000). Treatment of GAD: targeting intolerance of uncertainty in two types of worry. *Behaviour Modification*, **24**, 635–657.

Dugas, M. J., Buhr, K., & Ladouceur, R. (2004). The role of intolerance of uncertainty in etiology and maintenance. In: R. Heimberg, C. L. Turk, & D. S. Mennin (eds.) *Generalized Anxiety Disorder: Advances in Research and Practice*, pp. 143–163. New York: Guilford Press.

Dugas, M. J., Freeston, M. H., & Ladouceur, R. (1997). Intolerance of uncertainty and problem orientation in worry. *Cognitive Therapy and Research*, **21**, 593–606.

Dugas, M. J., Gagnon, F., Ladouceur, R., & Freeston, M. H. (1998). Generalized anxiety disorder: preliminary tests of a conceptual model. *Behaviour Research and Therapy*, **36**, 215–226.

Dugas, M. J., Gosselin, P., & Ladouceur, R. (2001). Intolerance of uncertainty and worry: investigating specificity in a nonclinical sample. *Cognitive Therapy and Research*, **25**, 551–558.

Dugas, M. J., Letarte, H., Rhéaume, J., Freeston, M. H., & Ladouceur, R. (1995). Worry and problem-solving: evidence of a specific relationship. *Cognitive Therapy and Research*, **19**, 109–120.

Dugas, M. J., Marchand, A., & Ladouceur, R. (2005). Further validation of a cognitive–behavioral model of generalized anxiety disorder: diagnostic and symptom specificity. *Journal of Anxiety Disorders*, **19**, 329–343.

Dugas, M. J., Schwartz, A., & Francis, K. (2004). Intolerance of uncertainty, worry, and depression. *Cognitive Therapy and Research*, **28**, 835–842.

Dunn, J. (1988). *The Beginnings of Social Understanding*. Oxford, UK: Blackwell.

Eisen, A. R. & Silverman, W. K. (1998). Prescriptive treatment for generalized anxiety disorder in children. *Behavior Therapy*, **29**, 105–121.

Evans, D. W., Milanak, M. E., Medeiros, B., & Ross, J. L. (2002). Magical beliefs and rituals in young children. *Child Psychiatry and Human Development*, **33**, 43–58.

Farrell, L. & Barrett, P. (2006). Obsessive–compulsive disorder across developmental trajectory: cognitive processing of threat in children, adolescents and adults. *British Journal of Psychology*, **97**, 95–114.

Field, A. P. & Lester, K. J. (2010a). Learning of information processing biases in anxious children and adolescents. In: J. A. Hadwin & A. P. Field (eds.) *Information Processing Biases and Anxiety: A Developmental Perspective*, pp. 253–278. Chichester, UK: Wiley-Blackwell.

Field, A. P. & Lester, K. J. (2010b). Is there room for 'development' in developmental models of information processing biases to threat in children and adolescents? *Clinical Child and Family Psychology Review*, **13**, 315–322. doi: 10.1007/s10567–010-0078–8

Fisher, P. L. & Wells, A. (2008). Meta-cognitive therapy for obsessive compulsive disorder: a case series. *Journal of Behavior Therapy and Experimental Psychiatry*, **39**, 117–132.

Flavell, J. H. (1999). Cognitive development: children's knowledge about the mind. *Annual Review of Psychology*, **50**, 21–45.

Freeston, M. H., Ladouceur, R., Gagnon, F., & Thibodeau, N. (1993). Beliefs about obsessional thoughts. *Journal of Psychopathology and Behavioral Assessment*, **15**, 1–21.

Gaskell, S., Wells, A., & Calam, R. (2001). An experimental investigation of thought suppression and anxiety in children. *British Journal of Clinical Psychology*, **40**, 45–56.

Gilboa-Schechtman, E., Foa, E. B., & Amir, N. (1999). Attentional biases for facial expressions in social phobia: the face-in-the-crowd paradigm. *Cognition and Emotion*, **13**, 305–318.

Gosselin, P., Langlois, F., Freeston, M. H., Ladouceur, R., Dugas, M. J., & Pelletier, O. (2002). Le questionnaire d'Evitement Cognitif (QEC): developpement et validation aupres d'adultes et d'adolescents. [The Cognitive Avoidance Questionnaire (CAQ): development and validation among the adult and adolescent samples.] *Journal de Therapie Comportmentale et Cognitive*, **12**, 24–37.

Gosselin, P., Langlois, F., Freeston, M. H., Ladouceur, R., Laberge, M., & Lemay, D. (2007). Cognitive variables related to worry among adolescents: avoidance strategies and faulty beliefs about worry. *Behaviour Research and Therapy*, **45**, 225–233.

Grave, J. & Blissett, J. (2004). Is cognitive behaviour therapy developmentally appropriate for young children? A critical review of the evidence. *Clinical Psychology Review*, **24**, 399–420.

Gwilliam, P., Wells, A., & Cartwright-Hatton, S. (2004). Does meta-cognition or responsibility predict obsessive compulsive disorder symptoms: a test of the meta-cognitive model. *Clinical Psychology and Psychotherapy*, **111**, 137–144.

Hackmann, A., Surawy, C., & Clark, D. M. (1998). Seeing yourself through others' eyes: a study of spontaneously occurring images in social phobia. *Behavioural and Cognitive Psychotherapy*, **26**, 3–12.

Hadwin, J. A. & Field, A. P. (eds.) (2010a). *Information Processing Biases and Anxiety: A Developmental Perspective*. Chichester, UK: Wiley-Blackwell.

Hadwin, J. A. & Field, A. P. (2010b). Theoretical and methodological issues in researching information processing biases in anxious children and adolescents. In: J. A. Hadwin & A. P. Field (eds.) *Information Processing Biases and Anxiety: A Developmental Perspective*, pp. 1–17. Chichester, UK: Wiley-Blackwell.

Hadwin, J. A., Garner, M., & Perez-Olivas, G. (2006). The development of information processing biases in childhood anxiety: a review and exploration of its origins in parenting. *Clinical Psychology Review*, **26**, 876–894. doi: 10.1016/j.cpr.2005.09.004

Hall, M. & Wilson, C. E. (2008). Thought control strategies and OCD in young people. Paper presented at the annual conference of the British Association of Behavioural and Cognitive Psychotherapies, Edinburgh, UK.

Harris, P. (1989). *Children and Emotion: The Development of Psychological Understanding*. Cambridge, MA: Blackwell.

Harris, P. L., Brown, E., Marriott, C., Whittall, S., & Harmer, S. (1991). Monsters, ghosts and witches: testing the limits of the fantasy reality distinction in young children. *British Journal of Developmental Psychology*, **9**, 105–123.

Harvey, A. G., Clark, D. M., Ehlers, A., & Rapee, R. M. (2000). Social anxiety and self-impression: cognitive preparation enhances the beneficial effects of video feedback following a stressful social task. *Behaviour Research and Therapy*, **38**, 1183–1192.

Harvey, J. M., Richards, J. C., Dziadosz, T., & Swindell, A. (1993). Misinterpretation of ambiguous stimuli in panic disorder. *Cognitive Therapy and Research*, **17**, 235–248.

Heimberg, R., Turk, C. L., & Mennin, D. S. (eds.) (2004). *Generalized Anxiety Disorder: Advances in Research and Practice*. New York: Guilford Press.

Hignett, E. & Cartwright-Hatton, S. (2008). Observer perspective in adolescence: the relationship with social anxiety and age. *Behavioural and Cognitive Psychotherapy*, **36**, 437–447.

Hirsch, C. R., Mathews, A., Clark, D. M., Williams, R., & Morrison, J. A. (2006). The causal role of negative imagery in social anxiety: a test in confident public speakers. *Journal of Behavior Therapy and Experimental Psychiatry*, **37**, 159–170.

Hodson, K. J., McManus, F. V., Clark, D. M., & Doll, H. (2008). Can Clark and Wells' (1995) cognitive model of social phobia be applied to young people? *Behavioural and Cognitive Psychotherapy*, **36**, 449–461. doi: 10.1017/s1352465808004487

Ivarrson, T. & Valderhaug, R. (2006). Symptom patterns in children and adolescents with obsessive compulsive disorder (OCD). *Behaviour Research and Therapy*, **44**, 1105–1116.

Janeck, A. S., Calamari, J. E., Riemann, B. C., & Heffelfinger, S. K. (2003). Too much thinking about thinking? Meta-cognitive differences in obsessive compulsive disorder. *Journal of Anxiety Disorders*, **17**, 181–195.

Kendall, P. C., Flannery-Schroeder, E., Panichelli-Mindel, S. M., Southam-Gerow, M., Henin, A., & Warman, M. (1997). Therapy for youths with anxiety disorders: a second randomized clinical trial. *Journal of Consulting and Clinical Psychology*, **65**, 366–380.

Kendall, P. C., Gosch, E., Furr, J. M., & Sood, E. (2008). Flexibility within fidelity. *Journal of the American Academy of Child and Adolescent Psychiatry*, **47**, 987–993.

Koerner, N. & Dugas, M. J. (2006). A cognitive model of generalized anxiety disorder: the role of intolerance of uncertainty. In: G. C. L. Davey & A. Wells (eds.) *Worry and its Psychological Disorders: Theory, Assessment and Treatment*, pp. 201–216. Chichester, UK: Wiley.

Ladouceur, R., Dugas, M. J., Freeston, M. H., Rhéaume, J., Blaise, F., Boisvert, J. M., et al. (1999). Specificity of generalized anxiety disorder symptoms and processes. *Behavior Therapy*, **30**, 191–207.

Ladouceur, R., Gosselin, P., & Dugas, M. J. (2000). Experimental manipulation of intolerance of uncertainty: a study of a theoretical model of worry. *Behaviour Research and Therapy*, **38**, 933–941.

Ladouceur, R., Rhéaume, J., Freeston, M. H., Aublet, F., Jean, K., & Lachance, S. (1995). Experimental manipulation of responsibility: an analogue test for models of obsessive-compulsive disorder. *Behaviour Research and Therapy*, **33**, 937–946.

Lagattuta, K. H. (2007). Thinking about the future because of the past: young children's knowledge about the causes of worry and preventative decisions. *Child Development*, **78**, 1492–1509.

Laguna, L. B., Ham, L. S., Hope, D. A., & Bell, C. (2004). Chronic worry as avoidance of arousal. *Cognitive Therapy and Research*, **28**, 269–281.

Laugesen, N. Dugas, M. J., & Bukowski, W. M. (2003). Understanding adolescent worry: the application of a cognitive model. *Journal of Abnormal Child Psychology*, **31**, 55–64.

Libby, S., Reynolds, S., Derisley, J., & Clark, S. (2004). Cognitive appraisals in young people with obsessive–compulsive disorder. *Journal of Child Psychology and Psychiatry*, **45**, 1076–1084.

Magnúsdóttir, I. & Smári, J. (1999). Social anxiety in adolescents and appraisal of negative events: specificity or generality of bias? *Behavioural and Cognitive Psychotherapy*, **27**, 223–230.

Magnúsdóttir, I. & Smári, J. (2004). Are responsibility attitudes related to obsessive–compulsive symptoms in schoolchildren? *Cognitive Behaviour Therapy*, **33**, 21–26.

Mancini, F., Gragnani, A., Orazi, F., & Pietrangeli, M. G. (1999). Obsession and compulsions: normative data on the Padua Inventory from an Italian non-clinical adolescent sample. *Behaviour Research and Therapy*, **37**, 919–925.

Mansell, W. & Clark, D. M. (1999). How do I appear to others? Social anxiety and processing of the observable self. *Behaviour Research and Therapy*, **37**, 419–434.

March, J. S. & Leonard, H. L. (1996). Obsessive compulsive disorder in children and adolescents: a review of the past 10 years. *Journal of the American Academy of Child and Adolescent Psychiatry*, **35**, 1265–1273.

Mather, A., & Cartwright-Hatton, S. (2004). Cognitive predictors of obsessive compulsive symptoms in adolescence: a preliminary investigation. *Journal of Clinical Child and Adolescent Psychology*, **33**, 743–749.

Matthews, L., Reynolds, S., & Derisley, J. (2007). Examining cognitive models of obsessive–compulsive disorder in adolescents. *Behavioural and Cognitive Psychotherapy*, **35**, 149–163.

Mellings, T. M. B. & Alden, L. E. (2000). Cognitive processes in social anxiety: the effects of self-focus, rumination and anticipatory processing. *Behaviour Research and Therapy*, **38**, 243–257.

Menzies, R. G., Harris, L. M., Cumming, S. R., & Epstein, D. A. (2000). The relationship between inflated personal responsibility and exaggerated danger expectancies in obsessive compulsive concerns. *Behaviour Research and Therapy*, **10**, 1029–1037.

Morgan, J. & Banerjee, R. (2006). Social anxiety and self-evaluation of social performance in a non-clinical sample of children. *Journal of Clinical Child and Adolescent Psychology*, **35**, 292–301.

Morris, L. W., Brown, N. R., & Halbert, B. L. (1977). Effects of symbolic modelling on the arousal of cognitive and affective components of anxiety in preschool children. In: C. D. Spielberger & I. G. Sarason (eds.) *Stress and Anxiety*, vol. 4, pp. 153–170. Washington, DC: Hemisphere.

Muris, P. (2007). *Normal and Abnormal Fear and Anxiety in Children and Adolescents.* Oxford, UK: Elsevier Science.

Muris, P., Hoeve, I., Meesters, C., & Mayer, B. (2004). Children's conception and interpretation of anxiety-related physical symptoms. *Journal of Behavior Therapy and Experimental Psychiatry*, **35**, 233–244.

Muris, P., Mayer, B., Vermeulen, L., & Hiemstra, H. (2007). Theory-of-mind, cognitive development, and children's interpretation of anxiety-related physical symptoms. *Behaviour Research and Therapy*, **45**, 2121–2132. doi: 10.1016/j.brat.2007.02.014

Muris, P., Meesters, C., Merckelbach, H., Sermon, A., & Zwakhalen, S. (1998). Worry in normal children. *Journal of the American Academy of Child and Adolescent Psychiatry*, **37**, 703–710.

Muris, P., Meesters, C., Rassin, E., Merckelbach, H., & Campbell, J. (2001). Thought–action fusion and anxiety disorders symptoms in normal adolescents. *Behaviour Research and Therapy*, **39**, 843–852.

Muris, P., Merckelbach, H., Gadet, B., & Moulaert, V. (2000). Fears, worries, and scary dreams in 4- to 12-year-old children: their content, developmental pattern, and origins. *Journal of Clinical Child Psychology*, **29**, 43–52.

Muris, P., Merckelbach, H., Meesters, C., & van den Brand, K. (2002). Cognitive development and worry in normal children. *Cognitive Therapy and Research*, **26**, 775–787.

Muris, P., Vermeer, E., & Horselenberg, R. (2008). Cognitive development and the interpretation of anxiety-related physical symptoms in 4- to 12-year-old non-clinical children. *Journal of Behavior Therapy and Experimental Psychiatry*, **39**, 73–86.

Nassif, Y. (1999). Predictors of pathological worry. Unpublished M.Phil. thesis, University of Manchester, UK. Cited in Wells (2006).

National Institute for Health and Clinical Excellence (2005). *Obsessive–Compulsive Disorder: Core Interventions in the Treatment of Obsessive-Compulsive Disorder and Body Dysmorphic Disorder.* London: National Institute for Clinical Excellence.

Parkinson, M. & **Creswell, C.** (2008). Worry and problem-solving in school-aged children. Paper presented at the annual conference of the British Association of Behavioural and Cognitive Psychotherapies, Edinburgh, UK.

Parr, C. & **Cartwright-Hatton, S.** (2009). Social anxiety in adolescents: the effect of video feedback on anxiety and the self-evaluation of performance. *Clinical Psychology and Psychotherapy*, **16** 46–54.

Patzelt, J., Gerlach A. L., Adam, S., Marschke, S., & **Melfsen, S.** (2008). Development and validation of a child version of the meta-cognitions questionnaire. Paper presented at the annual congress of the European Association of Behavioural and Cognitive Therapy, Helsinki, Finland.

Pauls, D. L., Alsobrook, J. P., Goodman, W., Rasmussen, S., & **Leckman, J.** (1995). A family study of obsessive–compulsive disorder. *American Journal of Psychiatry*, **152**, 76–84.

Piacentini, J., Bergman, L., Keller, O., & **McCracken, J.** (2003). Functional impairment in children and adolescents with obsessive–compulsive disorder. *Journal of Child and Adolescent Psychopharmacology*, **13**(Suppl. 1), 61–69.

Piaget, J. (1936/1953). *Origins of Intelligence in the Child.* London: Routledge & Kegan Paul.

Piaget, J. (1951). *Play, Dreams and Imitation in Childhood.* London: Routledge.

Piaget, J. & **Inhelder, B.** (1956). *The Child's Conception of Space.* London: Routledge & Kegan Paul.

Pollock, R. A. & **Carter, A. C.** (1999). The familial and developmental context of obsessive compulsive disorder. *Child and Adolescent Psychiatry Clinics of North America*, **8**, 461–479.

Purdon, C. (1999). Thought suppression and psychopathology. *Behaviour Research and Therapy*, **37**, 1029–1054.

Quakley, S., Coker, S., Palmer, K., & **Reynolds, S.** (2003). Can children distinguish between thoughts and behaviours? *Behavioural and Cognitive Psychotherapy*, **31**, 159–168.

Quakley, S., Reynolds, S., & **Coker, S.** (2004). The effect of cues on young children's abilities to discriminate among thoughts, feelings and behaviours. *Behaviour Research and Therapy*, **42**, 343–356. doi: 10.1016/s0005–7967(03)00145–1

Rachman, S. (1997). A cognitive theory of obsessions. *Behaviour Research and Therapy*, **35**, 793–802.

Rachman, S. & **Shafran, R.** (1999). Cognitive distortions: thought–action fusion. *Clinical Psychology and Psychotherapy*, **6**, 80–85.

Rapee, R. M. & **Heimberg, R. G.** (1997). A cognitive–behavioral model of anxiety in social phobia. *Behaviour Research and Therapy*, **35**, 741–756.

Rassin, E., Diepstraten, P., Merkelbach, H., & **Muris, P.** (2000). Thought–action fusion and thought suppression in obsessive compulsive disorder. *Behaviour Research and Therapy*, **39**, 757–764.

Rassin, E., Merckelbach, H., Muris, P., & **Spann, V.** (1999). Thought–action fusion as a causal factor in the development of intrusions. *Behaviour Research and Therapy*, **37**, 231–237.

Reeves, J., Reynolds, S., Coker, S., & **Wilson, C.** (2010). An experimental manipulation of responsibility in children: a test of the inflated responsibility model of obsessive–compulsive disorder. *Journal of Behavior Therapy and Experimental Psychiatry*, **41**, 228–233.

Reynolds, S., Girling, E., Coker, S., & **Eastwood, L.** (2006). The effect of mental health problems on children's ability to discriminate amongst thoughts, feelings and behaviours. *Cognitive Therapy and Research*, **30**, 599–607.

Rheingold, A. A., Herbert, J. D., & Franklin, M. E. (2003). Cognitive bias in adolescents with social anxiety disorder. *Cognitive Therapy and Research*, **27**, 639–655.

Roy, A. K., Vasa, R. A., Bruck, M., Mogg, K., Bradley, B. P., Sweeney, M., *et al.* (2008). Attention bias toward threat in pediatric anxiety disorders. *Journal of the American Academy of Child and Adolescent Psychiatry*, **47**, 1189–1196.

Saarni, C. (1999). *The Development of Emotional Competence*. New York: Guilford Press.

Salkovskis, P. M. (1985). Obsessional–compulsive problems: a cognitive–behavioural analysis. *Behaviour Research and Therapy*, **23**, 571–583.

Salkovskis, P. M. (1999). Understanding and treating obsessive–compulsive disorder. *Behaviour Research and Therapy*, **37**, 529–552.

Salkovskis, P. M., Richards, H. C., & Forrester, E. (1995). The relationship between obsessional problems and intrusive thoughts. *Behavioural and Cognitive Psychotherapy*, **23**, 281–299.

Salkovskis, P., Shafran, R., Rachman, S., & Freeston, M. (1999). Multiple pathways to inflated responsibility beliefs in obsessional problems: possible origins and implications for therapy and research. *Behaviour Research and Therapy*, **37**, 1055–1072.

Salkovskis, P., Wroe, A. L., Gledhill, N., Morrison, E., Forrester, C., Reynolds, M., *et al.* (2000). Responsibility attitudes and interpretations are characteristic of obsessive compulsive disorder. *Behaviour Research and Therapy*, **38**, 347–372.

Schraw, G. & Moshman, D. (1995). Metacognitive theories. *Educational Psychology Review*, **7**, 351–371.

Silverman, W. K., Kurtines, W. M., Ginsburg, G. S., Weems, C. F., Lumpkin, P. W., & Carmichael, D. H. (1999). Treating anxiety disorders in children with group cognitive–behavioral therapy: a randomized clinical trial. *Journal of Consulting and Clinical Psychology*, **67**, 995–1003.

Simonian, S. J., Beidel, D. C., Turner, S. M., Berkes, J. L., & Long, J. H. (2001). Recognition of facial affect by children and adolescents diagnosed with social phobia. *Child Psychiatry and Human Development*, **32**, 137–145.

Smári, J. & Holmsteinsson, E. H. (2001). Intrusive thoughts, responsibility attitudes, thought action fusion and chronic thought suppression in relation to obsessive compulsive symptoms. *Behavioural and Cognitive Therapy*, **29**, 13–21.

Spence, S. H., Donovan, C., & Brechman-Toussaint, M. (2000). The treatment of childhood social phobia: the effectiveness of a social skills training based, cognitive–behavioural intervention, with and without parental involvement. *Journal of Child Psychology and Psychiatry*, **41**, 713–726.

Spurr, J. M. & Stopa, L. (2003). The observer perspective: effects on social anxiety and performance. *Behaviour Research and Therapy*, **41**, 1009–1028.

Stallard, P. (2003). *Think Good – Feel Good: A Cognitive Behaviour Therapy Workbook for Children and Young People*. Chichester, UK: Wiley.

Thayer, J. T., Friedman, B. H., & Borkovec, T. D. (1996). Autonomic characteristics of generalized anxiety disorder and worry. *Biological Psychiatry*, **39**, 255–266.

Tracey, S. A., Chorpita, B. F., Douban, J., & Barlow, D. H. (1997). Empirical evaluation of DSM-IV generalized anxiety disorder criteria in children and adolescents. *Journal of Clinical Child Psychology*, **26**, 404–414.

Tullos, A. & Woolley, J. D. (2009). The development of children's ability to use evidence to infer reality status. *Child Development*, **80**, 101–114. doi: 10.1111/j.1467–8624.2008.01248.x

Vasey, M. W. (1993). Development and cognition in childhood anxiety: the example of worry. *Advances in Clinical Child Psychology*, **15**, 1–39.

Vasey, M. W. & Daleiden, E. L. (1994). Worry in children. In: G. C. L. Davey & F. Tallis (eds.) *Worrying: Perspectives on Theory, Assessment and Treatment*, pp. 185–207. Chichester, UK: Wiley.

Vasey, M. W., Crnic, K. A., & Carter, W. G. (1994). Worry in childhood: a developmental perspective. *Cognitive Therapy and Research*, **18**, 529–549.

Vassilopoulos, S. P. & Banerjee, R. (2008). Interpretations and judgments regarding positive and negative social scenarios in childhood social anxiety. *Behaviour Research and Therapy*, **46**, 870–876.

Vrana, S. R., Cuthbert, B. M., & Lang, P. J. (1986). Fear imagery and text processing. *Psychophysiology*, **23**, 247–253.

Watson, H. J. & Rees, C. S. (2008). Meta-analysis of randomized controlled trials for pediatric obsessive compulsive disorder. *Journal of Child Psychology and Psychiatry*, **49**, 489–498.

Weems, C. F., Silverman, W. K., & La Greca, A. M. (2000). What do youth referred for anxiety problems worry about? Worry and its relation to anxiety and anxiety disorders in children and adolescents. *Journal of Abnormal Child Psychology*, **28**, 63–72.

Wells, A. (1995). Meta-cognition and worry: a cognitive model of generalized anxiety disorder. *Behavioural and Cognitive Psychotherapy*, **23**, 301–320.

Wells, A. (1999). A metacognitive model and therapy for generalized anxiety disorder. *Clinical Psychology and Psychotherapy*, **6**, 86–95.

Wells, A. (2006). The metacognitive model of worry and generalized anxiety disorder. In: G. C. L. Davey & A. Wells (eds.) *Worry and Its Psychological Disorders: Theory, Assessment and Treatment*, pp. 179–199. Chichester, UK: Wiley.

Wells, A. & Carter, K. (2001). Further tests of a cognitive model of GAD: metacognitions and worry in GAD, panic disorder, social phobia and depression, and non-patients. *Behavior Therapy*, **32**, 85–102.

Wells, A. & Papageorgiou, C. (1998). Relationships between worry, obsessive–compulsive symptoms and meta-cognitive beliefs. *Behaviour Research and Therapy*, **36**, 899–913.

Wells, A., Clark, D. M., & Ahmad, S. (1998). How do I look with my minds eye: perspective taking in social phobic imagery. *Behaviour Research and Therapy*, **36**, 631–634.

Whittal, M. L., Thordarson, D. S., & McLean, P. D. (2005). Treatment of obsessive–compulsive disorder: cognitive behaviour therapy vs. exposure and response prevention. *Behaviour Research and Therapy*, **43**, 1559–1576.

Wilson, C. E. (2008). Worry and meta-cognition in children: developmental patterns. Paper presented at the annual conference of the British Association of Behavioural and Cognitive Psychotherapies, Edinburgh, UK.

Wilson, C. E. & Hughes, C. (2006). Why worry? Paper presented at the ESRC Seminar Series, Childhood Anxiety: Theory and Treatment, Norwich, UK.

Zucker, B. G., Craske, M. G., Barrios, V., & Holguin, M. (2002). Thought–action fusion: can it be corrected? *Behaviour Research and Therapy*, **40**, 653–664.

The biology of child and adolescent anxiety

8

The genetic basis of child and adolescent anxiety

Alice M. Gregory and Thalia C. Eley

Although the last edition of this book was published only a decade ago, there would be little point basing this narrative on the genetics chapter presented in the last edition – because the field has changed enormously. In particular, there has been a shift away from simply enquiring about the extent to which child and adolescent anxiety is due to genes and the environment, to focusing upon more detailed questions about how these estimates vary with regard to factors such as age and sex, as well as investigating other ways in which genetic and environmental influences upon anxiety are mediated and moderated. Addressing a wider range of issues has led to a body of literature that is too large to exhaustively review in this chapter. Hence, this chapter will focus on a selection of some of the most important research studies in the field. The chapter begins with a discussion of long-standing research methods and key early findings from which the field has developed. Novel findings and methods of investigation are then highlighted to provide the reader with knowledge about the types of issues that are likely to be addressed in chapters written on child and adolescent anxiety another 10 years from now.

How do we know about the genetic basis of anxiety?

By observing the world around us, it is clear that anxiety runs in families (i.e., is familial). Anxious children are met at the school gates by anxious parents, whereas carefree parents seem to produce children temperamentally similar to themselves. Supporting these observations are data from family studies, which show clearly that anxiety runs in families (see Creswell, Murray, Stacey, & Cooper, Chapter 14, this volume). For example, one study found that children of anxious parents are more likely to be diagnosed with an anxiety disorder as compared to children of parents with dysthymia or who have never been mentally ill (Turner, Beidel, & Costello, 1987).

Studying parents and children confirms our beliefs about the familiality of anxiety – but tells us nothing about the extent to which familiality is due to genetic and environmental factors. Different types of studies are used to address this issue, with twin studies constituting the major approach to examining the magnitude of genetic and environmental influences upon anxiety in children and adolescents.

Twin studies are based on the assumption that the only reason that identical (or monozygotic, MZ) twins are more similar to one another than non-identical (or dizygotic, DZ) twins is because they are more similar genetically. MZ twins are considered genetic clones

Anxiety Disorders in Children and Adolescents, 2nd edn, ed. W. K. Silverman and A. P. Field. Published by Cambridge University Press. © Cambridge University Press 2011.

of one another, whereas it is known that DZ twins share on average half of their segregating genes (i.e., those genes that account for differences between people). Of course, the resemblance within both MZ and DZ twin pairs is also due to environmental factors – but it is assumed that this influence accounts for similarity in both MZ and DZ twins equally. Taken together, this means that if MZ twins are more similar to one another than DZ twins with regard to their levels of anxiety, genetic influences are likely to be important.

In addition to providing information about genetic influences upon a trait, twin studies are able to provide information about the environment. Indeed, twin studies of anxiety typically involve splitting the variance of the phenotype (V_p) into three factors described as additive genetic influences (A), common or shared environmental influences (C), and non-shared environmental influences (E). Additive genetic influences can be defined as the effects of alleles (alternative forms of a gene) or loci (positions of specific sections of DNA on chromosomes) "adding up." Shared environmental influences refer to environmental influences that make family members alike. Certain aspects of parenting (e.g., controlling parenting which is known to be associated with anxiety in children: Ballash, Leyfer, Buckley, & Woodruff-Borden, 2006) could act so as to make children within a family alike, hence acting as a shared environmental influence for anxiety. However, there is also literature to suggest that parenting acts in a way that makes children within a family different (e.g., Pike, Reiss, Hetherington, & Plomin, 1996). When an environmental influence makes family members dissimilar it is classified as part of the non-shared environment.

Some basic equations are used to calculate genetic, shared, and non-shared environmental influences upon individual differences in anxiety. First, genetic, shared, and non-shared environmental influences upon variation in anxiety are represented as:

$$V_p = A + C + E. \tag{8.1}$$

Second, the resemblance within MZ twins is represented as:

$$rMZ = A + C. \tag{8.2}$$

Third, the resemblance within DZ twins is represented as:

$$rDZ = \tfrac{1}{2}A + C. \tag{8.3}$$

From equations (8.2) and (8.3) it is possible to estimate heritability as twice the difference between the MZ and DZ correlations:

$$A = 2(rMZ - rDZ). \tag{8.4}$$

Shared environment can be estimated as the difference between the MZ correlation (8.2) and heritability (8.4):

$$C = rMZ - A. \tag{8.5}$$

Non-shared environmental influence is often considered the only thing that makes identical twins differ from one another, and can therefore be calculated as the total phenotypic variance (8.1), which is usually standardized to 1 for simplicity of interpretation, minus the rMZ correlation (8.2):

$$E = 1 - rMZ. \tag{8.6}$$

Although twin studies are widely considered amongst the best available methods of investigating genetic and environmental influences upon anxiety, the assumptions underlying this approach are often challenged. For example, the equal environments assumption holds that MZ twins do not share a more similar environment than DZ twins. However, there are data to suggest otherwise. For example, a recent study investigated parental control assessed by rating an interaction between parents and children on a task involving cooperation (the Etch-a-sketch task) (Eley, Napolitano, Lau, & Gregory, 2010). Analyses revealed that if a parent demonstrated controlling behavior towards one twin they were more likely to show the same type of behavior to the co-twin if he/she was part of a MZ twin pair as compared to if he/she was part of a DZ twin pair. An alternative explanation for this finding is that MZ twins are genetically more similar than DZ twins and that the children are eliciting responses from their parents partly based on their genetic propensities. Indeed, there is research to suggest that when MZ twins are treated more similarly than DZ twins – this is due to their increased genetic resemblance. For example, research demonstrates that MZ twins mislabeled as DZ twins are treated as similarly as correctly labeled MZ twins (Goodman & Stevenson, 1991).

Further confidence in twin studies comes from noting that the other major approach used to estimate genetic and environmental influences upon anxiety – adoption studies – has a distinct set of limitations but yield similar results: once again suggesting that childhood anxiety is heritable and that both shared and non-shared environmental factors may also play a role. For a further discussion of the strengths and weaknesses of twin and adoption studies see elsewhere (Plomin, DeFries, McClearn & McGuffin, 2008; Rutter, 2006).

Once we have identified that a trait is genetically influenced, a next step is to search for the genes involved. Two main approaches are used for this purpose: linkage and association studies. Linkage refers to a technique in which the presence of a specific trait/disorder is traced alongside a particular section of deoxyribonucleic acid (DNA), which also occurs less frequently in individuals without the trait/disorder. This technique is powerful when focusing upon single-gene disorders, such as Huntington's disease, but is less appropriate for use with traits that are influenced by multiple genes of small effect size (or quantitative trait loci, QTL) and no single gene is necessary or sufficient to cause the disorder (Risch & Merikangas, 1996). Because anxiety is an example of a trait that is influenced by multiple genes and environmental influences (for another review of this issue see Gregory & Eley, 2007), linkage studies are rarely used to identify the genes influencing anxiety – although a number of important findings have been obtained using this approach (e.g., see Gelernter, Page, Stein & Woods, 2004; Middeldorp et al., 2008).

Association studies are perhaps considered the method of choice for identifying genes that play a role in the etiology of anxiety, as association provides a more powerful technique for identifying QTL (Plomin et al., 2008; Risch & Merikangas, 1996). Association involves comparing the frequencies of specific alleles in cases and controls. If we wanted to examine whether a certain version of a gene played a role in anxiety we could examine the frequency of that gene in those individuals with clinically significant anxiety and those without a history of anxiety. If the gene was involved in anxiety, we would expect it to occur more frequently in the anxious individuals as compared to the controls.

Although association and linkage studies can focus on candidate genes (genes hypothesized to be involved in the trait being investigated), genome-wide association and linkage studies (which focus on the entire sequence of DNA in the genome) are sometimes considered preferable in that they are systematic. Such studies therefore hold the potential to highlight novel genes influencing anxiety (for a brief commentary of the contribution of genome-wide association studies, see van Ommen, 2008).

How heritable is anxiety?

Even if we consider the techniques that are used to estimate genetic and environmental influences upon traits to be adequate, there are still difficulties in estimating the heritability of anxiety in children and adolescents. This is because heritability is a population statistic, meaning that it applies to the particular population under investigation (and can change depending on the population being studied). Indeed, anxiety can be considered a broad term spanning everything from shyness in an infant to post-traumatic stress disorder in an elderly war-veteran – and examining the heritability of anxiety in these two groups would likely yield differences. Given this, it is difficult to answer the question "How heritable is anxiety?" – although if the question is broken down, then a meaningful answer is more likely.

Different conceptualizations of anxiety

One way that we can split the literature is to look at various definitions of anxiety. Focusing on different types of anxiety has yielded different conclusions. For example, research suggests that symptoms of separation anxiety are influenced by genetic, shared, and non-shared environmental influences (Eley, Bolton, O'Connor, Perrin, Smith, & Plomin, 2003; Feigon, Waldman, Levy, & Hay, 2001; Silove, Manicavasagar, O'Connell, & Morris-Yates, 1995). In contrast, shared environmental influence may not play a role in the etiology of symptoms of overanxious disorder (e.g., Eaves *et al.*, 1997). It should be noted that this conclusion is tentative – and one study of child and adolescent twins and siblings found some evidence of shared environmental influence on lifetime generalized anxiety disorder – but not separation anxiety disorder (Ehringer, Rhee, Young, Corley, & Hewitt, 2006).

In addition to considering different subtypes of anxiety, this phenotype can be considered as an aspect of temperament or personality, a range of symptoms, or a disorder. Furthermore, "anxiety" can span mild shyness to anxiety so severe that clinical intervention is essential. Behavioral genetic research has considered various anxiety-related phenotypes. For example, twin studies have demonstrated genetic influence upon behavioral inhibition, which involves a fearful reaction when confronted with novelty (Robinson, Kagan, Reznick, & Corley, 1992), neuroticism (Thapar & McGuffin, 1996), shyness and emotionality (Saudino, Cherny, & Plomin, 2000), and emotional dysregulation (van Hulle, Lemery-Chalfant, & Goldsmith, 2007). Similarly, genes have been shown to play a role in symptoms of anxiety (Thapar & McGuffin, 1995; Topolski *et al.*, 1997) as well as disorders (Bolton *et al.*, 2006).

In addition to showing that anxiety of differing severity is influenced by genes, researchers have asked whether heritability estimates for childhood anxiety are similar at the extremes as in the full range. Findings indicate this to be the case for a range of different phenotypes including fear and anxiety symptoms (e.g., Goldsmith & Lemery, 2000; Stevenson, Batten, & Cherner, 1992). A recent study of children and adolescent twins compared heritability estimates for anxious/depressed behavior defined by the standard Child Behavior Checklist (CBCL) scale, and anxiety assessed as a CBCL DSM-oriented scale (Spatola, Fagnani, Pesenti-Gritti, Ogliari, Stazi, & Battaglia, 2007). The heritability estimates were almost identical, with genes accounting for 53% of the variance when using the first definition, and 54% of the variance when using the second.

Although much of the research has considered anxiety as a trait, it can also be examined as a temporary state. Studies that have compared the heritability of both trait and state anxiety in children and adolescents have found that whereas trait anxiety is best explained by genetic and non-shared environmental influences, state anxiety is better explained by shared and to a greater extent non-shared environmental influences (Lau, Eley, & Stevenson, 2006; Legrand, McGue, & Iacono, 1999). This latter finding could be due to genetic influence being overpowered by the shared environmental experience of testing twins in similar settings. The overlap between state and trait anxiety has also been examined and was found to be largely due to non-shared environmental influences – with smaller genetic and shared environmental influences (Lau *et al.*, 2006).

Age differences

As with differences with regard to the definition of anxiety being investigated, different heritability estimates also come from looking at participants of different ages. For example, some studies have found that heritability increases with age (e.g., Feigon *et al.*, 2001), although this pattern of results has not been reported in all studies (e.g., Boomsma, van Beijsterveldt, & Hudziak, 2005). Indeed, a recent report showed a decrease in the heritability of anxious/depressed symptoms from 3 to 12 years coupled with an increase in shared environmental influence (Bartels *et al.*, 2007).

Because DNA sequence is highly stable throughout life, it is not immediately obvious how to interpret developmental changes in heritability. However, genes may be "switched on" (functioning) or "switched off" (not functioning) at different stages of development. Studies focusing on gene expression (a process resulting in gene products) are likely to be important in explaining developmental changes in genetic influences upon anxiety. Furthermore, if genetic influences become more important over time (i.e., accounting for a larger proportion of the total variance of anxiety), it is a logical necessity that environmental influences become less important. The finding that shared environment in particular becomes less important with age chimes well with the observation that environmental factors making siblings alike – such as shared home environments – become less influential as children grow older and have more experiences outside of the home.

Sex differences

Another way the literature can be divided is to look at the sexes individually. Indeed, anxiety research often examines the sexes separately given the finding that most types of anxiety are more common in females than males, especially in post-pubertal populations (e.g., see sex ratios for anxiety in adults taking part in the Dunedin Multidisciplinary Health and Development Study: Gregory, Caspi, Moffitt, Koenen, Eley, & Poulton, 2007). Rather than looking at sex differences with regard to the prevalence of anxiety, behavioral genetic research can address questions about whether the magnitude of genetic and environmental influences is similar in males and females and whether the genetic and environmental influences accounting for individual differences in symptoms of anxiety in males are the same as those accounting for individual differences in symptoms of anxiety in females.

With regard to whether the magnitude of genetic and environmental influences is similar in males and females, several studies have demonstrated greater heritability for anxiety in girls as compared to boys (Eaves *et al.*, 1997; Feigon *et al.*, 2001). Fewer studies have addressed the issue of whether the genetic and environmental influences accounting for individual differences in symptoms of anxiety in males are the same as those accounting for individual differences in symptoms of anxiety in females. However, it appears that the genes involved in the anxious/depressed phenotype are likely to be similar in boys and girls (the correlations for DZ twins are similar whether focusing upon opposite- or same-sex twin pairs: Boomsma *et al.*, 2005).

Although genetic research has told us little about the post-pubertal sex differences in the prevalence of anxiety, it is likely that future genetic research will be useful. Indeed, it has been suggested that epigenetic research may inform this issue. Epigenetic research focuses upon heritable, but reversible, regulation of gene expression that does not involve a change in DNA sequence (Jirtle & Skinner, 2007). For example, it is possible that hormone changes occurring during puberty alter gene functioning and account for the emerging sex differences in anxiety prevalence. Epigenetic processes are discussed in greater detail later in this chapter (see section on mechanisms).

Rater differences

The estimates of genetic and environmental influences upon anxiety may also be influenced by the person rating the anxiety. Several studies have found that parent reports of children's anxiety suggest that genetic influences are more important than shared environmental influences; whereas children's self-reports suggest lower estimates of genetic influence and more substantial shared environmental influence (e.g., Thapar & McGuffin, 1995). It has been proposed that the discrepancy between parents' reports and children's self-reports is due to parents rating enduring traits while children are reporting upon their current state. However, a study of a community-based sample of boys and girls aged 8–16 years examined this hypothesis finding minimal support (parents' reports of their children's anxiety were not much more stable than children's self-reports of their own anxiety: Topolski *et al.*, 1999).

A further hypothesis for the finding of greater heritability estimates from parent as opposed to self-report is that parents may be exaggerating differences between DZ twins (contrast effects) or accentuating similarity between MZ twins (assimilation effects), both of which could artificially inflate estimates of genes on anxiety. Data on temperament in twins have supported this hypothesis – finding that whereas MZ correlations are typically moderate, DZ correlations are very low or negative (Plomin *et al.*, 1993; Stevenson & Fielding, 1985). Although this pattern of results is consistent with contrast effects, assimilation effects, and genetic dominance (where the effect of one copy of a gene depends on that of another), a study of infants found that the data were best explained by a model including contrast effects (Saudino *et al.*, 2000).

In addition to acknowledging differences between reports of anxiety provided by parents and children, behavioral genetic research has revealed differences between maternal and paternal reports. For example, it has been found that in addition to rating overlapping aspects of anxiety/depression in children, mothers and fathers also provide additional information about their children's symptoms from their own viewpoint (Boomsma *et al.*, 2005; see also Bartels *et al.*, 2007; van Hulle *et al.*, 2007).

Summary

In considering the heritability of anxiety, it is advantageous to decompose the large body of literature into different components. Anxiety is clearly heritable, but the precise heritability depends upon numerous factors including type of anxiety under investigation, the age and sex of the population under investigation, how anxiety is assessed, and whether anxiety is considered as a personality trait or a psychiatric disorder. This precise information may seem unimportant, but can in fact be useful in identifying genes involved in anxiety. To optimize the chances of specifying the genes involved in anxiety, it makes sense to focus upon the most heritable component of anxiety. So, if anxiety is genuinely more heritable in girls than boys, then we may have more success attempting to find anxiety genes in female-only samples.

Are genes important in explaining the persistence of anxiety from childhood to adolescence?

In addition to providing information about the heritability of child and adolescent anxiety, twin studies have shed light on the known persistence of anxiety throughout the life course (Gregory *et al.*, 2007; Pine, Cohen, Gurley, Brook, & Ma, 1998). A recent study that examined stability in anxious/depressed symptoms from early to late childhood (3 to 12 years) found that genetic and shared environmental influences were most important (Bartels *et al.*, 2007). Other studies have also addressed this issue focusing on different anxiety phenotypes – with one study highlighting important roles for genetic, shared, and non-shared environmental influences in explaining the moderate stability (in the $r = 0.5$ range) of obsessive–compulsive phenotypes from 7 to 12 years of age (van Grootheest, Bartels, Cath, Beekman, Hudziak, & Boomsma, 2007).

Are genes important in explaining comorbidity too?

So far we have considered anxiety in isolation. However, we know that anxiety co-occurs with other difficulties including depression, sleep disturbance, and conduct problems (e.g., see Angold, Costello, & Erkanli, 1999; Garland, 2001). The twin studies reviewed above have demonstrated that both genetic and environmental factors are important in explaining individual differences in anxiety. However, the studies provide little information about whether genes or aspects of the environment are most important in explaining comorbidity.

Twin studies are able to inform this issue by comparing cross-twin cross-trait correlations (e.g., anxiety in one twin and depression in the co-twin). If the correlation is higher within MZ pairs than DZ pairs it can be inferred that genetic factors are playing a role in the association between the two traits. Studies of this type focusing on the association between anxiety and depression in children have shown that genetic factors play a key role in accounting for the association (e.g., see Eley & Stevenson, 1999; Nelson *et al.*, 2000; Thapar & McGuffin, 1997). This finding is salient as a similar pattern of results is found when examining this issue in adults. Indeed, a recent review of the literature showed that anxiety and depression are genetically speaking the same disorder (genes that make us susceptible to anxiety also make us susceptible to depression and vice versa: see Middeldorp, Cath, van Dyck, & Boomsma, 2005). This review also highlighted an important role for the non-shared environment in accounting for the different manifestations of this underlying genetic risk. To provide a simple illustration of this point, a pair of identical twins may share genetic risk for developing an emotional problem. However, one may have increased experiences associated with anxiety (such as life events involving danger), which may lead to the development of anxiety. The other twin, in contrast, may have more experiences associated with depression (such as suffering humiliation), which make him/her more likely to suffer depression (for a discussion of life events associated with anxiety and depression see elsewhere, e.g., Kendler, Hettema, Butera, Gardner, & Prescott, 2003).

In addition to the concurrent correlation between anxiety and depression, there are longitudinal associations between these two phenotypes (e.g., see Moffitt *et al.*, 2007). Genetic research has been useful in explaining successive comorbidity and a study of this type demonstrated that symptoms of overanxious disorder experienced early in life are influenced by the same genes as depression symptoms experienced later in life (Silberg, Rutter, & Eaves, 2001). Amongst other interesting findings, this study also revealed an overlap between the environmental risks influencing separation anxiety symptoms and later depression.

Researchers have also investigated the links between anxiety and other difficulties and in one study of over 6000 twin pairs aged 3–4 years, the overlap between sleep problems and anxiety was mainly due to shared environmental influences (Gregory, Eley, O'Connor, Rijsdijk, & Plomin, 2005; see also van den Oord, Boomsma, & Verhulst, 2000). An important role for the shared environment was also found when the link between anxiety and conduct difficulties was examined in the same sample of twins (Gregory, Eley, & Plomin, 2004). Other teams have also addressed the overlap between internalizing and externalizing symptoms, and a recent study explored the role of early temperament on this association (Rhee, Cosgrove, Schmitz, Haberstick, Corley, & Hewitt, 2007). It was found that for boys, shared environmental influences on emotionality and shyness in infancy helped to explain the association between internalizing and externalizing problems in childhood. For the girls, shared environmental influences on emotionality helped to explain the subsequent association between internalizing and externalizing problems.

Other phenotypes have also been explored and longitudinal links between anxiety and eating disorders were found to be partially due to genetic influences in a sample of juvenile twin girls (Silberg & Bulik, 2005). The association between sub-threshold obsessive–compulsive disorder (OCD), other anxiety disorders, and tics in 6-year-olds was recently investigated (Bolton, Rijsdijk, O'Connor, Perrin, & Eley, 2007). A familial aggregation for OCD and tics and OCD and other anxiety was found, although given the diagnostically defined phenotypes, there was insufficient statistical power to establish whether genetic or shared environmental factors accounted for the familiality.

Moving on from bivariate studies, twin studies have also told us about why multiple difficulties co-occur. A study of child and adolescent twins examined the associations between DSM-oriented CBCL scales and found that a single genetic factor accounted for the associations between anxiety, affective, attention deficit hyperactivity, oppositional defiant, and conduct problems (Spatola *et al.*, 2007). In contrast, two separate non-shared environmental factors explained the covariance of difficulties within internalizing and externalizing domains.

The practical implications of genetic research focusing upon comorbidity are clear. For example, the aforementioned finding that the same genes influence anxiety and depression but that their different manifestations are largely explained by environmental factors has two sets of implications for designing studies to specify genes and environmental influences involved in these difficulties. First, these findings suggest which genetic and environmental influences should be focused upon. For example, if we have previously identified genes that play a role in the etiology of anxiety, then we know that they are likely to be good candidates to explore with regard to depression (and vice versa). Second, these results suggest the types of participants who should be focused on. Indeed, the results suggest that it is possible to pool individuals suffering from anxiety and depression when searching for genes involved in these difficulties, although when examining environmental influences, groups of individuals with anxiety and depression should be examined separately (e.g., Middeldorp *et al.*, 2005).

So, which genes are important in explaining anxiety?

Despite the wealth of literature documenting the heritability of anxiety, relatively little is known about the specific genes involved in this common difficulty. This is because, as with other complex difficulties, anxiety is influenced by numerous genes, most of which are likely to account for less than 1% of the variance. Despite this, there are several highly plausible candidate genes that deserve further attention.

Most research in this area has focused upon the serotoninergic system, based on the findings that dysregulation of this system is a core feature of anxiety and selective serotonin reuptake inhibitors (SSRIs) are successful for treating anxiety. Within the serotoninergic system the most widely explored polymorphism (section of DNA which varies between individuals) is the serotonin transporter polymorphism (5-HTTLPR). This is a variable number of tandem repeats (VNTR) polymorphism, which means that a section of DNA is repeated a greater number of times in certain individuals as compared to others. Individuals who have one or two short alleles (who have fewer repeats of this section of DNA) have been found to have higher anxiety-related personality scores than those with none (Lesch *et al.*, 1996). This finding has been the subject of considerable attempts at replication, some successful (e.g., Katsuragi *et al.*, 1999) and others not (Ball *et al.*, 1997; Jorm *et al.*, 1998; for meta-analyses see Sen, Burmeister, & Ghosh, 2004). Research focusing on children has also yielded mixed results. One study found that having two copies of the short 5-HTTLPR allele was associated with shyness in White children (mean age 8 years: Battaglia *et al.*, 2005); whereas another found that the long version of the 5-HTTLPR was associated with shyness in children (Arbelle, Benjamin, Golin, Kremer, Belmaker, & Ebstein, 2003). Further studies have reported no associations between the 5-HTTLPR gene and shyness as well as anxiety/depression (Schmidt, Fox, Rubin, Hu, & Hamer, 2002; Young, Smollen, Stallings, Corley, & Hewitt, 2003).

Genetic polymorphisms associated with other neurotransmitter systems have also been explored with regard to anxiety. For example, catechol-*O*-methyltransferase (COMT) is an enzyme involved in the inactivation of chemical compounds within both the serotonin and dopamine pathways. A single-nucleotide polymorphism (whereby there is a change in a single structural unit of DNA between individuals) has been associated with phobic anxiety (McGrath, Kawachi, Ascherio, Colditz, Hunter, & De Vivo, 2004) and OCD in males (Karayiorgou *et al.*, 1997). The dopamine receptor DRD4 has also been associated with anxiety and there was a report that the DRD4 two-repeat allele may be protective against OCD (Millet *et al.*, 2003). One study examined the joint effects of the serotonin transporter genes and the DRD4 seven-repeat allele and found that these polymorphisms moderated infants' response to novelty (Lakatos *et al.*, 2003).

Another neurotransmitter system that has been considered in association with anxiety and related phenotypes is the gamma-aminobutyric (GABA) system. A recent study investigated glutamic acid decarboxylase (GAD) which synthesizes GABA from glutamate. A number of polymorphisms in the GAD1 gene were found to contribute to risk for anxiety and mood disorders (Hettema *et al.*, 2006).

Corticotropin-releasing hormone (CRH) is released during the experience of fear and may alter the activity of fear circuits. Genes associated with CRH have therefore been considered in association with anxiety, with one study revealing an association between behavioral inhibition and the CRH gene (Smoller *et al.*, 2003; see also Smoller *et al.*, 2005). A further study focusing on CRH did not find an association between the CRH receptor and neuroticism (Tochigi *et al.*, 2006).

Other candidate genes for anxiety include those associated with brain-derived neuro-trophic factor (BDNF); this is a neuroprotective protein which has been associated with depression (e.g., Karege, Perret, Bondolfi, Schwald, Bertschy, & Aubry, 2002) and more recently, anxiety in mice (Chen *et al.*, 2006). The estrogen receptor (ESR) has also been considered as a candidate gene based on the finding that estrogen plays a role in mood and cognitive functioning. Polymorphisms of this gene have been found to account for between 1.6% and 2.8% of the variance in anxiety in children and adolescents (Prichard *et al.*, 2002). Estrogen has also been associated with anxiety in adults (e.g., Comings, Muhleman, Johnson, & Macmurray, 1999) and rats (Hiroi, McDevitt, & Neumaier, 2006). Finally, a new candidate gene is plexin A2 (PLXNA2), a semaphorin receptor. Semaphorins are involved in neuron growth in the hippocampus. As lithium (a commonly prescribed mood stabilizer) also enhances neuronal growth in the hippocampus, PLXNA2 was exam-ined in association with mood. Associations were found with anxiety, distress, neuroticism, and psychological distress (Wray *et al.*, 2007).

What about the environment?

Although this chapter has focused on the genetic basis of child and adolescent anxiety, quantitative genetic research has provided as much information about the environment as it has about genes. Arguably, it would have been equally appropriate to have included this chapter in the section of this book focusing on "Environmental influences on child and adolescent anxiety" as it is to include it in the section on "The biology of child and adolescent anxiety." Reconsidering the results of twin studies, it is possible to note that genes influence anxiety, but none of the studies suggests that genes explain all of the variance, demonstrating that environmental factors are clearly important too. In addition to telling us that the environment is important, the results of twin studies go further. They highlight types of environmental influences that may be important. As with most traits, twin studies of anxiety in children emphasize the importance of non-shared environmental influences.

In attempting to specify potential non-shared environmental influences upon anxiety in children, Asbury, Dunn, and Plomin (2006) considered teachers' reports of anxiety for over 1500 pairs of 7-year-old twins. They then interviewed the parents of the most dissimilar 19 pairs of twins (the children themselves were also interviewed, although their responses were found to be less informative). Parent reports suggested that amongst other things, negative school experiences, parent–child relationships, and neonatal life events may all be sources of non-shared environmental influences on anxiety (Asbury *et al.*, 2006).

In addition to non-shared environmental influence, and in contrast to research on most other phenotypes (including anxiety in adults: see Hettema, Neale, & Kendler, 2001, for a review), shared environmental influences appear to play a role in childhood anxiety. This information can help to design studies aimed at specifying environmental factors playing a role. The message is that factors likely to account for differences between siblings (e.g., peer relationships) and account for similarities (e.g., sharing similar neighborhoods) should all be considered. With regards to the latter type of influence, a study of 1887 female twin pairs aged 13–23 years examined associations between measured aspects of the shared environment (parental absence and socioeconomic disadvantage) and separation anxiety (Cronk, Slutske, Madden, Bucholz, & Heath, 2004). The researchers found that these shared environmental factors influenced separation anxiety symptom categories as defined in certain ways but not others. There is a clear need to continue specifying which aspects of the environment encourage the development of anxiety in children.

Although most twin studies are based on the implausible assumption that genes and environments act separately, some studies have examined the known reality that genes and environments interact. Indeed, it is now widely accepted that gene–environment correlations (referring to the phenomenon whereby people with certain genes are more likely to experience certain environments as compared to other people) and gene–environment interactions (referring to increased sensitivity to environmental experiences based on genetic propensities) influence many psychological traits (see Moffitt, Caspi, & Rutter, 2005). A pioneering study examining gene–environment interactions in relation to female adolescent anxiety found that genetic factors influenced sensitivity towards negative life events (Silberg, Rutter, Neale, & Eaves, 2001; see also Eaves, Silberg, & Erkanli, 2003). A further study demonstrated an interaction between the short version of the 5-HTTLPR allele and low social support for increased behavioral inhibition in children (Fox *et al.*, 2005).

Research of this type may benefit from focusing upon narrow age groups and definitions of anxiety. Indeed, one study examining subtypes of anxiety in two samples of twins (one child and the other adolescent), showed that in children, genetic effects on separation anxiety symptoms increase as a function of independent negative life events; and in adolescents, there was a gene–environment interaction for panic symptoms (Lau, Gregory, Goldwin, Pine, & Eley, 2007). Despite these informative preliminary studies, there is need for further research in this area, as indicated by the dedication of a special issue of the *European Archives of Psychiatry and Clinical Neuroscience* (March 2008) to the topic of identifying gene–environment interactions for different types of anxiety.

So, what are the mechanisms by which genes influence childhood anxiety?

Research to date is clear in indicating that genes and environments individually and interactively influence child and adolescent anxiety. The next step is to try to understand the mechanisms by which these factors lead to anxiety. One relatively new area of investigation is to explore the epigenome. Epigenetic changes are mediated through changes in DNA methylation (involving chemical modification of DNA) and chromatin structure (referring to the DNA and protein complex making up chromosomes). Epigenetic processes can be induced following exposure to a range of environmental insults (Feinberg, 2007) and so provide a direct mechanistic route by which the environment can interact with the genome to bring about changes in gene expression. Of note, epigenetic processes are developmentally regulated and highly dynamic and are therefore potentially a good starting point from which to explain developmental changes in the heritability of a trait.

Although there is limited research with regard to epigenetic factors and anxiety, one study suggested a way in which early life experiences can lead to later anxiety (Weaver *et al.*, 2004). In this study of rats, it was found that pups that were licked and groomed to a greater extent by their mothers were more stress-resistant as adults as compared to those that received less licking and grooming. This effect was found to be mediated by differences in terms of methylation of a site in the glucocorticoid receptor promoter in the hippocampus. The same team also demonstrated that the effects of maternal care could be reversed in adulthood (Weaver, Meaney, & Szyf, 2006). Researchers in the field of epigenetics are optimistic that epigenetic factors will offer new insights into non-Mendelian features of many psychiatric illnesses such as MZ twin discordance, sex effects, and parent-of-origin effects (for a review on epigenetics and complex diseases, see van Vliet, Oates, & Whitelaw, 2007).

Another way of considering mechanisms by which genes and environment influence child and adolescent anxiety is to focus on endophenotypes. Endophenotypes are phenotypes that lie in between genes and disorders (and are therefore closer to genes than are disorders themselves). It is possible to consider neuronal activity in response to fearful stimuli as an example of an endophenotype for anxiety. In adult samples, it has been demonstrated that the short allele of the 5-HTTLPR polymorphism is associated with higher levels of neuronal activity in the amygdala in response to the presentation of fearful stimuli (Hariri *et al.*, 2002). Consistent findings have been found in a sample of 8–9-year-old children, where cerebral visual-event-related potentials were examined in response to hostile and neutral faces (Battaglia *et al.*, 2005).

Endophenotypes can also be cognitive and one study investigated anxiety sensitivity (fear of the physical symptoms of anxiety) in association with panic symptoms in a sample of 8-year-old twins (Eley, Gregory, Clark, & Ehlers, 2007). There was moderate heritability for anxiety sensitivity, and a large genetic correlation between anxiety sensitivity and panic symptoms, which suggests that the genes influencing both are largely shared.

What next?

Decades of research have demonstrated what we have always known: anxiety is heritable. This research has of course told us much more than this simple fact, and has emphasized heterogeneity in terms of the heritability of anxiety depending upon numerous factors, including the subtype of anxiety being investigated and the age and sex of the participants. Reasons for comorbidity between childhood difficulties have also been explicated by genetic research. Perhaps most excitingly, specific genes and the mechanisms by which they influence childhood anxiety are now being identified. We predict that if this book is updated in another decade from now, this chapter will tell us a great deal more with regard to the pathways by which genes influence anxiety. This information needs to be integrated into testable models of childhood anxiety as has been done in the case of other phenotypes such as depression (Lau, Rijsdijk, Gregory, McGuffin, & Eley, 2007).

Increased interest in behavioral genetic research globally will also result in the current findings – which come largely from Europe, the USA and Australia – being supplemented by important findings from other geographical locations. This will allow for an examination of whether genes (and environmental factors too) influencing anxiety in one geographical location are the same as those influencing anxiety in other populations.

Another line of investigation is to examine the role of genes in treatment response. Although this issue has not previously been examined in relation to anxiety, examination of this issue with regard to other phenotypes suggests that this line of investigation may prove fruitful. For example, the authors of one study reported that a polymorphism in the glucocorticoid receptor was associated with speed of antidepressant treatment response (van Rossum *et al.*, 2006). One of the authors of this chapter (Thalia Eley) is currently involved in an international study examining whether there is genetic influence upon response to cognitive behavior therapy for childhood anxiety disorders. It is hoped that further knowledge of the involvement in genes in child and adolescent anxiety will eventually help us to predict and prevent its occurrence.

Acknowledgment

Alice M. Gregory is supported by a Research Fellowship from the Leverhulme Trust.

References

Angold, A., Costello, E., & Erkanli, A. (1999). Comorbidity. *Journal of Child Psychology and Psychiatry*, **40**, 57–87.

Arbelle, S., Benjamin, J., Golin, M., Kremer, I., Belmaker, R. H., & Ebstein, R. P. (2003). Relation of shyness in grade school children to the genotype for the long form of the serotonin transporter promoter region polymorphism. *American Journal of Psychiatry*, **160**, 671–676.

Asbury, K., Dunn, J., & Plomin, R. (2006). The use of discordant MZ twins to generate hypotheses regarding non-shared environmental influence on anxiety in middle childhood. *Social Development*, **15**, 564–570.

Ball, D. M., Hill, L., Freeman, B., Eley, T. C., Strelau, J., Riemann, R., *et al.* (1997). The serotonin transporter gene and peer-rated neuroticism. *NeuroReport*, **8**, 1301–1304.

Ballash, N., Leyfer, O., Buckley, A. F., & Woodruff-Borden, J. (2006). Parental control in the etiology of anxiety. *Clinical Child and Family Psychology Review*, **9**, 113–133.

Bartels, M., van Beijsterveldt, C. E. M., Derks, E. M., Stroet, T. M., Polderman, T. J. C., Hudziak, J. J., *et al.* (2007). Young Netherlands Twin Register (Y-NTR): a longitudinal multiple informant study of problem behaviour. *Twin Research and Human Genetics*, **10**, 3–11.

Battaglia, M., Ogliari, A., Zanoni, A., Citterio, A., Pozzoli, U., Giorda, R., *et al.* (2005). Influence of the serotonin transporter promoter gene and shyness on children's cerebral responses to facial expressions. *Archives of General Psychiatry*, **62**, 85–94.

Bolton, D., Eley, T. C., O'Connor, T. G., Perrin, S., Rabe-Hesketh, S., Rijsdijk, F., *et al.* (2006). Prevalence and genetic and environmental influences on anxiety disorders in 6-year-old twins. *Psychological Medicine*, **36**, 335–344.

Bolton, D., Rijsdijk, F., O'Connor, T. G., Perrin, S., & Eley, T. C. (2007). Obsessive–compulsive disorder, tics and anxiety in 6-year-old twins. *Psychological Medicine*, **37**, 39–48.

Boomsma, D. I., van Beijsterveldt, C. E. M., & Hudziak, J. J. (2005). Genetic and environmental influences on anxious/depression during childhood: a study from the Netherlands twin register. *Genes, Brain and Behavior*, **4**, 466–481.

Chen, Z. Y., Jing, D. Q., Bath, K. G., Ieraci, A., Khan, T., Siao, C. J., *et al.* (2006). Genetic variant BDNF (Val66Met) polymorphism alters anxiety-related behavior. *Science*, **314**, 140–143.

Comings, D. E., Muhleman, D., Johnson, P., & Macmurray, J. P. (1999). Potential role of the estrogen receptor gene (ESR1) in anxiety. *Molecular Psychiatry*, **4**, 374–377.

Cronk, N. J., Slutske, W. S., Madden, P. A. F., Bucholz, K. K., & Heath, A. C. (2004). Risk for separation anxiety disorder among girls: paternal absence, socioeconomic disadvantage, and genetic vulnerability. *Journal of Abnormal Psychology*, **113**, 237–247.

Eaves, L., Silberg, J., & Erkanli, A. (2003). Resolving multiple epigenetic pathways to adolescent depression. *Journal of Child Psychology and Psychiatry*, **44**, 1006–1014.

Eaves, L. J., Silberg, J. L., Meyer, J. M., Maes, H. H., Simonoff, E., Pickles, A., *et al.* (1997). Genetics and developmental psychopathology. II. The main effects of genes and environment on behavioral problems in the Virginia Twin Study of Adolescent Behavioral Development. *Journal of Child Psychology and Psychiatry*, **38**, 965–980.

Ehringer, M. A., Rhee, S. H., Young, S., Corley, R., & Hewitt, J. K. (2006). Genetic and environmental contributions to common psychopathologies of childhood and adolescence: a study of twins and their siblings. *Journal of Abnormal Child Psychology*, **34**, 1–17.

Eley, T. C. & Stevenson, J. (1999). Exploring the covariation between anxiety and depression symptoms: a genetic analysis of the effects of age and sex. *Journal of Child Psychology and Psychiatry*, **40**, 1273–1282.

Eley, T. C., Bolton, D., O'Connor, T. G., Perrin, S., Smith, P., & Plomin, R. (2003). A twin study of anxiety-related behaviours in pre-school children. *Journal of Child Psychology and Psychiatry*, **44**, 945–960.

Eley, T. C., Gregory, A. M., Clark, D. M., & Ehlers, A. (2007). Feeling anxious: a twin study of panic/somatic symptoms, anxiety sensitivity and heart-beat perception in children. *Journal of Child Psychology and Psychiatry*, **48**, 1184–1191.

Eley, T. C., Napolitano, M., Lau, J. Y. F., & Gregory, A. M. (2010). Does childhood anxiety evoke maternal control? A genetically informed study. *Journal of Child Psychology and Psychiatry*, **51**, 772–779.

Feigon, S. A., Waldman, I. D., Levy, F., & Hay, D. A. (2001). Genetic and environmental influences on separation anxiety disorder symptoms and their moderation by age and sex. *Behavior Genetics*, **31**, 403–411.

Feinberg, A. P. (2007). Phenotypic plasticity and the epigenetics of human disease. *Nature*, **447**, 433–440.

Fox, N. A., Nichols, K. E., Henderson, H. A., Rubin, K., Schmidt, L., Hamer, D., *et al.* (2005). Evidence for a gene–environment interaction in predicting behavioral inhibition in middle childhood. *Psychological Science*, **16**, 921–926.

Garland, J. E. (2001). Sleep disturbances in anxious children. In: G. Stores & L. Wiggs (eds.) *Sleep Disturbance in Children and Adolescents with Disorders of Development: Its Significance and Management*, pp. 155–160. Cambridge, UK: Cambridge University Press.

Gelernter, J., Page, G. P., Stein, M. B., & Woods, S. W. (2004). Genome-wide linkage scan for loci predisposing to social phobia: evidence for a chromosome 16 risk locus. *American Journal of Psychiatry*, **161**, 59–66.

Goldsmith, H. H. & Lemery, K. S. (2000). Linking temperamental fearfulness and anxiety symptoms: a behavior-genetic perspective. *Biological Psychiatry*, **48**, 1199–1209.

Goodman, R. & Stevenson, J. (1991). Parental criticism and warmth toward unrecognized monozygotic twins. *Behavioral and Brain Sciences*, **14**, 394–395.

Gregory, A. M. & Eley, T. C. (2007). Genetic influences on anxiety in children: what we've learned and where we're heading. *Clinical Child and Family Psychology Review*, **10**, 199–212.

Gregory, A. M., Caspi, A., Moffitt, T. E., Koenen, K., Eley, T. C., & Poulton, R. (2007). Juvenile mental health histories of adults with anxiety disorders. *American Journal of Psychiatry*, **164**, 301–308.

Gregory, A. M., Eley, T. C., O'Connor, T. G., Rijsdijk, F. V., & Plomin, R. (2005). Family influences on the association between sleep problems and anxiety in a large sample of pre-school aged twins. *Personality and Individual Differences*, **39**, 1337–1348.

Gregory, A. M., Eley, T. C., & **Plomin, R.** (2004). Exploring the association between anxiety and conduct problems in a large sample of twins aged 2–4. *Journal of Abnormal Child Psychology*, **32**, 111–122.

Hariri, A. R., Mattay, V. S., Tessitore, A., Kolachana, B., Fera, F., Goldman, D., *et al.* (2002). Serotonin transporter genetic variation and the response of the human amygdala. *Science*, **297**, 400–403.

Hettema, J. M., An, S. S., Neale, M. C., Bukszar, J., van den Oord, E. J. C. G., Kendler, K. S., *et al.* (2006). Association between glutamic acid decarboxylase genes and anxiety disorders, major depression, and neuroticism. *Molecular Psychiatry*, **11**, 752–762.

Hettema, J. M., Neale, M. C., & Kendler, K. S. (2001). A review and meta-analysis of the genetic epidemiology of anxiety disorders. *American Journal of Psychiatry*, **158**, 1568–1578.

Hiroi, R., McDevitt, R. A., & Neumaier, J. F. (2006). Estrogen selectively increases tryptophan hydroxylase-2 mRNA expression in distinct subregions of rat midbrain raphe nucleus: association between gene expression and anxiety behavior in the open field. *Biological Psychiatry*, **60**, 288–295.

Jirtle, R. L. & Skinner, M. K. (2007). Environmental epigenomics and disease susceptibility. *Nature Reviews Genetics*, **8**, 253–262.

Jorm, A. F., Henderson, A. S., Jacomb, P. A., Christensen, H., Korten, A. E., Rodgers, B., *et al.* (1998). An association study of a functional polymorphism of the serotonin transporter gene with personality and psychiatric symptoms. *Molecular Psychiatry*, **3**, 449–451.

Karayiorgou, M., Altemus, M., Galke, B. L., Goldman, D., Murphy, D. L., Ott, J., *et al.* (1997). Genotype determining low catechol-O-methyltransferase activity as a risk factor for obsessive-compulsive disorder. *Proceedings of the National Academy of Sciences of the USA*, **94**, 4572–4575.

Karege, F., Perret, G., Bondolfi, G., Schwald, M., Bertschy, G., & Aubry, J. M. (2002). Decreased serum brain-derived neurotrophic factor levels in major depressed patients. *Psychiatry Research*, **109**, 143–148.

Katsuragi, S., Kunugi, H., Sano, A., Tsutsumi, T., Isogawa, K., Nanko, S., *et al.* (1999). Association between serotonin transporter gene polymorphism and anxiety-related traits. *Biological Psychiatry*, **45**, 368–370.

Kendler, K. S., Hettema, J. M., Butera, F., Gardner, C. O., & Prescott, C. A. (2003). Life event dimensions of loss, humiliation, entrapment, and danger in the prediction of onsets of major depression and generalized anxiety. *Archives of General Psychiatry*, **60**, 789–796.

Lakatos, K., Nemoda, Z., Birkas, E., Ronai, Z., Kovacs, E., Ney, K., *et al.* (2003). Association of D4 dopamine receptor gene and serotonin transporter promoter polymorphisms with infants' response to novelty. *Molecular Psychiatry*, **8**, 90–97.

Lau, J. Y. F., Eley, T. C., & Stevenson, J. (2006). Examining the state–trait anxiety relationship: a behavioural genetic approach. *Journal of Abnormal Child Psychology*, **34**, 19–27.

Lau, J. Y. F., Gregory, A. M., Goldwin, M. A., Pine, D. S., & Eley, T. C. (2007). Assessing gene–environment interactions on anxiety symptom subtypes across childhood and adolescence. *Development and Psychopathology*, **19**, 1129–1146.

Lau, J. Y. F., Rijsdijk, F., Gregory, A. M., McGuffin, P., & Eley, T. C. (2007). Pathways to childhood depressive symptoms: the role of social, cognitive, and genetic risk factors. *Developmental Psychology*, **43**, 1402–1414.

Legrand, L. N., McGue, M., & Iacono, W. G. (1999). A twin study of state and trait anxiety in childhood and adolescence. *Journal of Child Psychology and Psychiatry*, **40**, 953–958.

Lesch, K. P., Bengel, D., Heils, A., Zhang Sabol, S., Greenburg, B. D., Petri, S., *et al.* (1996). Association of anxiety-related traits with a polymorphism in the serotonin transporter gene regulatory region. *Science*, **274**, 1527–1531.

McGrath, M., Kawachi, I., Ascherio, A., Colditz, G. A., Hunter, D. J., & De Vivo, I. (2004). Association between catechol-*O*-methyltransferase and phobic anxiety. *American Journal of Psychiatry*, **161**, 1703–1705.

Middeldorp, C. M., Cath, D. C., van Dyck, R., & Boomsma, D. I. (2005). The comorbidity of anxiety and depression in the perspective of genetic epidemiology: a review of twin and family studies. *Psychological Medicine*, **35**, 611–624.

Middeldorp, C. M., Hottenga, J. J., Slagboom, P. E., Sullivan, P. F., De Geus, E. J. C., Posthuma, D., *et al.* (2008). Linkage on chromosome 14 in a genome-wide linkage study of a broad anxiety phenotype. *Molecular Psychiatry*, **13**, 84–89.

Millet, B., Chabane, N., Delorme, R., Leboyer, M., Leroy, S., Poirier, M. F., *et al.* (2003). Association between the dopamine receptor D4 (DRD4) gene and obsessive–compulsive disorder. *American Journal of Medical Genetics, Part B, Neuropsychiatric Genetics*, **116**, 55–59.

Moffitt, T. E., Caspi, A., & Rutter, M. (2005). Strategy for investigating interactions between measured genes and measured environments. *Archives of General Psychiatry*, **62**, 473–481.

Moffitt, T. E., Harrington, H. L., Caspi, A., Kim-Cohen, J., Goldberg, D., Gregory, A. M., *et al.* (2007). Depression and generalized anxiety disorder: cumulative and sequential comorbidity in a birth cohort followed to age 32. *Archives of General Psychiatry*, **64**, 651–660.

Nelson, E. C., Grant, J. D., Bucholz, K. K., Glowinski, A., Madden, P. A. F., Reich, W., *et al.* (2000). Social phobia in population-based female adolescent twin sample: comorbidity and associated suicide-related symptoms. *Psychological Medicine*, **30**, 797–804.

Pike, A., Reiss, D., Hetherington, E. M., & Plomin, R. (1996). Using MZ differences in the search for nonshared environmental effects. *Journal of Child Psychology and Psychiatry*, **37**, 695–704.

Pine, D. S., Cohen, P., Gurley, D., Brook, J., & Ma, Y. J. (1998). The risk for early-adulthood anxiety and depressive disorders in adolescents with anxiety and depressive disorders. *Archives of General Psychiatry*, **55**, 56–64.

Plomin, R., DeFries, J. C., McClearn, G. E., & McGuffin, P. (2008). *Behavioral Genetics*, 5th edn. New York: Worth Publishers.

Plomin, R., Kagan, J., Emde, R. N., Reznick, J. S., Braungart, J. M., Robinson, J., *et al.* (1993). Genetic change and continuity from fourteen to twenty months: the MacArthur Longitudinal Twin Study. *Child Development*, **64**, 1354–1376.

Prichard, Z., Jorm, A. F., Prior, M., Sanson, A., Smart, D., Zhang, Y. F., *et al.* (2002). Association of polymorphisms of the estrogen receptor gene with anxiety-related traits in children and adolescents: a longitudinal study. *American Journal of Medical Genetics*, **114**, 169–176.

Rhee, S. H., Cosgrove, V. E., Schmitz, S., Haberstick, B. C., Corley, R. C., & Hewitt, J. K. (2007). Early childhood temperament and the covariation between internalizing and externalizing behavior in school-aged children. *Twin Research and Human Genetics*, **10**, 33–44.

Risch, N. & Merikangas, K. (1996). The future of genetic studies of complex human diseases. *Science*, **273**, 1516–1517.

Robinson, J. L., Kagan, J., Reznick, J. S., & Corley, R. (1992). The heritability of inhibited and uninhibited behavior: a twin study. *Developmental Psychology*, **28**, 1030–1037.

Rutter, M. (2006). *Genes and Behaviour*. Oxford, UK: Blackwell.

Saudino, K. J., Cherny, S. S., & Plomin, R. (2000). Parent ratings of temperament in twins: explaining the "too low" DZ correlations. *Twin Research*, **3**, 224–233.

Schmidt, L. A., Fox, N. A., Rubin, K. H., Hu, S., & Hamer, D. H. (2002). Molecular genetics of shyness and aggression in preschoolers. *Personality and Individual Differences*, **33**, 227–238.

Sen, S., Burmeister, M., & Ghosh, D. (2004). Meta-analysis of the association between a serotonin transporter promoter polymorphism (5-HTTLPR) and anxiety-related personality traits. *American Journal of Medical Genetics, Part B, Neuropsychiatric Genetics*, **127**, 85–89.

Silberg, J. L. & Bulik, C. M. (2005). The developmental association between eating disorders symptoms and symptoms of depression and anxiety in juvenile twin girls. *Journal of Child Psychology and Psychiatry*, **46**, 1317–1326.

Silberg, J. L., Rutter, M., & Eaves, L. (2001). Genetic and environmental influences on the temporal association between earlier anxiety and later depression in girls. *Biological Psychiatry*, **49**, 1040–1049.

Silberg, J., Rutter, M., Neale, M., & Eaves, L. (2001). Genetic moderation of environmental risk for depression and anxiety in adolescent girls. *British Journal of Psychiatry*, **179**, 116–121.

Silove, D., Manicavasagar, V., O'Connell, D., & Morris-Yates, A. (1995). Genetic factors in early separation anxiety: implications for the genesis of adult anxiety disorders. *Acta Psychiatrica Scandinavica*, **92**, 17–24.

Smoller, J. W., Rosenbaum, J. F., Biederman, J., Kennedy, J., Dai, D., Racette, S. R., et al. (2003). Association of a genetic marker at the corticotropin-releasing hormone locus with behavioral inhibition. *Biological Psychiatry*, **54**, 1376–1381.

Smoller, J. W., Yamaki, L. H., Fagerness, J. A., Biederman, J., Racette, S., Laird, N. M., et al. (2005). The corticotropin-releasing hormone gene and behavioral inhibition in children at risk for panic disorder. *Biological Psychiatry*, **57**, 1485–1492.

Spatola, C. A. M., Fagnani, C., Pesenti-Gritti, P., Ogliari, A., Stazi, M. A., & Battaglia, M. (2007). A general population twin study of the CBCL/6–18 DSM-oriented scales. *Journal of the American Academy of Child and Adolescent Psychiatry*, **46**, 619–627.

Stevenson, J. & Fielding, J. (1985). Ratings of temperament in families of young twins. *British Journal of Developmental Psychology*, **3**, 143–152.

Stevenson, J., Batten, N., & Cherner, M. (1992). Fears and fearfulness in children and adolescents: a genetic analysis of twin data. *Journal of Child Psychology and Psychiatry*, **33**, 977–985.

Thapar, A. & McGuffin, P. (1995). Are anxiety symptoms in childhood heritable? *Journal of Child Psychology and Psychiatry*, **36**, 439–447.

Thapar, A. & McGuffin, P. (1996). A twin study of antisocial and neurotic symptoms in childhood. *Psychological Medicine*, **26**, 1111–1118.

Thapar, A. & McGuffin, P. (1997). Anxiety and depressive symptoms in childhood: a genetic study of comorbidity. *Journal of Child Psychology and Psychiatry*, **38**, 651–656.

Tochigi, M., Kato, C., Otowa, T., Hibino, H., Marui, T., Ohtani, T., et al. (2006). Association between corticotropin-releasing hormone receptor 2 (CRHR2) gene polymorphism and personality traits. *Psychiatry and Clinical Neurosciences*, **60**, 524–526.

Topolski, T. D., Hewitt, J. K., Eaves, L., Meyer, J. M., Silberg, J. L., Simonoff, E., et al. (1999). Genetic and environmental influences on ratings of manifest anxiety by parents and children. *Journal of Anxiety Disorders*, **13**, 371–397.

Topolski, T. D., Hewitt, J. K., Eaves, L. J., Silberg, J. L., Meyer, J. M., Rutter, M., et al. (1997). Genetic and environmental influences on child reports of manifest anxiety and symptoms of separation anxiety and overanxious disorders: a community-based twin study. *Behavior Genetics*, **27**, 15–28.

Turner, S. M., Beidel, D. C., & Costello, A. (1987). Psychopathology in the offspring of anxiety disordered patients. *Journal of Consulting and Clinical Psychology*, **55**, 229–235.

van den Oord, E. J. C. G., Boomsma, D. I., & Verhulst, F. C. (2000). A study of genetic and environmental effects on the co-occurrence of problem behaviors in three-year-old twins. *Journal of Abnormal Psychology*, **109**, 360–372.

van Grootheest, D. S., Bartels, M., Cath, D. C., Beekman, A. T., Hudziak, J. J., & Boomsma, D. I. (2007). Genetic and environmental contributions underlying stability in childhood obsessive–compulsive behavior. *Biological Psychiatry*, **61**, 308–315.

van Hulle, C. A., Lemery-Chalfant, K., & Goldsmith, H. H. (2007). Genetic and environmental influences on socio-emotional behavior in toddlers: an initial twin study of the infant–toddler social and emotional assessment. *Journal of Child Psychology and Psychiatry*, **48**, 1014–1024.

van Ommen, G. J. B. (2008). GWAS here, last year. *European Journal of Human Genetics*, **16**, 1–2.

van Rossum, E. F. C., Binder, E. B., Majer, M., Koper, J. W., Ising, M., Modell, S., *et al.* (2006). Polymorphisms of the glucocorticoid receptor gene and major depression. *Biological Psychiatry*, **59**, 681–688.

van Vliet, J., Oates, N. A., & Whitelaw, E. (2007). Epigenetic mechanisms in the context of complex diseases. *Cellular and Molecular Life Sciences*, **64**, 1531–1538.

Weaver, I. C. G., Cervoni, N., Champagne, F. A., D'Alessio, A. C., Sharma, S., Seckl, J. R., *et al.* (2004). Epigenetic programming by maternal behavior. *Nature Neuroscience*, **7**, 847–854.

Weaver, I. C. G., Meaney, M. J., & Szyf, M. (2006). Maternal care effects on the hippocampal transcriptome and anxiety-mediated behaviors in the offspring that are reversible in adulthood. *Proceedings of the National Academy of Sciences of the USA*, **103**, 3480–3485.

Wray, N. R., James, M. R., Mah, S. P., Nelson, M., Andrews, G., Sullivan, P. F., *et al.* (2007). Anxiety and comorbid measures associated with PLXNA2. *Archives of General Psychiatry*, **64**, 318–326.

Young, S. E., Smolen, A., Stallings, M. C., Corley, R. P., & Hewitt, J. K. (2003). Sibling-based association analyses of the serotonin transporter polymorphism and internalizing behavior problems in children. *Journal of Child Psychology and Psychiatry*, **44**, 961–967.

9

The brain and behavior in childhood and adolescent anxiety disorders

Daniel S. Pine

Introduction

Chapter perspective

This chapter begins with an introduction that delineates the perspective adopted throughout the chapter, defines core terms, and outlines the plan for the remainder of the chapter. The purpose of the chapter is to examine relationships among brain function, emotional processes, and individual differences relevant to the classification of pediatric anxiety disorders. As such, the chapter summarizes current knowledge, on a relatively broad conceptual basis, that describes the manner in which measures of brain function relate to both normal and abnormal anxiety, particularly in children and adolescents. The chapter is not definitive, as the pace of research both on anxiety and on the brain is such that any summary becomes outdated shortly after it is written. However, the organizational approach to brain-based research summarized herein is likely to persist for some time, because the approach emerged gradually, organizes considerable ongoing work, and is likely to heavily inform future work.

The chapter is written from dual perspectives. First, a neuroscience perspective is adopted, which means that an emphasis is placed on charting the manner in which individual differences in the brain relate to individual differences in behavior. This perspective specifically focuses on affective neuroscience, brain-based work on emotional processes. Because research in neuroscience draws heavily on cross-species comparisons, a premium is placed on perspectives on behavior that can be applied with equal clarity to research with humans and with other mammals. Of course, humans possess unique panoplies of anxiety responses; the current brain-based perspective limits in-depth consideration of these features. This limitation is necessary so that insights can emerge through the scientific advantages afforded by working in animal-model systems. Second, a developmental perspective is adopted, which means that individual differences in anxiety, manifest at any age, are recognized as reflecting ontogeny. Such a perspective appears particularly relevant for anxiety: perhaps in no other area relevant to mental disorders have developmental–neuroscience perspectives been more informative.

Defining terms

Attempts to chart cross-species parallels benefit from precise definitions equally applicable across diverse species. Thus, the term *emotion* is used here specifically to define brain states elicited by stimuli for which organisms will extend effort to approach or avoid.

Anxiety Disorders in Children and Adolescents, 2nd edn, ed. W. K. Silverman and A. P. Field. Published by Cambridge University Press. © Cambridge University Press 2011.

The brain-based processes through which emotionally evocative stimuli are processed and responded to are defined as *information-processing functions*, and much of the current chapter focuses on delineation of specific information-processing functions elicited by dangerous scenarios, those that are capable of harming the organism.

Fear is defined as the specific brain state elicited by an immediately present, highly salient, *overt threat*, a discrete danger that the organism avoids. Fear and its associated triggers can be dissociated from the related emotion of anxiety, based both on the nature of the triggers and the chronometry of the resulting brain state. Thus, whereas fear is triggered by acute, abruptly appearing, overt threats, *anxiety* is defined as the brain state triggered by more sustained threats that less precisely predict onset of danger in terms of either temporal or spatial aspects of the threat. Of note, some investigators working in animal model systems have suggested that measures of "fear" might index "normal," "adaptive," or "healthy" responding to danger, whereas "anxiety" might index "abnormal" responding to danger (Davis, 1998). However, both fear and anxiety can be considered either "normal" or "abnormal," based on the degree to which the associated brain state facilitates or impedes adaptive functioning.

Finally, the occurrence of an emotion, as reflected in a neural response and associated behavioral or cognitive changes, differs from processes designed to regulate emotions. From the perspective of neuroscience research with children and adolescents, far more work examines the neural correlates of emotional responses than attempts to regulate these responses. Accordingly, the current chapter largely summarizes research examining neural correlates of emotional responses, but it does not review data on neural correlates of emotional regulation.

Chapter outline

Following this introduction, this chapter proceeds in three subsequent stages. The immediately proceeding section reviews the manner in which brain-based research characterizes anxiety, both in terms of species-typical responses and individual differences. Next, the chapter describes the utility of neuroscience for informing research on human individual differences; key findings in neuroscience are highlighted, and neuroscience methods applicable to children are delineated. Particular focus is placed on the role of specific information-processing functions in bridging research on the brain and behavior. Finally, the chapter highlights select findings focused on pediatric anxiety that have examined information-processing functions amenable to cross-species neuroscience approaches.

Behaviors examined in brain-based research

Investigators focusing on the mammalian response to danger have adopted various perspectives. A large body of work focuses on the typical response that most organisms exhibit when confronting danger; other investigators focus on the nature of individual differences. Care must be taken to distinguish these approaches. Just because brain structures within a particular circuit mediate species-typical response does not imply that the same set mediates individual differences (Davis, 1998).

Species-typical responding

Organisms possessing behavioral features that lead to successful responses to danger are expected to benefit, in terms of survival, from an evolutionary perspective. This should lead these features to become integrated into the core behavioral repertoire of the species, and the selective advantages afforded should contribute to cross-species conservation of behavior. As a result, certain aspects of fear and anxiety are viewed as general characteristics of all organisms within a species; these features also are expected to show strong cross-species parallels. Within a diverse array of mammals, strong similarities emerge in various aspects of threat-response behaviors (Darwin, 1998; Davis & Whalen, 2001; LeDoux, 2000). This includes the nature of changes in motor programs, autonomic physiology, measures of information processing, and activity within specific brain structures. Moreover, data also establish that fear and anxiety are probably best viewed as families of related but clearly separable brain states. This view stems from the fact that fears of different situations differ based on the nature of the underlying brain circuitry (Blanchard, Griebel, Henrie, & Blanchard, 1997; Davis, 1998).

Cross-species similarities extend to humans. For example, humans living in diverse cultures exhibit striking similarities in the things they fear (Ollendick, Yang, King, Dong, & Akande, 1996); similar cross-cultural similarity emerges for developmental phenomena. As in other mammals, human fear and anxiety represent collections of developmentally dissociable states. Young children typically fear separation before they fear small animals or other discrete sources of danger, such as thunderstorms or darkness (see Muris & Field, Chapter 4, this volume). These fears are later replaced by fears associated with social experiences or abstract threats, such as humiliation (Ollendick, Langley, Jones, & Kephart, 2001; Pine, Helfinstein, Bar-Haim, Nelson, & Fox, 2009; Stattin, 1984). These differences parallel culturally consistent patterns of gender differences, whereby girls report more fears than boys (Ollendick *et al.*, 1996).

Classification of individual differences

Attempts to delineate neural correlates of species-typical behavior can be differentiated from attempts to delineate neural correlates of individual differences. The current chapter focuses most directly on individual differences. Brain systems underlying individual differences encompass similar structures mediating species-typical behavior, but the functional correlates of typical and atypical responding differ. Individual differences can be viewed from either categorical or dimensional perspectives; children can be arranged along a continuum in terms of their responses to threat exposure, or children who show particularly high levels of fear can be distinguished as a unique group, relative to children who show typical levels of fear. Of course, these perspectives are complementary in that a continuous scale can be used to rank children in their threat-response profile, and those scoring particularly high on this scale can be categorically separated as unique (Kraemer, 2007).

Considerable debate surrounds these alternative perspectives, because the categorical perspective has advantages when trying to allocate services to those children most in need. However, the dimensional approach accommodates data from longitudinal and family-based studies suggesting that fears lie along continua in children (Biel *et al.*, 2008; Kraemer, 2007; Pine, Cohen, & Brook, 2001). This review emphasizes categories because most work on neural correlates in children adopts a categorical perspective. Nevertheless, the true nature of relationships between biology and individual differences is revealed by research charting the relationship between these two constructs across large populations to determine if the relationship is truly continuous or categorical. Such research is many years away.

Closely related debates focus on temperament and psychopathology (see Lonigan, Phillips, Wilson, & Allan, Chapter 10, this volume). At one level, these two constructs can be readily distinguished. Temperament refers to early-emerging extreme patterns of responding to specific stimuli; work on one specific temperament, behavioral inhibition, shows that a relatively small group of children exhibit early tendencies to respond with fear, apprehension, and wariness when confronted with novelty, particularly social novelty (Fox, Henderson, Marshall, Nichols, & Ghera, 2005; Kagan, 1994). Children can be arranged along continua in terms of their levels of inhibition, though some suggest discontinuity emerges in these data supporting a categorical view (Kagan, 1994). Regardless, temperament is viewed as a form of normal variation. Research on clinical forms of anxiety, in contrast, delineates the degree to which fears are associated with perturbed function.

At another level, this distinction can be seen as artificial: both temperament and clinical anxiety can be measured similarly. Most research on associated neural circuitry examines either temperamental groups or individuals with disorders, considered in isolation; few studies compare groups cross-classified on both constructs. Since studies of behavioral inhibition and anxiety disorders find comparable associations with measures of brain function, it remains unclear the degree to which the two sets of studies examine distinguishable, as opposed to identical associations. As with questions on distinctions between categories and continua, currently available data cannot clarify the true nature of these relationships.

Risk versus behavior

Based on longitudinal or family-genetic data (Rosenbaum, Biederman, Bolduc, Hirshfeld, Faraone, & Kagan, 2000; Schwartz, Snidman, & Kagan, 1999), some view behavioral inhibition as a risk factor for anxiety disorders. This work demonstrates an association between behavioral inhibition in children and anxiety disorders in these same children followed prospectively or in their parents. However, both anxiety and inhibition classifies children based on their behavior. Other schemes classify children based on risk factors less closely tied to children's behavior.

Probably the most comprehensive literature considers measures of parental psychopathology (see Creswell, Murray, Stacey, & Cooper, Chapter 14, this volume). Here, parental history of panic disorder or major depression predicts risk for anxiety disorders as well as patterns of biological correlates in children (Grillon *et al.*, 2005; Pine, 2007; Pine *et al.*, 2005). For both parental risk profiles, patterns of responding on anxiety-related phenotypes are independent of symptoms in the child. Other risk factors include direct measures of genotype or stress exposure (see Gregory & Eley, Chapter 8, this volume), which shape risk through interactions (Rutter, Moffitt, & Caspi, 2006). While this work is only beginning, emerging findings link both genetics and stress exposure to children's brain function (Lau *et al.*, 2008; Pine & Cohen, 2002).

Affective neuroscience

Neuroscience incorporates data from animal models and children. Figure 9.1 depicts an affective neuroscience framework for the current chapter; related frameworks can be found in similar publications (Pine, 2007). This framework is mutually informed by studies in rodents, non-human primates, and humans; it illustrates relationships between individual differences in brain function, as depicted in the left-hand margin (box A), and individual differences in behavior, as depicted in the right-hand margin (box C). As described in the

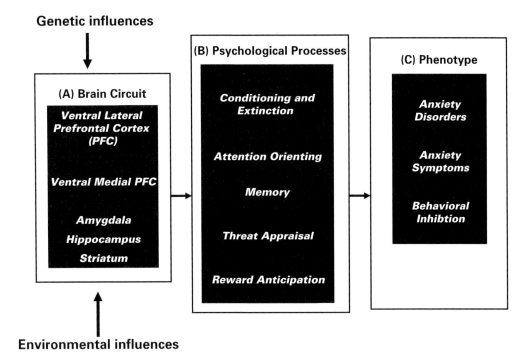

Genetic influences

(B) Psychological Processes

(C) Phenotype

(A) Brain Circuit

Ventral Lateral Prefrontal Cortex (PFC)

Ventral Medial PFC

Amygdala

Hippocampus

Striatum

Conditioning and Extinction

Attention Orienting

Memory

Threat Appraisal

Reward Anticipation

Anxiety Disorders

Anxiety Symptoms

Behavioral Inhibtion

Environmental influences

Figure 9.1 Framework for integrating research on gene/environmental influences as brain circuitry (box A) with research on individual differences in behavior, or "phenotypes" (box C). Central to this framework is a focus on psychological processes (box B) as intermediaries between measures of brain function and behavior (boxes A and C). Figure 9.1 emphasizes five sets of psychological processes around which considerable neuroscience-related work in pediatric anxiety disorders can be organized.

next section, box B depicts fear-related processes conceptualized from an information-processing-function perspective. Constructs in box B bridge brain- and behavior-focused research.

Individual differences in brain function (box A) are shaped by the dual influences of genes and the environment; these individual differences, in turn, shape individual differences in information processing (box B), which mediate individual differences in behavior (box C). Thus, individual differences in mammals are viewed through various lenses, focusing on an increasingly broad level of analysis.

Animal models of anxiety

Research in animal models delineates neural architecture engaged during the processing of threats, an architecture typically labeled as the "fear circuit." Like the architecture associated with most complex behavioral repertoires, the fear circuit encompasses relatively large collections of brain structures. At a minimum, as listed in Figure 9.1, this includes ventral expanses of the prefrontal cortex (PFC) on both medial and lateral (vmPFC and vlPFC) sides of the brain, as well as the amygdala, lying within the medial temporal lobes. Although disagreement persists for other structures, the hippocampus and striatum, also listed in Figure 9.1, are occasionally included as components of the fear circuit, as is the ventral cingulate cortex, which sometimes is considered to be part of the vmPFC.

One key to extending work from animal models to the clinic involves focusing on the manner in which these brain structures mediate particular, narrowly defined behaviors and their associated information-processing functions. The next five subsections describe such work in five areas. In one sense, these areas provide distinct targets of separate scientific lines of investigation. In another sense, however, many of the areas show strong relationships among each other, both in terms of conceptual definitions and associated neural circuitry.

Fear conditioning

In fear conditioning, a neutral conditioned stimulus (CS+), such as a light or tone, is paired with an aversive unconditioned stimulus, such as shock or a loud sound (US). Following such pairing, the CS+ acquires the capacity to elicit behaviors, information-processing functions, and physiologic changes previously associated only with the US. Organisms also develop fear of the contexts within which the CS+ is presented, a process known as "context conditioning" or "occasion setting," and organisms also can learn to withhold fear responses, through a process called "extinction," if the CS+ is repeatedly presented in the absence of the US. While other processes beyond extinction also modulate the organism's response to the CS+ over time, translational research tends to focus more on extinction than these other processes. As a result, the current chapter focuses only on extinction.

Considerable work delineates the underlying neural architecture engaged during fear conditioning. Full discussion of these details and their developmental correlates are found elsewhere (Davis, 1998; LeDoux, 2000; Pine *et al.*, 2009). This work establishes the fact that specific brain structures play comparable roles in diverse mammalian species. Thus, the amygdala is necessary for an organism to form CS+–US associations, possibly by modulating attention responses (Davis & Whalen, 2001). The hippocampus is necessary for context conditioning, and the vmPFC is necessary for extinction (Quirk & Mueller, 2008). The striatum allows CS+–US association to influence behavior. Interestingly, individual differences in humans as well as rodents tend to relate less strongly to the most robust measures of fear conditioning and their associated neural changes than to more subtle measures, such as conditioning to ambiguous cues, and their unique neural changes (Pine *et al.*, 2009). For example, anxious and healthy subjects may exhibit similar increases in fear responding when the responses to overtly dangerous and ambiguous cues are compared. However, anxious subjects may exhibit more robust increases when the response to either the dangerous or the ambiguous cue is compared with the response to an overtly non-dangerous cue. This observation represents one of the above noted instances where neural correlates of species-typical behavior can be differentiated from correlates of individual differences.

Attention orienting

The mammalian brain is said to be "capacity-limited," meaning that it cannot simultaneously process all features of the environment. Attention is the information-processing function through which mammals prioritize one or another stimulus feature for particularly detailed processing. Attention is most accurately described as a suite of processes, and stimulus features associated with threats or danger impact on many of these (Davis & Whalen, 2001). In terms of cross-species research on individual differences, the most detailed work focuses on attention orienting, the process whereby one or another specific feature in the environment has the capacity to engage neural resources and produce associated changes in behavior. Relative to neutral stimuli, both CS+ and innately threatening stimuli show an enhanced capacity to "capture" attention, as organisms tend to orient towards threats.

Research on the neural circuitry mediating orienting has been reviewed elsewhere (Corbetta, Patel, & Shulman, 2008; Davis & Whalen, 2001; Pine *et al.*, 2009). As with fear conditioning, this work demonstrates strong cross-species parallels in brain–behavior associations. This circuitry involves three interacting components. First, the amygdala is immediately engaged when attention is captured by threats, through a path that extends directly from the periphery, to the thalamus, and to the amygdala. Second, this pathway diverges at the thalamus to include a second, slower pathway, through the posterior ventral cortex, which provides slower but more elaborately processed signals. Finally, information in the amygdala is fed to the vlPFC, which interacts with the striatum and cortically based nodes to regulate the orienting of attention towards or away from specific environmental components.

Memory

As with attention, memory involves a collection of diverse but related processes, each allowing organisms to adapt through experience dependent changes in the brain. From this perspective, fear conditioning represents one form of memory. Many other forms of memory show distinct features from conditioning, in terms of the psychological characteristics and associated anatomy. Thus, declarative memory, as usually studied in humans, relates to forms of so-called explicit memory, in animals (Squire & Kandel, 1999). Relative to conditioning, these forms of memory allow mammals to form more flexible associations among key features of specific stimuli. Particular types of memories form for stimuli that are particularly important for survival: mammals better remember emotionally evocative than neutral scenarios (Phelps & LeDoux, 2005). Unique types of memory also may occur specifically for social stimuli (Young & Wang, 2004).

The circuitry underlying emotionally modulated memory also is reviewed elsewhere (Cahill, 1999; Phelps & LeDoux, 2005; Young & Wang, 2004). This circuitry encompasses many structures implicated in conditioning and attention orienting, though the hippocampus, through interactions with the amygdala, probably plays a particularly strong and broad role in emotional memory, whereas the striatum may play a similarly strong role in social memory.

Threat appraisal

Appraisal refers to the process whereby emotionally salient stimuli are categorized based on an organism's tendency to approach or avoid them (Pine, 2007; Scherer, 2001). In humans, appraisal is typically assessed by participants' reports of the behavior they would exhibit when confronted by the stimulus, though an unambiguous appraisal typically involves both a report and a corresponding, manifest behavior (Pine, 2007). In animal models, appraisal is usually indexed based on behavior, with threat appraisal manifesting in avoidance. Across species, however, appraisals allow organisms to consistently make relatively subtle classifications, in terms of a stimulus's potential to harm. The circuitry through which appraisal is instantiated involves many of the same structures implicated in the four other processes described above (Pine, 2007; Scherer, 2001). However, the circuitry has been less comprehensively delineated, and the specific psychological components have been less precisely delineated, relative to conditioning, attention, and memory.

Reward processing

Considerable work distinguishes neural circuits engaged by threats and rewards, stimuli which, respectively, motivate avoidance or approach. In terms of research relevant to anxiety, reward-related behavior can be separated into evaluative components, which have been shown to be highly relevant to individual differences in anxiety, and consummatory components, which have been less consistently linked to anxiety (Ernst, Pine, & Hardin, 2006; Guyer *et al.*, 2006). Much as organisms have evolved complex, conserved architecture for handling threats, they have a similarly elaborative circuitry that detects rewards and organizes approach behavior. The amygdala plays a role in this circuitry, mediating attention to rewards, but more research on reward-related processes focuses on the role of the striatum, through interactions with the vmPFC, than the amygdala (Holland & Gallagher, 2004). As noted above, the vmPFC and the vlPFC represent two components of PFC circuitry implicated in humans' emotional processing. The most extensive research on vmPFC function in human anxiety focuses on the role of this structure in extinction, though considerable work also implicates the structure in regulation of reward processing. Current conceptualizations view the striatum as central to a circuit that detects errors related to the expected value of environmental stimuli in terms of their capacity to predict reward (Schultz, 2001). This provides signals that modulate motor plans designed to secure rewards.

Environmental and genetic influences on development

The focus on cross-species similarities in brain–behavior associations carries unique advantages when trying to delineate the mechanisms that give rise to these associations. Animal-model systems provide unique opportunities for precise experimental control and in-depth probing of neural function, allowing scientists to establish causal chains of events that shape individual differences. Such work demonstrates that individual differences in anxiety emerge from mutually reinforcing interactions between genes and the environment, all evolving in a developmental context.

Environmental effects

Studies in both rodents and non-human primates demonstrate that individual differences in the rearing environment produce robust individual differences in fear-circuitry function, associated information-processing functions, and behaviors (Coplan, Rosenblum, & Gorman, 1995; Meaney, 2001; Pine, 2003). By randomly assigning animals to distinct rearing conditions, this work shows that environments exert direct, causal influences on threat processing. This work has used diverse manipulations to study environmental influences. This includes studies manipulating species-typical grooming behavior of rat pups, studies of relatively subtle early-life stress through brief separations in various species, or studies of more extreme and extensive stress, through longer separations. Moreover, work using such manipulations in rodents demonstrates that these environmental influences engage molecular processes, such as gene methylation, which produce changes in genetic function that also are passed on to offspring. In both rodents and non-human primates, these environmental effects occur during specific developmental time points: environmental events permanently alter the organism's response to threats in ways that do not occur in maturity. Early emerging individual differences in rodents and non-human primates, much as they do in humans, show robust associations with lifelong patterns of threat-response behavior (Pine, 2003).

Genetic effects

Genetic manipulations also show a unique ability to alter patterns of threat-response behavior in immature, relative to mature, rodents. These effects appear particularly strong for genes controlling the actions of serotonin (5-HT) (Gross & Hen, 2004). Thus, both for manipulations of the genes for the 5-HT1a receptor and 5-HT transporter, effects on anxiety occur selectively for early-life manipulations. Such manipulations are possible in rodents, through advances in techniques of genetic engineering. These techniques provide scientists with the tools to selecting introduce or eliminate various genes into an embryo. Moreover, these genes can be selectively turned on or off, by modulating the natural regulators of gene activity.

Affective neuroscience applications with children

Clinical applications of neuroscience ultimately require studies directly with children. Such research occurs at multiple levels organized in Figure 9.1. From the perspective of genes and environmental risk factors, studies can document the manner in which these factors map onto individual differences in brain function, information processing, or behavior manifest in children's daily lives. Considerable work pursues these themes, and readers are referred to these reviews for more comprehensive summaries of this work (Pine, 2003; Pine & Klein, 2008). Other work examines individual differences in peripheral physiology (Pine & Klein, 2008). For example, some studies examine startle response, cardiovascular regulation, or respiratory physiology. In each instance, individual differences in physiology are thought to reflect the downstream effects on the periphery emanating from functional differences in the circuitry appearing in Figure 9.1, box A. In other situations, studies have examined the relationship between individual differences in hormones or neurochemistry, such as measures that are influenced by 5-HT function, such as densities of 5-HT receptors or levels of neurochemicals influenced by 5-HT. In these instances, individual differences in hormones or chemicals are thought to shape circuitry functions (Nelson, Leibenluft, McClure, & Pine, 2005). While most biological research on pediatric anxiety focuses on peripheral measures of physiology, none of this work is reviewed in depth in this chapter.

Instead of a focus on peripheral physiology, genes, or environmental risk, the final chapter section focuses on one particular area of affective neuroscience inquiry that provides particularly fruitful opportunities to link research on brain–behavior associations in humans with research on brain–behavior associations in other mammals. This work involves the engagement of an information-processing function depicted in box B of Figure 9.1 and relates these functions to individual differences in anxiety. To achieve the most comprehensive integration with studies using animal models, ideally, this work is completed within the context of a brain imaging experiment. Moreover, functional magnetic resonance imaging (fMRI) provides a particularly important tool, because it possesses the best combination of temporal and spatial resolution for charting functional aspects of relevant neural circuitry, directly mapping relationships among brain function, information processing, and behavior, linking the three boxes depicted in Figure 9.1.

Brain–behavior associations in pediatric anxiety

Research described in this final section provides particularly promising avenues for integrating basic and clinical research. An increasing amount of work uses fMRI to chart species-typical developmental changes in the amygdala and associated components of the brain's fear circuit. As noted above, work on species-typical neural responses often finds unique associations, relative to work on individual differences. This also applies to fMRI. As this chapter focuses on individual differences, work on normal development is mentioned briefly.

Normal development

The search for functional differences in the amygdala probably represents the most consistent theme in research on development of the fear circuit. While the data are quite complex, a consistent story is emerging. Thus, human amygdala fMRI activation varies based on the attention processes engaged during scanning, and attention requirements of many cognitive tasks place distinct demands on children, adolescents, and adults (Beesdo et al., 2009; Guyer, Lau, et al., 2008; Guyer, Monk, et al., 2008). Therefore, developmental studies of amygdala function using different cognitive tasks generate different conclusions. Similar concerns apply to studies of gender influences, whereby the effects of both age and attention also have been shown to uniquely influence amygdala responding in males and females. For example, before maturity, adolescent males and females may respond similarly to threat stimuli, at least under certain attention-constraining circumstances. In maturity, however, women and men may respond differently under these same circumstances. When each factor is considered, data consistently document immature amygdala function well into adolescence, both among anxious children and adolescents, as well as among healthy ones. Other research demonstrates similar findings in other components of neural circuitry relevant to anxiety, particularly the PFC (Steinberg, 2008).

Fear conditioning and extinction

Attempts to study fear conditioning in children confront unique ethical issues. This is because an ethically permissible US must be chosen that will not unduly frighten the child, but the US must be sufficiently frightening to support fear conditioning. Electric shock is the most frequently employed US in adults but typically is not used in children or adolescents. Although a range of US has been used, consistent data are beginning to emerge with mildly aversive sounds (Craske et al., 2008; Lau, Lissek, et al., 2008; Pine et al., 2009). These data generate findings comparable to those found in adults and animal models.

Individual differences in anxiety show the most consistent associations with perturbed classification of CS+. Both in people and rodents, individual differences emerge for responses to an ambiguous CS+ that is difficult to classify as either safe or threatening, as opposed to an overtly threatening CS+ (Pine et al., 2009). Figure 9.2 depicts data emerging from a fear-conditioning paradigm used to demonstrate associations between clinical anxiety and fear-conditioning responses in adolescents. In this paradigm, one stimulus, depicting a woman, serves as a CS+ through pairings with an aversive sound, and a similar unpaired stimulus serves as a CS−. Relative to healthy adolescents, anxious patients exhibit increased fear responding on this paradigm. However, prior findings in adults suggest that such patients would exhibit even greater differences from healthy adolescents when viewing ambiguous stimuli (Lissek et al., 2008). For example, Figure 9.2, in the recall of extinction paradigm, shows three stimuli. These comprise an original CS+, an original CS−, and a novel, "morphed" stimulus, shown between the CS+ and the CS−. As shown, this morphed stimulus incorporates 50% of the physical features of the CS+ and 50% of the features of the CS−. Thus, the morphed stimulus incorporates features of

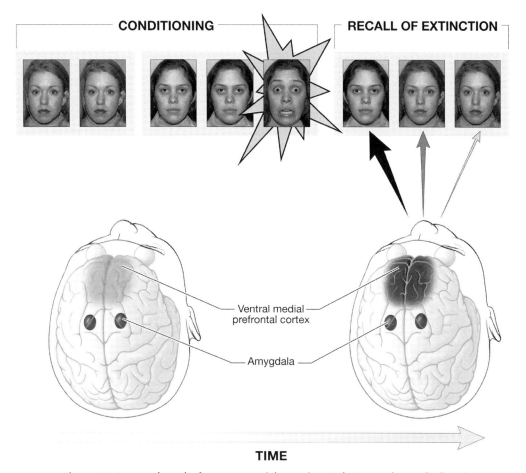

Figure 9.2 Expected results from a potential experiment that extends two findings in recent fear-conditioning experiments. First, in one study, individual difference in conditioning emerged when subjects were exposed to facial photographs, as appearing in the left-hand side of the figure, whereby one neutral facial photograph is paired with an aversive sound (Lau, Lissek, *et al.*, 2008). While this study did not collect neuroimaging data, this between-group difference would be expected to reflect between-group differences in amygdala function. Second, in this study as well as other work, data suggest that anxious adolescents are likely to exhibit modest differences from healthy adolescents when they are exposed to the two previously used conditioned stimuli, though both groups of adolescents are expected to exhibit strong fear responses to the conditioned stimulus (first photograph under "recall of extinction") (Lau, Lissek, *et al.*, 2008; Lissek *et al.*, 2008; Pine *et al.*, 2009). While data have not been obtained when adolescents are exposed to a morphed photograph incorporating some features of both the conditioned and non-conditioned stimulus, previous work suggests that individual differences are likely to be particularly large to this stimulus (second photograph under "recall of extinction"). Finally, while no imaging data have been collected here, these between-group differences at recall of extinction are expected to reflect between-group differences in both amygdala and ventral medial prefrontal cortex function.

both the CS+ and CS−. This stimulus would be expected to elicit greater between-group differences than the CS+ itself, which would be expected, in contrast, to elicit the greatest fear in both healthy and anxious adolescents. Hence, the response to the CS− would be relatively low in both anxious and healthy adolescents; similarly, the response to the CS+ would be relatively high in both anxious and healthy adolescents. However, the response to the ambiguous, morphed stimulus would be moderately high in the anxious subjects, higher than to the CS−, lower than to the CS+, but higher than to the morphed stimulus in the healthy subjects. The process of extinction represents another instance where a CS+ is rendered ambiguous, as this is a stimulus that used to be dangerous but is currently not associated with danger. As with morphed stimuli, a strong anxiety-related relationship with extinguished CS+ would be expected.

Studies using fMRI on fear conditioning in adults generate hypotheses on the neural structure that might mediate these anxiety-related differences manifest during fear conditioning (Phelps & LeDoux, 2005). This work suggests that both the amygdala and vmPFC are likely to be involved, as also illustrated in Figure 9.2. However, direct tests of this hypothesis require studies in anxious children and adolescents.

Attention orienting

The dot-probe paradigm represents the most consistently used measure in research on threat-related perturbations in attention orienting (see Garner, 2010, for a review). The paradigm generates consistent between-group differences in anxious and non-anxious individuals across a wide age range (Bar-Haim, Lamy, Pergamin, Bakermans-Kranenburg, & van IJzendoorn, 2007). Recent fMRI studies successfully extend this paradigm to the neuroimaging environment (Pine *et al.*, 2009). This work links adolescent individual differences in anxiety to individual differences in fear-circuitry function.

Much like in work among rodents and non-human primates, orienting to threats in humans involves the amygdala and vlPFC. Thus, studies in adolescents establish that anxiety-related individual differences in amygdala function emerge for very briefly presented threats, emphasizing the role of amygdala-based circuitry in the immediate response to threats. Differences in vlPFC function, a region centrally involved in the control of attention, become apparent for stimuli that are presented for more sustained time periods. Importantly, this work has been completed directly in human adolescents, and it can be readily integrated with a larger body of work in adult humans and in rodents or non-human primates of various ages. In these instances, work using the dot-probe paradigm importantly demonstrates the manner in which fMRI charts relationships among brain function, information processing, and individual differences in anxiety.

Memory

Considerable work examines individual differences in emotionally modulated memory as it relates to individual differences in psychopathology. This work fits within the broader context of neuroscience-focused investigations charting the manner in which particularly brain regions mediate memory for emotional and non-emotional stimuli. Nevertheless, from an individual difference standpoint, memory-related perturbations relate more strongly to individual differences in mood as opposed to anxiety (Roberson-Nay *et al.*, 2006). Pediatric anxiety disorders typically involve normal emotional memory, and these findings contrast with data in major depression, where consistent associations with perturbed emotionally modulated memory emerge. Some correlates of these findings related to amygdala function may be best captured using emotional memory tasks, administered in the fMRI scanner. Since these findings are more relevant to the differences between pediatric anxiety and depression than the specific correlates of pediatric anxiety, comprehensive review of material in this area is beyond the scope of the current chapter.

Threat appraisal

More work relates individual differences in threat appraisal and anxious behavior to individual differences in neural responding than for any other information-processing function (Pine, 2007). However, as noted above, work in neuroscience using rodents or non-human primates explicitly examines threat appraisal less comprehensively than fear conditioning, attention orienting, or memory, though many processes, including fear conditioning, would also be expected to engage threat-appraisal processes. Hence, the questions that arise on appraisal contrast with those that arise in fear conditioning, where considerable work is needed using fMRI-based fear-conditioning paradigms that extend work from rodents and non-human primates. For threat appraisal, work is needed that extends fMRI findings in children to rodents and non-human primates. Such an extension would allow experimental work in rodents and non-human primates to inform more directly clinical studies in children.

Many initial fMRI studies of pediatric anxiety relied on paradigms that are difficult to classify in terms of the information-processing functions that they engaged. These studies typically employed block-design paradigms, where multiple different stimuli drawn from a common class would be presented for relatively long intervals, lasting on the order of minutes. These studies often allowed patient participants to passively view these blocks of stimuli, providing no online data concerning the degree to which particular information-processing functions were engaged. Nevertheless, discussions of results from these studies often emphasized the relevance of threat appraisal, whereby patients were expected implicitly and automatically to classify the stimuli encountered during imaging in terms of the degree to which they should be approached or avoided. This is reasonable.

In the first such imaging investigation, Thomas et al. (2001) found anxious children selected from a clinic to show signs of enhanced amygdala responding to fear faces, relative to both depressed and healthy children, the latter two of whom, curiously, actually showed no amygdala responses to fear faces, contrasting with considerable data in adults (Thomas et al., 2001). Similarly, Schwartz and colleagues used a related paradigm to examine the neural correlates of behavioral inhibition among formerly inhibited children who had been followed prospectively into adulthood (Schwartz, Wright, Shin, Kagan, & Rauch, 2003). In this work, novel faces were contrasted with familiar faces, familiarized to subjects through experimental manipulations. In this paradigm, all faces appeared neutral, but differential threat appraisal was expected to be engaged in formerly inhibited versus other individuals during viewing of novel-face blocks. As with Thomas et al.'s findings in pediatric anxiety, this study also found enhanced amygdala responding, here in the formerly inhibited, relative to the other individuals. Other related block-design studies generally confirmed these findings. Thus, individual differences in anxiety relate to individual differences in amygdala function, as manifest over relatively long periods of time, probed through block-design fMRI experiments.

More recent fMRI investigations have begun to use event-related designs, whereby neural responses to briefly presented stimuli can be evaluated. These designs also allow threat appraisal to be explicitly elicited, monitored, and contrasted with other information-processing functions. For example, Beesdo *et al.* (2009) had healthy adolescents and adolescents presenting for treatment of a mood or anxiety disorder view a series of faces drawn from one of four face-emotion categories and perform distinct ratings on these faces at specific points in time. In this study, threat appraisal was specifically engaged by requiring participants to attend towards the subjective level of anxiety they experienced. Behavioral data collected during scanning confirmed that participants were in fact engaging such appraisal processes at the required time points. Other processes also were engaged, as confirmed through behavioral data collected during scanning. This study extended earlier block-design paradigms by finding amygdala hyperactivation in anxious relative to healthy adolescents specifically when participants directly appraised faces based on their anxiety-provoking capacity. Interestingly, in contrast to the data for emotional memory tasks, this study also showed that amygdala hyperactivation during threat appraisal occurs in both adolescent anxiety and adolescent depression.

Studies with fMRI on threat appraisal also provide an opportunity to examine commonalities and differences in the neural correlates of specific anxiety disorders. Data in rodents and non-human primates suggest that anxiety states can be distinguished based on their neural correlates and their precipitators (Pine, 2007). Studies with fMRI of appraisal extend these findings to human adolescents. Demonstration of specificity actually has been a consistent theme in pediatric anxiety disorder research, even prior to widespread application of fMRI in developmental neuroscience investigations. Thus, prior work shows that specific threats have the unique capacity to elicit extreme fear in specific pediatric anxiety disorders, with the most comprehensive data demonstrating a double dissociation between social anxiety and separation anxiety disorders, as reviewed elsewhere (Pine, 2007). This work shows that separation anxiety but not social anxiety disorder is characterized by hypersensitivity to respiratory threat, consistent with other work in panic disorder and its connection to separation anxiety disorder. Social anxiety disorder, in contrast to separation anxiety disorder, is characterized by hypersensitivity to social threats. As shown in Figure 9.3, recent fMRI work has begun to extend this line of investigation by charting the brain regions engaged by social threat appraisal events that are expected to be particularly salient for the adolescent (Guyer, Lau, *et al.*, 2008). Other work using this same fMRI paradigm demonstrates dissociations among typical and atypical responding in the circuit mediating social threat appraisal.

Reward anticipation

As noted, studies in animals demonstrate both associations and dissociations in the circuitry mediating approach to rewards and avoidance of threats. Whereas imaging studies of threat in anxiety focus on the amygdala, imaging studies of reward in various contexts focus on the striatum and its interactions with the ventral PFC. This includes imaging studies of both normal and atypical developmental variation in reward-related behavior (Ernst *et al.*, 2006). Although relatively few imaging studies examine reward-related processes in pediatric anxiety disorders, this area is emerging as a potentially important avenue for understanding the commonalities and differences in correlates of pediatric anxiety and depressive disorders. As summarized above, studies of threat processing, somewhat surprisingly, find similar perturbations in amygdala function in anxious and depressed adolescents, relative to their healthy peers (Beesdo *et al.*, 2009). Studies of reward processing, in contrast, find signs of specific perturbations in the two families of syndromes, with signs of enhanced responses in anxiety and reduced responses in depression, again, relative to in

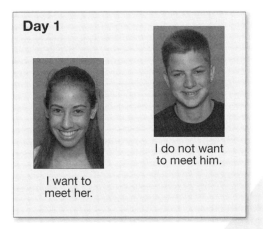

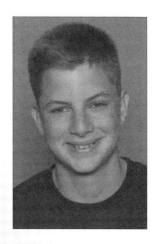

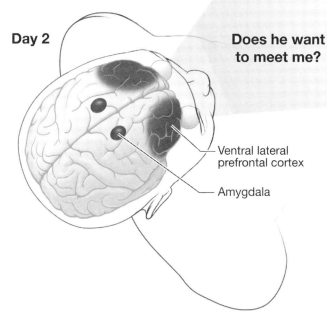

Figure 9.3 Results from a brain imaging experiment conducted in socially anxious and healthy adolescents (Guyer *et al.*, 2008). In this experiment, on Day 1, both anxious and healthy adolescents initially rate perceived levels of desirability for a series of photographs depicting adolescents that the research participants expect to meet, through an internet "chatroom" at a later date. Two weeks later, on Day 2, research participants return and are placed in an MRI scanner where they are told they will learn how the peers depicted in the photographs on Day 1 had rated the research participant. Through this process, adolescents believe they will be paired with a specific peer. When adolescent research participants view photographs on Day 2 of peers rated as undesirable on Day 1, socially anxious adolescents, but not healthy adolescents, exhibit robust amygdala activation as well as associated activations in the ventral lateral prefrontal cortex.

healthy peers (Beesdo *et al.*, 2009; Pine, 2007). These perturbations occur specifically when subjects anticipate receipt of reward. Thus, the striatum in anxious adolescents appears to respond more robustly to such anticipatory events than the striatum of healthy adolescents, whereas the striatum of depressed adolescents appears to respond less robustly than that of healthy adolescents.

Conclusions

This chapter summarized current research on brain–behavior associations related to individual differences in pediatric anxiety. The chapter provides a broad, conceptually focused perspective, emphasizing insights that have emerged from the dual theoretical schools of neuroscience and developmentally focused investigations of psychopathology. The core ideas in the chapter reflect three themes, each covered in a distinct chapter section. The first section reviewed the type of individual differences and associated features around which research on anxiety has been organized. The second section reviewed the core ideas emerging in neuroscience, focusing on information-processing functions implicated in developmental research on anxiety. The final section, focusing on findings from fMRI studies, described the manner in which research in neuroscience has been extended through work in individual differences in fear circuitry function and its relationship to individual differences in anxiety. Clearly, the material presented in this section is far more relevant to ongoing research in pediatric anxiety than current clinical practice, either as it relates to diagnosis or treatment. However, the material reviewed here is at least indirectly relevant to clinical settings. This is because novel treatments for pediatric anxiety disorders may arise from the insights emerging from the data reviewed in the current chapter.

References

Bar-Haim, Y., Lamy, D., Pergamin, L., Bakermans-Kranenburg, M. J., & van IJzendoorn, M. (2007). Threat-related attentional bias in anxious and nonanxious individuals: a meta-analytic study. *Psychology Bulletin*, **133**, 1–24.

Beesdo, K., Lau, J., McClure-Tone, E. B., Guyer, A. E., Monk, C. S., Nelson, E. E., *et al.* (2009). Common and specific amygdala-function perturbations in depressed versus anxious adolescents. *Archives of General Psychiatry*, **66**, 275–285.

Biel, M. G., Klein, R. G., Manuzza, S., Roizen, E. R., Tmong, N. L., Roberson-Nay, R., *et al.* (2008). Does major depressive disorder in parents predict specific fears and phobias in offspring? *Depression and Anxiety*, **25**, 379–382.

Blanchard, R. J., Griebel, G., Henrie, J. A., & Blanchard, D. C. (1997). Differentiation of anxiolytic and panicolytic drugs by effects on rat and mouse defense test batteries. *Neuroscience and Biobehavior Review* **21**, 783–789.

Cahill, L. (1999). A neurobiological perspective on emotionally influenced, long-term memory. *Seminars in Clinical Neuropsychiatry*, **4**, 266–273.

Coplan, J. D., Rosenblum, L. A., & Gorman, J. M. (1995). Primate models of anxiety: longitudinal perspectives. *Psychiatry Clinics of North America*, **18**, 727–743.

Corbetta, M., Patel, G., & Shulman, G. L. (2008). The reorienting system of the human brain: from environment to theory of mind. *Neuron*, **58**, 306–324.

Craske, M. G., Waters, A. M., Lindsey Bergman, R., Naliboff, B., Lipp, O. V., Negoro, H., *et al.* (2008). Is aversive learning a marker of risk for anxiety disorders in children? *Behaviour Research and Therapy*, **46**, 954–967.

Darwin, C. (1998). *The Expression of the Emotions in Man and Animals*, 3rd edn. New York: Oxford University Press.

Davis, M. (1998). Are different parts of the extended amygdala involved in fear versus anxiety? *Biological Psychiatry*, **44**, 1239–1247.

Davis, M. & Whalen, P. J. (2001). The amygdala: vigilance and emotion. *Molecular Psychiatry*, **6**, 13–34.

Ernst, M., Pine, D. S., & Hardin, M. (2006). Triadic model of the neurobiology of motivated behavior in adolescence. *Psychological Medicine*, **36**, 299–312.

Fox, N. A., Henderson, H. A., Marshall, P. J., Nichols, K. E., & Ghera, M. M. (2005). Behavioral inhibition: linking biology and behavior within a developmental framework. *Annual Review of Psychology*, **56**, 235–262.

Garner, M. (2010). Assessment of attentional bias using the dot-probe task in anxious children and adolescents. In **J. Hadwin** & **A. P. Field** (eds.) *Information Processing Biases and Anxiety: A Developmental Perspective*, pp. 77–108. Chichester, UK: Wiley-Blackwell.

Grillon, C., Warner, V., Hille, J., Merikangas, K. R., Bruder, G. E., Tenke, C. E., *et al.* (2005). Families at high and low risk for depression: a three-generation startle study. *Biological Psychiatry*, **57**, 953–960.

Gross, C. & Hen, R. (2004). The developmental origins of anxiety. *Nature Reviews Neuroscience*, **5**, 545–552.

Guyer, A. E., Lau, J. Y. F., McClure-Tone, E. B., Parrish, J., Shiffrin, N. D., Reynold, R. C., *et al.* (2008). Amygdala and ventrolateral prefrontal cortex function during anticipated peer evaluation in pediatric social anxiety. *Archives of General Psychiatry*, **65**, 1303–1312.

Guyer, A. E., Monk, C. S., McClure-Tone, E. B., Nelson, E. E., Roberson, Nay, R., *et al.* (2008). A developmental examination of amygdala response to facial expressions. *Journal of Cognitive Neuroscience*, **20**, 1565–1582.

Guyer, A. E., Nelson, E. E., Perez-Edgar, K., Hardin, M. G., Roberson-Nay, R., Monk, C. S., *et al.* (2006). Striatal functional alteration in adolescents characterized by early childhood behavioral inhibition. *Journal of Neuroscience*, **26**, 6399–6405.

Holland, P. C. & Gallagher, M. (2004). Amygdala-frontal interactions and reward expectancy. *Current Opinion in Neurobiology*, **14**, 148–155.

Kagan, J. (1994). *Galen's Prophecy*. New York: Basic Books.

Kraemer, H. C. (2007). DSM categories and dimensions in clinical and research contexts. *International Journal of Methods in Psychiatric Research*, **16**(Suppl. 1), S8–S15.

Lau, J. Y., Goldman, D., Buzas, B., Fromm, S. J., Guyer, A. E., Hodgkinson, C., *et al.* (2008). Amygdala function and 5HTT gene variants in adolescent anxiety and major depressive disorder. *Biological Psychiatry*, **65**, 349–355.

Lau, J. Y., Lissek, S., Nelson, E. E., Lee, Y., Roberson-Nay, R., Poeth, K., *et al.* (2008). Fear conditioning in adolescents with anxiety disorders: results from a novel experimental paradigm. *Journal of the American Academy of Child and Adolescent Psychiatry*, **47**, 94–102.

LeDoux, J. E. (2000). Emotion circuits in the brain. *Annual Review of Neuroscience*, **23**, 155–184.

Lissek, S., Biggs, A. L., Rabin, S. J., Cornwell, B. R., Alvarez, R. P., Pine, D. S., *et al.* (2008). Generalization of conditioned fear-potentiated startle in humans: experimental validation and clinical relevance. *Behaviour Research and Therapy*, **4b**, 678–687.

Meaney, M. J. (2001). Maternal care, gene expression, and the transmission of individual differences in stress reactivity across generations. *Annual Review of Neuroscience*, **24**, 1161–1192.

Nelson, E. E., Leibenluft, E., McClure, E. B., & Pine, D. S. (2005). The social re-orientation of adolescence: a neuroscience perspective on the process and its relation to psychopathology. *Psychological Medicine*, **35**, 163–174.

Ollendick, T. H., Langley, A. K., Jones, R. T., & Kephart, C. (2001). Fear in children and adolescents: relations with negative life events, attributional style, and avoidant coping. *Journal of Child Psychology and Psychiatry*, **42**, 1029–1034.

Ollendick, T. H., Yang, B., King, N. J., Dong, Q., & Akande, D. (1996). Fears in American, Australian, Chinese, and Nigerian children and adolescents: a cross-cultural study. *Journal of Child Psychology and Psychiatry*, **37**, 213–220.

Phelps, E. A. & LeDoux, J. E. (2005). Contributions of the amygdala to emotion processing: from animal models to human behavior. *Neuron*, **48**, 175–187.

Pine, D. S. (2003). Developmental psychobiology and response to threats: relevance to trauma in children and adolescents. *Biological Psychiatry*, **53**, 796–808.

Pine, D. S. (2007). Research review: a neuroscience framework for pediatric anxiety disorders. *Journal of Child Psychology and Psychiatry*, **48**, 631–648.

Pine, D. S. & Cohen, J. A. (2002). Trauma in children and adolescents: risk and treatment of psychiatric sequelae. *Biological Psychiatry*, **51**, 519–531.

Pine, D. S. & Klein, R. G. (2008). Anxiety disorders. In: M. Rutter, D. Bishop, D. S. Pine, S. Scott, J. Stevenson, E. Taylor, A. Thapar (eds.) *Rutter's Child and Adolescent Psychiatry*, 5th edn, pp. 628–647. Oxford, UK: Blackwell.

Pine, D. S., Cohen, P., & Brook, J. (2001). Adolescent fears as predictors of depression. *Biological Psychiatry*, **50**, 721–724.

Pine, D. S., Helfinstein, S. M., Bar-Haim, Y., Nelson, E., & Fox, N. A. (2009). Challenges in developing novel treatments for childhood disorders: lessons from research on anxiety. *Neuropsychopharmacology*, **34**, 213–228.

Pine, D. S., Klein, R. G., Roberson-Nay, R., Mannuzza, S., Moulton, J. L., Woldehawariat, G., *et al.* (2005). Response to 5% carbon dioxide in children and adolescents: relationship to panic disorder in parents and anxiety disorders in subjects. *Archives of General Psychiatry*, **62**, 73–80.

Quirk, G. J. & Mueller, D. (2008). Neural mechanisms of extinction learning and retrieval. *Neuropsychopharmacology*, **33**, 56–72.

Roberson-Nay, R., McClure, E. B., Monk, C. S., Nelson, E. E., Guyer, A. E., Fromm, S. J., *et al.* (2006). Increased amygdala activity during successful memory encoding in adolescent major depressive disorder: an FMRI study. *Biological Psychiatry*, **60**, 966–973.

Rosenbaum, J. F., Biederman, J., Bolduc, E. A., Hirshfeld, D. R., Faraone, S. V., & Kagan, J. (2000). A controlled study of behavioral inhibition in children of parents with panic disorder and depression. *American Journal of Psychiatry*, **157**, 2002–2010.

Rutter, M., Moffitt, T. E., & Caspi, A. (2006). Gene–environment interplay and psychopathology: multiple varieties but real effects. *Journal of Child Psychology and Psychiatry*, **47**, 226–261.

Scherer, K. R. (2001). Appraisal considered as a process of multilevel sequential checking. In: K. R. Scherer, A. Schorr, & T. Johnstone (eds.) *Appraisal Processes in Emotion: Theory, Methods, Research*, pp. 92–120. Oxford, UK: Oxford University Press.

Schultz, W. (2001). Reward signaling by dopamine neurons. *Neuroscientist*, **7**, 293–302.

Schwartz, C. E., Snidman, N., & Kagan, J. (1999). Adolescent social anxiety as an outcome of inhibited temperament in childhood. *Journal of the American Academy of Child and Adolescent Psychiatry*, **38**, 1008–1015.

Schwartz, C. E., Wright, C. I., Shin, L. M., Kagan, J., & Rauch, S. L. (2003). Inhibited and uninhibited infants "grown up": adult amygdalar response to novelty. *Science*, **300**, 1952–1953.

Squire, L. R. & Kandel, E. R. (1999). *Memory: From Mind to Molecules*. New York: Scientific American Press.

Stattin, H. (1984). Developmental trends in the appraisal of anxiety-provoking situations. *Journal of Personality*, **52**, 46–57.

Steinberg, L. (2008). A neurobehavioural perspective on adolescent risk-taking. *Developmental Review*, **28**, 78–106.

Thomas, K. M., Drevets, W. C., Dahl, R. E., Ryan, N. D., Birmaher, B., Eccard, C. H., *et al.* (2001). Amygdala response to fearful faces in anxious and depressed children. *Archives of General Psychiatry*, **58**, 1057–1063.

Young, L. J. & Wang, Z. (2004). The neurobiology of pair bonding. *Nature Neuroscience*, **7**, 1048–1054.

10

Temperament and anxiety in children and adolescents

Christopher J. Lonigan, Beth M. Phillips, Shauna B. Wilson, and Nicholas P. Allan

Problematic anxiety and anxiety disorders are common forms of emotional disturbance affecting children and adolescents. Estimates of the prevalence of anxiety disorders in child and adolescent populations range from 3% to 25%, depending on the specific anxiety disorder diagnosis, the classification system used, and whether or not a stringent functional impairment criterion is employed (e.g., Costello, Egger, & Angold, 2005; Costello, Egger, Copeland, Erkanli, & Angold, Chapter 3, this volume). Although anxiety disorders in childhood often remit within 3 to 4 years (Last, Perrin, Hersen, & Kazdin, 1996), some cases of childhood anxiety disorder have a chronic course (Keller, Lavori, Wunder, Beardslee, Schwartz, & Roth, 1992; Last *et al.*, 1996; Orvaschel, Lewinsohn, & Seeley, 1995), and many adult anxiety disorders may have their onset in childhood or adolescence (Burke, Burke, Regier, & Rae, 1990; Kendler, Neale, Kessler, Heath, & Eaves, 1992). Moreover, even when a specific anxiety disorder in youth does not persist, it may represent significant risk for other disorders, particularly other anxiety disorders, depression, and substance abuse (Kendall, Safford, Flannery-Schroeder, & Webb, 2004; Last *et al.*, 1996; Lewinsohn, Zinbarg, Seeley, Lewinsohn, & Sack, 1997; Moffitt *et al.*, 2007; Orvaschel *et al.*, 1995; Woodward & Fergusson, 2001). These findings indicate that anxiety disorders in children and adolescents are both common and associated with significant negative sequelae. Consequently, there is significant need to understand factors that are associated with the development and maintenance of anxiety.

The purpose of this chapter is to review theoretical propositions and empirical findings concerning the relations between temperament and anxiety pathology in children and adolescents. As reviewed below, there is no doubt that at a broad level, temperament is related to anxiety and anxiety disorders in children and adolescents. At a number of deeper levels of specification, however, there are many questions concerning the definitions of the underlying constructs as well as questions concerning the match between the underlying constructs and the measures used to operationalize them. Hence, when attempting to determine the various empirical relations between the constructs, one is left questioning which construct is temperament, which construct is personality, and which construct is psychopathology? At some level, the distinctions are arbitrary. For instance, if personality is conceptualized as the ultimate realization of temperament, then the point at which temperament ends and personality begins depends on how one distinguishes temperamental variability versus emerging personality, or depends on a determination that at some age sufficient development or neurobiological maturation has taken place to declare

Anxiety Disorders in Children and Adolescents, 2nd edn, ed. W. K. Silverman and A. P. Field. Published by Cambridge University Press. © Cambridge University Press 2011.

the behavioral, cognitive, and emotional characteristics of an individual personality. If psychopathology is conceptualized on a continuum, the underlying dimensions apply to individuals with or without psychopathology, and individuals have more or less of some characteristic or characteristics that, at the extreme, are labeled a disorder.

Although a number of measurement problems concerning the assessment of psychopathology in children and adolescents have been addressed over the past decade, there are still some questions, and many studies continue to use older measures. Development and validation of self- and parent-report measures like the Revised Children's Anxiety and Depression Scales (RCADS: Chorpita, Yim, Moffitt, Umemoto, & Francis, 2000), with subscales that correspond to symptoms of specific anxiety disorders, represent advances over older self-report measures like the Revised Children's Manifest Anxiety Scales (RCMAS: Reynolds & Richmond, 1978) that appear to be measures of broader constructs like internalizing problems (Lonigan, Carey, & Finch, 1994). Refinement and validation of structured clinical interviews for children and adolescents (e.g., Silverman & Albano, 1996) provide validated standards for assessment of clinical anxiety disorders.

With respect to temperament, in an earlier summary concerning the relations between temperament and anxiety in children (Lonigan & Phillips, 2001), we noted several issues concerning the assessment of temperament. Whereas there have been advances in the assessment of temperament subsequently, there are still many significant issues related to measurement that remain unanswered and unresolved. As summarized below, although there is now general consensus on higher-order dimensions of temperament, many researchers utilize measures designed for the assessment of lower-order dimensions and interpret associations between these lower-order dimensions and other constructs, like psychopathology, despite limited evidence that these subscales represent valid indices of these lower-order dimensions.

Not your father's (or mother's) temperament

There is a rich descriptive literature concerning aspects of the static and changing nature of children's development in areas related to behavior, emotion, and regulation. The study of temperament has a long history, dating to the early Greek and Greco-Roman physicians (Diamond, 1974). In more recent times, Allport, who might be described as the father of modern temperament, defined temperament as:

The characteristic phenomenon of an individual's emotional nature, including his susceptibility to emotional stimulation, his customary speed and strength of response, the quality of his prevailing mood, and all the peculiarities of fluctuation and intensity of mood; this phenomenon being regarded as dependent on constitutional make-up. (Allport, 1937, p. 54)

What is temperament?

There are many definitions and conceptualizations of temperament. Whereas many people would be satisfied with the broad definition of temperament provided by Allport (1937), there is less agreement among temperament theorists about key aspects of temperament. Most researchers now agree that temperament concerns biologically based, largely heritable, individual differences that contribute to the disposition or behavior of a person. Among the current and recent-past lines of temperament research, there are varying degrees of agreement regarding the heritability of temperament, the role of neurophysiological structures, and the stability of temperament as a person ages. There is debate about the timeline for the emergence of temperamental dimensions, the status of temperament as categorical versus dimensional, and the appropriate lower-order variables to include (e.g., Nigg, 2006; Rothbart & Bates, 2006; Shiner & Caspi, 2003).

It is beyond the scope of this chapter to provide a comprehensive review of the many facets of models of temperament. Interested readers should consult alternate works for both historical and more detailed explanation of more recent temperament theories (e.g., Buss & Plomin, 1984; Goldsmith & Campos, 1982; Goldsmith *et al.*, 1987; Nigg, 2006; Rothbart & Bates, 2006; Shiner & Caspi, 2003). Herein we briefly highlight the areas of overlap and distinctiveness of temperament theories and provide a description of models of temperament. We detail how some issues have been resolved to form a more unified theoretical template of temperament, and we offer models that provide possible pathways for observed links between temperament, personality, and symptoms of psychopathology.

Evolution of the temperament construct

The description of temperament that is probably familiar to most is that of Thomas and Chess (e.g., Thomas, Chess, & Birch, 1996), who developed one of the first modern descriptions of temperament. They based their model on observations and parent reports of a small group of infants. Within their model, temperament was conceptualized as the "stylistic" (the how) component of behavior, excluding abilities (the what), content (how well), and motivation (why). Thomas and Chess distinguished nine categories of temperamental behavior, including activity level, approach or withdrawal from novel stimuli, adaptability, sensory threshold, dominant quality of mood, intensity of mood expression, persistence/attention span, distractibility, and rhythmicity. Additionally, they identified three temperamental patterns, including "easy temperament" (i.e., infants who display mild or moderate approach/withdrawal, high adaptability to change, and quickly develop regular patterns of behavior, such as sleeping and eating), "difficult temperament" (i.e., infants with extreme scores on approach/withdrawal, mood, intensity, adaptability, and rhythmicity), and "slow-to-warm-up temperament" (i.e., a combination of negative, mild responses to novelty, and a slow-to-adapt style even after repeated exposure).

Other temperament theories have been constructed to address perceived shortcomings of the Thomas and Chess model. Buss and Plomin (e.g., 1984; Goldsmith *et al.*, 1987) merged the pediatric approach of Thomas and Chess with personality research. They also stressed the genetic component of temperament. Buss and Plomin defined temperament as a set of inherited traits that appear early in life. Goldsmith and Campos (e.g., 1982; Goldsmith *et al.*, 1987) provided an alternative model of temperament in which temperament was defined as being comprised of individual differences in the probability of experiencing and expressing the primary emotions (e.g., Ekman, Friesen, & Ellsworth, 1972). They excluded examinations of motivation, biology, and heritability as useful temperamental markers.

Rothbart and colleagues (e.g., Derryberry & Rothbart, 1984; Rothbart & Bates, 2006) developed what has come to be the most widely accepted and empirically supported model of temperament to date. Their model extends beyond the behavioral style of the Thomas and Chess model to include predispositions and reactions. The importance of individual differences in emotional susceptibility is included in their model, but their model is not limited to emotionality like that of Goldsmith and Campos (1982). Moreover, in their model, consideration of emotion is not limited to negatively valenced emotions, as in the Buss and Plomin (1984) model. Within this model, temperament is defined as the constitutionally based individual differences in emotional, motor, and attentional reactivity, as well as the ability to self-regulate automatic reactions to the environment. The constitutionally based aspect of the definition refers to a relatively enduring biological basis for temperament due to genetics, maturation, and experience (Rothbart, Ahadi, Hershey, & Fisher, 2001). The model of temperament contains both higher-order and lower-order dimensions. The 15 lower-order dimensions include aspects of behavior and emotion such as activity level, shyness, fear, anger/frustration, sadness, attentional focusing, positive anticipation, and soothability. The two higher-order reactive dimensions are negative affectivity (NA) and extraversion/surgency, and the higher-order regulative dimension is effortful control (EC) (e.g., Ahadi, Rothbart, & Ye, 1993; Rothbart, Ahadi, & Hershey, 1994; Rothbart et al., 2001).

The reactive temperament factors of NA and extraversion/surgency fit well with models of reactive motivational systems involving both inhibitory systems and approach or activation systems. Delineation of these motivational systems is typically related to Gray's (e.g., 1982) model. According to Gray, two neural systems serve to motivate behavior: the Behavioral Inhibition System (BIS) and the Behavioral Activation System (BAS). Activation of the BIS is associated with sensitivity to signals of punishment, frustrative non-reward, and novelty. The behavioral effects of the BIS include inhibition of ongoing behavior, increased attention, and increased arousal. Thus, the BIS is aligned with the dimension of NA. In contrast, activation of the BAS is associated with sensitivity to signals of both reward and relief from punishment. The behavioral effects of the BAS include appetitive approach behavior. Thus, the BAS is aligned with the dimension of extraversion/surgency. Aspects of these reactive systems have been shown to be heritable (e.g., Goldsmith & Lemery, 2000) and related to various underlying neurobiological systems (e.g., see Whittle, Allen, Lubman, & Yücel, 2006).

In contrast to the reactive dimensions of temperament, EC involves the capacity to regulate reactive processes. Effortful control functions in conjunction with the reactive dimensions by moderating reactive responses in the service of more long-term goals or socialized behavior (Posner & Rothbart, 2000; Rothbart, 1989; Rothbart & Bates, 1998). A hallmark of EC is the "ability to inhibit a dominant response to perform a subdominant response" (Rothbart & Bates, 1998, p. 137). It allows for flexible responding to environmental stimuli and is capable of exerting a significant impact on behavior (Ahadi & Rothbart, 1994; Posner & Rothbart, 2000). For instance, children who possess high levels of EC are capable of overriding a reactive disposition to avoid negative stimuli and instead may develop more strategic coping responses when encountering fear-producing stimuli. Data suggest that EC is heritable (e.g., Fan, Wu, Fossella, & Posner, 2001; Lemery-Chalfant, Doelger, & Goldsmith, 2008) and it has been connected with executive attention networks in the brain, particularly those involving the anterior cingulate gyrus and other frontal areas (e.g., see Rothbart, Sheese, & Posner, 2007).

Measuring temperament

Despite convergence around a model of temperament in children, there are significant issues concerning measurement of specific dimensions of temperament that relate to demonstrations of convergence of different measures of the same temperament constructs, discrimination between measures of different temperament constructs, and stability in specific temperament dimensions within individuals across time or situation in which stability is expected. Although many studies have demonstrated moderate cross-time stability across the lower-order dimensions of temperament (e.g., Putnam, Rothbart, & Gartstein, 2008), strong evidence of the validity of lower-order dimensions is scarce (e.g., evidence of convergent and discriminant properties). Such construct underspecification at the measurement level may restrict the yield of studies that attempt to relate specific lower-order temperament constructs to other developmental outcomes (e.g., Eisenberg *et al.*, 2009; Oldehinkel, Hartman, Ferdinand, Verhulst, & Ormel, 2007).

Measures of temperament have often been developed following a conceptual, rather than an empirical, approach. Although subscales within these measures that are intended to measure specific temperament dimensions have evidence of at least moderate internal consistency, there is less evidence that these scales have adequate discriminant properties. For instance, Rothbart *et al.* (2001) reported results of multiple analyses of the Children's Behavior Questionnaire (CBQ). Across analyses, Cronbach's alpha coefficients for the 15 CBQ lower-order dimensions ranged from 0.67 to 0.94 (*M* alpha across scales = 0.77). In factor analyses of the subscale scores, however, substantial cross-loadings of the lower-order dimensions onto the three higher-order dimensions often emerge, suggesting substantial overlap of construct variance of the lower-order dimensions across the three higher-order factors. Some degree of scale interrelatedness might be expected because from a broader perspective (e.g., Tellegen, Watson, & Clark, 1999); NA and extraversion/surgency are hypothesized to be dimensions of temperament that are largely orthogonal to each other, and EC is hypothesized to be a separate but correlated construct. Specifically, with respect to EC, correlations between EC and positive and negative reactivity are likely – at least at the level of measurement – because EC is not activated (and hence not observed) except under conditions that activate reactive temperament factors.

Results of other studies also call into question aspects of the construct validity of measures of the lower-order temperament dimensions. For instance, Oldehinkel *et al.* (2007) reported that the three hypothesized facets of EC (attention control, inhibitory control, activation control) did not emerge as separate components in a factor analysis of the Early Adolescent Temperament Questionnaire (EAT-Q: Capaldi & Rothbart, 1992). Muris and Meesters (2009) reported results on the EAT-Q with a large sample of Dutch children and adolescents. Although a scale-level factor analysis recovered three higher-order factors, roughly corresponding to NA, extraversion/surgency, and EC, there were some substantial cross-loadings (e.g., fearfulness loaded across all factors). Moreover, there was not a clear pattern of expected results in a correlation analysis of lower-order EAT-Q factors and a measure of BIS and BAS (i.e., factors associated with extraversion/surgency did not consistently correlate with BAS and factors associated with NA did not consistently correlate with BIS). Majdandžić, van den Boom, and Heesbeen (2008) found, at best, modest associations between parent-ratings on the CBQ and observed temperament on the Laboratory Temperament Assessment Battery (Goldsmith, Reilly, Lemery, Longley, & Prescott, 1995).

Hierarchical models of psychopathology, personality, and temperament

Hierarchical models of psychopathology

Comorbidity between diagnostic categories of psychopathology is the norm, not the exception, for both adults (e.g., Brown, 2007; Clark, 2005; Kessler *et al.*, 1994) and children (e.g., Brady & Kendal, 1992; Essau, Conradt, & Petermann, 2000; Last, Strauss, & Francis, 1987; Verduin & Kendall, 2003). Not only is there significant diagnostic comorbidity among the anxiety disorders, there is significant diagnostic comorbidity between the anxiety disorders and other disorders, particularly depression (Costello *et al.*, 2005; Lewinsohn *et al.*, 1997;

Moffitt *et al.*, 2007; Costello, Egger, Copeland, Erkanli, & Angold, Chapter 3, this volume). To account for this diagnostic comorbidity, a variety of hierarchical models have been proposed that partition shared and unique components of the disorders. One model that has received substantial empirical support is the Tripartite Model of Anxiety and Depression (Clark & Watson, 1991). In this model, (high) NA is viewed as a general factor associated with both anxiety and depression, (low) positive affectivity (PA) is viewed as a factor that is unique to depression, and (high) physiological hyperarousal (PH) is viewed as a factor that is unique to anxiety. As summarized below, at the symptom cluster level, the expected pattern of relations between NA and PA with anxiety and depression has been supported. In contrast, PH seems to be a factor that is specific to panic disorder, rather than anxiety disorders in general (e.g., Brown, Chorpita, & Barlow, 1998; Chorpita, Albano, & Barlow, 1998).

Watson (2005) proposed a revised quantitative hierarchical model to account for comorbidity and heterogeneity among disorders. The model, based on observed patterns of interrelations between disorders, has three hierarchical levels: (a) an overarching diagnostic category of emotional (or internalizing) disorder, (b) a secondary diagnostic categorization for bipolar, distress, and fear disorders, and (c) a tertiary diagnostic categorization of specific mood and anxiety disorder diagnoses. The model differs from traditional conceptualizations of separate mood and anxiety disorder clusters. Major depression, dysthymia, generalized anxiety disorder (GAD), and post-traumatic stress disorder (PTSD) are categorized as distress disorders, whereas panic, agoraphobia, social phobia, and specific phobia are categorized as fear disorders. Consistent with earlier hierarchical models, this model suggests that a single general factor, like general distress or NA, is responsible for observed patterns of comorbidity. Disorders with strong components of general distress/NA are more likely to be comorbid than disorders with less strong components of general distress/NA.

Support for this model has been reported in adult community and clinical samples (Selbom, Ben-Porath, & Bagby, 2008). In two large community samples of children and adolescents, Lahey and colleagues (Lahey, Applegate, Waldman, Loft, Hankin, & Rick, 2004; Lahey *et al.*, 2008) reported results similar to this hierarchical model, but with a somewhat different organization of specific diagnostic groupings. Lonigan and Phillips (unpublished data) recently tested Watson's model in a community sample of children and adolescents who completed the RCADS as a part of a larger study. Although a multifactor hierarchical model provided the best fit to the data, symptoms of depression and symptoms of anxiety were accounted for by different factors. A more differentiated model, approximating the model proposed by Watson, was obtained when examining only the adolescents, and a simple depression–anxiety model was obtained when examining only the children. These results suggest that the specific hierarchical structure of emotional (internalizing) disorders is age-dependent.

Hierarchical models of personality and temperament

Hierarchical models also have assumed a dominant position within theories of adult personality. Many personality psychologists agree that individual differences in adults, as measured by rating scales and questionnaire items, are almost completely described by five broad factors, labeled Surgency/Extraversion, Agreeableness, Conscientiousness, Emotional Stability/Neuroticism, and Openness to Experience (i.e., the Big Five Model of Personality: McCrae & Costa, 1987). These five higher-order personality traits differentiate into mid-level traits that yield a still more differentiated set of personality facets (e.g., see Clark, 2005; Tellegen & Waller, 2008).

Studies indicate substantial overlap between dimensions of temperament and the factors of the Big Five Model of Personality in children and adolescents (e.g., Ahadi *et al.*, 1993; Digman, 1994) and adults (e.g., Angleitner & Ostendorf, 1994). Watson, Clark, and Harkness (1994) demonstrated that dimensions consistent with PA and NA mapped onto the Surgency and Neuroticism factors, respectively, of the Big Five Model in adults. Other work suggests that a three-factor model, similar to that representing positive and negative reactive components and a regulatory component underlie the Big Five traits (Clark, 2005; Markon, Krueger, & Watson, 2005; see also Caspi & Silva, 1995). Within this hierarchical structure, temperament can be conceptualized as the precursor to adult personality. Several longitudinal studies have found significant associations between temperament ratings in early childhood and personality ratings in middle childhood (Hagekull & Bohlin, 1998), adolescence (John, Caspi, Robins, Moffitt, & Stouthamer-Loeber, 1994), and adulthood (Angleitner & Ostendorf, 1994; Caspi & Silva, 1995).

Results of studies with children and adolescents demonstrate specific overlap between the constructs of NA and PA and higher-order reactive dimensions of temperament (Anthony, Lonigan, Hooe, & Phillips, 2002; Lonigan & Dyer, 2000, described in Lonigan & Phillips, 2001). For instance, Anthony *et al.* had a group of 290 5th to 11th grade children complete the Positive and Negative Affectivity Scales (Watson, Clark, & Tellegen, 1988) and a modified version of the adult self-report Emotionality, Activity, and Sociability Scales (EAS: Buss & Plomin, 1984). Factor analysis of the modified EAS revealed five lower-order factors identical to those found with adults (Distress, Fear, Anger, Activity, and Sociability). A scale-level factor analysis of the modified EAS yielded two orthogonal (i.e., $r = 0.04$) higher-order factors, Negative Temperament (consisting of the lower-order factors Distress, Fear, and Anger) and Positive Temperament (consisting of the lower-order factors Sociability and Activity). Correlations between the Negative Temperament factor and the NA scale of the Positive and Negative Affectivity Schedule (PANAS) ($r = 0.62$) and between the Positive Temperament factor and the PA scale of the PANAS ($r = 0.40$) indicated moderate overlap of the constructs. Similarly, Lonigan and Dyer (2000; cited in Lonigan & Phillips, 2001) reported that the NA and PA scales of the PANAS loaded on the appropriate higher-order factors in a scale-level factor analysis of the CBQ completed by parents of 4–6-year-old children. Thus, affect and temperament are characterized by the higher-order factors of Negative Affectivity/Neuroticism (hereinafter referred to as NA/N) and Positive Affectivity/Surgency (hereinafter referred to as PA/S).

Integrative hierarchical models

It is possible that temperament, personality, and psychopathology all fit together in an integrative hierarchical model. A significant body of research suggests that the NA/N and PA/S dimensions of the Tripartite Model of Anxiety and Depression (Clark & Watson, 1991) reflect core temperament traits in addition to the common and unique state components of anxiety and depression. Given the overlap between and within DSM Axis I and Axis II disorders, the connections between personality and psychopathology, and evidence for broad-band hierarchical structures of personality, Clark (2005) argued for the interconnectedness of temperament, personality, and psychopathology. According to Clark, one explanation of these interconnections could be that temperament underlies both personality and psychopathology.

There are four major models of how temperament and psychopathology can be interrelated (e.g., see Akiskal, Hirschfeld, & Yerevanian, 1983; Clark, 2005; Clark, Watson, &

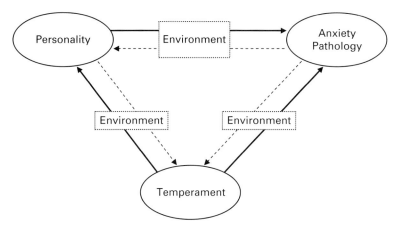

Figure 10.1 Simplified integrative model for the relations between temperament, personality, and anxiety pathology in which temperament underlies both personality and psychopathology. As outlined in the text, the model has direct and indirect (i.e., mediated or moderated by the environment) bidirectional effects (e.g., predisposition, pathoplasticity, complication, continuity models) between constructs.

Mineka, 1994). First, temperament may serve as a *predisposition* for a disorder, playing a direct causal role in the development of psychopathology. The common version of the predisposition model, the diathesis–stress model, suggests that a relevant stressor, in combination with a temperament predisposition, is needed to trigger the onset of the disorder. Second, temperament may serve to moderate the expression or course of a disorder without having a direct causal role in its onset. This *pathoplasticity* model includes situations in which temperament plays a role in shaping the environment of the individual (e.g., temperament is responsible for shaping a parent's "protective" reactions to a child that serve to maintain an anxiety disorder by inhibiting exposure to anxiety-provoking situations). Third, temperament itself may be altered by the experience of a disorder. In this *complication* model, the disorder can cause enduring changes ("scar model") in temperament factors by fundamentally altering them or the disorder can cause transient changes ("complication model") in temperament factors because of residual symptoms of the disorder. Effects within this model can be both direct and indirect (i.e., through changes in the environment because of the disorder). Finally, a disorder may reflect the extreme of some dimension of temperament. In this *continuity* model, both temperament and disorder reflect the same underlying process. Evidence of shared genetic factors between temperament and anxiety (e.g., Goldsmith & Lemery, 2000; Lemery-Chalfant *et al.*, 2008) are consistent with this model.

These models of the relation between temperament and psychopathology are not mutually exclusive across or within individuals. It is possible that temperament can predispose to a disorder, influence the symptoms and course of the disorder once present, and be modified by the experience of the disorder. Consistent with Clark's (2005) summary, there appear to be two general models of how the development of psychopathology is influenced by temperament. Figure 10.1 represents a model consistent with Clark's proposal that temperament underlies both personality and psychopathology. This model includes the dynamic and bidirectional influences between temperament, personality, and

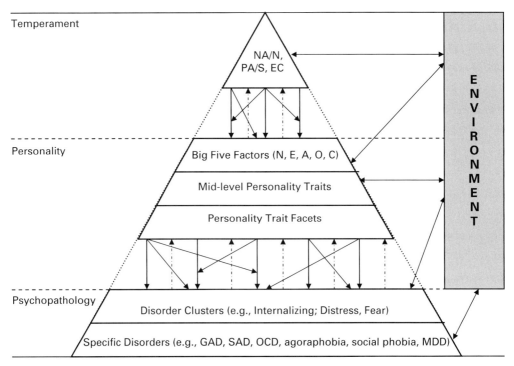

Figure 10.2 Integrated hierarchical model for the relations between temperament, personality, and psychopathology in which each construct is organized as higher- and lower-order dimensions reflecting greater differentiation of the construct, as a result of variable levels of influence of higher-order dimensions and interactions between higher-order dimensions. As outlined in the text, there are both direct and indirect (i.e., mediated or moderated by the environment) bidirectional effects (e.g., predisposition, pathoplasticity, complication, continuity models) between constructs. NA/N, Negative Affectivity/Neuroticism; PA/S, Positive Affectivity/Surgency; EC, Effortful Control; N, Neuroticism; E, Extraversion; A, Agreeableness; O, Openness; C, Conscientiousness; GAD, generalized anxiety disorder; SAD, separation anxiety disorder; OCD, obsessive–compulsive disorder; MDD, major depressive disorder.

psychopathology (e.g., predisposition and complication models). Additionally, this model includes a role for the environment in moderating or mediating the influences of temperament on personality and psychopathology (e.g., pathoplasticity, predisposition models) as well as effects of psychopathology on temperament and personality moderated or mediated by the environment (e.g., complication model).

Figure 10.2 represents the integrated hierarchical model. In this model, there is increasing differentiation of temperament, personality, and psychopathology. Across domains (e.g., temperament, psychopathology), there are connections between factors at the higher-order levels (e.g., NA/N is associated with internalizing disorders). Connections between lower-order levels across domains are likely the product of several aspects of a domain as well as interactions between these facets (e.g., distress disorders reflect a strong influence of NA/N and low levels of EC). As with the model in Figure 10.1, effects can be mediated or moderated by the environment, and effects between domains can be bidirectional.

A model for the linkages between temperament and problematic anxiety

Building on the work of Rothbart and colleagues (e.g., Rothbart, Posner, & Hershey, 1995), Lonigan and Phillips (2001; see also Lonigan, Vasey, Phillips, & Hazen, 2004) hypothesized that in addition to direct effects of NA/N and EC on the development of psychopathology generally and anxiety in particular, the interaction of NA/N and EC was important. That is, whereas NA/N has clear links to anxiety, the specific level of risk for an individual with higher levels of NA/N would be moderated by the individual's level of EC. Therefore, both higher levels of NA/N and lower levels of EC are required to predispose individuals to anxiety.

Within this model of temperamental risk for problematic anxiety, although anxiety is characterized by reactive control (e.g., inhibition of behavior) and is NA/N motivated, individuals with high levels of EC have the capacity to deploy self-regulatory processes that prevent or reduce the experience of significant distress in the face of aversive stimulation. Significant anxious behavior and negative emotional dysregulation occurs in the context of aversive stimulation because of a combination of significant temperamental negative reactivity, high situational demands (e.g., significant aversive stimulation, prolonged aversive situation, fatigue), or low temperamental capacity to engage in self-regulative processes. Those with temperamentally high levels of NA/N have more of a need for higher levels of EC because they experience more stimuli than average as aversive, react more negatively than average to aversive stimuli, or both. Therefore, similar to the model proposed by Rothbart and colleagues (e.g., Rothbart *et al.*, 1995) this model suggests that both high NA/N and low EC should be related to both more anxiety and more severe anxiety. However, the model also suggests that although high NA/N is a necessary condition for the development of anxiety pathology, it is not sufficient – except, perhaps, at the most extreme levels of NA/N. Instead, the model proposes that a dynamic combination of high NA/N and low EC is required for the emergence of significant anxiety pathology. Stated differently, EC moderates the impact of NA/N on anxiety pathology.

Empirical relations between temperament and anxiety

A large number of studies have demonstrated a substantial link between measures of NA/N and anxiety or anxiety disorders with both adults and youth. Many of these studies have been conducted within the theoretical framework of the Tripartite Model of Anxiety and Depression (Clark & Watson, 1991). For instance, Watson, Clark, and Carey (1988) examined the overlap of anxiety and depressive disorders in adults and found that they could be discriminated by measures of NA/N and PA/S. Individuals with either an anxiety or a depressive disorder reported high levels of NA/N; however, only individuals with a depressive disorder reported low levels of PA/S. Brown *et al.* (1998) reported similar results in a large sample of adults diagnosed with anxiety disorders. Both anxiety disorders and depression were associated with NA/N. Hence, in adults, there is consistent evidence that anxiety and anxiety disorders are associated with high levels of NA/N.

Similar findings within the framework of the Tripartite Model have emerged for children and adolescents. In a sample of 233 child inpatients suffering from anxiety or depression, Lonigan *et al.* (1994) found that whereas measures indicative of low PA/S (i.e., low interest or low motivation) discriminated between children diagnosed with a depressive disorder and children diagnosed with an anxiety disorder, anxious and depressed children were indistinguishable on more general indices of NA/N. Using child and parent report with a group of clinically anxious children, Chorpita *et al.* (1998) conducted a scale-level analysis on the tripartite structure of symptoms of anxiety and depression and found that a model with three factors that were analogous to NA/N, PA/S, and physiological hyperarousal provided the best fit to the data. Other investigations have reported similar findings (e.g., Joiner, Catanzaro, & Laurent, 1996; Lonigan, Hooe, David, & Kistner, 1999; Phillips, Lonigan, Driscoll, & Hooe, 2002) with both clinical and community samples of children and adolescents.

In addition to the role of NA/N in explaining structural relations between symptoms of psychopathology associated with anxiety, studies have demonstrated linkages between measures of NA/N as temperament or personality and measures of anxiety symptoms or anxiety diagnoses. Chorpita and Daleiden (2002) found that measures of NA/N and PA/S were predictive of diagnostic status in a clinical sample of children and adolescents. Lonigan *et al.* (1999) found that children's responses to the PANAS (Watson *et al.*, 1988) yielded the expected relations with measures of depression and anxiety. Austin and Chorpita (2004) demonstrated that the expected relations of NA/N and PA/S with anxiety and depression held across five ethnic groups (White, Chinese American, Japanese American, Filipino American, Native Hawaiian) in a large community sample of 1155 children and adolescents.

Other research indicates that measures of NA/N and PA/S index trait vulnerabilities to psychopathology, including anxiety. Clark *et al.* (1994) reviewed the influence of personality factors on psychopathology in adults and concluded that NA/N represented a risk factor for both anxiety and depression, whereas PA/S represented a risk factor for depression. For instance, clinically anxious patients who show little improvement tend to have higher NA/N scores than patients who do improve. Other work with adults extends these findings to non-patient samples and prospective studies (e.g., Krueger, Caspi, Moffitt, Silva, & McGee, 1996; Trull & Sher, 1994). In a recent study of a large clinical sample of adults seeking treatment for anxiety, Brown (2007) demonstrated that initially high levels of NA/N predicted less improvement in measures of generalized anxiety disorder and social phobia, after controlling for initial symptom severity levels, over a 24-month period. Moreover, Brown found evidence for mood-state dependent elevations of NA/N, consistent with a complication model (see also Kasch, Rottenberg, Arnow, & Gotlieb, 2002).

Research involving children and adolescents also supports the conclusion that NA/N and PA/S operate as trait vulnerabilities for anxiety- and depression-related psychopathology. For example, Lonigan, Phillips, and Hooe (2003) longitudinally studied a community sample of 270 4th through 11th grade children over the course of 7 months and found that high NA/N was predictive of increases in anxiety and low PA/S was predictive of increases in depression. Joiner and Lonigan (2000) found that the combination of NA/N and PA/S predicted changes in the severity of symptoms experienced by a group of child and adolescent psychiatric inpatients.

A smaller, but still substantial, number of studies have examined the linkage between both NA/N and EC dimensions of temperament and anxious psychopathology. Studies relating NA/N and EC dimensions of temperament to psychopathology with child or adolescent populations tend to fall into two distinct subgroups. In one group of studies, measures of temperament are generally based on a variation of Rothbart and colleagues' CBQ (Rothbart *et al.*, 2001) or EAT-Q (Capaldi & Rothbart, 1992) and psychopathology is measured by assessments of broad-band psychopathology (e.g., internalizing problems), such as the Child Behavior Checklist (CBCL: Achenbach, 1991a) or Youth Self-Report (YSR: Achenbach, 1991b). In the second group of studies, measures of temperament tend to reflect the higher-order dimensions (e.g., the Attentional Control Scale [ACS]: Derryberry & Reed, 2002) and psychopathology tends to be measured by assessments specific to a form of psychopathology (e.g., RCADS).

Relations of temperament factors with broad-band psychopathology

Eisenberg and colleagues (Eisenberg *et al.*, 2001, 2005, 2009) examined the concurrent and longitudinal relations of reactive and regulative dimensions of temperament with children's internalizing and externalizing problems. In their study, a group of 214 children were recruited when they were between 55 and 97 months of age. Children were assessed at study entry and at both 2 and 4 years following initial recruitment. Children's mothers, fathers, and teachers completed ratings of temperament, using subscales of the CBQ, and problem behaviors, using the CBCL. Children were classified categorically as control, internalizing, externalizing, or both internalizing and externalizing based on whether internalizing and externalizing *T*-scores on the CBCL were equal to/greater than or below 60. At both the initial and follow-up assessments, Eisenberg *et al.* found that aspects of NA/N and aspects of EC were associated with both internalizing and externalizing problems, and they also found that changes in status of internalizing and externalizing problems were associated with aspects of both NA/N and EC.

Similar findings were reported by Oldehinkel and colleagues in a large population sample of Dutch children ($n = 2230$; mean age 11.1 years at recruitment) known as the Tracking Adolescents' Individual Lives Survey (TRAILS). Oldehinkel, Hartman, De Winter, Veenstra, and Ormel (2004) classified children categorically as control, internalizing, externalizing, or both internalizing and externalizing based on whether their internalizing and externalizing scores on the CBCL and YSR were more than one standard deviation above the mean. Temperament was measured with the short version of the Early Adolescent Temperament Questionnaire–Revised (EATQ-R: Ellis & Rothbart, 2001), which was completed by both children and parents. Their analyses indicated that temperament factors associated with high NA/N and low EC distinguished between children classified as control and both children classified as internalizing and children classified as both internalizing and externalizing.

In a longitudinal analysis of the TRAILS sample, Oldehinkel *et al.* (2007) reported results on 1800 of the children (mean age of sample at Time 2 was 13.6 years) approximately $2\frac{1}{2}$ years after initial recruitment. They found that fearfulness and EC, as measured by parent-report on the EATQ-R, as well as the interaction of fearfulness and EC was correlated with internalizing problems, as measured by the CBCL and YSR, at the initial assessment. Higher initial levels of fearfulness and lower initial levels of EC also predicted increases in internalizing symptoms over time; however, the interaction between fearfulness and EC was not significantly related to changes in internalizing symptoms. In an analysis of this same sample, Ormel *et al.* (2005) demonstrated that the parent reports of temperament predicted psychopathology even when rates of familial psychopathology were controlled.

Relations of temperament factors with specific anxiety measures

In addition to evidence summarized above demonstrating a strong link between NA/N and anxiety (broadly defined), there is now consistent evidence that EC and anxiety are related concurrently (Muris & Meesters, 2009; Muris, Mayer, van Lint, & Hofman, 2008; Muris, Meesters, & Rompelberg, 2006; Muris, van der Penne, Sigmond, & Mayer, 2008). Other studies of the concurrent relations between temperament and anxiety support the hypothesized connections between NA/N, EC, and the interaction of NA/N and EC with anxiety. For instance, Vasey, Lonigan, Hazen, Ho, Hirai, and Anderson (2002) had 200 adolescents complete the PANAS, the ACS, and a measure of anxiety symptoms (i.e., the RCMAS). Their analyses showed that RCMAS scores were significantly and uniquely predicted by both NA/N (i.e., PANAS-NA) and EC (i.e., ACS), and that these main effects were modified by a significant interaction between NA/N and EC. Adolescents with high levels of NA/N on the PANAS had high levels of anxiety on the RCMAS if they also reported low levels of EC on the ACS; however, for adolescents who reported high levels of EC on the ACS, similarly high levels of NA/N were associated with lower levels of anxiety on the RCMAS than that reported by adolescents who had lower levels of EC.

In several studies with Dutch children and adolescents, Muris and colleagues have reported similar results using a variety of measures of temperament and anxiety. Muris (2006) collected data on temperament and psychopathology on a sample of 173 12–15-year-olds and found that higher levels of NA/N, measured by the Big Five Questionnaire for Children (Barbaranelli, Caprara, Rabasca, & Pastorelli, 2003), lower levels of EC, measured by a modified version of the ACS, and the interaction of NA/N and EC predicted higher levels of both emotional problems (i.e., anxiety, depression, eating problems) and behavioral problems (disruptive behavior, substance abuse) as measured by the Psychopathology Questionnaire for Youths (Hartman *et al.*, 2001).

Meesters, Muris, and van Rooijen (2007) examined the influence of NA/N, measured using the short version of the Junior Eysenck Personality Questionnaire (JEPQ: Eysenck & Eysenk, 1975), and EC, measured using the modified ACS, aspects of temperament on concurrent self-reports of anxiety, measured using the Screen for Child Anxiety and Related Emotional Disorders (SCARED: Birmaher *et al.*, 1997), in a community sample of 409 children and adolescents. They found that both NA/N and EC were independent predictors of anxiety, and that the interaction of NA/N and EC accounted for additional unique variance in reported anxiety. Moreover, they found no evidence that age moderated the relations of NA/N and EC with anxiety. Muris, Meesters, and Blijlevens (2007) collected self-report data on a group of 208 children who averaged 10.9 years of age. They found that both NA/N and EC, both measured using EATQ-R, contributed unique variance to the prediction of internalizing symptoms on the YSR. For internalizing symptoms overall, the interaction of NA/N and EC was marginally significant; however, when the anxiety/depression scale of the YSR was examined alone, the interaction of NA/N and EC was statistically significant.

Whereas the connection of both NA/N and EC with anxiety is a consistent finding across studies, the hypothesized moderating role of EC on NA/N is not always found. For instance, Muris, de Jong, and Engelen (2004) measured NA/N (JEPQ), EC (modified ACS), and anxiety (SCARED) in a sample of 303 8–13-year-old children, and they reported that both NA/N and EC made unique concurrent predictions to self-reported anxiety but that the interaction of NA/N and EC was not a significant unique predictor of anxiety (see also Oldehinkel *et al.*, 2007). In some of our own work, we also have failed to find a significant moderating role of EC on NA/N. For instance, in a community sample of children and adolescents (*n* = 430; average age 14.2 years), Lonigan (2007) found that both NA/N, measured using the PANAS, and EC, measured using the Effortful Control Scale (ECS:

Lonigan, 1998) were significant unique predictors of increases in reported anxiety on the RCMAS over one year; however, the interaction between NA/N and EC did not predict increases in anxiety for this sample.

We have completed a recent analysis with results indicating that the linkage between NA/N, EC, and the interaction of NA/N with EC is dependent on the anxiety disorder type. In this study (Lonigan & Phillips, unpublished data), 450 children and adolescents (average age 14.3 years) completed the PANAS, the ECS, the RCADS, and the RCMAS. It was found that NA/N, EC, and their interaction were significantly associated with the overall RCADS score; however, the strength of the association between the temperament measures and anxiety was dependent on the specific cluster of anxiety symptoms. For instance, symptoms of GAD were more strongly correlated with NA/N than were symptoms of specific phobia, separation anxiety disorder (SAD), or obsessive–compulsive disorder (OCD). Additionally, whereas the interaction of NA/N with EC was a significant unique predictor of symptoms of GAD, SAD, and panic/agoraphobia, it was not a significant unique predictor of symptoms of OCD, specific phobia, or overall anxiety as measured by the RCMAS.

These results from studies of children and adolescents demonstrate significant linkages between both reactive and regulative dimensions of temperament and psychopathology. These linkages have been shown in concurrent and longitudinal studies using broad-band measures of psychopathology, categorical classification of psychopathology, specific measures of anxiety, measures of lower-order temperament dimensions, and measures of the higher-order dimensions of temperament. Consequently, it is unlikely that the demonstrated relations between temperament and anxiety or internalizing psychopathology are the result of specific measurement operations, populations, or statistical procedures. Children and adolescents with higher levels of anxiety have higher levels of NA/N and lower levels of EC. Moreover, high NA/N and low EC predict risk for the development of anxiety and other internalizing psychopathology. In cases in which it has been tested, it has typically been found that EC moderates the influence of NA/N on anxiety; however, recent results suggest that the role of EC (and perhaps the role of NA/N) is, in part, dependent on the specific anxiety disorder, with symptoms of more global or more severe anxiety disorders more related to both NA/N and EC.

Behavioral inhibition and risk for anxiety

A substantial amount of research has been conducted on a particular variant of early childhood temperament known as behavioral inhibition (BI: see Degnan & Fox, 2007; Oosterlaan, 2001, for reviews). Children are categorized as being in the BI category if they demonstrate, in infancy or as toddlers, an extreme presentation of inhibition, uncertainty, and physiological arousal when confronted with novel objects, people, or events (Kagan, Snidman, & Arcus, 1998; Kagan, Snidman, Arcus, & Reznick, 1994). Using a categorical framework in which children are allocated to BI and non-BI extreme group clusters and remaining children with moderate observation scores receive no category, researchers have estimated the prevalence of BI to be 10–15% of the early childhood population and indicated that BI appears to be moderately heritable (Hirschfeld-Becker, Biederman, Calltharp, Rosenbaum, Faraone, & Rosenbaum, 2003; Kagan, Reznick, & Snidman, 1987; Kagan et al., 1994).

A series of short-term longitudinal studies using both Kagan's original cohorts of children, first assessed at ages 21 or 31 months, and a number of newer cohorts has indicated that BI categorization has a moderate degree of cross-time stability (Biederman *et al.*, 2001; Hirshfeld-Becker *et al.*, 2003; Kagan *et al.*, 1994; Scarpa, Raine, Venables, & Mednick, 1995). Across several of these studies, children who were the most extreme at initial assessment were the children most likely to retain their group membership. Children were more likely to move from being BI to being moderate or non-BI than to move into the BI extreme group (Biederman *et al.*, 1993; Degnan & Fox, 2007; Hirshfeld *et al.*, 1992). Evidence also suggests that after infancy, BI may be best conceptualized as a characteristic response exclusively occurring within social contexts (Fox, Henderson, Rubin, Calkins, & Schmidt, 2001).

Association between behavioral inhibition and anxiety disorders

Although not all children with BI end up with an anxiety disorder, children categorized as BI are more likely than non-BI children to develop problematic anxiety (Biederman *et al.*, 2001; Hirshfeld-Becker *et al.*, 2007; Schwartz, Snidman, & Kagan, 1999). A relatively consistent finding is the specificity of BI as a predictor of social anxiety, rather than of all anxiety types. For example, in a study of children first assessed at $1\frac{1}{2}$ to 6 years of age, data from a 5-year follow-up linked initial BI status to social anxiety in middle childhood (i.e., social phobia or avoidant disorder: Hirshfeld-Becker *et al.*, 2007). Despite this linkage between BI and anxiety, particularly social anxiety, the fact that the majority of these studies were completed on a small number of child samples, often selected based on high-risk status, additional studies are needed to clarify the nature of BI's relationship to anxiety and to determine if this relation is robust across diverse populations.

Alternative conceptualizations of behavioral inhibition

Whereas most research on BI has held to the categorical conceptualization, a related strand of longitudinal research on behavioral inhibition in social contexts as a dimensional construct also indicates developmental stability that is greatest at the extremes, with links to other temperament variables, and some relations to internalizing problems in middle childhood (e.g., Bengtsgard & Bohlin, 2001; Sanson, Pedlow, Cann, Prior, & Oberklaid, 1996). Studies that have used retrospective measures of BI also have demonstrated significant relations with adolescent or adult measures of internalizing psychopathology (e.g., Hayward, Killen, Kraemer, & Taylor, 1998; Reznick, Hegeman, Kaufman, Woods, & Jacobs, 1992). However, no study has demonstrated that these questionnaire measures identify a BI construct that is isomorphic with the BI construct measured by laboratory and parent report assessments in younger children or whether children categorized as BI by the traditional methods would develop into adolescents or adults who would self-identify as BI on these questionnaires.

Connections between behavioral inhibition and broader temperament models

The concept of BI has substantial overlap with the triadic model of temperament. Children exhibiting the BI constellation of behaviors appear to be high in NA/N (i.e., as manifest in their inhibited response to novel stimuli and their active distress) and low in EC, in that they appear to be less capable than other children in overriding their NA/N-motivated inhibition to allow adaptation to and increased comfort with the novel context (Degnan & Fox, 2007; Muris & Meesters, 2002). Despite the overlapping profiles, it is not yet clear whether BI may be a direct manifestation of the interaction between these temperament variables, a separate behavioral characteristic that, along with risk factors such as insecure attachment and particular parenting behaviors, mediates between temperament and anxiety disorders, or perhaps a subclinical manifestation of the psychopathology itself (e.g., Muris & Meesters, 2002; van Brakel, Muris, Bögels, & Thomassen, 2006). Across time, BI children who are unable to quell their inhibited reactions may be less competent at regulating their own affect and behavior; therefore, they may be more likely to demonstrate inhibition in their next social encounter and to have limited opportunities to actually acquire social competence (e.g., Oosterlaan, 2001; Rubin & Burgess, 2001; Shamir-Essakow, Ungerer, & Rapee, 2005). It seems likely that social reticence and poor competence contribute directly to the development of childhood anxiety and that both are consequences of an underlying inhibited temperament profile (e.g., Rubin, Coplan, & Bowker, 2009).

Other factors shaping the linkage between temperament and anxiety

The evidence summarized above provides clear evidence of the linkage between temperament and the development of anxiety in children and adolescents. Lonigan and Phillips (2001) outlined several possible routes by which the influence of temperamental risk for anxiety could be mediated or moderated by other factors such as parenting, attachment, cognition, or coping strategies. In contrast to the growing body of research establishing the link between temperament and psychopathology, there has been far less research conducted examining the influence of these other factors. In this section, we briefly highlight some of this research.

Environmental stressors

Vasey and Dadds (2001) suggested that respondent conditioning was one route to the acquisition of anxiety pathology. It is likely, however, that such potential conditioning events are ubiquitous and only result in heightened levels of anxiety or anxiety disorders when they are very severe, frequent, or occur in combination with temperamentally high NA/N, low EC, or both (e.g., see Chorpita & Barlow, 1998; Mineka & Zinbarg, 1995). Evidence supports the notion that anxiety disorders in children are often preceded by severe life events or chronic adversity (Allen, Rapee, & Sandberg, 2008). Similarly, Field and colleagues (Field, 2006; Field, Lawson, & Banerjee, 2008) have shown that avoidance as a consequence of verbal threat information is moderated by increased BIS sensitivity (i.e., NA/N).

A study by King, Molina, and Chassin (2008) offers another intriguing possibility for a role of temperament with respect to such acquisition of anxiety. King *et al.* studied high- and low-risk samples of adolescents with respect to stressful life events using latent variable modeling of a state–trait model in which stressful life events over three assessment intervals were modeled as both time-varying and stable components, and they found evidence of a sizeable trait component. That is, there was a stable, individual-specific tendency for adolescents to experience higher or lower levels of stressful events. Significantly, King *et al.* found that the adolescents' NA/N and EC dimensions of temperament (measured by the EASI) predicted this trait-like stress dimension. Hence, research suggests that temperament has a role not only in shaping children's responses to stressful environment events but also in shaping the likelihood of experiencing stressful environmental events.

Cognitive factors

Within explanatory models of anxiety, there have been a host of cognitive factors proposed, such as attributional style, emotional memory networks, and schematic processing of environmental events. One area that has received significant attention concerns the role of attentional biases associated with anxiety and anxiety disorders. Anxious individuals, including children (e.g., Vasey, Daleiden, Williams, & Brown, 1995), tend to display attentional biases toward threat cues (see Bar-Haim, Lamy, Pergamin, Bakermans-Kranenburg, & van IJzendoorn, 2007, for review). It is possible that attention selectively influences children's subsequent emotional and cognitive process, thus shaping children's developing cognitive representations of themselves, others, and the larger environmental context (e.g., Derryberry & Reed, 2002; Derryberry & Rothbart, 1997). Not all individuals with high levels of NA/N or trait anxiety display these attentional biases, however, and differences in attentional bias toward threat are more pronounced under conditions when it would be possible to engage strategic control of attention (e.g., at longer intervals of presentation).

Lonigan and Vasey (2009) recently tested the hypothesis that EC played a significant role in attentional bias toward threat. In this study, a community sample of children and adolescents were selected to represent four groups corresponding to high versus low levels of NA/N crossed with high versus low EC. Only participants with both high NA/N and low EC displayed biased attention toward threat; participants with high NA/N and high EC did not evidence this bias. In conjunction with other research (e.g., Muris, van der Penne, *et al.*, 2008), these findings suggest that attentional biases toward threat specifically – and not attention generally or cognitive interpretative bias – may mediate the influence of temperament on the development of anxiety pathology.

Parenting

There is a clear association between parenting style and anxiety in children (McLeod, Wood, & Weisz, 2007; Creswell, Murray, Stacey, & Cooper, Chapter 14, this volume). For example, higher levels of parental control are associated with higher levels of child anxiety. Hudson, Comer, and Kendall (2008), using a laboratory task in which anxious or non-anxious children were likely to display negative emotions, found that mothers (but not fathers) of children with an anxiety disorder were more likely to display higher levels of intrusive involvement when their children were experiencing negative emotions. Moreover, this effect was moderated by the mothers' own anxiety disorders such that intrusive involvement was highest for mothers of anxious children who themselves had an anxiety disorder. Degnan, Henderson, Fox, and Rubin (2008) indicated an interaction between infant negative reactivity and maternal characteristics such that high infant negative reactivity predicted social reticence at 7 years of age only when their mothers reported high negativity (i.e., neuroticism and symptoms of depression). A similar interaction was found between social reticence and maternal over-solicitousness at 4 years of age predicting high social wariness at age 7 years.

In the context of BI and clear evidence that BI is not a stable dimension for many children, a number of researchers have been intrigued by what factors might influence which children remain stably inhibited and which develop more typical approach and interaction behavioral styles. One suggested contributor to the maintenance of BI is an overprotective parenting style, in which one or both parents, when confronted with a child's distress around unfamiliar peers or adults, step in to shield the child from the perceived threatening situation by either removing them or by intrusively directing the child's behavior. Such parenting actions may both reinforce the behavioral pattern of inhibition and withdrawal from social interaction, and simultaneously prevent the child from developing more adaptive coping skills and competence within social contexts (e.g., Hudson *et al.*, 2008; Rubin, Burgess, & Hastings, 2002). For example, Rubin *et al.* demonstrated that children showed greater stability in inhibition and social reticence across the toddler to preschool time period when their mothers displayed an overly solicitous and protective parenting style.

Whereas these studies suggest there may be a role of parenting in the development of anxiety disorders, there are many unanswered questions about the direction and mechanism of the effect (e.g., see Silverman, Kurtines, Jaccard, & Pina, 2009). More studies are needed that explore the role that temperament may play in how reactive individual children are to different types of parenting behaviors (e.g., Lindhout, Markus, Hoogendijk, & Boer, 2009; McLeod *et al.*, 2007) and how much shared genetics may explain the association between parenting, parental personality, and child temperament, and risk for anxiety pathology (Wood, McLeod, Sigman, Hwang, & Chu, 2003). Regardless, as noted by McLeod *et al.* (2007), extant studies support, at best, a very modest association between parenting and child anxiety. Therefore, efforts to identify the origins of problematic anxiety are unlikely to find that parenting factors account for a significant component of the variance – particularly when common genetic and environmental factors are taken into account.

Conclusions

Throughout this chapter, we have highlighted ways in which temperament may influence the development of problematic anxiety in children and adolescents as well as the evidence supporting some of these potential paths of influence. We believe that the evidence is strong for a significant connection between anxiety and the higher-order temperament dimensions of NA/N and EC, and that the evidence supports a model in which the interaction of these two temperament factors provides an important explanatory mechanism for problematic anxiety. In addition to models in which these temperament factors predispose children to anxiety or anxiety represents an extreme manifestation of temperament traits, there is emerging evidence that these higher-order dimensions of temperament have influences on environmental and cognitive factors that may mediate or moderate the relation between temperament and anxiety.

Emerging evidence across child, adolescent, and adult populations suggests that temperament, personality, and psychopathology can be conceptualized as an integrated hierarchical model. Across constructs, higher-order dimensions differentiate into more fine-grained dimensions through variable levels of influence and interactions among the higher-order dimensions, maturation, and experiential factors. There are significant and established connections between the high-order dimensions of each construct (e.g., NA/N, neuroticism, internalizing [emotional] disorders), and there are likely predictable connections between lower-order dimensions and specific subtypes of psychopathology (e.g., GAD, social phobia).

Whereas the evidentiary framework for such an integrated hierarchical model currently exists, additional research is needed to probe the exact nature of the interrelations between higher- and lower-order dimensions within and between constructs. Specifically, we believe that greater specification of the lower-order dimensions of temperament is needed. As noted above, current support for many of these dimensions exists at the conceptual level without strong empirical support. Given the potential importance of understanding how these lower-order dimensions may interact with each other to bring about risk for specific forms of psychopathology, such measurement work seems a high priority. Additionally, there is now a wealth of studies demonstrating concurrent links between temperament and anxiety. Longitudinal studies will not only provide information for how temperament factors operate over time to bring about risk for anxiety, but they will allow the possibility of disentangling cause and consequence not only between temperament and anxiety but between temperament and other potential mediating and moderating factors (e.g., parenting, cognitive processes). Finally, within a hierarchical model of internalizing disorders, it seems clear that temperament factors may play a greater or lesser role depending on the specific disorder. Examining these linkages at a level beyond internalizing versus externalizing seems warranted.

References

Achenbach, T. M. (1991a). *Manual for the Child Behavior Checklist/4–18 and 1991 profile.* Burlington, VT: University of Vermont Department of Psychiatry.

Achenbach, T. M. (1991b). *Manual for the Youth Self-Report.* Burlington, VT: University of Vermont Department of Psychiatry.

Ahadi, S. A. & Rothbart, M. K. (1994). Temperament, development, and the Big Five. In: C. F. Halverson, Jr., G. A. Kohnstamm, & R. P. Martin (eds.) *The Developing Structure of Temperament and Personality from Infancy to Adulthood,* pp. 189–207. Hillsdale, NJ: Erlbaum.

Ahadi, S. A., Rothbart, M. K., & Ye, R. (1993). Children's temperament in the US and China: similarities and differences. *European Journal of Personality,* **7,** 359–377.

Akiskal, L. Y., Hirschfeld, R. M. A., & Yerevanian, B. J. (1983). The relationship of personality to affective disorders. *Archives of General Psychiatry,* **40,** 801–810.

Allen, J. L., Rapee, R. M., & Sandberg, S. (2008). Severe life events and chronic adversities as antecedents to anxiety: a matched control study. *Journal of Abnormal Child Psychology,* **26,** 1047–1056.

Allport, G. W. (1937). *Personality: A Psychological Interpretation.* New York: Holt.

Angleitner, A. & Ostendorf, F. (1994). Temperament and the big five factors of personality. In: C. F. Halverson, Jr., G. A. Kohnstamm, & R. P. Martin (eds.) *The Developing Structure of Temperament and Personality from Infancy to Adulthood,* pp. 69–90. Hillsdale, NJ: Erlbaum.

Anthony, J. L., Lonigan, C. J., Hooe, E. S., & Phillips, B. M. (2002). An affect based, hierarchical model of temperament and its relations with internalizing symptomatology. *Journal of Clinical Child and Adolescent Psychology,* **31,** 480–490.

Austin, A. A. & Chorpita, B. F. (2004). Temperament, anxiety, and depression: comparisons across five ethnic groups of children. *Journal of Clinical Child and Adolescent Psychology,* **33,** 216–226.

Bar-Haim, Y., Lamy, D., Pergamin, L., Bakermans-Kranenburg, M. J., & van IJzendoorn, M. H. (2007). Threat-related attentional bias in anxious and nonanxious individuals: a meta-analytic study. *Psychological Bulletin,* **133,** 1–24.

Barbaranelli, C., Caprara, G. V., Rabasca, A., & Pastorelli, C. (2003). A questionnaire for measuring the Big Five in late childood. *Personality and Individual Differences,* **34,** 645–664.

Bengtsgard, K. & Bohlin, G. (2001). Social inhibition and overfriendliness: two-year follow-up and observational validation. *Journal of Clinical Child Psychology,* **30,** 364–375.

Biederman, J., Hirshfeld-Becker, D. R., Rosenbaum, J. F., Herot, C., Friedman, D., Snidman, N., *et al.* (2001). Further evidence of association between behavioral inhibition and social anxiety in children. *American Journal of Psychiatry,* **158,** 1673–1679.

Biederman, J., Rosenbaum, J. F., Bolduc-Murphy, E. A., Faraone, S. V., Chaloff, J., Hirshfeld, D. R., *et al.* (1993). A three-year follow-up of children with and without behavioral inhibition. *Journal of the American Academy of Child and Adolescent Psychiatry,* **32,** 814–821.

Birmaher, B., Khetarpal, S., Brent, D., Cully, M., Balach, L., Kaufman, J., *et al.* (1997). The Screen for Child Anxiety Related Emotional Disorders (SCARED): scale construction and psychometric characteristics. *Journal of the American Academy of Child and Adolescent Psychiatry*, **36**, 545–553.

Brady, E. U. & Kendall, P. C. (1992). Comorbidity of anxiety and depression in children and adolescents. *Psychological Bulletin*, **111**, 244–255.

Brown, T. A. (2007). Temporal course and structural relationships among dimensions of temperament and DSM-IV anxiety and mood disorder constructs. *Journal of Abnormal Psychology*, **116**, 313–328.

Brown, T. A., Chorpita, B. F., & Barlow, D. H. (1998). Structural relations among dimensions of the DSM-IV anxiety and mood disorders and dimensions of negative affect, positive affect, and autonomic arousal. *Journal of Abnormal Psychology*, **107**, 179–192.

Burke, C. B., Burke, J. D., Regier, D. A., & Rae, D. S. (1990). Age at onset of selected mental disorders in five community populations. *Archives of General Psychiatry*, **47**, 511–518.

Buss, A. H. & Plomin, R. (1984). *Temperament: Early Developing Personality Traits*. Hillsdale, NJ: Wiley & Sons.

Capaldi, D. M. & Rothbart, M. K. (1992). Development and validation of an early adolescent temperament measure. *Journal of Early Adolescence*, **12**, 153–173.

Caspi, A. & Silva, P. A. (1995). Temperamental qualities at age three predict personality traits in young adulthood: longitudinal evidence from a birth cohort. *Child Development*, **66**, 486–498.

Chorpita, B. F. & Barlow, D. H. (1998). The development of anxiety: the role of control in the early environment. *Psychological Bulletin*, **124**, 3–21.

Chorpita, B. F. & Daleiden, E. L. (2002). Tripartite dimensions of emotion in a child clinical sample: measurement strategies and implications for clinical utility. *Journal of Consulting and Clinical Psychology*, **70**, 1150–1160.

Chorpita, B. F., Albano, A. M., & Barlow, D. H. (1998). The structure of negative emotions in a clinical sample of children and adolescents. *Journal of Abnormal Psychology*, **107**, 74–85.

Chorpita, B. F., Yim, L., Moffitt, C., Umemoto, L. A., & Francis, S. E. (2000). Assessment of symptoms of DSM-IV anxiety and depression in children: a revised child anxiety and depression scale. *Behaviour Research and Therapy*, **38**, 835–855.

Clark, L. A. (2005). Temperament as a unifying basis for personality and psychopathology. *Journal of Abnormal Psychology*, **114**, 505–521.

Clark, L. A. & Watson, D. (1991). Tripartite model of anxiety and depression: psychometric evidence and taxonomic implications. *Journal of Abnormal Psychology*, **100**, 316–336.

Clark, L.A., Watson, D., & Mineka, S. (1994). Temperament, personality, and the mood and anxiety disorders. *Journal of Abnormal Psychology*, **103**, 103–116.

Costello, E. J., Egger, H. L., & Angold, A. (2005). The developmental epidemiology of anxiety disorders: phenomenology, prevalence, and comorbidity. *Child and Adolescent Psychiatric Clinics of North America*, **14**, 631–648.

Degnan, K. A. & Fox, N. A. (2007). Behavioral inhibition and anxiety disorders: multiple levels of a resilience process. *Development and Psychopathology*, **19**, 729–746.

Degnan, K. A., Henderson, H. A., Fox, N. A., & Rubin, K. H. (2008). Predicting social wariness in middle childhood: the moderating roles of childcare history, maternal personality and maternal behavior. *Social Development*, **17**, 471–487.

Derryberry, D. & Reed, M. A. (2002). Anxiety-related attentional biases and their regulation by attentional control. *Journal of Abnormal Psychology*, **111**, 225–236.

Derryberry, D. & Rothbart, M. K. (1984). Emotion, attention, and temperament. In: H. C. Izard, J. Kagan, & R. Zajonc (eds.) *Emotion, Cognition, and Behavior*, pp. 132–166. Cambridge, UK: Cambridge University Press.

Derryberry, D. & Rothbart, M. K. (1997). Reactive and effortful processes in the organization of temperament. *Development and Psychopathology*, **9**, 633–652.

Diamond, S. (1974). *The Roots of Psychology: A Sourcebook in the History of Ideas.* New York: Basic Books.

Digman, J. M. (1994). Child personality and temperament: does the five-factor model embrace both domains? In: C. F. Halverson, Jr., G. A. Kohnstamn, & R. P. Martin (eds.) *The Developing Structure of Temperament and Personality from Infancy to Adulthood*, pp. 323–338. Hillsdale, NJ: Erlbaum.

Eisenberg, N., Cumberland, A., Spinrad, T. L., Fabes, R. A., Shepard, S. A., Reiser, M., *et al.* (2001). The relations of regulation and emotionality to children's externalizing and internalizing problem behavior. *Child Development*, **72**, 1112–1134.

Eisenberg, N., Sadovsky, A., Spinrad, T. L., Fabes, R. A., Losoya, S. H., Valiente, C., *et al.* (2005). The relations of problem behavior status to children's negative emotionality, effortful control, and impulsivity: concurrent relations and prediction of change. *Developmental Psychology*, **41**, 193–211.

Eisenberg, N., Valiente, C., Spinrad, T. L., Cumberland, A., Liew, J., Reiser, M., *et al.* (2009). Longitudinal relations of children's effortful control, impulsivity, and negative emotionality, and co-occurring behavior problems. *Developmental Psychology*, **45**, 988–1008.

Ekman, P., Friesen, W. V., & Ellsworth, P. (1972). *Emotion in the Human Face.* New York: Pergamon.

Ellis, L. K. & Rothbart, M. K. (2001). Revision of the early adolescent temperament questionnaire. Poster presented at the biennial meeting of the Society for Research in Child Development, Minneapolis, MN.

Essau, C. A., Conradt, J., & Petermann, F. (2000). Frequency, comorbidity, and psychosocial impairment of anxiety disorders in German adolescents. *Journal of Anxiety Disorders*, **14**, 263–279.

Eysenck, H. J. & Eysenck, S. B. G. (1975). *Manual of the Eysenck Personality Questionnaire (Adult and Junior).* London: Hodder & Stoughton.

Fan, J., Wu, Y., Fossella, J. A., & Posner, M. I. (2001). Assessing the heritability of attentional networks. *BMC Neuroscience*, **3**, 14.

Field, A. P. (2006). The behavioral inhibition system and the verbal information pathway to children's fears. *Journal of Abnormal Psychology*, **115**, 742–752.

Field, A. P., Lawson, J., & Banerjee, R. (2008). The verbal threat information pathway to fear in children: the longitudinal effects on fear cognitions and the immediate effects on avoidance behavior. *Journal of Abnormal Psychology*, **117**, 214–224.

Fox, N. A., Henderson, H. A., Rubin, K. H., Calkins, S. D., & Schmidt, L. A. (2001). Continuity and discontinuity of behavioral inhibition and exuberance: psychophysiological and behavioral influences across the first four years of life. *Child Development*, **72**, 1–21.

Goldsmith, H. H. & Campos, J. J. (1982). Toward a theory of infant temperament. In: R. N. Emde & R. J. Harmon (eds.) *The Development of Attachment and Affiliative Systems*, pp. 161–193. New York: Plenum Press.

Goldsmith, H. H. & Lemery, K. S. (2000). Linking temperamental fearfulness and anxiety symptoms: a behavior-genetic perspective. *Biological Psychiatry*, **48**, 1199–1209.

Goldsmith, H. H., Buss, A., Plomin, R., Rothbart, M. K., Thomas, A., Chess, S., *et al.* (1987). Roundtable: What is temperament? Four approaches. *Child Development*, **58**, 505–529.

Goldsmith, H. H., Reilly, J., Lemery, K. S., Longley, S., & Prescott, A. (1995). *Preliminary Manual for the Preschool Laboratory Temperament Assessment Battery, Version 0.5.* Madison, WI: University of Wisconsin Department of Psychology.

Gray, J. A. (1982). *The Neuropsychology of Anxiety: An Enquiry into the Functions of the Septo-Hippocampal System.* New York: Oxford University Press.

Hagekull, B. & Bohlin, G. (1998). Preschool temperament and environmental factors related to the five-factor model of personality in middle childhood. *Merrill-Palmer Quarterly*, **44**, 194–215.

Hartman, C. A., Hox, J., Mellenbergh, G. J., Boyle, M. H., Offord, D. R., Racine, Y., et al. (2001). DSM-IV internal construct validity: when a taxonomy meets data. *Journal of Child Psychology and Psychiatry*, **42**, 817–836.

Hayward, C., Killen, J. D., Kraemer, H. C., & Taylor, C. B. (1998). Linking self-reported childhood behavioral inhibition to adolescent social phobia. *Journal of the American Academy of Child and Adolescent Psychiatry*, **37**, 1308–1316.

Hirshfeld, D. R., Rosenbaum, J. F., Biederman, J., Bolduc, E. A., Faraone, S. V., Snidman N., et al. (1992). Stable behavioral inhibition and its association with anxiety disorder. *Journal of the American Academy of Child and Adolescent Psychiatry*, **31**, 103–111.

Hirshfeld-Becker, D. R., Biederman, J., Calltharp, S., Rosenbaum, E. D., Faraone, S. V., & Rosenbaum, J. F. (2003). Behavioral inhibition and disinhibition as hypothesized precursors to psychopathology: implications for pediatric bipolar disorder. *Biological Psychiatry*, **53**, 985–999.

Hirshfeld-Becker, D. R., Biederman, J., Henin, A., Faraone, S. V., Davis, S., Harrington, K., et al. (2007). Behavioral inhibition in preschool children at risk is a specific predictor of middle childhood social anxiety: a five-year follow-up. *Journal of Developmental and Behavioral Pediatrics*, **28**, 225–233.

Hudson, J. L., Comer, J. S., & Kendall, P. C. (2008). Parental responses to positive and negative emotions in anxious and nonanxious children. *Journal of Clinical Child and Adolescent Psychology*, **37**, 303–313.

John, O. P., Caspi, A., Robins, R. W., Moffitt, T. E., & Stouthamer-Loeber, M. (1994). The "little five": exploring the nomological network of the five-factor model of personality in adolescent boys. *Child Development*, **65**, 160–178.

Joiner, T. E., Jr. & Lonigan, C. J. (2000). Tripartite model of depression and anxiety in youth psychiatric inpatients: relations with diagnostic status and future symptoms. *Journal of Clinical Child Psychology*, **29**, 372–382.

Joiner, T. E., Jr., Catanzaro, S., & Laurent, J. (1996). The tripartite structure of positive and negative affect, depression, and anxiety in child and adolescent psychiatric inpatients. *Journal of Abnormal Psychology*, **105**, 401–409.

Kagan, J., Reznick, J. S., & Snidman, N. (1987). The physiology and psychology of behavioral inhibition in children. *Child Development*, **58**, 1459–1473.

Kagan, J., Snidman, N., & Arcus, D. (1998). Childhood derivatives of high and low reactivity in infancy. *Child Development*, **69**, 1483–1493.

Kagan, J., Snidman, N., Arcus, D., & Reznick, S. J. (1994). *Galen's Prophecy: Temperament in Human Nature.* New York: Basic Books.

Kasch, K. L., Rottenberg, J., Arnow, B. A., & Gotlieb, I. H. (2002). Behavioral activation and inhibition systems and the severity and course of depression. *Journal of Abnormal Psychology*, **111**, 589–597.

Keller, M. B., Lavori, P. W., Wunder, J., Beardslee, W. R., Schwartz, C. E., & Roth, J. (1992). Chronic course of anxiety disorders in children and adolescents. *Journal of the American Academy of Child and Adolescent Psychiatry*, **31**, 595–599.

Kendall, P. C., Safford, S., Flannery-Schroeder, E., & Webb, A. (2004). Child anxiety treatment: outcomes in adolescence and impact on substance use and depression at 7.4-year follow-up. *Journal of Consulting and Clinical Psychology*, **72**, 276–287.

Kendler, K. S., Neale, M. C., Kessler, R. C., Heath, A. C., & Eaves, L. J. (1992). The genetic epidemiology of phobias in women: the interrelationship of agoraphobia, social phobia, situational phobia, and simple phobia. *Archives of General Psychiatry*, **49**, 273–281.

Kessler, R. C., McGonagle, K. A., Zhao, S., Nelson, C. B., Hughes, M., Eshleman, S., *et al.* (1994). Lifetime and 12-month prevalence of DSM-III-R psychiatric disorders in the United States: results from the National Comorbidity Survey. *Archives of General Psychiatry*, **51**, 8–19.

King, K. M., Molina, B. S. G., & Chassin, L. (2008). A state-trait model of negative life event occurrence in adolescence: predictors of stability in the occurrence of stressors. *Journal of Clinical Child and Adolescent Psychology*, **37**, 848–859.

Krueger, R. F., Caspi, A., Moffitt, T. E., Silva, P. A., & McGee, R. (1996). Personality traits are differentially linked to mental disorders: a multitrait–multidiagnosis study of an adolescent birth cohort. *Journal of Abnormal Psychology*, **105**, 299–312.

Lahey, B. B., Applegate, B., Waldman, I. D., Loft, J. D., Hankin, B. L., & Rick, J. (2004). The structure of child and adolescent psychopathology: generating new hypotheses. *Journal of Abnormal Psychology*, **113**, 358–385.

Lahey, B. B., Rathouz, P. J., Van Hulle, C., Urbano, R. C., Krueger, R. F., Applegate, B., *et al.* (2008). Testing structural models of DSM-IV symptoms of common forms of child and adolescent psychopathology. *Journal of Abnormal Child Psychology*, **36**, 187–206.

Last, C. G., Perrin, S., Hersen, M., & Kazdin, A. E. (1996). A prospective study of childhood anxiety disorders. *Journal of the American Academy of Child and Adolescent Psychiatry*, **35**, 1502–1510.

Last, C. G., Strauss, C. C., & Francis, G. (1987). Comorbidity among childhood anxiety disorders. *Journal of Nervous and Mental Disease*, **175**, 726–730.

Lemery-Chalfant, K., Doelger, L., & Goldsmith, H. H. (2008). Genetic relations between effortful and attentional control and symptoms of psychopathology in middle childhood. *Infant and Child Development*, **17**, 365–385.

Lewinsohn, P. M., Zinbarg, R., Seeley, J. R., Lewinsohn, M., & Sack, W. H. (1997). Lifetime comorbidity among anxiety disorders and between anxiety disorders and other mental disorders in adolescents. *Journal of Anxiety Disorders*, **11**, 377–394.

Lindhout, I. E., Markus, M. M., Hoogendijk, T. H., & Boer, F. (2009). Temperament and parental child-rearing style: unique contributions to clinical anxiety disorders in childhood. *European Child and Adolescent Psychiatry*, **18**, 439–446.

Lonigan, C. J. (1998). Development of a measure of effortful control in school-age children. Unpublished raw data, Florida State University, Tallahassee, FL.

Lonigan, C. J. (2007). Temperamental influences on the development of internalizing psychopathology in children and adolescents: the role of reactive and effortful processes. Keynote paper given at the Conference on Temperament and Psychopathology, Katholieke Universiteit Leuven, Leuven, Belgium.

Lonigan, C. J. & Phillips, B. M. (2001). Temperamental influences on the development of anxiety disorders. In: M. W. Vasey & M. R. Dadds (eds.) *The Developmental Psychopathology of Anxiety*, pp. 60–91. New York: Oxford University Press.

Lonigan, C. J. & Vasey, M. W. (2009). Negative affectivity, effortful control, and attention to threat-relevant stimuli. *Journal of Abnormal Child Psychology*, **37**, 387–399.

Lonigan, C. J., Carey, M. P., & Finch, A. J., Jr. (1994). Anxiety and depression in children and adolescents: negative affectivity and the utility of self-reports. *Journal of Consulting and Clinical Psychology*, **62**, 1000–1008.

Lonigan, C. J., Hooe, E. S., David, C. F., & Kistner, J. A. (1999). Positive and negative affectivity in children: confirmatory factor analysis of a two-factor model and its relation to symptoms of anxiety and depression. *Journal of Consulting and Clinical Psychology*, **67**, 374–386.

Lonigan, C. J., Phillips, B. M., & Hooe, E. S. (2003). Tripartite model of anxiety and depression in children: evidence from a latent variable longitudinal study. *Journal of Consulting and Clinical Psychology*, **71**, 465–481.

Lonigan, C. J., Vasey, M. W., Phillips, B. M., & Hazen, R. A. (2004). Temperament, anxiety, and the processing of threat-relevant stimuli. *Journal of Clinical Child and Adolescent Psychology*, **33**, 8–20.

Majdandžić, M., van den Boom, D. C., & Heesbeen, D. G. M. (2008). Peas in a pod: biased in the measurement of sibling temperament? *Developmental Psychology*, **44**, 1354–1368.

Markon, K. E., Krueger, R. F., & Watson, D. (2005). Delineating the structure of normal and abnormal personality: an integrative hierarchical approach. *Journal of Personality and Social Psychology*, **88**, 139–157.

McCrae, R. R. & Costa, P. T. (1987). Validation of the five factor model across instruments and observers. *Journal of Personality and Social Psychology*, **49**, 710–727.

McLeod, B. D., Wood, J. J., & Weisz, J. R. (2007). Examining the association between parenting and child anxiety: a meta-analysis. *Clinical Psychology Review*, **27**, 155–172.

Meesters, C., Muris, P., & van Rooijen, B. (2007). Relations of neuroticism and attentional control with symptoms of anxiety and aggression in non-clinical children. *Journal of Psychopathology and Behavioral Assessment*, **29**, 149–158.

Mineka, S. & Zinbarg, R. (1995). Conditioning and ethological models of social phobia. In: R. G. Heinberg, M. R. Liebowitz, D. A. Hope, & F. R. Schneider (eds.) *Social Phobia: Diagnosis, Assessment, and Treatment*, pp. 134–162. New York: Guilford Press.

Moffitt, T. E., Harrington, H., Caspi, A., Kim-Cohen, J., Goldberg, D., Gregory, A. M., *et al.* (2007). Depression and generalized anxiety disorder: cummulative and sequential comorbidity in a birth cohort followed prospectively to age 32 years. *Archives of General Psychiatry*, **64**, 651–660.

Muris, P. (2006). Unique and interactive effects of neuroticism and effortful control on psychopathological symptoms in non-clinical adolescents. *Personality and Individual Differences*, **20**, 1409–1419.

Muris, P. & Meesters, C. (2002). Attachment, behavioral inhibition, and anxiety disorders symptoms in normal adolescents. *Journal of Psychopathology and Behavioral Assessment*, **24**, 97–106.

Muris, P. & Meesters, C. (2009). Reactive and regulative temperament in youths: psychometric evaluation of the Early Adolescent Temperament Questionnaire–Revised. *Journal of Psychopathology and Behavioral Assessment*, **31**, 7–19.

Muris, P., de Jong, P. J., & Engelen, S. (2004). Relationships between neuroticism, attentional control, and anxiety disorders symptoms in non-clinical children. *Personality and Individual Differences*, **37**, 789–797.

Muris, P., Mayer, B., van Lint, C., & Hofman, S. (2008). Attentional control and psychopathological symptoms in children. *Personality and Individual Differences*, **44**, 1495–1505.

Muris, P., Meesters, C., & Blijlevens, P. (2007). Self-reported reactive and regulative temperament in early adolescence: relations to internalizing and externalizing problem behavior and "Big Three" personality factors. *Journal of Adolescence*, **30**, 1035–1049.

Muris, P., Meesters, C., & Rompelberg, L. (2006). Attention control in middle childhood: relations to psychopathological symptoms and threat perception distortions. *Behaviour Research and Therapy*, **45**, 997–1010.

Muris, P., van der Penne, E., Sigmond, R., & Mayer, B. (2008). Symptoms of anxiety, depression, and aggression in non-clinical children: relationships with self-report and performance-based measures of attention and effortful control. *Child Psychiatry and Human Development*, **39**, 455–467.

Nigg, J. T. (2006). Temperament and developmental psychopathology. *Journal of Child Psychology and Psychiatry*, **47**, 395–422.

Oldehinkel, A. J., Hartman, C. A., De Winter, A. F., Veenstra, R., & Ormel, J. (2004). Temperament profiles associated with internalizing and externalizing problems in preadolescence. *Development and Psychopathology*, **16**, 421–440.

Oldehinkel, A. J., Hartman, C. A., Ferdinand, R. F., Verhulst, F. C., & Ormel, J. (2007). Effortful control as a modifier of the association between negative emotionality and adolescents' mental health problems. *Development and Psychopathology*, **19**, 523–539.

Oosterlaan, J. (2001). Behavioral inhibition and the development of childhood anxiety disorders. In: **W. K. Silverman** & **P. D. A. Treffers** (eds.) *Anxiety Disorders in Children and Adolescents: Research, Assessment, and Intervention*, pp. 45–71. Cambridge, UK: Cambridge University Press.

Ormel, J., Oldehinkel, A. J., Ferdinand, R. F., Hartman, C. A., De Winter, A. F., Veenstra, R., *et al.* (2005). Internalizing and externalizing problems in adolescence: general and dimension-specific effects of familial loadings and preadolescent temperament traits. *Psychological Medicine*, **35**, 1825–1835.

Orvaschel, H., Lewinsohn, P. M., & Seeley, J. R. (1995). Continuity of psychopathology in a community sample of adolescents. *Journal of the American Academy of Child and Adolescent Psychiatry*, **34**, 1525–1535.

Phillips, B. M., Lonigan, C. J., Driscoll, K., & Hooe, E. S. (2002). Positive and negative affectivity in children: a multitrait–multimethod evaluation. *Journal of Clinical Child and Adolescent Psychology*, **31**, 465–479.

Posner, M. R. & Rothbart, M. K. (2000). Developing mechanisms of self-regulation. *Development and Psychopathology*, **12**, 427–441.

Putnam, S. P., Rothbart, M. K., & Gartstein, M. A. (2008). Homotypic and heterotypic continuity of fine-grained temperament during infancy, toddlerhood, and early childhood. *Infant and Child Development*, **17**, 387–405.

Reynolds, C. R. & Richmond, B. O. (1978). What I think and feel: a revised measure of children's manifest anxiety. *Journal of Abnormal Child Psychology*, **6**, 271–280.

Reznick, J., Hegeman, I., Kaufman, E., Woods, S., & Jacobs, M. (1992). Retrospective and concurrent self-report of behavioral inhibition and their relation to adult mental health. *Developmental Psychopathology*, **4**, 301–321.

Rothbart, M. K. (1989). Temperament and development. In: **G. A. Kohnstamm, J. E. Bates,** & **M. K. Rothbart** (eds.) *Temperament in Childhood*, pp. 187–247. New York: Wiley & Sons.

Rothbart, M. K. & Bates, J. E. (1998). Temperament. In: **W. Damon** & **N. Eisenberg** (eds.) *Handbook of Child Psychology*, vol. 3, *Social, Emotional, and Personality Development*, 5th edn, pp. 105–176. New York: Wiley & Sons.

Rothbart, M. K. & Bates, J. E. (2006). Temperament in children's development. In: **W. Damon** & **R. Lerner** (eds.) *Handbook of Child Psychology*, vol. 3, *Social, Emotional, and Personality Development*, 6th edn, pp. 99–166. New York: Wiley & Sons.

Rothbart, M. K., Ahadi, S. A., & Hershey, K. L. (1994). Temperament and social behavior in childhood. *Merrill-Palmer Quarterly*, **40**, 21–39.

Rothbart, M. K., Ahadi, S. A., Hershey, K. L., & Fisher, P. (2001). Investigation of temperament at three to seven years: the Children's Behavior Questionnaire. *Child Development*, **72**, 1394–1408.

Rothbart, M. K., Posner, M. I., & Hershey, K. L. (1995). Temperament, attention, and developmental psychology. In: **D. Cicchetti** & **D. J. Cohen** (eds.) *Developmental Psychopathology*, vol. 1, *Theory and Methods*, pp. 315–340. New York: Wiley & Sons.

Rothbart, M. K., Sheese, B. E., & Posner, M. I. (2007). Executive attention and effortful control: linking temperament, brain networks, and genes. *Child Development Perspectives*, **1**, 2–7.

Rubin, K. H. & Burgess, K. B. (2001). Social withdrawal and anxiety. In: **M. W. Vasey** & **M. R. Dadds** (eds.) *The Developmental Psychopathology of Anxiety*, pp. 407–434. New York: Oxford University Press.

Rubin, K. H., Burgess, K. B., & Hastings, P. D. (2002). Stability and social–behavioral consequences of toddlers' inhibited temperament and parenting behaviors. *Child Development*, **73**, 483–495.

Rubin, K. H., Coplan, R. J., & Bowker, J. C. (2009). Social withdrawal in childhood. *Annual Review of Psychology*, **60**, 141–171.

Sanson, A., Pedlow, R., Cann, W., Prior, M., & Oberklaid, F. (1996). Shyness ratings: stability and correlates in early childhood. *International Journal of Behavioral Development*, **19**, 705–724.

Scarpa, A., Raine, A., Venables, P. H., & Mednick, S. A. (1995). The stability of inhibited/uninhibited temperament from ages 3 to 11 years in Mauritian children. *Journal of Abnormal Child Psychology*, **23**, 607–618.

Schwartz, C. E., Snidman, N., & Kagan, J. (1999). Adolescent social anxiety as an outcome of inhibited temperament in childhood. *Journal of the American Academy of Child and Adolescent Psychiatry*, **38**, 1008–1015.

Selbom, M., Ben-Porath, Y., & Bagby, R. M. (2008). On the hierarchical structure of mood and anxiety disorders: confirmatory evidence and elaboration of a model of temperament markers. *Journal of Abnormal Psychology*, **117**, 576–590.

Shamir-Essakow, G., Ungerer, J. A., & Rapee, R. M. (2005). Attachment, behavioral inhibition, and anxiety in preschool children. *Journal of Abnormal Child Psychology*, **33**, 131–143.

Shiner, R. & Caspi, A. (2003). Personality differences in childhood and adolescents: measurement, development, and consequences. *Journal of Child Psychology and Psychiatry*, **44**, 2–32.

Silverman, W. K. & Albano, A. M. (1996). *Anxiety Disorders Interview Schedule for Children–IV: Child and Parent Versions*. San Antonio, TX: The Psychological Corporation.

Silverman, W. K., Kurtines, W. M., Jaccard, J., & Pina, A. A. (2009). Directionality of change in youth anxiety treatment involving parents: an initial examination. *Journal of Consulting and Clinical Psychology*, **77**, 474–485.

Tellegen, A. & Waller, N. G. (2008). Exploring personality through test construction: development of the Multidimensional Personality Questionnaire. In: **G. J. Boyle, G. Matthews, & D. H. Saklofske** (eds.) *The SAGE Handbook of Personality Theory and Assessment*, vol. 2, *Personality Measurement and Testing*, pp. 261–292. Thousand Oaks, CA: Sage Publications.

Tellegen, A., Watson, D., & Clark, L. A. (1999). On the dimensional and hierarchical structure of affect. *Psychological Science*, **10**, 297–303.

Thomas, A., Chess, S., & Birch, S. D. (1996). *Temperament and Behavior Disorders in Children*. New York: New York University Press.

Trull, T. J. & Sher, K. J. (1994). Relationship between the five-factor model of personality and axis I disorders in a nonclinical sample. *Journal of Abnormal Psychology*, **103**, 350–360.

van Brakel, A. M. L., Muris, P., Bögels, S. M., & Thomassen, C. (2006). A multifactorial model for the etiology of anxiety in non-clinical adolescents: main and interactive effects of behavioral inhibition, attachment and parental rearing. *Journal of Child and Family Studies*, **15**, 569–579.

Vasey, M. W. & Dadds, M. R. (2001). An introduction to the developmental psychopathology of anxiety. In: **M. W. Vasey** & **M. R. Dadds** (eds.) *The Developmental Psychopathology of Anxiety*, pp. 3–26. New York: Oxford University Press.

Vasey, M. W., Daleiden, E. L., Williams, L. L., & Brown, L. M. (1995). Biased attention in childhood anxiety disorders: a preliminary study. *Journal of Abnormal Child Psychology*, **23**, 267–279.

Vasey, M. W., Lonigan, C. J., Hazen, R., Ho, A., Hirai, K., & Anderson, M. (2002). Effortful control as a moderator of risk for internalizing and externalizing symptoms in early adolescence. Paper presented at the 36th Annual Convention of the Association for the Advancement of Behavior Therapy, Reno, NV.

Verduin, T. L. & Kendall, P. C. (2003). Differential occurrence of comorbidity within childhood anxiety disorders. *Journal of Clinical Child and Adolescent Psychology*, **32**, 290–295.

Watson, D. (2005). Rethinking mood and anxiety disorders: a quantitative hierarchical model for DSM-V. *Journal of Abnormal Psychology*, **114**, 522–536.

Watson, D., Clark, L. A., & Carey, G. (1988). Positive and negative affectivity and their relation to anxiety and depressive disorders. *Journal of Abnormal Psychology*, **97**, 346–353.

Watson, D., Clark, L. A., & Harkness, A. R. (1994). Structures of personality and their relevance to psychopathology. *Journal of Abnormal Psychology*, **103**, 18–31.

Watson, D., Clark, L. A., & Tellegen, A. (1988). Development and validation of brief measures of positive and negative affect: the PANAS scales. *Journal of Personality and Social Psychology*, **54**, 1063–1070.

Whittle, S., Allen, N. B., Lubman, D. I., & Yücel, M. (2006). The neurobiologiocal basis of temperament: towards a better understanding of psychopathology. *Neuroscience and Biobehavioral Reviews*, **30**, 511–525.

Wood, J. J., McLeod, B. D., Sigman, M., Hwang, W. C., & Chu, B. C. (2003). Parenting and childhood anxiety: theory, empirical findings, and future directions. *Journal of Child Psychology and Psychiatry*, **44**, 134–151.

Woodward, L. J. & Fergusson, D. M. (2001). Life course outcome of young people with anxiety disorders in adolescence. *Journal of the American Academy of Child and Adolescent Psychiatry*, **40**, 1086–1093.

Environmental influences on child and adolescent anxiety

11

The role of learning in the etiology of child and adolescent fear and anxiety

Andy P. Field and Helena M. Purkis

Hush little baby, don't say a word; And never mind that noise you heard.
It's just the beast under your bed. In the closet, in your head.

(Metallica, 1991, track 1)

Children are so prone to fear that it has been seen as a normal part of childhood development (see Muris & Field, Chapter 4, this volume). These normal fears are likely to be the precursors of more persistent and severe anxiety (Field & Davey, 2001) because the age of onset of anxiety disorders broadly follows the developmental pattern of non-clinical fears. As reviewed by Muris and Field, infants tend to fear novel stimuli within their immediate environment such as loud noise, objects, and separation from a caretaker (Campbell, 1986), in mid-childhood (6–8 years old) fears are focused towards ghosts and animals, then self-injury in late childhood (Bauer, 1976), and social evaluation in pre-adolescence and adolescence (Westenberg, Drewes, Goedhart, Siebelink, & Treffers, 2004). Similarly, phobias concerning environmental threats (e.g., heights, water) typically originate in infancy (Menzies & Clarke, 1993a, 1993b), then specific phobias emerge in middle childhood (5–6 years) followed by generalized anxiety in late childhood and social anxiety in pre-adolescence (Costello, Egger, Copeland, Erkanli, & Angold, Chapter 3, this volume). This broad correspondence between normal fears and the onset of anxiety disorders raises three questions pertinent to explaining the etiology of anxiety disorders: (1) are these normal fears innate or learnt? (2) What process underlies whether a fear develops into an anxiety disorder? And (3) what variables moderate this process? This chapter attempts to explore these questions by evaluating the contribution of learning processes in the development of both normal fears and anxiety disorders.

What are fear and anxiety?

Lang, Davis, and Öhman (2000) characterize fear as a reaction to a specific threat, with increasing proximity resulting in escape or avoidance; anxiety, however, is characterized by a more diffuse state with less explicit, more generalized cues and involves increased physiological arousal but without necessarily leading to organized functional behavior. Throughout this chapter, we talk primarily about models of "fear" because it is convenient to describe the mechanisms of acquisition as operating at an individual stimulus level. The difference between whether a child acquires "fear" or "anxiety" lies in the extent to which

Anxiety Disorders in Children and Adolescents, 2nd edn, ed. W. K. Silverman and A. P. Field. Published by Cambridge University Press. © Cambridge University Press 2011.

they have learning experiences about a specific group of related stimuli (fear) or a diffuse array of situations (anxiety). However, the underlying mechanisms are similar. There is also a distinction to be made between the intensity of "normal" fear and anxiety responses and those that characterize anxiety disorders.

According to Lang (1968) an emotion consists of three response systems: (1) subjective states and cognitions associated with those states (verbal–cognitive responses); (2) behavioral changes; and (3) physiological states. This tripartite model is well accepted as a theoretical model but is also the scaffolding for a recent formulation of treatment for child anxiety (Davis & Ollendick, 2005). As such, models of how fears develop during childhood have to explain how each of these three response systems might be changed during the course of development.

Pathways to fear

More than 30 years ago, Rachman (1977, 1991) proposed a theoretical model for the acquisition of fears and phobias that consisted of three main routes. The first pathway is direct, classical conditioning. The conditioning model is the foundation of many contemporary theories of fear acquisition and has been validated as a pathway for fear in numerous laboratory and real-world situations (see Davey, 1997; Field, 2006a; Mineka & Zinbarg, 2006; Öhman & Mineka, 2001). The second pathway is modeling or vicarious learning, whereby fear is acquired by observing another person's fearful reaction to a stimulus or situation. The third pathway is fear acquired through the transmission of verbal threat information, in which fear is acquired on the basis of negative information regarding a stimulus or situation. Rachman (1977) maintained that this pathway is particularly relevant for understanding the origins of childhood fears and phobias: "Information-giving is an inherent part of child-rearing and is carried on by parents and peers in an almost unceasing fashion, particularly in the child's earliest years" (p. 384).

In a review of seven studies that looked at self-reported attributions of fear (King, Gullone, & Ollendick, 1998), 94% of children or parents endorsed one or more of Rachman's (1977) three pathways to fear. We will overview the empirical support that changes to cognitive, behavioral, and physiological (Lang's three emotional response systems) components of the fear emotion can occur via each of Rachman's (1977) three pathways.

The verbal information pathway to fear

> *Beware the Jabberwock, my son! The jaws that bite, the claws that catch!*
> *Beware the Jubjub bird, and shun the frumious Bandersnatch!*
>
> (Carroll, 1872)

Threat information forms an intrinsic part of culture, folklore, and society (Ragan, 2006). Whether gathered around fires, huddled in houses, or at the bedside, people have recounted folk tales both as allegories of real danger and as ways to turn fear into hope or action (Ragan, 2006; Zipes, 1979). Though fairy tales often provide brutal, frightening, and at times unrealistic portrayals of the world (Sale, 1978), arguably these tales have served an adaptive function in teaching children to cope with fear. Threat information permeates not just bedtime stories, but everyday conversations and the media (see Comer & Kendall, 2007, for a review).

Children experience a great deal of culturally transmitted information about which objects might be scary and this information not only guides their normative fears but provides a basis for future phobias. Nursery rhymes often transmit information about things to be feared: Little Miss Muffett was an exemplary spider phobic, and Little Red Riding Hood was afraid of the "big bad wolf" (fear of dogs). Children's literature contains many examples of scary stimuli and situations; the *Goosebumps* book series for instance (popular in many countries such as the USA and UK) readily endorse ghosts and all things dead as being scary. Children's television programs provide further information about what to fear; from evil robots, monsters, and aliens in *Transformers*, *Gremlins*, and *Ben10*, through the varied criminals in cartoons such as *Batman* and the *Powerpuff Girls*, to combative enemies in anime such as *Naruto* and *Dragonball Z.*

There is a great deal of retrospective evidence from anxious adults that they attribute their anxieties to verbal threat information in childhood (see King *et al.*, 1998; Muris & Field, 2010, for reviews). However, data from these studies are potentially prone to memory bias and because of their correlational nature cannot be used to determine the causal status of verbal threat information as a pathway to fear (Field, Argyris, & Knowles, 2001). Field and colleagues have used experimental methods to look at the causal impact of threat information about novel animals on children's fear responses. In the first study, 7–9-year-old school children were given either positive or threat verbal information about previously unencountered toy monsters (Field *et al.*, 2001). The children's self-reported fear beliefs for the monster about which they had received negative information significantly increased. In many subsequent studies, Field and colleagues adapted his paradigm to include more "factual" type information about real, but novel, animals (three Australian marsupials: the quoll, quokka, and cuscus). The cognitive component of fear has been measured both directly through self-report and indirectly using an implicit association task (IAT). In schoolchildren typically aged between 6 and 10 years, verbal threat information (compared to positive and no information) about a novel animal has been shown consistently to increase the cognitive component of fear (Field, 2006a, 2006c; Field & Lawson, 2003, 2008; Field & Price-Evans, 2009; Field & Schorah, 2007; Field & Storksen-Coulson, 2007; Field *et al.*, 2001; Field, Ball, Kawycz, & Moore, 2007; Field, Lawson, & Banerjee, 2008; Muris, Bodden, Merckelbach, Ollendick, & King, 2003; Price-Evans & Field, 2008). Verbal threat information also creates an attentional bias for the animal (Field, 2006c). The behavioral component of fear has typically been measured using two tasks: (1) the time taken for children to place their hands in pet boxes that they believe contains an animal, the "touch box task" (Field & Lawson, 2003); or (2) the "nature reserve task" (Field & Storksen-Coulson, 2007) in which children place a Lego figure representing themselves onto a board dressed to look like a nature reserve with model animals living in certain areas – the toy's distance from these models is taken as a proxy of the child's avoidance. Using these tasks on 6–10-year-old schoolchildren, verbal threat information consistently promotes avoidance of the novel animals (Field, 2006a; Field & Lawson, 2003; Field *et al.*, 2008; Kelly, Barker, Field, Wilson, & Reynolds, 2010). Finally, the physiological component of fear can be measured by recording heart rates during the touch box task, and these too are causally influenced by verbal threat information about an animal before the child approaches (Field & Price-Evans, 2009; Field & Schorah, 2007). Similar results have been found for subjective fear beliefs about novel social situations (Field, Hamilton, Knowles, & Plews, 2003; Lawson, Banerjee, & Field, 2007), but there are no data yet to show whether verbal information about social situations creates behavioral avoidance and changes in physiology.

The changes in children's fear beliefs have been shown to last beyond the initial experimental situation; the effects are maintained at 1 week (Muris *et al.*, 2003) and up to 6 months (Field *et al.*, 2008). Temperament and context seem to moderate the effects of verbal threat information. The effects of verbal threat information on avoidance, attentional bias, and heart rate increase as a function of trait anxiety (Field, 2006a; Field & Price-Evans, 2009). With respect to context, in 6–9-year-old schoolchildren a punitive maternal parenting style and a greater number of negative interactions with fathers (but not mothers) increased the impact of verbal threat information on fear beliefs about novel animals (Field *et al.*, 2007). Also, Price-Evans and Field (2008) found that a neglectful maternal parenting style interacts with the verbal information pathway to affect the child's physiological response to verbal threat information. Although these results are inconsistent in that different parenting styles emerged as interacting with verbal threat information, these studies show that the child's everyday environment is a context within which they process verbal threat information. If that context is negative then threat information is likely to have a greater impact.

This brief review (see Muris & Field, 2010, for a more extensive one) shows that verbal threat information, in isolation, is powerful enough to change all three response systems of the fear emotion. However, it is worth noting that the fears induced in these studies were not at clinical levels (and nor would the experimenters want them to be for ethical reasons). Therefore, although these studies are important in demonstrating the causal impact of this pathway, work needs to be done to explain how these induced fears might magnify to clinical levels.

Learning through others' reactions

> *Don't show your fear, keep it out of site,*
> *Don't lose your place in here and you might be all right.*
> (Motörhead, 2002, track 1)

It is now more than 40 years since Rachman (1968) and Bandura (1969) suggested that individuals can acquire fear vicariously by witnessing another individual's fear. From an evolutionary perspective such a learning mechanism is advantageous, because it means avoidance of a potentially dangerous stimulus can be learnt without having a direct, life-threatening encounter with it. Despite widespread acceptance of vicarious (or observational) learning as a theory, until recently there was little experimental evidence in human children to support the proposition that childhood fears and phobias can be acquired in this way (see Askew & Field, 2008, for a review of vicarious learning as a pathway to fear).

Some of the most persuasive evidence for vicarious learning as a pathway to fear comes from a series of observational learning studies conducted with rhesus monkeys (*Macaca mulatta*) by Mineka, Cook, and colleagues (e.g., Cook & Mineka, 1989, 1990; Mineka & Cook, 1986, 1993; Mineka, Davidson, Cook, & Keir, 1984). In contrast to wild-reared monkeys, laboratory-reared rhesus monkeys seemingly have little fear of snakes. This observation implies that fear of snakes is not innate in rhesus monkeys (Joslin, Emlen, & Fletcher, 1964; Mineka *et al.*, 1984; Mineka, Keir, & Price, 1980), and therefore wild monkeys might acquire fear by observing other monkeys display fear in the presence of snakes (Joslin *et al.*, 1964; Mineka *et al.*, 1984).

In the initial study (Mineka *et al.*, 1984), laboratory-reared, non-snake-fearful monkeys (observers) observed their wild-reared, snake-fearful parents (models) interact with a variety of real, toy, and model snakes. Five of the six monkeys acquired a fear of snakes and demonstrated fear and avoidance behavior with snakes and snake-like stimuli following the observation session. The fear was still present after 3 months and was not context specific. These findings were replicated using unrelated monkeys and demonstrated fear responses in two of Lang's (1968) three fear-response systems: behavioral avoidance and signs of distress (Cook, Mineka, Wolkenstein, & Laitsch, 1985). Moreover, Cook *et al.* (1985) showed that the observer monkeys could act as models in a subsequent session, although fear acquired by the subsequent observers was not as robust as was acquired by the observers in the original learning session.

Cook and Mineka (1987) investigated several additional characteristics of observational learning with monkeys that had already acquired fear in previous observational learning experiments. A striped box that was presented together with a snake also came to evoke a fear response in observers via its association with snakes, demonstrating second-order conditioning (Rescorla, 1980), a well-established feature of conditioning. Thus a fear response associated with one stimulus via observational learning can be elicited by a second stimulus if this stimulus is presented contiguously with the first, even though the second stimulus is never experienced together with an aversive event.

The studies from Mineka, Cook, and colleagues have made a strong case for vicarious/ observational learning as a mechanism for the acquisition of fear. However, the environment of laboratory-reared monkeys can be strictly controlled, whereas humans gain exposure to numerous stimuli during development. Mineka and Cook (1986) proposed that whilst their monkeys had little prior exposure to the experimental stimuli (snakes), human children may have had previous exposure to potentially fear-evoking stimuli before observing a fearful parent interacting with that stimulus. Prior experience of a stimulus can inhibit conditioning during a subsequent learning event, a process called latent inhibition (Lubow, 1989; Siddle, Remington, & Churchill, 1985). In a study in which monkeys were exposed to models interacted positively with snakes prior to the observational learning procedure, six out of eight observer monkeys showed little to no acquisition of snake fear (Mineka & Cook, 1986). This finding suggests that either non-fearful vicarious experience of a stimulus may inhibit future fear learning or infants and younger children are particularly susceptible to vicarious learning because of their relatively limited prior experience of stimuli.

Until relatively recently, there was little human research on vicarious learning as a pathway to fear. A few early studies demonstrated that adults could learn emotional responses by observing models in aversive conditioning procedures, even though they did not directly experience the aversive stimulus themselves (e.g., Bandura & Rosenthal, 1966; Berger, 1962; Brown, 1974; Vaughan & Lanzetta, 1980). In Berger's (1962) study, participants observed a model move their arm in response to (apparent) electric shocks that followed a buzzer sound. Participants showed increased skin conductance responding during observation, and to the buzzer when it was presented alone, suggesting that conditioning had occurred; participants had associated the buzzer with the negative response to the electric shocks supposedly delivered to the models (see also Bandura & Rosenthal, 1966; Olsson & Phelps, 2004).

In a further experiment Berger (1962) used three additional control conditions: the model received a shock but did not move their arm; the model did not receive a shock but moved their arm; and the model did not receive a shock or move their arm. Observer responses were significantly greater in the condition where the model moved their arm in response to the shock. Berger believed that vicarious conditioning relied on the observer responding emotionally to the model's response and not solely to what they saw and their interpretation of the model's emotional state (see also Kravetz, 1974). Berger's methodology used deceit to imply that a model was physically hurt, which implies some limitations for vicarious learning outside of the laboratory: though vicarious fear learning in the real world may occasionally involve physical harm (e.g., someone burns their hand on a stove), often the model might respond fearfully to a stimulus without actually being harmed (e.g., a parent might show caution around a hot stove without actually burning themselves). Mineka and Cook's studies demonstrated vicarious learning without overt harm to which the model is responding, and this has been shown in humans too – as we shall see – therefore, it is likely that fear can be acquired both with or without overt consequences for the model.

The only evidence for vicarious learning in infants was, until recently, provided by studies of social referencing. Such studies present infants with an ambiguous situation and examine how a caregiver's emotional signaling influences the infant's behavior. Sorce, Emde, Campos, and Klinnert (1985) used the "visual cliff" (Gibson & Walk, 1960) in which infants crawl towards their parent across a sheet of glass that, on one side, spans an abrupt drop. In Sorce *et al.*'s (1985) adaptation of the task, the mothers of infants (aged 12 months) stood at the far end of the apparent drop and were instructed to show facial expressions of fear, happiness, interest, or anger, without using sounds or gestures. None of the infants who observed their mother display a fearful face crossed the cliff, whereas 14 of the 19 crossed the cliff when observing their mother display a happy face. This research suggested that an infant's avoidance behavior in an ambiguous situation could be influenced by the mother's facial expression. Similarly, infants have been shown to play less with toys toward which their mothers displayed negative facial expressions (Hornik, Risenhoover, & Gunnar, 1987), and avoid objects towards which they had seen actors on television display negative emotional responses (Mumme & Fernald, 2003). These effects are stronger when accompanied by vocal signals (Mumme, Fernald, & Herrera, 1996).

Gerull and Rapee (2002) used social referencing to investigate the observational learning of fear in toddlers (aged 15–20 months). Toddlers were shown a toy snake or spider while their mothers talked to them about the stimulus and displayed either a negative (fearful/disgusted) face, or a positive (happy/encouraging) face. The children's behavior was rated for affective response and approach/avoidance behavior during modeling and on two subsequent sessions in which they were exposed to the stimuli while their mother presented a neutral face. Increased fear expression and stimulus avoidance was observed in children who observed their mothers expressing a negative face toward the stimulus, and this behavior remained 10 minutes later. This finding was replicated with fear-irrelevant stimuli in addition to fear-relevant stimuli; however, fear and avoidance did not persist after 10 minutes for either stimulus type (Dubi, Rapee, Emerton, & Schniering, 2008). In addition, Egliston and Rapee (2007) replicated the aforementioned finding from rhesus monkeys that positive modeling could prevent fear acquisition in subsequent observational learning trials. These basic findings translate to social anxiety too: infants (aged 12–14 months) were more fearful with strangers after observing their mothers acting in a socially anxious manner with a stranger relative to interacting normally (de Rosnay, Cooper,

Tsigaras, & Murray, 2006; Murray, Cooper, Creswell, Schofield, & Sack, 2007; Murray *et al.*, 2008)

Askew and Field (2007) conducted an experimental study with schoolchildren (aged 7–9 years) in which images of three novel Australian marsupials (the quoll, quokka, and cuscus) were presented on a computer screen alongside images of faces portraying fear or happiness (or no face as a control). Children's fear beliefs, as indicated on questionnaires and an affective priming task, increased significantly for animals paired with scared faces compared to animals paired with no faces. This effect remained at a 1-week and 3-months (affective priming only) follow-up. In addition, response times from the touch box task described earlier indicated that children were slower to approach an animal they had previously seen paired with scared faces. This procedure confirms that children can acquire fear beliefs and avoidance behavior (two of Lang's response systems) in a controlled vicarious learning episode in the laboratory. Causal inferences could be made about the role of vicarious learning in creating fears because of the use of trials in which no facial expression was used. Moreover, because Askew and Field used three versions of each of the three animals paired randomly with 10 versions of each type of face (scared, happy), the results suggested associations had been formed between the conceptual representation of each animal and the emotional representation evoked by the faces, rather than associations between specific images.

To sum up, there is considerable evidence from adults, monkeys, children, and infants that subjective and behavioral components of fear can be acquired vicariously; adult studies also demonstrate the acquisition of physiological changes. As such, there is support for vicarious learning as a causal mechanism in the creation of all components of fear responses (see Askew & Field, 2008, for a more thorough review).

Direct traumatic experiences

> *And one day as the boy lay sleeping in the sunshine*
> *Of a half remembered afternoon*
> *A cloud of bees with no particular aim, and no brain*
> *Found the boy, decided that his time had come*
> *Came down out of the sky, Stung him in the face, Again and again*
> (Marillion, 1997, track 8)

A century ago, John Watson conceived that anxiety disorders could be understood in terms of conditioned emotional responses (Watson, 1916) and his empirical demonstration of this theory has gone down in psychological folklore as the "Little Albert" study (Watson & Rayner, 1920). In this study, Watson and Rayner pre-tested a 9-month-old child, Albert B, to ensure that he was not initially fearful of several stimuli including a rat (which acted as a conditioned stimulus, CS), but that he was fearful of a loud noise made by banging a claw hammer on an iron bar (which acted as an aversive unconditioned stimulus, US). In subsequent testing sessions, whenever Albert touched the rat, Watson hit the iron bar, thus scaring the infant. After several pairings of the rat with the loud noise, Albert began to cry or show signs of distress when the rat was presented without the loud noise. Although Watson himself did not formulate a coherent theory of phobia acquisition, the implication from the study was that excessive and persistent fear (i.e., a phobia) could be acquired through direct experience with a CS in temporal proximity to some fear-inducing or traumatic event. Although the Little Albert study is very much of its era and, by today's standards, has many well-documented limitations and methodological inadequacies, its influence on theories and treatments of anxiety resonates to this day (Field & Nightingale, 2009).

There are some studies that confirm that directly fear-inducing or traumatic experiences during childhood can lead to extreme and persistent fear. Dollinger, O'Donnell, and Staley (1984) studied 29 children (aged 10 to 13), survivors of a severe lightning-strike and found that these children showed more numerous and intense fear of thunderstorms, lightning, and tornadoes than control children. In a similar study, Yule, Udwin, and Murdoch (1990) studied 25 teenage girls (aged 14 to 16) who survived the sinking of the cruise ship *Jupiter.* Compared to control participants of the same age, these girls showed an excess of fears relating to ships, water travel, swimming, and water, and this fear even generalized to other modes of transport. Both of these studies support the idea that a single traumatic event can lead to intense fears of objects related to the trauma and change in Lang's cognitive and behavioral response systems.

There is evidence that traumatic experiences can affect the physiological response system too. One of the criteria for diagnosis of post-traumatic stress disorder (PTSD) is being physically responsive, such as experiencing a surge in your heart rate or sweating, when reminded of the traumatic event (American Psychiatric Association, 1994). There is consistent evidence that PTSD emerges from direct traumatic experience: a meta-analysis that pooled data from 2697 children and adolescents who experienced traumatic events (across 34 studies) found that 36% were diagnosed with PTSD (Fletcher, 1996). However, although this shows that exposure to a traumatic event may be necessary to develop PTSD, it might not be sufficient: rates of PTSD following trauma vary from 0% to 100% across studies (Dalgleish, Meiser-Stedman, & Smith, 2005).

As well as these field studies, there is ample evidence from the laboratory that fears can be acquired through direct experience with trauma. There are around 747 published papers with "Fear Conditioning" in their title in the period 1959–2010;[1] direct conditioning as a mechanism for fear acquisition has been well and truly established. These include some recent studies showing that non-anxious and anxious children (aged 7 to 12 years) can acquire physiological and subjective fear responses to previously neutral stimuli through contiguous presentations with aversive noises and shocks (Craske *et al.*, 2008), and that this acquired physiological response is harder to extinguish in anxious (8–12-year-old) children (Waters, Henry, & Neumann, 2009).

Moreover, there is good evidence that fear learning can be acquired on the basis of one intensely aversive experience. In a study that paired a neutral tone with an injection of scoline, a curare derivate that induces transient respiratory paralysis, a conditioned fear response was established to the tone in only one trial. This fear response did not extinguish and actually became stronger across 100 extinction trials (Campbell, Sanderson, & Laverty, 1964). Similar results have been obtained using illness and shock as an aversive consequence (Garcia, McGowan, & Green, 1972; Izquierdo, Barros, Ardenghi, *et al.*, 2000; Izquierdo, Barros, Medina, & Izquierdo, 2000), and one-trial learning to both fear-relevant (snakes) and fear-irrelevant (houses) stimuli was observed when these were paired with an intense shock (Öhman, Eriksson, & Olofsson, 1975).

---

[1] Source: PubMed (www.ncbi.nlm.nih.gov/pubmed).

Fear conditioning and the neural systems involved in fear responses have been thoroughly mapped in animal subjects. There is now a substantial body of work that translates this work to humans (e.g., Delgado, Olsson, & Phelps, 2006). This work has established that the amygdala is central to the automatic processing of emotional, and particularly fear- or threat-related information (LeDoux, 2003; Morris, Öhman, & Dolan, 1998; Phelps, 2006; Phelps & LeDoux, 2005). Other work has demonstrated that a stimulus that signals an aversive event, such as a shock, will, regardless of its valence, induce a physiological profile consistent with defensive activation (Bradley, Moulder, & Lang, 2005). In addition, fear conditioning changes the valence of a CS from positive to negative measured both explicitly and implicitly (Purkis & Lipp, 2009).

To sum up, as with the other pathways to fear, there is considerable evidence from adults and children in both laboratory and field studies that subjective, behavioral, and physiological components of fear can be acquired through direct traumatic experiences.

Combined pathways to fear

The three pathways that Rachman (1977) identified do not operate in isolation: real-life experiences can rarely be neatly decomposed into verbal, vicarious, and direct experiences. One illustration of interconnectedness between Rachman's pathways is televised and film media, which may combine verbal information, visual representations of people's reactions to events, and images or events that are in themselves directly fear-evoking.

There is evidence that televised media can change cognitive and behavioral components of fear, but there is as yet little direct evidence of changes to physiology (Muris & Field, 2010). For example, 90% of adult undergraduates remembered being frightened by a television program or movie that they watched as a child, and that these fears bothered them for years afterward (Harrison & Cantor, 1999). A significant number (26.1%) still experienced residual fear in relation to the event, and some still avoided the stimulus or situation depicted in the program (see also Hoekstra, Harris, & Helmick, 1999). Studies based on reports from both adults (e.g., Cantor & Nathanson, 1996) and children (Valkenburg, Cantor, & Peeters, 2000; van der Molen & Bushman, 2008) show that around one-third of children experience fear reactions in response to threat information displayed on television or in films (for a review see Cantor, 1998).

It is not only fictional media that has an impact; numerous studies have looked at the effect of real world news stories presented in the media. Terr and colleagues (Terr, Bloch, Michel, Shi, Reinhardt, & Metayer, 1999) examined children's fears and post-traumatic stress symptoms following the *Challenger* space shuttle explosion in January 1986. More than 60% of the young participants in the study feared at least one stimulus related to the *Challenger* within the first 2 months after the explosion. Children who had followed the news about the event via television were more symptomatic than children with less media exposure. Comparable findings have been obtained from children after watching news about the Iraq War (Smith & Moyer-Gusé, 2006), and the September 11 (9/11) terrorist attacks (Holmes, Creswell, & O'Connor, 2007; Hoven *et al.*, 2005; Otto, Henin, Hirshfeld-Becker, Pollack, Biederman, & Rosenbaum, 2007). These effects are not proximal – children as far away as London showed PTSD symptoms after watching coverage of the 9/11 attacks (Holmes *et al.*, 2007) – and younger children (under 10) are often more affected than older children (Otto *et al.*, 2007). There is also evidence that in 7–12-year-old schoolchildren perceived available social support and use of coping strategies predicts the changes in state anxiety created by watching disaster-related television clips (Ortiz, Silverman, Jaccard, & La Greca, 2010).

Only two studies have attempted to look at the interactions between Rachman's pathways experimentally through systematically manipulating children's exposure to different pathways. Field and Storksen-Coulson (2007) asked 6–8-year-old schoolchildren to place their hands into two pet boxes each of which that they believed contained a novel animal (Australian marsupials). Prior to this task, children were given threatening information about one of the animals. During the box task, one of the boxes moved suddenly as the child placed their hand inside, startling the child. The animal in the scary box and the animal about which information was given were crossed over so Field and Storksen-Coulson could dissociate the effects of verbal information alone, the scary experience alone, and also their combined effect. Data showed that the threatening information (without a subsequent negative experience) and the direct negative experience (without prior information) had comparable fear-enhancing effects. However, the combination of the two pathways (verbal threat information followed by a direct negative experience) yielded a magnified effect. The extent to which the verbal information changed the child's fear beliefs (expectancies) fully mediated the effect that the direct negative experience had on that child. This mediation effect is particularly interesting because it fully supports conditioning models of the etiology of anxiety, which predict that cognitive expectancies about what will happen when a stimulus is encountered should affect the strength of association formed during a subsequent negative conditioning experience (Davey, 1997).

A second study looked at the effect of verbal information on the vicarious learning pathway rather than direct conditioning (Askew, Kessock-Philip, & Field, 2008). Across three experiments, verbal threat information was given to 7–9-year-old schoolchildren before, during, or after vicarious learning experiences similar to those in Askew and Field (2007 – described above). Consistent with Field and Storksen-Coulson's (2007) results, prior verbal threat information significantly facilitated the effects of negative vicarious learning experiences on children's fear beliefs; however, verbal information after vicarious learning did not enhance fear learning, which is inconsistent with conditioning models, which predict that verbal information should enhance an already acquired conditioned response (Davey, 1997).

Theoretical models of the development of fears and anxiety

The basic conditioning model of fear

We have already briefly described Watson's idea that emotional responses could be conditioned. In subsequent years, with the increased interest in and understanding of Pavlovian conditioning (Pavlov, 1927), conditioning models of the etiology and treatment of fear responses evolved (e.g., Eysenck, 1979; Mowrer, 1960; Wolpe, 1961).

The main premise of Pavlovian conditioning is that the pairing of a neutral conditional stimulus, CS, with a reaction-evoking unconditional stimulus, US, will lead the conditional stimulus to evoke a conditioned response, CR (e.g., fear when the US is fear-evoking). For example, presentation of an electric shock, US, elicits a fear response whenever it is presented. If a neutral tone, CS, that does not normally evoke a response, is presented together with the electric shock, then presentation of the tone, CS, alone will come to elicit a fear response.

The fear response elicited by the CS may differ in its characteristics from the fear response elicited by the US, but nonetheless, it represents a response that has been conditioned via pairing of CS and US. For example, rats respond with behaviors such as increased heart rate, squeaking, and jumping to an aversive shock but show anticipatory responses (opposite to the behaviors elicited by the US) such as a decrease in heart rate and "freezing" to a CS that has been previously paired with a shock (Black, 1971). The nature of the CS also determines the CR: a tone that predicts a shock is likely to elicit freezing behavior, whereas a localized prod that predicts a shock is likely to elicit behaviors that try to bury the prod (Pinel & Treit, 1979). Thus CRs to the same US can differ depending on the nature of the CS. Moreover, although most fear-conditioning paradigms use repeated pairings of CS and US to achieve conditioning, the CS–US pairing itself is not sufficient for conditioning: the information about the occurrence of the US that the CS provides is what matters (Rescorla, 1988).

What is learned during conditioning?

Conditioning is often referred to as associative learning,[1] reflecting that CS–US associations mediate conditioning. This definition is acknowledged in both the learning (e.g., Davey, 1989a; Mackintosh, 1983) and anxiety literatures (e.g., Davey, 1989b, 1997; Field, 2006b; Field & Davey, 2001; Mineka & Zinbarg, 2006). Associative learning reflects a mental linking of the relevant events and stimuli encountered during a learning episode (Hall, 2002; Pearce & Bouton, 2001). There are two main competing theories about the specific associations formed during associative learning: (1) stimulus–response (S–R), an association is formed between the CS and the UR (i.e., between a previously neutral stimulus and a reaction to an aversive stimulus); or (2) stimulus–stimulus (S–S), an association is formed between the CS and the US (i.e., between the previously neutral stimulus and the aversive stimulus itself). The latter explanation is endorsed with two converging streams of evidence.

First, in studies where the response to the aversive stimulus is prevented, conditioning still occurs. For instance when the drug curare, which blocks all skeletal responses, is used during associative learning, conditioned skeletal responses to the CS are present once the drug has worn off (Solomon & Turner, 1962). Second, revaluing the US affects the conditioned response. In studies in which a response is conditioned using a weak aversive US but then a more intense version of this US is presented in the absence of the CS, subsequent presentations of the CS elicit stronger CRs than were previously observed (Rescorla, 1974).

The processes involved in associative learning are far more complex than a simple CS–US association model suggests. Learning is not simply the association of two stimuli but is influenced by past learning and contextual variables. During a learning episode, associations are formed between representations of multiple events (including relationships generated by other associations). Conditioning, far from being a simple association between two events, is a complex process that provides a highly detailed representation of the environment. We will now outline a few of these complexities, but there are more extensive reviews elsewhere (Field, 2006b; Field & Purkis, 2011; Mineka & Zinbarg, 2006; Rescorla, 1988).

---

[1] The observant among you will have noticed that we have already used the terms interchangeably in this chapter.

The complexity of conditioning

Early formulations of conditioning assumed that CRs were overt responses, which in the case of anxiety would mean that a person shows overt signs of distress when faced with a traumatic event. However, we will now discuss several phenomena that demonstrate conditioning in the absence of any overt behavioral signs that learning has occurred. These phenomena illustrate both that (1) learning situations are more complex than a simple association being formed between a discrete stimulus and a traumatic outcome; and (2) humans and animals do not enter conditioning episodes as *tabulae rasae*, but bring with them prior experiences with a variety of stimuli and situations, and have numerous, pre-existing associations between stimuli and consequences.

Learning history and cue competition

Cue competition reflects that when several different cues are predictive of the same US, the learning histories of the various cues will determine which cues generate the strongest conditioned responses. In the case of anxiety disorders this means that in the face of trauma, the stimulus that enters into an association with trauma will depend upon what's happened in the past. *Blocking* (Kamin, 1968) is a good illustration. A standard blocking experiment consists of two phases of learning. First, a stimulus, such as a light, predicts a consequence, such as a shock. Second, a compound stimulus that includes the first stimulus, such as a light and a tone, predicts the same consequence, the shock. Compared to a group that experiences only the second phase, the compound stimulus followed by the shock, the blocking group will have reduced conditioning to the tone. For this group, the light already predicts the shock; as such the tone does not add new information about the occurrence of the shock and learning to the tone is "blocked" in this group. The group that experiences only the second, compound learning phase, will have equal learning to both the light and tone, because each provide some information about the occurrence of the shock. In this scenario, learning will be different to tone and light only if one of these stimuli is significantly more salient than the other. In that case, more learning is observed with the more salient cue (*overshadowing*).

Stimuli can also enter into inhibitory relationships in which they predict the *absence* of an event (e.g., trauma). Imagine a three-phase experiment. In the first phase, a stimulus such as a light is presented with a consequence, such as a shock. In the second phase, a compound stimulus (the light accompanied by a tone) is presented in the absence of the shock. In this case the animal learns that, given that the light predicts the shock, the tone must predict the absence of the shock (an inhibitory relationship). In the third phase, the tone is presented in compound with another stimulus, such as a buzzer, and this new tone and buzzer compound is presented with the shock. The new stimulus, the buzzer, will acquire a magnified CR compared to a group that experiences only buzzer–shock pairings. This magnified CR occurs because, if the tone predicts the absence of the shock, but the buzzer and the tone together predict the shock, then the buzzer must be a strong predictor of the shock. This phenomenon is called *super-learning* or *super-conditioning* (Aitken, Larkin, & Dickinson, 2000; Rescorla, 1971). Other forms of cue competition can be achieved through altering the extent to which different cues are predictive of consequences.

The presentation of a stimulus in the absence of consequences will make it more difficult to learn to associate that stimulus with a consequence. This phenomenon is called *latent inhibition*, and results from CS pre-exposure: presentations of the CS in absence of the

US prior to conditioning. It has been well established that conditioning takes significantly longer after CS pre-exposure than when there is no pre-exposure of the CS (Lubow, 1973; Lubow & Moore, 1959). Thus it may be more difficult to condition a particular response to a familiar stimulus than to a novel stimulus. Studies with fear of dogs and fear of dentists (Doogan & Thomas, 1992) suggest that the acquisition of fear is less likely after a history of non-traumatic experiences (see also Bond & Siddle, 1996, for an important experimental study involving pictures of facial expressions).

The uncorrelated presentation of cues and consequences will also make it more difficult to learn to associate the cue and consequence that have been experienced. This phenomenon is called *learned irrelevance* (or learned helplessness in operant terms), and results from the pre-exposure of uncorrelated presentations of CSs and USs prior to conditioning. This kind of pre-exposure retards the subsequent conditioning of correlated CS–US presentations (Mackintosh, 1973). Latent inhibition and learned irrelevance are similar, but in latent inhibition the animal learns that a particular CS is not predictive of consequences, whereas in learned irrelevance, it learns that a particular CS is not predictive of a particular consequence.

Both latent inhibition and learned irrelevance demonstrate that predictive power of a CS is crucial (in both cases the overall correlation between the CS and US is reduced). Moreover, it is possible to learn about the absence of relationships and respond accordingly (Mackintosh, 1973, for example, believed that during pre-exposure to uncorrelated CS–US presentations, what is learned is that the CS is irrelevant). Thus conditioning is affected by prior experience and pre-existing relationships between CSs and USs.

The effect of context on conditioning

Some of the aforementioned phenomena (e.g., blocking) allude to the fact that conditioning is context dependent. In some circumstances, conditioned responding can become contingent on the presence or absence of a predictive cue, in addition to the CS. Rescorla (1991) demonstrated that if a CS was reinforced only when accompanied by another stimulus (called a "feature") the CR would occur only if that feature was present. A similar pattern is observed if the CS is reinforced only in absence of another stimulus (feature), and in this case the feature will inhibit a CR. *Feature modulation* (also known as *occasion setting*) differs from cue competition, in that the feature can precede the presentation of the CS and the stimuli do not need to overlap.

Conditioned responding also depends on the extent to which a given CS resembles the most salient aspects of the CS that was involved in conditioning. A good example is overshadowing (see above), which can be understood by thinking about eating a meal that subsequently makes you ill. It is usual to attribute the illness to the most distinctive, salient, or novel flavor that was present in the meal, because this overshadows the other flavors (in combination with latent inhibition for flavors that have been eaten previously without incident). There is a tendency to assume that conditioning takes place between one stimulus (viewed as a whole) and another stimulus (also viewed as a whole). This is not the case: a given stimulus is a combination of many features (in the way that a meal is made up of many distinct flavors).

This brief overview illustrates the complexity of conditioning: it reflects the association of multiple stimulus features with multiple other stimulus features, and takes into account contextual cues and learning history. A fear response can be elicited by specific features of a stimulus and the elicitation of such a response may, therefore, reflect the extent to which those features are present in a particular example of the feared stimulus. For example, in PTSD flashbacks are often triggered by very specific smells, sounds, or images (Brewin & Holmes, 2003); a victim of a nocturnal road traffic accident, for example, might have flashbacks triggered by a bright light that reminds them of a car headlight but these flashbacks will not be triggered by cars in general. The phenomena described in this section also go a long way towards explaining why not all people develop a persistent fear in response to a traumatic event: prior learning and contextual cues might mitigate against an association being formed (or strengthened) between a cue and the trauma (Field, 2006b).

Conditioning does not depend upon contiguity

Though conditioning will often be described as occurring on the basis of contiguous CS–US pairings, contiguity is neither necessary nor sufficient for associative learning to occur (Rescorla, 1968). Conditioning relies on the base rate of the US and therefore the predictive power of the CS, which is not the same thing as contiguity. If conditioning depended on contiguity, then phenomena that rely on conditioned inhibition could not occur. In situations in which the US is presented alone, nothing would be learned, but as we have demonstrated above, this is not the case. The truth is that even in the absence of CS–US contiguity, information is being acquired concerning stimuli and their associations. This may explain why not all phobia sufferers remember a traumatic event, because the trauma might not have occurred contiguously with the stimulus that is feared.

Extinction does not break the CS–US association

An association between a CS and US can be formed very quickly, but when it comes to eliminating this association, things are not so straightforward. Though it was once thought that unreinforced presentations of the CS (*extinction*) eliminated the original CS–US association, we now know that this is not the case. In a conditioning paradigm that contains random presentations of CS and US, responses are initially evoked by the CS, however these quickly diminish as more random presentations are experienced. Nonetheless, Rescorla (2000) demonstrated that CS–US associations were formed and remained intact after such training. The association between CS and US forms rapidly during training, however when the CS and US occurrence was random, the CS quickly lost its power to evoke a CR.

In an extinction paradigm, the CS is presented alone and this exposure results in a gradual decline in the CR until the presentation of the CS no longer evokes any response. Given that CS–US associations survive random presentations, it is probably no surprise that they also survive extinction (even if the CR is extinguished). Conditioning-based models of fear are often criticized because they predict extinction of fear responses, yet this extinction does not seem to occur with people who experience phobic levels of fear (Rachman, 1977). However, this criticism arises to a large extent from the misconception that extinction is forever. Research has now demonstrated that CS–US associations not only survive subsequent random CS–US presentations, they also survive extinction procedures (Bouton, 1994).

There are several factors that affect extinction. As we have already seen, conditioning is context dependent and so too is extinction: when CRs are trained in one context, and extinguished in a different context, presentation of the CS in the original context will evoke a response. This is called *renewal*, because the response is seemingly renewed.

Time can also be viewed as a context (Bouton & Swartzentruber, 1991): weak conditioned responses will also be displayed to the CS merely after the passage of a sufficient amount of time. If time is viewed as a context then in this situation conditioning and extinction occur in different contexts. Though the CS cannot be experienced in the same temporal context after conditioning, it can be experienced in a new temporal context that differs from conditioning and extinction contexts. This is sufficient to produce the weak renewal of response known as *spontaneous recovery*.

Conditioned responses will also reappear if the US is presented again on its own. This is termed *reinstatement*, because the experience of the US reinstates responding to the CS. As with renewal, reinstatement is context dependent and the CS must be experienced in the same context as the reinstating stimulus (the US) for conditioned responses to be reinstated.

Therefore, the extent to which fear extinction is successful depends strongly on context: CS–US associations remain even after responses to the CS have seemingly extinguished, and conditioned responses can be re-elicited after context change or re-experiencing the US. These phenomena have obvious implications for treatment: extinction to reduce fear responses should be attempted in a variety of contexts to maximize generalization of extinguished responses and reduce the risks of renewal and reinstatement once the client leaves therapy.

The nature of the CS and US

Classic conceptualizations of conditioning imply that the CS and US are real events, and that the US is biologically significant. However, this simplification has led to misconceptions about the etiology of fear: for example, why some phobic individuals cannot remember experiencing a traumatic event (Davey, 1992), and why phobic fears of some stimuli are more common than others (Seligman, 1971). Conditioning depends on the very nature of the stimuli between which associations are formed.

Preparedness theory

Seligman (1971) proposed that associations, such as taste and nausea, which have an obvious survival benefit, are biologically "prepared" to be learned. He proposed that phobias represent instances of highly prepared learning. Seligman argued that phobias differed from conditioned fear reactions; they were selective, occurred often to a limited range of stimuli, were irrational, and were resistant to extinction, and that phobias might therefore be special instances of fear conditioning that occurred when fear was conditioned to stimuli that were prepared to enter into a fear association. As such, "fear-relevant" stimuli would be those that tend to be commonly associated with phobia, such as snakes, spiders, or heights.

The predictions derived from Seligman's theory have been tested extensively (see Öhman & Mineka, 2001, for a review). An early series of studies demonstrated greater resistance to extinction in electrodermal responding following conditioning with pictures of fear-relevant stimuli, snakes, compared to pictures of non-fear-relevant stimuli, houses and faces, when a fear-evoking electric shock was used as the US. Moreover this enhanced conditioning seemed restricted to fear associations, supporting the notion of selectivity (Öhman *et al.*, 1975). In addition, vicariously learnt responses appear to be very difficult to extinguish when the CSs are fear-relevant, but not when they are fear-irrelevant (Hygge & Öhman, 1978).

Further support for preparedness was provided in several experiments which used edited video to present monkeys with films of other monkeys interacting fearfully with fear-relevant stimuli (snakes and a toy crocodile) or fear-irrelevant stimuli (flowers and a toy rabbit). The choice of stimuli was based on the observation that wild-reared rhesus monkeys fear crocodiles but not rabbits. The vicarious acquisition of fear responses was demonstrated for fear-relevant but not for fear-irrelevant stimuli (Cook & Mineka, 1989, 1990) supporting preparedness theory.

Compelling as this evidence for preparedness seems, culturally fear-relevant stimuli, such as pointed guns, are also more effective CSs than control stimuli; furthermore, the effect of fear relevance on conditioning does not seem to differ between phylogenetic and ontogenetic fear-relevant stimuli (Hugdahl & Johnsen, 1989). Also, much of the evidence reviewed for vicarious and verbal information pathways to fear suggests children can readily acquire fears for fear-irrelevant stimuli (e.g., Askew & Field, 2007; Dubi *et al.*, 2008; Field & Lawson, 2003, 2008; Field & Schorah, 2007; Field *et al.*, 2001, 2008; Gerull & Rapee, 2002). Therefore, though there is some evidence that the nature of the CS plays a role in the ease with which fear can be conditioned, it may be that the so-called preparedness of the CS reflects factors in individual learning history rather than any evolved predisposition to fear certain things.

Conditioning without "real" stimuli

Conditioning is the mental linking of relevant events and stimuli during a learning episode (Hall, 2002), which means that behavior is elicited on the basis of a mental representation of an association between stimuli. Consistent with this idea, conditioning can occur with an imaginary CS and/or US. Much research has demonstrated that CRs can be acquired without the presence of the actual CS or US at the time of learning, but rather with mental representations of these stimuli. First, when a mental representation of a CS (in the absence of the actual CS) is paired with a US, the actual CS acquires a CR. Thus, fear can be conditioned to a stimulus without the presence of the actual stimulus, but merely with the thought of that stimulus. Second, if a stimulus (CS1) is paired with a US, then subsequently a mental representation of a second stimulus (CS2) is paired with CS1, the actual CS2 stimulus will acquire a CR. In both cases, a mental representation of the CS is paired with a mental representation of the US, and therefore learning has occurred in the absence of the actual CS and US (Dwyer, 1999, 2001, 2003; Dwyer, Mackintosh, & Boakes, 1998).

Moreover, a CS can act as a US for a second CS, a phenomenon called *second-order conditioning* (Rescorla, 1980). For instance, if a light is paired with a shock, and the light comes to elicit a response, then a tone presented with the light may also come to elicit a response. This response suggests that the tone has formed an association with the shock, despite never having been paired directly with it. There is some evidence in humans that devaluing the US after second-order conditioning eliminates the conditional response to the second CS (Davey & McKenna, 1983). Moreover, a US representation can be used in place of an actual US to produce a fear response. These lines of evidence support that mental representations of CS and US are sufficient for learning to occur.

The biological significance of the US

Finally, humans can also readily associate stimuli with other stimuli that do not evoke unconditional responses. Causal learning paradigms involve the learning of predictive relationships between neutral stimuli (De Houwer & Beckers, 2002; Dickinson, 2001; Shanks, Holyoak, & Medin, 1996). Typical paradigms include predicting whether pictures of butterflies will mutate when exposed to radiation (Collins & Shanks, 2002; Lober & Shanks, 2000), whether certain foods predict an allergic reaction (Aitken *et al.*, 2000; Le Pelley & McLaren, 2003; Matute, Vegas, & De Marez, 2002), and whether chemicals affect the survival of different strains of bacteria (Tangen & Allan, 2004). Though the US does not evoke an unconditional response in the traditional sense, humans readily learn these contingencies (e.g., they can make accurate predictions after several trials on which they receive feedback about whether their predictions are correct). These learnt associations also follow many of the rules of conditioning found when biologically significant USs are used (Dickinson, 2001).

The fact that CSs and USs can simply be imagined stimuli or events and need not be biologically significant opens the doors for complex associative networks that form the basis of fear learning. For example, a fear could develop not from a real trauma, but from thoughts that are distressing; equally, a feared stimulus need never have been paired with an actual trauma; it would be sufficient for the person to have thought of that stimulus when the trauma occurred. These ideas can readily explain why some clinically anxious people cannot remember a specific event when they experienced both the source of their fear and a traumatic event. However, another explanation is that a relatively innocuous association has been formed between two stimuli that is revalued through subsequent experience.

The CS–US association can be manipulated by other experiences

As we have seen, conditioning reflects an association between the mental representation of a CS and the representation of a US. These representations are somewhat open to reinterpretation, and subsequent experiences can cause them to be reevaluated. The representation of a US can be revalued, on the basis of a subsequent encounter or new information, as more or less threatening and this may affect conditioned responses to any CS with which the US is associated.

When the US is revalued as more negative, stronger conditioned responses are observed on subsequent presentations of the CS. In Rescorla (1974), rats were conditioned with a weak shock. They were then presented with a strong shock in absence of the CS. Subsequent presentations of the CS elicited stronger conditioned responses than were obtained during conditioning, because the US had been subsequently revalued as more threatening. White and Davey (1989) presented participants with a CS paired with an innocuous tone US. After the aversiveness of the tone was inflated by presenting it alone at an increased volume, participants showed increased skin conductance responses to the CS when that was later presented on its own, suggesting that the CS had become more negative. When the US is revalued as more positive, then weaker conditioned responses are observed on subsequent presentations of the CS. In a study by Davey and McKenna (1983), habituation of the US following conditioning resulted in a more favorable assessment of the US and in reduced conditioned responses on subsequent presentations of the CS. Davey, de Jong, and Tallis (1993) report three case studies of people who had USs revalued (including a girl whose parents inflated the aversiveness of an encounter with a spider by telling her all the potentially bad things that could have happened). Thus in fear conditioning, a strong fear response may be elicited by a CS that did not elicit a strong response during initial conditioning.

The CS–US association can also be affected by events prior to the association being formed. For example, a conscious expectancy that a negative outcome (US) will follow a CS will aid the learning of CS–US associations in a subsequent aversive conditioning episode (Davey, 1997; Field & Davey, 2001). Both negative vicarious learning and verbal threat information have been shown to create these expectancies in non-anxious children (e.g., Askew & Field, 2007; Field & Lawson, 2003, 2008; Field *et al.*, 2001, 2008) and expectancies created by verbal information have been shown to affect the strength of learning following a mildly traumatic event (Field & Storksen-Coulson, 2007).

Personality

Humans are a complex combination of genetic and environmental influences. The acquisition of fear and anxiety, like any psychological process, is affected by personality. It has been theorized that maladaptive or abnormal behavior, such as clinical levels of fear and anxiety, may reflect underlying predispositions that are triggered by particular life experiences or environmental stressors: e.g., the diathesis–stress model (Monroe & Simons, 1991; Zuckerman, 1999); the biological sensitivity to context model (Boyce & Ellis, 2005); and the differential susceptibility to environment model (Belsky & Pluess, 2009). Certain individuals are disproportionately likely to be adversely affected by environmental stress, and this is reflected in the component of personality referred to as temperament. The physiological correlate of temperament is reactivity (Strelau, 1983) which indexes individual differences in the intensity of response to stimulation (Boyce & Ellis, 2005). Higher reactivity is associated with less gating of internal information from external events; thus more reactive individuals are susceptible to weaker environmental signals, have comparatively low optimal levels of arousal, and are less able to endure strong stimulation for prolonged periods (Strelau, 1983). Reactivity is strongly related to certain personality traits, whereby high-reactivity individuals (introverts, sensation avoiders) tend to avoid strong stimulation and arousal, whereas low-reactivity individuals (extraverts, sensation seekers) are predisposed to seek out arousing situations and activities (Strelau & Eysenck, 1987).

Personality factors are likely to mediate fear conditioning through the speed that different associations are processed and perceptions of aversive stimuli (reactive individuals should find a given US relatively more threatening). There is some evidence that trait anxiety does influence associative learning: first, trait anxiety is positively related to the speed of acquisition of punishment expectancies (Zinbarg & Mohlman, 1998); second, verbal threat information has a greater impact on high-trait-anxious children (Field, 2006a; Field & Price-Evans, 2009). These findings suggest that trait-anxious individuals may be more susceptible to developing new fears.

Contemporary models of fear acquisition

Davey's and Mineka and Zinbarg's models

Several modern models of fear acquisition have conditioning processes at their core but also acknowledge the complexity of learning events in the real world. Davey (1997) and Mineka and Zinbarg (2006) have both developed models of fear acquisition that have a basic CS–US association at their core, but incorporate contemporary knowledge about conditioning processes. These models share many common features and Figure 11.1 represents these commonalities rather than focusing on the minor differences. Both models suggest that clinical fear and anxiety are learned through conditioning experiences, but that humans

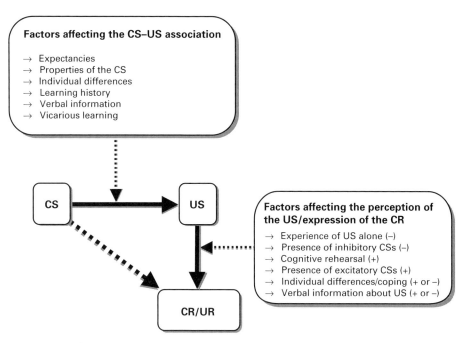

Figure 11.1 Schematic representation of the core components of Davey (1997) and Mineka and Zinbarg's (2006) conditioning models of fear acquisition (see text for details).

coming into such experiences could bring with them past knowledge and experience of both the CS and US, expectancies about what will happen, genetic and temperamental differences, and prior verbal information and vicarious learning. They also both acknowledge that following a learning episode, experiences such as positive information, experience alone with the US, the presence of inhibitory stimuli and coping abilities could devalue the US and negative information, cognitive rehearsal, the presence of excitatory stimuli, and poor coping skills may serve to inflate the aversiveness of the US (and hence the CR). As such, both models neatly tie together contemporary wisdom of conditioning theory (which we have just described in detail) around a basic CS–US association, which drives the fear response.

An elaboration on Field's model

Field (2006b) described a very similar model, which differs only in how he sees the CS and US (Figure 11.2). Like Davey and Zinbarg and Mineka, Field views the fear response as being driven by a mental connection between a CS and US, and that the formation and strength of this connection can be influenced by learning history, the context in which learning occurs, the properties of the CS, and individual sensitivity to conditioning. The expression of the CR is, likewise, affected by the context, personality, and factors that inflate or devalue the aversiveness of the US. However, Field's model has some important differences.

First, Field acknowledges recent research showing that the CS and US can themselves be representations rather than physical stimuli. He argues that this frees the model from needing any kind of direct conditioning experience (in the traditional use of that phrase).

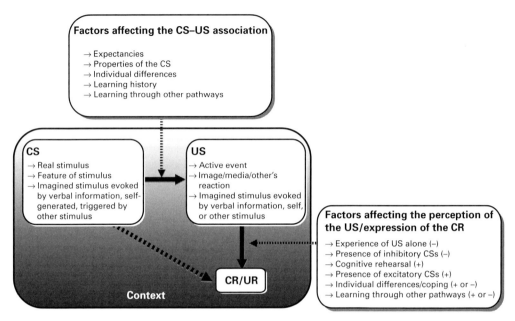

Figure 11.2 An elaborated representation of Field's (2006b) model of fear acquisition (see text for details).

Instead, he argues that experiences from all of Rachman's (1977) pathways can be conceptualized as "conditioning episodes" in which a CS becomes mentally connected with a US. For example, informational learning reflects a conditioning experience in which a stimulus (CS) such as a novel animal becomes associated with threat information (US) or a representation of threat (and its related qualia). Vicarious learning can be similarly viewed as a conditioning episode in which the response of the model is the US (Mineka & Cook, 1993) or a representation of threat that the reaction evokes in the individual experiencing it.

Davey and Mineka and Zinbarg put direct traumatic experiences at the center of conditioning models, and verbal information and vicarious learning act as either vulnerability factors (they create expectancies prior to conditioning) or modifying factors after conditioning (such as verbal information devaluing the US). In contrast, Field suggests that all three pathways can create a mental link between a stimulus and a traumatic outcome. That link can be created through any one of the three pathways, and any one of the three pathways can strengthen or weaken that link. Clinical levels of fear develop not just from a single traumatic experience, but evolve through sustained learning experiences through each of the three pathways.

Support for this idea comes from the fact that implicit associations between novel animals and threat can be formed through both verbal information and vicarious learning (Askew & Field, 2007; Field & Lawson, 2003; Field et al., 2008), and that verbal information and vicarious learning alone are sufficient to create changes in all three of Lang's response systems (Askew & Field, 2007; Field & Lawson, 2008; Field & Schorah, 2007; Mineka et al., 1984).

Field's model offers a single underlying mechanism to explain how all three pathways to fear operate. The CS–US link can be formed through any pathway, but its strength will depend on the many factors already discussed. For example, a completely novel stimulus experienced with a very traumatic active event (i.e., a trauma in which the person is directly involved) will result in a strong CS–US link; in contrast, the link formed by hearing some threatening information may be relatively weaker. The extent to which verbal information and indirect experiences (such as mass media) create or strengthen the CS–US link depends on its intrinsic threat value and its power to evoke images or representations of threat. This model is accompanied by clear predictions that CS–US links created through verbal information and vicarious learning should behave in the same way as those created by direct conditioning. Although there is some evidence that this is true for vicarious learning (Mineka & Cook, 1986), more research is needed.

Throughout our description of Field's model we have referred to a CS–US link, rather than a CS–US association. This is because of recent challenges to the long-accepted idea that conditioning is associative learning. Simple conditioning has been convincingly demonstrated in very simple organisms, such as sea slugs. Early models of conditioning assumed that human conditioning was a more evolved form of the same basic learning system. However, as we have shown, conditioning has more advanced properties (such as cue competition, and occasion setting), and its definition now includes associations between representations of CS and US rather than requiring the overlapping experience of an actual CS and US. Moreover, in humans, fear conditioning seems to rely heavily on awareness of the CS–US contingency (see Lovibond & Shanks, 2002, for a review). Such developments have led some to question the CS–US association which has, for many years, been the foundation of conditioning theory. It is argued that conditioning in humans does not utilize the same mechanism as in other animals; instead it is based on propositional reasoning, and thus CRs in humans are entirely dependent on high-level cognitive processes (De Houwer, 2009; Mitchell, De Houwer, & Lovibond, 2009a). The authors even go so far as to suggest that the removal of the primitive learning mechanism during human evolution may have been adaptive, because in a complex organism, a system that automatically makes associations between stimuli might lead to an overload of associations and result in chaotic behavior (Mitchell, De Houwer, & Lovibond, 2009b). Not everyone is in agreement with this perspective, however; the learning camp is split into endorsees of a propositional-only mechanism, and dual theorists, who believe in two systems, a low-level association-based mechanism working in conjunction with a high-level propositional system (see Shanks, 2010, for a review of the current evidence for independent explicit and implicit learning systems).

The elaboration of Field's model described here leaves the issue of whether the CS–US link is an association or a proposition unresolved. When conditioning does not involve the direct experience of a CS and aversive US (e.g., direct conditioning with mental representations, or verbal or vicarious learning without experiencing a traumatic US), then it necessarily requires propositional learning processes. Learning on the basis of direct experience could involve both a primitive system that creates a mental link between the stimuli, and a more complex system that requires the cognitive appraisal of the CS and US before an association is encoded. Either way, there is good evidence that conditioning reflects changes that occur at the neural/cellular level (Schultz & Dickinson, 2000; Waelti, Dickinson, & Schultz, 2001). Given that conditioning can occur with representations, this implies that cellular changes can be made on the basis of information acquired at the representational level.

Though a full understanding of the underlying system is of theoretical interest, the main point is that conditioning can occur through many different pathways with the same end result. Conditioning causes changes in patterns of activation of the neuronal level, which result in fear responses to stimuli that previously did not evoke a response. This process is mediated by factors as diverse as personality and context. Future research should focus on using the wealth of information on fear acquisition to find new avenues for the treatment and prevention of severe fears and phobia.

Summary

This chapter has reviewed the evidence that children can acquire fears through three basic pathways: verbal threat information, vicarious experience, and direct conditioning. By looking at the characteristics of conditioning we have shown that learning is a complex process in which a mental link is made between a previously neutral stimulus and a real or imagined threat outcome. We have also shown that this process can be used to conceptualize the underlying mechanisms of all three pathways. The strength of the mental link and the expression of the response that it drives is affected by numerous variables including past experience, personality, the context of learning, the presence of competing stimuli, and the intrinsic properties of the stimuli themselves.

Acknowledgment

Andy Field was funded by Economic and Social Research Council grant number RES-062–23-0406 while writing this chapter.

References

Aitken, M. R. F., Larkin, M. J. W., & Dickinson, A. (2000). Super-learning of causal judgements. *Quarterly Journal of Experimental Psychology, Section B, Comparative and Physiological Psychology*, **53**, 59–81.

American Psychiatric Association (1994). *Diagnostic and Statistical Manual of Mental Disorders*, 4th edn. Washington, DC: American Psychiatric Association.

Askew, C. & Field, A. P. (2007). Vicarious learning and the development of fears in childhood. *Behaviour Research and Therapy*, **45**, 2616–2627. doi: 10.1016/j.brat.2007.06.008

Askew, C. & Field, A. P. (2008). The vicarious learning pathway to fear 40 years on. *Clinical Psychology Review*, **28**, 1249–1265. doi: 10.1016/j.cpr.2008.05.003

Askew, C., Kessock-Philip, H., & Field, A. P. (2008). Interaction between the indirect pathways to fear in children: what happens when verbal threat information and vicarious learning combine? *Behavioural and Cognitive Psychotherapy*, **36**, 491–505.

Bandura, A. (1969). Social-learning theory of identificatory processes. In: **D. A. Gostin** (ed.) *Handbook of Socialization Theory and Research*, pp. 213–262. Chicago, IL: Rand-McNally.

Bandura, A. & Rosenthal, T. L. (1966). Vicarious classical conditioning as a function of arousal level. *Journal of Personality and Social Psychology*, **3**, 54–64.

Bauer, D. H. (1976). An exploratory study of developmental changes in children's fears. *Journal of Child Psychology and Psychiatry*, **17**, 69–74.

Belsky, J. & Pluess, M. (2009). Beyond diathesis stress: differential susceptibility to environmental influences. *Psychological Bulletin*, **135**, 885–908. doi: 10.1037/a0017376

Berger, S. M. (1962). Conditioning through vicarious instigation. *Psychological Review*, **69**, 450–466.

Black, A. H. (1971). Autonomic aversive conditioning in infrahuman subjects. In: **F. R. Brush** (ed.) *Aversive Conditioning and Learning*, pp. 3–104. New York: Academic Press.

Bond, N. W. & Siddle, D. A. T. (1996). The preparedness account of social phobia: some data and alternative explanations. In: **R. Rapee** (ed.) *Current Controversies in the Anxiety Disorders*, pp. 291–316. New York: Guilford Press.

Bouton, M. E. (1994). Context, ambiguity, and classical conditioning. *Current Directions in Psychological Science*, **3**, 49–53.

Bouton, M. E. & Swartzentruber, D. (1991). Sources of relapse after extinction in Pavlovian and instrumental learning. *Clinical Psychology Review*, **11**, 123–140.

Boyce, W. T. & Ellis, B. J. (2005). Biological sensitivity to context. I. An evolutionary–developmental theory of the origins and functions of stress reactivity. *Development and Psychopathology*, **17**, 271–301. doi: 10.1017/s0954579405050145

Bradley, M. M., Moulder, B., & Lang, P. J. (2005). When good things go bad: the reflex physiology of defense. *Psychological Science*, **16**, 468–473.

Brewin, C. R. & Holmes, E. A. (2003). Psychological theories of posttraumatic stress disorder. *Clinical Psychology Review*, **23**, 339–376. doi: 10.1016/s0272–7358(03)00033–3

Brown, I. (1974). Effects of perceived similarity on vicarious emotional conditioning. *Behaviour Research and Therapy*, **12**, 165–173.

Campbell, D., Sanderson, R. E., & Laverty, S. G. (1964). Characteristics of a conditioned response in human subjects during extinction trials following a single traumatic conditioning trial. *Journal of Abnormal and Social Psychology*, **68**, 627–639.

Campbell, S. B. (1986). Developmental issues in childhood anxiety. In: **R. Gittelman** (ed.) *Anxiety Disorders of Childhood*, pp. 24–57. New York: Guilford Press.

Cantor, J. (1998). *Mommy I'm Scared: How TV and Movies Frighten Children and What We Can Do to Protect Them*. San Diego, CA: Harcourt Brace.

Cantor, J. & Nathanson, A. I. (1996). Children's fright reactions to television news. *Journal of Communication*, **46**, 139–152.

Carroll, L. (1872). *Through the Looking Glass and What Alice Found There*. London: Macmillan.

Collins, D. J. & Shanks, D. R. (2002). Momentary and integrative response strategies in causal judgment. *Memory and Cognition*, **30**, 1138–1147.

Comer, J. S. & Kendall, P. C. (2007). Terrorism: the psychological impact on youth. *Clinical Psychology – Science and Practice*, **14**, 179–212.

Cook, M. & Mineka, S. (1987). 2nd-order conditioning and overshadowing in the observational conditioning of fear in monkeys. *Behaviour Research and Therapy*, **25**, 349–364.

Cook, M. & Mineka, S. (1989). Observational conditioning of fear to fear-relevant versus fear-irrelevant stimuli in rhesus monkeys. *Journal of Abnormal Psychology*, **98**, 448–459.

Cook, M. & Mineka, S. (1990). Selective associations in the observational conditioning of fear in rhesus monkeys. *Journal of Experimental Psychology – Animal Behavior Processes*, **16**, 372–389.

Cook, M., Mineka, S., Wolkenstein, B., & Laitsch, K. (1985). Observational conditioning of snake fear in unrelated rhesus monkeys. *Journal of Abnormal Psychology*, **94**, 591–610.

Craske, M. G., Waters, A. M., Bergman, R. L., Naliboff, B., Lipp, O. V., Negoro, H., *et al.* (2008). Is aversive learning a marker of risk for anxiety disorders in children? *Behaviour Research and Therapy*, **46**, 954–967. doi: 10.1016/j.brat.2008.04.011

Dalgleish, T., Meiser-Stedman, R., & Smith, P. (2005). Cognitive aspects of posttraumatic stress reactions and their treatment in children and adolescents: an empirical review and some recommendations. *Behavioural and Cognitive Psychotherapy*, **33**, 459–486. doi: Doi 10.1017/S1352465805002389

Davey, G. C. L. (1989a). *Ecological Learning Theory.* London: Routledge.

Davey, G. C. L. (1989b). UCS revaluation and conditioning models of acquired fears. *Behaviour Research and Therapy*, **27**, 521–528.

Davey, G. C. L. (1992). Characteristics of individuals with fear of spiders. *Anxiety Research*, **4**, 299–314.

Davey, G. C. L. (1997). A conditioning model of phobias. In: **G. C. L. Davey** (ed.) *Phobias: A Handbook of Theory, Research and Treatment*, pp. 301–322. Chichester, UK: Wiley & Sons.

Davey, G. C. L. & McKenna, I. (1983). The effects of postconditioning revaluation of CS1 and UCS following Pavlovian second-order electrodermal conditioning in humans. *Quarterly Journal of Experimental Psychology, Section B, Comparative and Physiological Psychology*, **35**, 125–133.

Davey, G. C. L., de Jong, P. J., & Tallis, F. (1993). UCS inflation in the etiology of a variety of anxiety disorders: some case histories. *Behaviour Research and Therapy*, **31**, 495–498.

Davis, T. E. & Ollendick, T. H. (2005). Empirically supported treatments for specific phobia in children: do efficacious treatments address the components of a phobic response? *Clinical Psychology – Science and Practice*, **12**, 144–160. doi: 10.1093/clipsy/bpi018

De Houwer, J. (2009). The propositional approach to associative learning as an alternative for association formation models. *Learning and Behavior*, **37**, 1–20. doi: 10.3758/lb.37.1.1

De Houwer, J. & Beckers, T. (2002). A review of recent developments in research and theories on human contingency learning. *Quarterly Journal of Experimental Psychology, Section B, Comparative and Physiological Psychology*, **55**, 289–310.

de Rosnay, M., Cooper, P. J., Tsigaras, N., & Murray, L. (2006). Transmission of social anxiety from mother to infant: an experimental study using a social referencing paradigm. *Behaviour Research and Therapy*, **44**, 1165–1175. doi: 10.1016/j.brat.2005.09.003

Delgado, M. R., Olsson, A., & Phelps, E. A. (2006). Extending animal models of fear conditioning to humans. *Biological Psychology*, **73**, 39–48. doi: 10.1016/j.biopsycho.2006.01.006

Dickinson, A. (2001). Causal learning: an associative analysis. *Quarterly Journal of Experimental Psychology, Section B, Comparative and Physiological Psychology*, **54**, 3–25.

Dollinger, S. J., O'Donnell, J. P., & Staley, A. A. (1984). Lightning-strike disaster: effects on children's fears and worries. *Journal of Consulting and Clinical Psychology*, **52**, 1028–1038.

Doogan, S. & Thomas, G. V. (1992). Origins of fear of dogs in adults and children: the role of conditioning processes and prior familiarity with dogs. *Behaviour Research and Therapy*, **30**, 387–394.

Dubi, K., Rapee, R. M., Emerton, J. L., & Schniering, C. A. (2008). Maternal modeling and the acquisition of fear and avoidance in toddlers: influence of stimulus preparedness and child temperament. *Journal of Abnormal Child Psychology*, **36**, 499–512. doi: 10.1007/s10802–007–9195–3

Dwyer, D. M. (1999). Retrospective revaluation or mediated conditioning? The effect of different reinforcers. *Quarterly Journal of Experimental Psychology, Section B, Comparative and Physiological Psychology*, **52**, 289–306.

Dwyer, D. M. (2001). Mediated conditioning and retrospective revaluation with LiCl then flavour pairings. *Quarterly Journal of Experimental Psychology, Section B, Comparative and Physiological Psychology*, **54**, 145–165.

Dwyer, D. M. (2003). Learning about cues in their absence: evidence from flavour preferences and aversions. *Quarterly Journal of Experimental Psychology, Section B, Comparative and Physiological Psychology*, **56**, 56–67.

Dwyer, D. M., Mackintosh, N. J., & Boakes, R. A. (1998). Simultaneous activation of the representations of absent cues results in the formation of an excitatory association between them. *Journal of Experimental Psychology – Animal Behavior Processes*, **24**, 163–171.

Egliston, K. A. & Rapee, R. M. (2007). Inhibition of fear acquisition in toddlers following positive modelling by their mothers. *Behaviour Research and Therapy*, **45**, 1871–1882. doi: 10.1016/j.brat.2007.02.007

Eysenck, H. J. (1979). The conditioning model of neurosis. *Behavioral and Brain Sciences*, **2**, 155–166.

Field, A. P. (2006a). The behavioral inhibition system and the verbal information pathway to children's fears. *Journal of Abnormal Psychology*, **115**, 742–752. doi: 10.1037/0021–843x.115.4.742

Field, A. P. (2006b). Is conditioning a useful framework for understanding the development and treatment of phobias? *Clinical Psychology Review*, **26**, 857–875. doi: 10.1016/j.cpr.2005.05.010

Field, A. P. (2006c). Watch out for the beast: fear information and attentional bias in children. *Journal of Clinical Child and Adolescent Psychology*, **35**, 431–439.

Field, A. P. & Davey, G. C. L. (2001). Conditioning models of childhood anxiety. In: **W. K. Silverman** & **P. A. Treffers** (eds.) *Anxiety Disorders in Children and Adolescents: Research, Assessment and Intervention*, pp. 187–211. Cambridge, UK: Cambridge University Press.

Field, A. P. & Lawson, J. (2003). Fear information and the development of fears during childhood: effects on implicit fear responses and behavioural avoidance. *Behaviour Research and Therapy*, **41**, 1277–1293. doi: 10.1016/s0005–7967(03)00034–2

Field, A. P. & Lawson, J. (2008). The verbal information pathway to fear and subsequent causal learning in children. *Cognition and Emotion*, **22**, 459–479. doi: 10.1080/02699930801886532

Field, A. P. & Nightingale, Z. C. (2009). What if Little Albert had escaped? *Clinical Child Psychology and Psychiatry*, **14**, 343–351.

Field, A. P. & Price-Evans, K. (2009). Temperament moderates the effect of the verbal threat information pathway on children's heart rate responses to novel animals. *Behaviour Research and Therapy*, **47**, 431–436. doi: 10.1016/j.brat.2009.01.020

Field, A. P. & Purkis, H. M. (2011). Associative learning and phobias. In: **M. Haselgrove** & **L. Hogarth** (eds.) *Clinical Applications of Learning Theory*. Hove, UK: Psychology Press.

Field, A. P. & Schorah, H. (2007). The verbal information pathway to fear and heart rate changes in children. *Journal of Child Psychology and Psychiatry*, **48**, 1088–1093. doi: 10.1111/j.1469–7610.2007.01772.x

Field, A. P. & Storksen-Coulson, H. (2007). The interaction of pathways to fear in childhood anxiety: a preliminary study. *Behaviour Research and Therapy*, **45**, 3051–3059. doi: 10.1016/j.brat.2007.09.001

Field, A. P., Argyris, N. G., & Knowles, K. A. (2001). Who's afraid of the big bad wolf: a prospective paradigm to test Rachman's indirect pathways in children. *Behaviour Research and Therapy*, **39**, 1259–1276.

Field, A. P., Ball, J. E., Kawycz, N. J., & Moore, H. (2007). Parent–child relationships and the verbal information pathway to fear in children: two preliminary experiments. *Behavioural and Cognitive Psychotherapy*, **35**, 473–486. doi: 10.1017/s1352465807003736

Field, A. P., Hamilton, S. J., Knowles, K. A., & Plews, E. L. (2003). Fear information and social phobic beliefs in children: a prospective paradigm and preliminary results. *Behaviour Research and Therapy*, **41**, 113–123.

Field, A. P., Lawson, J., & Banerjee, R. (2008). The verbal threat information pathway to fear in children: the longitudinal effects on fear cognitions and the immediate effects on avoidance behavior. *Journal of Abnormal Psychology*, **117**, 214–224. doi: 10.1037/0021–843x.117.1.214

Fletcher, K. E. (1996). Childhood posttraumatic stress disorder. In: **E. J. Mash** & **R. Barkley** (eds.) *Child Psychopathology*, pp. 242–276. New York: Guilford Press.

Garcia, J., McGowan, B. K., & Green, K. F. (1972). Biological constraints on conditioning. In: A. H. Black & W. F. Prokasy (eds.) *Classical Conditioning II: Current Research and Theory*, pp. 3–27. New York: Appleton-Century-Crofts.

Gerull, F. C. & Rapee, R. M. (2002). Mother knows best: effects of maternal modelling on the acquisition of fear and avoidance behaviour in toddlers. *Behaviour Research and Therapy*, **40**, 279–287.

Gibson, E. J. & Walk, R. D. (1960). The "visual cliff." *Scientific American*, **202**, 64–72.

Hall, G. (2002). Associative structures in Pavlovian and instrumental conditioning. In: C. R. Gallistel (ed.) *Stevens' Handbook of Experimental Psychology*, 3rd edn., vol. 3, pp. 1–45. New York: Wiley & Sons.

Harrison, K. & Cantor, J. (1999). Tales from the screen: enduring fright reactions to scary media. *Media Psychology*, **1**, 97–116. doi: 10.1207/s1532785xmep0102_1

Hoekstra, S. J., Harris, R. J., & Helmick, A. L. (1999). Autobiographical memories about the experience of seeing frightening movies in childhood. *Media Psychology*, **1**, 117–140. doi: 10.1207/s1532785xmep0102_2

Holmes, E. A., Creswell, C., & O'Connor, T. G. (2007). Posttraumatic stress symptoms in London school children following September 11, 2001: an exploratory investigation of peri-traumatic reactions and intrusive imagery. *Journal of Behavior Therapy and Experimental Psychiatry*, **38**, 474–490. doi: 10.1016/j.jbtep.2007.10.003

Hornik, R., Risenhoover, N., & Gunnar, M. (1987). The effects of maternal positive, neutral, and negative affective communications on infant responses to new toys. *Child Development*, **58**, 937–944.

Hoven, C. W., Duarte, C. S., Lucas, C. P., Wu, P., Mandell, D. J., Goodwin, R. D., *et al.* (2005). Psychopathology among New York city public school children 6 months after September 11. *Archives of General Psychiatry*, **62**, 545–552.

Hugdahl, K. & Johnsen, B. H. (1989). Preparedness and electrodermal fear-conditioning: ontogenetic vs phylogenetic explanations. *Behaviour Research and Therapy*, **27**, 269–278.

Hygge, S. & Öhman, A. (1978). Modeling processes in acquisition of fears: vicarious electrodermal conditioning to fear-relevant stimuli. *Journal of Personality and Social Psychology*, **36**, 271–279.

Izquierdo, L. A., Barros, D. M., Ardenghi, P. G., Pereira, P., Rodrigues, C., Choi, H., *et al.* (2000). Different hippocampal molecular requirements for short- and long-term retrieval of one-trial avoidance learning. *Behavioural Brain Research*, **111**, 93–98.

Izquierdo, L. A., Barros, D. H., Medina, J. H., & Izquierdo, I. (2000). Novelty enhances retrieval of one-trial avoidance learning in rats 1 or 31 days after training unless the hippocampus is inactivated by different receptor antagonists and enzyme inhibitors. *Behavioural Brain Research*, **117**, 215–220.

Joslin, J., Emlen, J., & Fletcher, H. (1964). A comparison of the responses to snakes of lab- and wild-reared rhesus monkeys. *Animal Behaviour*, **12**, 348–352.

Kamin, L. J. (1968). "Attention-like" processes in classical conditioning. In: M. R. Jones (ed.) *Miami Symposium on the Prediction of Behavior: Aversive Stimulation*, pp. 9–32. Coral Gables, FL: University of Miami Press.

Kelly, V. L., Barker, H., Field, A. P., Wilson, C., & Reynolds, S. (2010). Can Rachman's indirect pathways be used to un-learn fear? A prospective paradigm to test whether children's fears can be reduced using positive information and modelling a non-anxious response. *Behaviour Research and Therapy*, **48**, 164–170. doi: 10.1016/j.brat.2009.10.002

King, N. J., Gullone, E., & Ollendick, T. (1998). Etiology of childhood phobias: current status of Rachman's three pathways theory. *Behaviour Research and Therapy*, **36**, 297–309.

Kravetz, D. F. (1974). Heart rate as a minimal cue for the occurrence of vicarious classical conditioning. *Journal of Personality and Social Psychology*, **29**, 125–131.

Lang, P. J. (1968). Fear reduction and fear behavior: problems in treating a construct. In: **J. M. Schlien** (ed.) *Research in Psychotherapy*, vol. 3, pp. 90–103. Washington, DC: American Psychological Association.

Lang, P. J., Davis, M., & Öhman, A. (2000). Fear and anxiety: animal models and human cognitive psychophysiology. *Journal of Affective Disorders*, **61**, 137–159.

Lawson, J., Banerjee, R., & Field, A. P. (2007). The effects of verbal information on children's fear beliefs about social situations. *Behaviour Research and Therapy*, **45**, 21–37. doi: 10.1016/j.brat.2006.01.007

Le Pelley, M. E. & McLaren, I. P. L. (2003). Learned associability and associative change in human causal learning. *Quarterly Journal of Experimental Psychology, Section B, Comparative and Physiological Psychology*, **56**, 68–79.

LeDoux, J. E. (2003). The emotional brain, fear, and the amygdala. *Cellular and Molecular Neurobiology*, **23**, 727–738.

Lober, K. & Shanks, D. R. (2000). Is causal induction based on causal power? Critique of Cheng (1997). *Psychological Review*, **107**, 195–212.

Lovibond, P. F. & Shanks, D. R. (2002). The role of awareness in Pavlovian conditioning: empirical evidence and theoretical implications. *Journal of Experimental Psychology – Animal Behavior Processes*, **28**, 3–26.

Lubow, R. E. (1973). Latent inhibition. *Psychological Bulletin*, **79**, 398–407.

Lubow, R. E. (1989). *Latent Inhibition and Conditioned Attention Theory*. Cambridge, UK: Cambridge University Press.

Lubow, R. E. & Moore, A. U. (1959). Latent inhibition: the effect of nonreinforced pre-exposure to the conditional stimulus. *Journal of Comparative and Physiological Psychology*, **52**, 415–419.

Mackintosh, N. J. (1973). Stimulus selection: learning to ignore stimuli that predict no change in reinforcement. In: **R. A. Hinde** & **L. S. Hinde** (eds.) *Constraints of Learning*, pp. 75–96. London: Academic Press.

Mackintosh, N. J. (1983). *Conditioning and Associative Learning*. Oxford, UK: Oxford University Press.

Marillion (1997). *This Strange Engine* [CD]. London: EMI.

Matute, H., Vegas, S., & De Marez, P. J. (2002). Flexible use of recent information in causal and predictive judgments. *Journal of Experimental Psychology – Learning Memory and Cognition*, **28**, 714–725. doi: 10.1037//0278–7393.28.4.714

Menzies, R. G. & Clarke, J. C. (1993a). The etiology of childhood water phobia. *Behaviour Research and Therapy*, **31**, 499–501.

Menzies, R. G. & Clarke, J. C. (1993b). The etiology of fear of heights and its relationship to severity and individual response patterns. *Behaviour Research and Therapy*, **31**, 355–365.

Metallica (1991). *Metallica* [CD]. London: Vertigo.

Mineka, S. & Cook, M. (1986). Immunization against the observational conditioning of snake fear in rhesus monkeys. *Journal of Abnormal Psychology*, **95**, 307–318.

Mineka, S. & Cook, M. (1993). Mechanisms involved in the observational conditioning of fear. *Journal of Experimental Psychology – General*, **122**, 23–38.

Mineka, S. & Zinbarg, R. (2006). A contemporary learning theory perspective on the etiology of anxiety disorders: it's not what you thought it was. *American Psychologist*, **61**, 10–26.

Mineka, S., Davidson, M., Cook, M., & Keir, R. (1984). Observational conditioning of snake fear in rhesus monkeys. *Journal of Abnormal Psychology*, **93**, 355–372.

Mineka, S., Keir, R., & **Price, V.** (1980). Fear of snakes in wild-reared and laboratory-reared rhesus monkeys (*Macaca mulatta*). *Animal Learning and Behavior*, **8**, 653–663.

Mitchell, C. J., De Houwer, J., & **Lovibond, P. F.** (2009a). The propositional nature of human associative learning. *Behavioral and Brain Sciences*, **32**, 183–198. doi: 10.1017/s0140525x09000855

Mitchell, C. J., De Houwer, J., & **Lovibond, P. F.** (2009b). Link-based learning theory creates more problems than it solves. *Behavioral and Brain Sciences*, **32**, 230–246. doi: 10.1017/s0140525x09001186

Monroe, S. M. & **Simons, A. D.** (1991). Diathesis stress theories in the context of life stress research: implications for the depressive disorders. *Psychological Bulletin*, **110**, 406–425.

Morris, J. S., Öhman, A., & **Dolan, R. J.** (1998). Conscious and unconscious emotional learning in the human amygdala. *Nature*, **393**, 467–470.

Motörhead (2002). *Hammered* [CD]. London: Sanctuary.

Mowrer, O. H. (1960). *Learning Theory and Behaviour*. New York: Wiley & Sons.

Mumme, D. L. & **Fernald, A.** (2003). The infant as onlooker: learning from emotional reactions observed in a television scenario. *Child Development*, **74**, 221–237.

Mumme, D. L., Fernald, A., & **Herrera, C.** (1996). Infants' responses to facial and vocal emotional signals in a social referencing paradigm. *Child Development*, **67**, 3219–3237.

Muris, P. & **Field, A. P.** (2010). The role of verbal threat information in the development of childhood fear: "Beware the Jabberwock!" *Clinical Child and Family Psychology Review*, **13**, 129–150. doi: 10.1007/s10567–010–0064–1

Muris, P., Bodden, D., Merckelbach, H., Ollendick, T. H., & **King, N.** (2003). Fear of the beast: a prospective study on the effects of negative information on childhood fear. *Behaviour Research and Therapy*, **41**, 195–208. doi: 10.1016/s0005–7967(01)00137–1

Murray, L., Cooper, P., Creswell, C., Schofield, E., & **Sack, C.** (2007). The effects of maternal social phobia on mother–infant interactions and infant social responsiveness. *Journal of Child Psychology and Psychiatry*, **48**, 45–52. doi: 10.1111/j.1469–7610.2006.01657.x

Murray, L., de Rosnay, M., Pearson, J., Bergeron, C., Schofield, E., Royal-Lawson, M., *et al.* (2008). Intergenerational transmission of social anxiety: the role of social referencing processes in infancy. *Child Development*, **79**, 1049–1064.

Öhman, A. & **Mineka, S.** (2001). Fears, phobias, and preparedness: toward an evolved module of fear and fear learning. *Psychological Review*, **108**, 483–522.

Öhman, A., Eriksson, A., & **Olofsson, C.** (1975). One-trial learning and superior resistance to extinction of autonomic responses conditioned to potentially phobic stimuli. *Journal of Comparative and Physiological Psychology*, **88**, 619–627.

Öhman, A., Erixon, G., & **Lofberg, I.** (1975). Phobias and preparedness: phobic versus neutral pictures as conditioned stimuli for human autonomic responses. *Journal of Abnormal Psychology*, **84**, 41–45.

Olsson, A. & **Phelps, E. A.** (2004). Learned fear of "unseen" faces after Pavlovian, observational, and instructed fear. *Psychological Science*, **15**, 822–828.

Ortiz, C. D., Silverman, W. K., Jaccard, J., & **La Greca, A. M.** (2010). Children's anxiety in reaction to disaster media cues: a preliminary test of a multivariate model. *Psychological Trauma: Theory, Research, Practice, and Policy*, in press.

Otto, M. W., Henin, A., Hirshfeld-Becker, D. R., Pollack, M. H., Biederman, J., & **Rosenbaum, J. F.** (2007). Posttraumatic stress disorder symptoms following media exposure to tragic events: impact of 9/11 on children at risk for anxiety disorders. *Journal of Anxiety Disorders*, **21**, 888–902.

Pavlov, I. P. (1927). *Conditioned Reflexes*. Oxford, UK: Oxford University Press.

Pearce, J. M. & **Bouton, M. E.** (2001). Theories of associative learning in animals. *Annual Review of Psychology*, **52**, 111–139.

Phelps, E. A. (2006). Emotion and cognition: insights from studies of the human amygdala. *Annual Review of Psychology*, **57**, 27–53. doi: 10.1146/annurev.psych.56.091103.070234

Phelps, E. A. & LeDoux, J. E. (2005). Contributions of the amygdala to emotion processing: from animal models to human behavior. *Neuron*, **48**, 175–187. doi: 10.1016/j.neuron.2005.09.025

Pinel, J. P. J. & Treit, D. (1979). Conditioned defensive burying in rats: availability of burying materials. *Animal Learning and Behavior*, **7**, 392–396.

Price-Evans, K. & Field, A. P. (2008). A neglectful parenting style moderates the effect of the verbal threat information pathway on children's heart rate responses to novel animals. *Behavioural and Cognitive Psychotherapy*, **36**, 473–482. doi: 10.1017/s1352465808004396

Purkis, H. M. & Lipp, O. V. (2009). Are snakes and spiders special? Acquisition of negative valence and modified attentional processing by non-fear-relevant animal stimuli. *Cognition and Emotion*, **23**, 430–452. doi: 10.1080/02699930801993973

Rachman, S. (1968). *Phobias: Their Nature and Control*. Springfield, IL: Charles C. Thomas.

Rachman, S. (1977). Conditioning theory of fear acquisition: critical examination. *Behaviour Research and Therapy*, **15**, 375–387.

Rachman, S. (1991). Neo-conditioning and the classical theory of fear acquisition. *Clinical Psychology Review*, **11**, 155–173.

Ragan, K. (2006). *Outfoxing Fear: Folktales from around the World*. New York: W.W. Norton.

Rescorla, R. A. (1968). Probability of shock in presence and absence of CS in fear conditioning. *Journal of Comparative and Physiological Psychology*, **66**, 1–15.

Rescorla, R. A. (1971). Variations in the effectiveness of reinforcement following prior inhibitory conditioning. *Learning and Motivation*, **2**, 113–123.

Rescorla, R. A. (1974). Effect of inflation of unconditioned stimulus value following conditioning. *Journal of Comparative and Physiological Psychology*, **86**, 101–106.

Rescorla, R. A. (1980). *Pavlovian Second-Order Conditioning: Studies in Associative Learning*. Hillsdale, NJ: Erlbaum.

Rescorla, R. A. (1988). Pavlovian conditioning: It's not what you think it is. *American Psychologist*, **43**, 151–160.

Rescorla, R. A. (1991). Combinations of modulators trained with the same and different target stimuli. *Animal Learning and Behavior*, **19**, 355–360.

Rescorla, R. A. (2000). Associative changes with a random CS–US relationship. *Quarterly Journal of Experimental Psychology, Section B, Comparative and Physiological Psychology*, **53**, 325–340.

Sale, R. (1978). *Fairy Tales and After*. Cambridge, MA: Harvard University Press.

Schultz, W. & Dickinson, A. (2000). Neuronal coding of prediction errors. *Annual Review of Neuroscience*, **23**, 473–500.

Seligman, M. E. P. (1971). Phobias and preparedness. *Behavior Therapy*, **2**, 307–320.

Shanks, D. R. (2010). Learning: from association to cognition. *Annual Review of Psychology*, **61**, 273–301. doi: 10.1146/annurev.psych.093008.100519

Shanks, D. R., Holyoak, K. J., & Medin, D. L. (eds.) (1996). *The Psychology of Learning and Motivation*, vol. 34, *Causal Learning*. San Diego, CA: Academic Press.

Siddle, D. A. T., Remington, B., & Churchill, M. (1985). Effects of conditioned stimulus pre-exposure on human electrodermal conditioning. *Biological Psychology*, **20**, 113–127.

Smith, S. L. & Moyer-Gusé, E. (2006). Children and the War on Iraq: developmental differences in fear responses to television news coverage. *Media Psychology*, **8**, 213–237.

Solomon, R. L. & Turner, L. H. (1962). Discriminative classical conditioning in dogs paralyzed by curare can later control discriminative avoidance responses in the normal state. *Psychological Review*, **69**, 202–219.

Sorce, J. F., Emde, R. N., Campos, J., & Klinnert, M. D. (1985). Maternal emotional signaling: its effect on the visual-cliff behavior of 1-year-olds. *Developmental Psychology*, **21**, 195–200.

Strelau, J. (1983). *Temperament Personality Activity*. New York: Academic Press.

Strelau, J. & Eysenck, H. J. (1987). *Personality Dimensions and Arousal*. New York: Plenum Press.

Tangen, J. M. & Allan, L. G. (2004). Cue interaction and judgments of causality: contributions of causal and associative processes. *Memory and Cognition*, **32**, 107–124.

Terr, L. C., Bloch, D. A., Michel, B. A., Shi, H., Reinhardt, J. A., & Metayer, S. (1999). Children's symptoms in the wake of Challenger: a field study of distant traumatic effects and an outline of related conditions. *American Journal of Psychiatry*, **156**, 1536–1544.

Valkenburg, P. M., Cantor, J., & Peeters, A. L. (2000). Fright reactions to television: a child survey. *Communication Research*, **27**, 82–99.

van der Molen, J. H. W. & Bushman, B. J. (2008). Children's direct fright and worry reactions to violence in fiction and news television programs. *Journal of Pediatrics*, **153**, 420–424. doi: 10.1016/j.jpeds.2008.03.036

Vaughan, K. B. & Lanzetta, J. T. (1980). Vicarious instigation and conditioning of facial expressive and autonomic responses to a models expressive display of pain. *Journal of Personality and Social Psychology*, **38**, 909–923.

Waelti, P., Dickinson, A., & Schultz, W. (2001). Dopamine responses comply with basic assumptions of formal learning theory. *Nature*, **412**, 43–48.

Waters, A. M., Henry, J., & Neumann, D. L. (2009). Aversive Pavlovian conditioning in childhood anxiety disorders: impaired response inhibition and resistance to extinction. *Journal of Abnormal Psychology*, **118**, 311–321. doi: 10.1037/a0015635

Watson, J. B. (1916). Behavior and the concept of mental disease. *Journal of Philosophy, Psychology, and Scientific Methods*, **13**, 589–597.

Watson, J. B. & Rayner, R. (1920). Conditioned emotional reactions. *Journal of Experimental Psychology*, **3**, 1–14.

Westenberg, P. M., Drewes, M. J., Goedhart, A. W., Siebelink, B. M., & Treffers, P. D. A. (2004). A developmental analysis of self-reported fears in late childhood through mid-adolescence: social-evaluative fears on the rise? *Journal of Child Psychology and Psychiatry*, **45**, 481–495.

White, K. & Davey, G. C. L. (1989). Sensory preconditioning and UCS inflation in human fear conditioning. *Behaviour Research and Therapy*, **27**, 161–166.

Wolpe, J. (1961). The systematic desensitization treatment of neurosis. *Journal of Nervous Mental Disease*, **132**, 189–203.

Yule, W., Udwin, O., & Murdoch, K. (1990). The *Jupiter* sinking: effects on children's fears, depression and anxiety. *Journal of Child Psychology and Psychiatry and Allied Disciplines*, **31**, 1051–1061.

Zinbarg, R. E. & Mohlman, J. (1998). Individual differences in the acquisition of affectively valenced associations. *Journal of Personality and Social Psychology*, **74**, 1024–1040.

Zipes, J. (1979). *Breaking the Magic Spell: Radical Theories of Folk and Fairy Tales*. New York: Routledge.

Zuckerman, M. (1999). *Vulnerability to Psychopathology: A Biosocial Model*. Washington, DC: American Psychological Association.

12

Traumatic events

Patrick Smith, Sean Perrin, and William Yule

Introduction

The concept of post-traumatic stress disorder (PTSD) as "a normal reaction to an abnormal event" is appealing in its simplicity, but does not do justice to the complexity of children's responses to traumatic events. Recent epidemiological investigations have confirmed that far from being "abnormal," exposure to trauma in childhood and adolescence is all too common (Costello, Erkanli, Fairbank, & Angold, 2002). Moreover, PTSD is rare, occurring only in a minority of those exposed to trauma (Copeland, Keeler, Angold, & Costello, 2007). To complicate matters further, PTSD is not the sole outcome of exposure trauma: a broad range of reactions is possible, and comorbidity of other disorders with PTSD is the norm (Bolton, Ryan, Udwin, Boyle, & Yule, 2000).

What is known about the nature of traumatic events in childhood and adolescence – their frequency, distribution, and the risks for exposure? What are the common psychiatric sequelae associated with trauma? What is the role of traumatic events in triggering the onset of, or increasing long-term liability for, a variety of anxiety disorders, including PTSD, depression, separation anxiety, generalized anxiety, and even some conduct disorders? Finally, what are the implications for treatment? This chapter addresses these issues from a developmental perspective.

Traumatic events

Definitions

The official American Psychiatric Association definition of what constitutes a traumatic event has altered considerably since PTSD was first included in the *Diagnostic and Statistical Manual* (DSM-III) in 1980. Initially, the Criterion A event in PTSD was "a recognisable stressor that would evoke considerable distress in almost anyone" (American Psychiatric Association, 1980). The next major revision, DSM-III-R, added that the event is "outside the range of usual human experience" (American Psychiatric Association, 1987). The current diagnostic criteria for PTSD in DSM-IV-TR define the extreme traumatic stressor somewhat differently: "the person experienced, witnessed, or was confronted with an event or events that involved actual or threatened death or serious injury, or a threat to the physical integrity of self or others; [and] the person's response involved intense fear helplessness or horror (or disorganised or agitated behavior in children)" (American

Anxiety Disorders in Children and Adolescents, 2nd edn, ed. W. K. Silverman and A. P. Field. Published by Cambridge University Press. © Cambridge University Press 2011.

Psychiatric Association, 2000). Hopefully any changes suggested in DSM-V will be informed by more empirical work with children and young people.

Two important changes are reflected in these shifting definitions. First, traumatic events are not necessarily "outside the range of usual human experience" – on the contrary, exposure to trauma is almost commonplace. Second, individual differences in responses at the time of exposure are fundamental.

This change in definition has widened the variety of traumatic events (Breslau & Kessler, 2001), which now include: violent personal assault (such as sexual assault, physical attack, robbery, mugging); being kidnapped or taken hostage; terrorist attack; torture, incarceration as a prisoner of war; natural or man-made disasters; severe traffic accidents; and witnessing or learning about the injury or unnatural death of others (American Psychiatric Association, 2000).

It is clear from the DSM-IV-TR definition, and from the examples listed above, that traumatic events involve intense threat. This feature of the diagnosis was operationalized early on by Rachman (1980) who, although not concerned directly with PTSD, listed stimulus characteristics that were likely to give rise to difficulties in emotional processing. Events that were sudden, intense, dangerous, uncontrollable, and unpredictable were thought to cause particular difficulties. Such factors broadly characterize what are now considered to be potentially traumatic events.

But traumatic events cannot be defined in terms of stimulus characteristics alone. Janoff-Bulman (1985) argued that traumatic events are those that "shatter" individuals' basic assumptions about themselves and the world. Three specific fundamental assumptions were proposed: (1) the world is benevolent; (2) the world is meaningful; and (3) the self is worthy (Janoff-Bulman, 1985, p. 16). The nature of traumatic events is such that they are incompatible with these basic assumptions. This argument was developed further by Foa and colleagues (e.g., Foa & Kozak, 1986; Foa, Steketee, & Olasov-Rothbaum, 1989), who emphasized that traumatic events violate our basic concepts of safety. More recently, Bolton and Hill (1996) have suggested that traumatic events are those that may violate a broader set of basic assumptions: that the world is safe enough, predictable enough, and satisfies enough needs; and that the self is competent enough (to act).

There are key differences between these approaches to characterizing extreme traumatic stressors, and varying degrees of empirical support for each. However, the general idea is the same: it is discrepancies between the meaning attributed to the trauma on the one hand, and the content of pre-existing mental representations (assumptions, beliefs, schema) about the world or the self on the other hand, that give rise to emotional distress, including PTSD (Dalgleish & Power, 2004; also see Dalgleish, 2004).

Roughly then, traumatic stressors are events which, because they are perceived as being extremely threatening, do not accord with our fundamental ideas about how the world works and our place in it. Recent research, discussed in more detail below, shows that these cognitive factors and appraisal processes are key to understanding the development of (and recovery from) PTSD in children.

Post-traumatic stress reactions

Clinical and diagnostic features

Post-traumatic stress reactions in children and adolescents have been reported following a wide range of traumatic events, including violent assaults, traffic accidents, shooting, serious illness, natural and man-made disasters, war, terrorist attacks, and physical or sexual abuse. This literature, and clinical experience, suggests that children's reactions tend to cluster around symptoms of re-experiencing, avoidance, and physiological overarousal.

Intrusive and distressing recollections of aspects of the traumatic event are the cardinal symptoms of post-traumatic stress. These can occur at any time of day and are notable for their vividness and "here and now" quality. Usually, the child "sees" the event or its worst moments replaying over and over again, but this can be accompanied by repetitive memories in any of the sensory modalities – sound, smell, touch, and motion. Some children who have sustained injury may re-experience physical pain when reminded of the trauma, despite there being no organic cause. Occasionally, children will report that the experience is so vivid that it feels as if it is happening all over again, as in dissociative flashbacks. When asleep, intrusions may occur in the form of frightening and vivid nightmares. These might be replays of what happened (often, the child will wake up at the worst moment), or variations on what actually occurred.

Many children try to cope with these upsetting intrusive recollections by pushing them out of mind, or by staying away from any trauma reminders. Children often report that they can keep intrusive memories at bay as long as they remain busy, but that upsetting recollections intrude into consciousness as soon as they relax, such as when trying to drop off to sleep. Some child survivors experience a pressure to talk about what happened, but paradoxically find it difficult to talk to parents and peers. Anecdotally, many children report that they do not want to upset their parents when they talk about what happened and so they keep their feelings to themselves – parents may not be aware of the full extent of the child's suffering. When avoidant coping becomes pervasive, children may lose interest in seeing friends, or in continuing with previously enjoyed activities or hobbies. Older adolescents may feel that no one else can understand what they have been through, and so feel cut off from peers. Survivors have learned that life is fragile. This can lead to a loss of faith in the future, a sense of foreshortened future, or a premature awareness of their mortality.

Unwanted memories can be so upsetting that children will fight against sleep and try to stay awake. It is ironic that children who are extremely tired still try to remain awake with the obvious consequence that they become tired, irritable, and unable to concentrate. The irritability can lead on to anger that can be difficult to deal with. Young trauma survivors are usually alert to danger in their environment, and continually on the lookout for potential threat. Children may report feeling on edge, wound up, or jumpy.

These sorts of symptoms were first officially recognized as forming a tripartite syndrome by the American Psychiatric Association in 1980 when the diagnostic label "post-traumatic stress disorder" (PTSD) was coined. Based on work with veterans of the Vietnam War, it was seen that what had variously been called nervous shock, railway spine, battle fatigue, and so on consisted essentially of the three symptom clusters outlined above. At first, the applicability to children and adolescents was unclear, but by the time of the revisions DSM-III-R (American Psychiatric Association, 1987), DSM-IV (American Psychiatric Association, 1994), and DSM-IV-TR (American Psychiatric Association, 2000) it was accepted that younger people could also develop PTSD. However, it must be emphasized that the application of the diagnosis was originally a downward extension from work with adults and considerable empirical study is still needed to pinpoint the nature and extent of stress reactions in children. Under the proposed changes to the diagnosis in DSM-V (due for publication in 2013), Criterion A and the symptom clusters of intrusive recollections and physiological arousal are retained in revised form. However, the avoidance symptom cluster is substantially reduced, while a fourth symptom cluster – "alterations in mood and cognition" – is introduced. At the time of writing, phase 1 field trials for these latest revisions to the DSM are about to begin, and guidelines on developmental manifestations of PTSD are being developed. Slightly different criteria for PTSD have been agreed by the World Health Organization in its official *International Classification of Diseases*, 10th edition (ICD-10) (World Health Organization, 1991). The WHO is also revising its diagnostic guidelines, with publication of the ICD-11 due in 2014.

According to DSM-IV, 4 weeks must have elapsed since the trauma before a diagnosis can be considered, and so a separate diagnostic category, acute stress disorder (ASD) is available for reactions occurring in the first month after a traumatic event. (ICD-10 is less prescriptive about the length of time since trauma, noting that "the latency period may range from a few weeks to months.") The ASD criteria are similar to those of PTSD, but fewer symptoms are required overall. The main difference is that an ASD diagnosis requires the presence of dissociative symptoms, such as numbing, reduced awareness, derealization, depersonalization, and dissociative amnesia. Research shows that children can experience (and report on) dissociative symptoms in the aftermath of traumatic events, and may suffer from a diagnosable ASD (e.g., Kassam-Adams & Winston, 2004). However, the utility of the diagnosis, especially the emphasis on dissociation, has been called into question (Dalgleish *et al.*, 2008; Meiser-Stedman, Dalgleish, Smith, Yule, & Glucksman, 2007; Meiser-Stedman, Yule, Smith, Glucksman, & Dalgleish, 2005).

Frequency of exposure

Among adults, exposure to traumatic events is common. Most people will experience at least one traumatic event during their lifetime. For example, in the National Women's Survey, 69% of respondents reported experiencing a traumatic event at some point in their lives (Resnick, Kilpatrick, Dansky, Saunders, & Best, 1993), while the US National Co-morbidity Survey found that 61% of men and 51% of women had experienced a trauma (Kessler, Sonnega, Bromet, Hughes, & Nelson, 1995). The Detroit Area Survey found an even higher overall lifetime trauma exposure rate of 89% (Breslau, Kessler, Chilcoat, Schultz, Davis, & Andreski, 1998). A similar picture is emerging for children and adolescents. Schwabb-Stone, Ayers, Kasprow, Voyce, Barone, Shriver, *et al.* (1995) found that more than 40% of 2248 11–15-year-old American schoolchildren had witnessed a shooting or stabbing in the past year. In a large national telephone survey of rates of exposure to violent victimization, Boney-McCoy and Finkelhor (1995) found that 40% of 10–16-year-old Americans had experienced some form of physical or sexual violence.

One of the first studies to investigate rates of exposure to a broad range of trauma among a young community sample found that 43% of 384 urban American adolescents had experienced a trauma by the age of 18 years (Giaconia, Reinherz, Silverman, Pakiz, Frost, & Cohen, 1995). Some events were more common than others: witnessing violence was more common (13%) than rape (2%) or being involved in a natural disaster (1%). More recently, Costello *et al.* (2002) found that 25% of a large representative rural cohort of young people ($n = 1420$, the Great Smoky Mountains Study) had experienced one or more DSM-listed traumatic events by the age of 16 years old. Further analyses of later annual waves of data from the same study revealed higher rates of exposure: more than two-thirds of the sample had experienced at least one traumatic event by the age of 16 (Copeland *et al.*, 2007). The higher rates found by Copeland *et al.* may reflect methodological refinements.

Participants were interviewed at least four times during childhood and adolescence about the immediate past; both parents and young people were interviewed; and interviewees were asked specifically about each of 17 traumatic events. Broadly in line with these high rates, Breslau *et al.*'s (Breslau, Lucia, & Alvarado, 2006) study of an older cohort reported that 75% of a representative sample of 17-year-olds had experienced at least one traumatic event.

Traumatic events are more frequent in some populations. Children living through war are at particular risk. For example, in a population survey ($n = 2976$) of 9–14-year-olds living in Bosnia, Smith, Perrin, Yule, Hacam, and Stuvland (2002) found that more than two-thirds had been in a situation where they thought they would be killed, 78% had experienced shooting at close range, and more than 90% had been under mortar attacks. Bayer, Klasen, and Adam (2007) reported that among child soldiers in Uganda and DR Congo, 93% had witnessed shooting, 90% had witnessed violent wounding, and 84% had themselves been beaten. Consequently, young refugees from war zones often have histories characterized by multiple chronic and repeated exposure to horrific traumatic events (e.g., Sack, Him, & Dickason, 1999).

In summary, methodologically rigorous epidemiological investigations show that trauma is common in childhood and adolescence, with between a quarter to three-quarters of young people experiencing at least one traumatic event by the age of 17. Some traumatic events are more common than others. Some populations are more at risk of exposure than others.

Risks for exposure

Although we tend to think of traumatic events as chance occurrences, they are generally not randomly distributed among the population. Knowledge of risks for exposure can therefore be of practical help in identifying at-risk young people. Investigations of exposure risk can also help in elucidating more clearly the causal role of traumatic events in relation to later psychiatric sequelae. Apparent association between exposure and psychopathology found in cross-sectional studies may (in principle) be due to a common third factor which puts children at risk for both. Prospective longitudinal cohort studies can address these issues directly.

In adults, a handful of epidemiological studies have identified a number of socio-demographic and personal vulnerability factors that are associated with risk for exposure to traumatic events. In general, men are at greater risk of exposure than women, but women are at greater risk for some types of trauma such as rape and sexual assault (Kessler *et al.*, 1995). In the Detroit Area Survey (Breslau *et al.*, 1998), rates of exposure to violent assault were higher in racially disadvantaged minorities, in people without a college education, and in people with a low income. A history of depression also appears to increase the risk for trauma exposure in adults (Breslau, Davis, Peterson, & Schultz, 2000).

In contrast, among adolescents, Giaconia *et al.*'s (1995) cross-sectional survey found that males and females were equally likely to have experienced a trauma (although risks varied for certain trauma types), and that socioeconomic status was not related to risk of exposure.

More recent work has utilized a long-term prospective cohort design (from age 6 to 17) to examine risks of exposure (Breslau *et al.*, 2006; Storr, Ialongo, Anthony, & Breslau, 2007). Overall, adolescents living in urban environments experienced more trauma than those from suburban homes. Exposure to violent assault (but not other traumas) by age 17 was more common in those who at 6 years had been rated by teachers as being disruptive or aggressive, or who had had concentration problems. Conversely, children who at 6 years were assessed as having a Full Scale IQ score of 115 or more, and who were in the top quartile for reading ability, were at significantly lower risk of exposure to trauma.

In another large prospective cohort study, Copeland *et al.* (2007) found that a history of depression, parenting problems, and environmental adversity predicted trauma exposure at age 16. In an earlier report, Costello *et al.* (2002) showed that there was a linear relation between these sorts of predictors (i.e., parental psychopathology, family relationship problems, and family environment problems) and trauma exposure among 16-year-olds. However, this applied only to certain types of trauma. Sexual abuse, and learning about events that had happened to others in the child's network, were strongly associated with vulnerability factors; whereas bereavement, illness, accidents, and physical violence were unrelated to vulnerability factors. Importantly, traumatic events also clustered with non-traumatic stressful life events. Trauma exposure was twice as likely among those young people who had experienced stressful events such as pregnancy, moving home, or parental divorce (Costello *et al.*, 2002).

Finally, age is consistently related to trauma exposure. Exposure is more common among 14–16-year-olds compared to 9–13-year-olds (Copeland *et al.*, 2007; Giaconia *et al.*, 1995). Breslau *et al.* (1998) showed that the peak age for trauma exposure is 16 to 20 years.

These community studies show that traumatic events generally occur against a background of personal and environmental vulnerability factors, and are often accompanied by additional stressful events. That is, traumas are rarely one-off events occurring in isolation. Secondary consequences may be just as significant as the traumatic event itself. Accidents can entail hospital stays, medical procedures, and time off school, for example. Assaults may have legal consequences. Violence and abuse within the family might mean a change of carer. The importance of the context of the trauma – both the events preceding it, and its secondary consequences – is illustrated by the finding that parental divorce generally carries a greater psychopathological risk than the loss of a parent through death (see Sandberg & Rutter, 2008).

In summary, although some traumatic events may be seen as unpredictable "acts of fate," many others show significant associations with risk and vulnerability factors. These differ by trauma type, but include: age, gender, a history of depression or of disruptive behavior problems in early childhood, and parental psychopathology, family relationship problems and/or parenting difficulties, and family adversity. Such factors appear to increase the risk for exposure to non-traumatic stressful life events as well as for trauma exposure, and these two sorts of events seem to cluster together in time. This social context of trauma exposure – specifically the clustering together of chronic adversity, stressful life events, and traumatic events – is especially relevant when considering broad outcomes. For example, many of the events associated with trauma include "exit events" (Goodyer, Herbert, Tamplin, & Altham, 2000) such as losses or personal disappointments which are strongly associated with adolescent depression, discussed in more detail below.

Developmental issues

Two reviews have examined the impact of development on reactions to trauma (Meiser-Stedman, 2002; Salmon & Bryant, 2002), addressing in some detail how language development, cognitive capacity, and memory encoding and retrieval play important roles in children's adjustment to trauma.

The diagnostic criteria for PTSD were developed initially for adults, and have been uneasily extended down the age range. Such downward application of adult criteria can be problematic for the reasons outlined in Cartwright-Hatton, Reynolds, and Wilson (Chapter 7, this volume). Of the three DSM-IV symptom clusters, it is symptoms of avoidance that remain the most adult-oriented. Many young people who present with cardinal intrusive symptoms, physiological overarousal, and clear impairment in functioning fail to reach DSM-IV diagnostic threshold because they present with insufficient avoidance symptoms. This applies to teenagers, but is especially true of younger children.

Very young children may not be able to report the sorts of symptoms described above. Instead, re-experiencing in the young child may be expressed in repetitive and trauma-thematic play. Likewise, although vivid nightmares involving the theme of the trauma are common in children of all ages, younger children may experience an increase in dreams that are not about the traumatic event as such, but which are nonetheless frightening. Dreams involving monsters, being chased, getting lost, or other threats to the self or loved ones are common.

In addition to differences in the way that some symptoms are expressed, very young children show a broader response to trauma, including behavior problems, new phobias (unrelated to the traumatic event), and clinginess. The clinical presentation of trauma-exposed preschool children is sufficiently different that Scheeringa and colleagues (Scheeringa, Peebles, Cook, & Zeanah, 2001; Scheeringa, Wright, Hunt, & Zeanah, 2006; Scheeringa, Zeanah, Drell, & Larrieu, 1995; Scheeringa, Zeanah, Myers, & Putnam, 2003) have developed and evaluated an alternative algorithm for diagnosing PTSD in preschool children, based on parent report of observations of children's behavior. Under Scheeringa *et al.*'s (2003) criteria, the number of symptoms required for each cluster is reduced, and an additional set of symptoms including new separation anxiety, new fears, and new aggression is added. Carefully conducted studies from Scheeringa's group and others (Ippen, Briscoe-Smith, & Lieberman, 2004; Meiser-Stedman, Smith, Glucksman, Yule, & Dalgleish, 2008; Ohmi *et al.*, 2002) suggest that these criteria are a sensitive, reliable, and valid means of diagnosing very young children's traumatic stress responses.

Cultural issues

Awareness of cultural aspects of mental health is crucial in planning services, and in individual assessment and treatment provision. Given the population diversity in many countries, this is relevant to all aspects of child and adolescent mental health. It is particularly important in relation to PTSD because traumatic events such as war and disaster occur globally. If appropriate help is to be provided for culturally diverse populations, the validity of Western frameworks for assessment and intervention should be investigated.

First, symptoms of post-traumatic stress have been reported in children from a variety of backgrounds, cultures, countries, and continents including Europe (e.g., Giannopoulou, Strouthos, Smith, Dikaiakou, Galanopoulou, & Yule, 2006), North America (e.g., Pynoos *et al.*, 2008), South America (e.g., Arroyo & Eth, 1985), the Middle East (e.g., Thabet, Karim, & Vostanis, 2006), Africa (e.g., Masinda & Muhesi, 2004), southeast Asia (Neuner, Schauer, Catani, Ruf, & Elbert, 2006), Australasia (e.g., Bryant, Salmon, Sinclair, & Davidson, 2007), and elsewhere (Perrin, Smith, & Yule, 2000).

Second, in an effort to address the debate about whether PTSD "transcends cultural barriers" (Sack, Seely, & Clarke, 1997), researchers have examined the factor structure of PTSD symptoms. It is reasoned that while differences in absolute scores between culturally diverse groups are to be expected, measurement instruments should possess similar under-lying factor structures when used with different populations if they are measuring the same construct. In studies to date, among Cambodian refugee youth (Sack *et al.*, 1997; Sack, Seeley, Him, & Clarke, 1998), Croatian children (Dyregrov, Kuterovac, & Barath, 1996), and children from Bosnia (Smith *et al.*, 2002), the factor structure of interview schedules and self-report measures closely resembled the structure of the same instruments when used with American and British children. As better child data sets are gathered, these issues can be properly addressed using confirmatory factor analysis as well as examining the construct validity of the scales used.

Third, ethnographic approaches have been used. In contrast to using self-report instru-ments, which may bias responses (and leave no room for respondents to report problems that do not fit neatly into the researchers' framework), ethnographic approaches employ open-ended methods, providing as little information as possible about what the interviewer is expecting. Using these methods, Bolton (2001) found that adult Rwandans' descriptions of post-genocide symptoms were very close to those described in the DSM-IV for PTSD (and depression), as well as to those described by Western patients. Further work using such an approach would be useful with children.

Although further research is needed, the available evidence suggests that post-traumatic stress reactions are not culture-bound. With some discrepancies, post-traumatic stress reactions in children and adolescents appear to be more similar across cultures than they are different.

Incidence, prevalence, and course

A handful of epidemiological investigations of childhood PTSD have been carried out. Methodology varies between studies, and a range of prevalence estimates for PTSD have been reported. Giaconia *et al.*'s (1995) early community survey found a lifetime prevalence of 6% by the age of 18, somewhat lower than the 8% lifetime prevalence reported for young adults in a large representative cohort study (Kessler *et al.*, 1995). Broadly in line with this, Elkit (2002) estimated 9% lifetime prevalence in a national sample of 8th grade Danish students. By contrast, a recent UK report, the National Survey of Mental Health (Meltzer, Gatward, Goodman, & Ford, 2003) found a point prevalence of 0.4% among 11–15-year-olds. Reporting on the Great Smoky Mountains Study of 9–16-year-olds, Copeland *et al.* (2007) reported a lifetime prevalence of 0.4%, and a 3-month prevalence of 0.1%. These authors suggest that the developmental insensitivity of the DSM-IV diagnostic criteria (as discussed above) may account in part for these much lower rates. Future community-based studies will help to clarify the issue, but for now it seems likely that at any one time point, up to 1% of children are likely to be suffering from PTSD (National Institute for Clinical Excellence, 2005) – a significant level of community morbidity.

These large-scale studies reveal that rates of PTSD in young people are far lower than the rates of trauma exposure outlined earlier. In other words, at a community level, most children exposed to trauma do not develop PTSD. This implies that trauma exposure alone is insufficient to explain the development of PTSD.

These findings are borne out in studies of at-risk children. Incidence rates among trauma-exposed young people in the studies above ranged from 15% (Giaconia *et al.*, 1995) to 3% for "subclinical PTSD" (Copeland *et al.*, 2007). In follow-up studies of children and adolescents involved in road traffic accidents or assaults, rates of between 20% and 30% are reported (Stallard, Salter, & Velleman, 2004; Meiser-Stedman *et al.*, 2007).

Studies of child survivors of large-scale disasters such as earthquakes, floods, hurricanes, and terrorist attacks report incidence rates ranging from 10% to 80% (Giannopoulou *et al.*, 2006, Green *et al.*, 1991; Pfefferbaum, DeVoe, Stuber, Schiff, Klein, & Fairbrother, 2004; Pynoos *et al.*, 1993; Vernberg, La Greca, Silverman, & Prinstein, 1996). This wide range of incidence estimates probably reflects various methodological variations between studies, including different informants, measurement instruments, and time elapsed since trauma, but the message is clear: generally, only a minority of children who are exposed to trauma develop PTSD.

Finally, of those who develop PTSD, a proportion will recover spontaneously. For example, when assessed 14 days after attending hospital, almost 25% of young people aged 10 to 18 who had been assaulted or involved in a traffic accident met criteria for PTSD (except the 1-month duration criterion). Six months later, although none of the young people had received treatment, this figure had halved to 12% (Meiser-Stedman *et al.*, 2005). These findings are in line with studies of adults exposed to trauma, which show the most substantial natural recovery occurring in the first 6 months (e.g., Breslau *et al.*, 1998). Although some young people will recover spontaneously, PTSD can last for many years in a significant minority of children if left untreated. Yule and colleagues' (Yule, Bolton, Udwin, Boyle, O'Ryan, & Nurrish, 2000) follow-up of teenagers involved in a shipping accident found that of the 51% who develop PTSD initially, one-third continued to meet diagnostic criteria 5–8 years later. A long-term 33-year follow-up of child survivors of the Aberfan disaster (in which a coal heap collapsed onto a primary school, killing 116 children) showed that PTSD can persist for decades, into adulthood, for a significant minority of trauma-exposed children (Morgan, Scourfield, Williams, Jasper, & Lewis, 2003).

In summary, most children exposed to trauma do not develop PTSD. Of those who do, a proportion will recover spontaneously. This implies that trauma exposure is necessary for PTSD to occur, but that it is not sufficient. What other factors influence who will go on to develop a persistent PTSD following exposure to traumatic events?

Dose–response relationship

Several studies have addressed the "dose–response" issue of whether there is a quantifiable relationship between the type, number, and severity of traumatic events, and later PTSD.

Type of traumatic event

Despite methodological differences between studies, it is clear that some events result in higher rates of PTSD than others. Highest rates are found for rape, physical assault, and violent death of a loved one; lowest rates are found for witnessing or learning about events that have happened to others (Copeland *et al.*, 2007; Giaconia *et al.*, 1995).

Number of traumatic events

Among adults, prior exposure to traumatic events is consistently found to be a significant risk for developing PTSD in relation to the most recent traumatic event (Brewin, Andrews, & Valentine, 2000; Ozer, Best, Lipsey, & Weiss, 2003). That is, exposure seems to have a sensitizing rather than an inoculating effect in adults. Elkit (2002) found the same to be true in a sample of young teenagers: those who had been exposed to more than one event were at greater risk than those who had been exposed to one event. Copeland *et al.* (2007) found that the prognosis in older teenagers after exposure to a first lifetime traumatic event was generally favorable, whereas those reporting PTSD symptoms were more likely to have had previous exposure to trauma. Among a particularly high-risk population – children living through war – Smith, Perrin, Dyregov, and Yule (2003) found a significant relation between the number of traumatic war experiences and children's level of PTSD symptoms.

Severity of traumatic events

The severity of children's exposure to traumatic events is also related to the risk for developing PTSD. For example, Pynoos et al. (1993) studied three large groups of children following an earthquake in Armenia – one from a town at the epicenter where buildings were totally destroyed; one from a town on the periphery; and one from a city outside the affected area. A clear relation was demonstrated, with those close to the epicenter showing more PTSD symptoms. Vernberg et al. (1996) studied the effects on children exposed to a severe hurricane. Using a specially developed Hurricane-Related Traumatic Experiences questionnaire and the children's post-traumatic stress reaction ratings, the authors found that greater exposure to the hurricane was strongly associated with more PTS symptoms. Giannopoulou et al. (2006) confirmed a similar relation among children exposed to an earthquake in Greece.

Although there is now fairly consistent evidence, using a variety of methodologies, that the type, number, and severity of exposure to traumatic events is related to children's risk for later PTSD (and the severity of PTS symptoms), these trauma-related factors explain only a modest proportion of the variance in outcome. Recent work has therefore attempted to discover additional factors that will help to explain who develops persistent PTSD in the face of trauma.

Other risk and maintaining factors

A growing number of studies have addressed this issue in adults, with two recent meta-analyses reporting broadly compatible findings. Brewin et al. (2000) included 77 studies to examine the effect of demographic and other factors on the risk for persistent PTSD. Each of 14 potential risk factors was significant, although risk factors showed a range of effect sizes, and there was considerable heterogeneity in the size of the effect depending on the trauma type. The strongest effect overall was for post-trauma social support. Ozer et al. (2003) investigated the role of seven potential risk factors in a meta-analysis of 68 studies. Small but significant effects were found for pre-trauma risk factors such as prior trauma exposure, previous psychological adjustment, and family history of mental health problems. Larger effects were found for peri-traumatic factors such as perceived life threat, peri-traumatic dissociation, and peri-traumatic emotional responses, and for social support in the aftermath of the trauma.

Fewer studies have been carried out with children (see Pine and Cohen, 2002, for a review). To date, a variety of approaches have been used. Retrospective (e.g., Udwin, Boyle, Yule, Bolton, & O'Ryan, 2000) and longitudinal epidemiological studies (e.g., Copeland, et al., 2007) have investigated demographic risks and personal vulnerability factors for developing post-traumatic stress symptoms following exposure to traumatic events. Prospective studies (e.g., Bryant et al., 2007; Meiser-Stedman et al., 2007) have investigated post-trauma memory processes and cognitive factors in exposed young people.

Demographic risks and personal vulnerability factors

Mirroring Brewin et al.'s (2000) meta-analysis with adults, conditional risks for young people to develop PTSD following trauma differ according to trauma type and study characteristics. Some consistent themes emerge from the relatively small literature. Age and gender are significant predictors, with females and adolescents being at higher risk than males and younger children (e.g., Copeland *et al.*, 2007; Kilpatrick, Ruggiero, Acierno, Saunders, Resnick, & Best, 2003; Udwin *et al.*, 2000). A history of psychological difficulties, especially anxiety problems (e.g., Breslau *et al.*, 2006; Copeland *et al.*, 2007; La Greca, Silverman, & Wasserstein, 1998; Udwin *et al.*, 2000; Weems, Pina, Costa, Watts, Taylor, & Cannon, 2007), and to a lesser extent depression and low self-esteem (e.g., Lengua, Long, Smith, & Meltzoff, 2005) or behavioral difficulties (e.g., Breslau *et al.*, 2006) also predict later PTSD. An adverse family environment, indexed by coming from an impoverished or poorly educated home (Copeland *et al.*, 2007), family drug and alcohol use problems (Kilpatrick *et al.*, 2003), or maternal symptoms of PTSD and depression (e.g., Meiser-Stedman, Yule, Dalgleish, Smith, & Glucksman, 2006), also appear to influence children's trauma responses. In line with adult risk factors, availability and quality of social support post-trauma shows fairly robust moderating influences (Laor, Wolmer, & Cohen, 2001; Udwin *et al.*, 2000).

Cognitive factors

Recent prospective studies have tested the applicability of adult cognitive models in explaining children's PTSD reactions (Dalgleish, Meiser-Stedman, & Smith, 2005). Such models have been fruitful in understanding adults' post-traumatic stress reactions, and have led to effective treatments (e.g., Ehlers, Clark, Hackmann, McManus, & Fennell, 2005). Ehlers and Clark's (2000) cognitive model of PTSD has generated considerable interest. Under this model, persistent PTSD arises when a sense of "current threat" is generated as a function of two key factors: (1) a disjointed and heavily sensory laden trauma memory and (2) idiosyncratic misappraisals of the trauma and reactions to it. These in turn lead to a variety of unhelpful coping strategies such as cognitive and behavioral avoidance, rumination, and use of safety behaviors.

There is now growing evidence that cognitive factors are important in children's reactions to trauma. For example, in a prospective study of 10–16-year-olds who attended hospital following an assault or road traffic accident, Meiser-Stedman *et al.* (2006, 2007) found that the presence of sensory-based memories at 2–4 weeks post-trauma was related to the severity of later PTSD symptoms at 6 months post-trauma. This work requires replication (e.g., see Stallard *et al.*, 2004; Stallard & Smith, 2007 for negative findings) and extension to younger samples; but appears promising. Idiosyncratic misappraisals of the trauma and sequelae also have been shown to play a key role in several recent studies (Ehlers, Mayou, & Bryant, 2003; Lengua, Long, & Meltzoff, 2006; Meiser-Stedman *et al.*, 2007; Stallard & Smith, 2007). Salmon, Sinclair, and Bryant (2007) found that misappraisals measured by the children's Post Traumatic Cognitions Inventory (cPTCI) (Meiser-Stedman *et al.*, 2009) accounted for 44% of the variance in ASD symptoms among 7–13-year-old children who had been hospitalized after traumatic injury. When this group of children was followed up at 6 months post-trauma, the majority of the variance in post-traumatic stress symptom severity was accounted for by negative appraisals about future harm (Bryant *et al.*, 2007). With regard to unhelpful coping strategies, there is evidence from retrospective (Udwin *et al.*, 2000) and prospective studies of children (Meiser-Stedman, 2002; Stallard, 2003) that cognitive and behavioral avoidance, and thought control strategies such as rumination and thought suppression, serve to maintain post-traumatic stress symptoms in children and young people.

In summary, a variety of factors explain why only a minority of children go on to develop persistent PTSD in the face of trauma. These include demographic and personal vulnerability factors. Recent work shows that theoretically derived cognitive factors play a key role, explaining the majority of the variance in outcome in several studies. This in turn has led to the development and evaluation of effective interventions (see below).

Arousal physiology

Exposure to traumatic events may also lead to changes in arousal physiology in children (see also Pine, Chapter 9, this volume). Contemporary neuroscience accounts of fear and stress have focused on two major stress systems – the catecholamine system and the hypothalamic–pituitary–adrenal (HPA) axis (see Cohen, Perel, DeBellis, Friedman, & Putnam, 2002; DeBellis, 2001; Pine, 2003 for reviews).

First, there is converging evidence that the catecholamine system is disrupted in traumatized children. For example, DeBellis et al. (DeBellis, Baum, et al., 1999; DeBellis, Chrousos, et al., 1994; DeBellis, Keshavan, et al., 1999) reported significantly increased urinary dopamine and increased 24-hour urinary adrenaline and noradrenaline (or their metabolites) in sexually abused girls, and in maltreated children with PTSD. Consistent with a malfunctioning adrenergic response, Perry (1994) found that abused children with PTSD had greater increases in heart rate when exposed to a physiological challenge, compared to non-PTSD control children. Scheeringa, Zeanah, Myers, and Putnam (2004) found that preschool children with PTSD also showed increased heart rate in response to trauma reminders, compared to non-traumatized controls. Acute changes in such peripheral physiology may predict later symptoms of post-traumatic stress in children. For example, Kassam-Adams and Winston (2004) reported that among children involved in road traffic accidents, acute heart rate (measured in hospital within hours of the accident) was significantly associated with severity of post-traumatic stress symptoms some 6 months later.

Second, investigations of HPA axis functioning in traumatized children show that this system works in a rather complex manner. In acutely traumatized children, there is evidence for hypersecretion of cortisol (e.g., Carrion, Weems, Ray, Glaser, Hessl, & Reiss, 2002). In contrast, investigations of children with chronic PTSD reveal lower baseline levels of cortisol (e.g., Goenjian et al., 1996) and a blunted corticotrophin response (DeBellis et al., 1994). It is plausible that compensatory downregulation of the HPA axis occurs in children with chronic PTSD, resulting in an increasingly maladaptive response over time. In addition, children with a history of severe maltreatment plus concurrent exposure to new stressors showed an increased corticotrophin response in one study (Kaufman et al., 1997), suggesting that individuals with history of chronic PTSD may demonstrate a hyperresponsive HPA axis when encountering new stressors. Evidence for disruption to the HPA axis has led to the administration of low-dose cortisol to treat symptoms of PTSD in adults (Aerni et al., 2004), but similar treatments have not yet been tested in children.

There is growing evidence that children with symptoms of PTSD may show alterations to a number of interrelated neurophysiological systems. Further research to develop a better understanding of the complex interplay between physiological and psychological responses to traumatic events is needed.

Broad reactions to trauma

All available data show that risk for a broad range of psychiatric disorders in children and adolescents is increased following trauma exposure, and that PTSD as the sole outcome of trauma exposure is rare. For example, Copeland et al.'s (2007) report of the Great Smoky Mountains Study showed that children exposed to trauma had almost double the rates of a broad range of disorders compared to those who were not exposed; and that 60% of those with significant post-traumatic stress symptoms met criteria for another psychiatric disorder. Bolton *et al.*'s (2000) follow-up study of teenagers involved in a shipping accident also found that survivors showed significantly higher rates of general psychopathology compared to non-exposed controls; and that more than 80% of those with PTSD met criteria for another disorder. The USA National Survey of Adolescents (Kilpatrick *et al.*, 2003) found that almost 75% of those with PTSD also met criteria for another disorder.

Other anxiety disorders

Giaconia *et al.* (1995) reported raised rates of specific phobia and social anxiety in adolescents exposed to trauma compared to those who were not exposed. Among a large community sample, rates of anxiety disorders including separation anxiety, generalized anxiety, and social anxiety were between twice (social anxiety) and six times (separation anxiety) as likely in those exposed to trauma compared to the non-exposed group (Copeland *et al.*, 2007). Bolton *et al.* (2000) found that 40% of over 200 adolescent survivors of a shipping accident met criteria for an anxiety disorder other than PTSD; rates of specific phobia (24%), panic disorder (12%), and separation anxiety (7%) were significantly higher in the survivors compared to controls. It is also likely that there are developmental differences in presentation, with for example separation anxiety being common in young children exposed to trauma, and social anxiety for example being relatively more common in teenagers.

The high rates of comorbidity in Bolton *et al.*'s (2000) follow-up study meant that most of those with an anxiety disorder also met criteria for a diagnosis of PTSD. This led to the suggestion that the increased rates of phobia may be conceptualized as a subset of PTSD symptoms; that increased separation anxiety (among the adolescent sample) may be an example of trauma-related regression; and that increased rates of panic disorder may be a complication of trauma-related changes in arousal physiology, as discussed above. Additionally, increased rates of anxiety disorders may occur in the absence of PTSD: here, learning theory and conditioning models may be useful in understanding various pathways from trauma exposure to anxiety disorder (see Field & Purkis, Chapter 11, this volume). Cognitive models on the other hand (e.g., see Dalgleish & Power, 2004) might imply that basic assumptions regarding attachment and security can be violated by exposure to trauma, leading to separation anxiety, and so on. While traumatic events are "threat" events known to be associated with a range of anxiety difficulties (e.g., Eley & Stevenson, 2000), further work will help to clarify the mechanisms and pathways involved.

Depression

Rates of depressive disorders are also raised among trauma-exposed young people compared to non-exposed groups; and depression is often comorbid with PTSD. Copeland *et al.* (2007) found depression to be more than three times as common in trauma-exposed adolescents compared to those who were not exposed; and more than seven times as common in those with significant PTSD symptoms compared to those without such symptoms. Bolton *et al.* (2000) reported that rates of depression among adolescent survivors of a shipping accident were almost as high (38%) as rates of anxiety disorders (other than PTSD). Nearly two-thirds of those with PTSD also met criteria for an affective disorder. Similarly, Giaconia *et al.* (1995) found far higher rates of depression among those adolescents with

PTSD (42%) compared to those who did not develop PTSD following exposure (9%) and to those who were not exposed to traumatic events (6%).

Several accounts of these raised rates of affective disorders have been suggested. First, given the high comorbidity, it is important to note that there is some symptom overlap between the two disorders: many of the symptoms of avoidance in PTSD could be endorsed as symptoms of depression; and many people with depression show intrusive thinking and related cognitive avoidance (e.g., Brewin, Hunter, Carroll, & Tata, 1996). Second, depression may arise as a secondary consequence of PTSD: trauma-related avoidance may mean that young people have less opportunity to be engaging in pleasurable or rewarding activities, for example. Third, while trauma-related appraisals often have to do with extreme threat, they may also concern loss. This may be related to loss of future goals or "cherished ideas" (Brown & Harris, 1978) as well as loss of a relationship or the death of friends or family. Dalgleish and Power (2004) have detailed how trauma-related appraisals of loss or failure may lead to depression when they are sufficiently discrepant from pre-existing schema or beliefs. Fourth, there is an extensive literature on the role of negative life events in the onset of depression in adults (Brown & Harris, 1978) and adolescents (Goodyer et al., 2000). Given that acute life events – constituting losses, disappointments, and "exit events" (Goodyer et al., 2000) – tend to cluster with traumatic events, then high rates of depression following trauma are to be expected. Last, there may be common mechanisms that maintain both disorders, such as ruminative thinking (Kuyken, Watkins, Holden, & Cook, 2006; Nolen-Hoeksema, 2000).

Other disorders

There is mixed evidence for raised rates of other disorders, beyond anxiety and affective disorders. Higher rates of substance use disorder were found by Giaconia et al. (1995) in a sample of urban adolescents with PTSD. In line with this, Kilpatrick et al. (2003) found that exposure to interpersonal violence increased significantly the risk for substance use disorders, after controlling for demographic and family risk factors. In contrast, elevated rates of substance abuse/dependence were not found in Copeland et al.'s (2007) Great Smoky Mountain Study, nor in the Jupiter shipping accident follow-up study (Bolton et al., 2000).

Disruptive behavior disorder, specifically conduct disorder, was found to be around twice as common in trauma-exposed young people compared to non-exposed groups by Copeland et al. (2007). As with PTSD, the risk for behavior problems was raised incrementally with increasing exposure to a greater number of traumatic events. Shaw et al. (1995) also reported an association between oppositional defiant disorder and post-traumatic stress symptoms among elementary school age children who had been exposed to a hurricane.

Traumatic grief reactions may result when the traumatic event includes the death of a loved one (Dyregrov, 2008). In such cases, unresolved grief reactions such as yearning or searching for the dead person, or a lack of acceptance of the death may occur alongside post-traumatic stress reactions (Cohen, Mannarino, & Staron, 2006). Intrusive memories often are of the violent sudden death itself: the young person may become overwhelmed by such intrusive memories, which in turn impedes the normal resolution of grief issues (Dyregrov, 2008; Layne et al., 2001). This syndrome has been termed childhood traumatic grief (CTG) by Cohen and colleagues (e.g., Cohen, Mannarino, Greenberg, Padlo, & Shipley, 2002; Cohen et al., 2006), and is a promising area for future research.

Treatment

With increasing understanding of children's and adolescents' reactions to traumatic events, the development and evaluation of effective interventions has continued. Recent reviews have highlighted the growing evidence for cognitive–behavioral therapy (CBT) for childhood post-traumatic stress reactions (Feeny, Foa, Treadwell, & March, 2004; National Institute for Clinical Excellence, 2005; Silverman *et al.*, 2008; Stallard, 2006). A variety of approaches is used, but common elements include psycho-education about the nature of PTSD and its treatment, imaginal exposure to the traumatic event, in vivo exposure to traumatic reminders, relaxation training, cognitive restructuring, and work with parents (Silverman *et al.*, 2008; Smith, Perrin, Yule, & Clark, 2010).

The largest evidence base is for the treatment of post-traumatic stress reactions (including PTSD symptoms and externalizing problems) in children who have been sexually abused (reviewed by Ramchandani & Jones, 2003). For example, pioneering work by Deblinger, Cohen and colleagues led to a series of studies that demonstrated that trauma-focused CBT (TF-CBT) is effective in treating the broad psychological effects of sexual abuse among 3–16-year-old children and adolescents (e.g., Cohen, Deblinger, Mannarino, & Steer, 2004; Cohen, Mannarino, & Knudsen, 2005).

There is also evidence that both group (e.g., Stein, Jaycox, Kataoka, Wong, Tu, & Elliott, 2003) and individual CBT (e.g., Smith, Yule, Perrin, Tranah, Dalgleish, & Clark, 2007) are effective in treating PTSD that has arisen from single-event trauma such as interpersonal violence and accidents. It is interesting to note that in both of these randomized controlled trials, there was significant improvement in comorbid conditions such as anxiety and depression when PTSD was specifically targeted and successfully treated. A modified CBT approach for preschool children has been developed by Scheeringa, Salloum, Arnberger, Weems, Amaya-Jackson, and Cohen (2007), with promising results.

Encouraging results also have been reported for a modified individual CBT protocol to treat children presenting with traumatic grief reactions (Cohen *et al.*, 2004, 2006). This approach combines treatment of PTSD symptoms followed by grief-focused interventions.

For children affected by war and disaster, group approaches have been preferred. For example, following a devastating earthquake in Armenia, Goenjian and colleagues (Goenjian, Walling, Steinberg, Karayan, Najarian, & Pynoos, 2005) showed that an eclectic model of treatment using group approaches supplemented by individual sessions was effective in reducing symptoms of PTSD and depression. Using a somewhat different approach for children affected by an earthquake in Greece, Giannoupoulou, Dikaiakou, and Yule (2006) found that a short-term group CBT intervention (available at www.childrenandwar.org) was effective in reducing symptoms of PTSD and depression – treatment gains were maintained at 18-month and 4-year follow-up. Layne *et al.* (2008) found that for children affected by war, classroom-based interventions and group therapy were both associated with reductions in PTSD and depression symptoms; group therapy was associated with improvement in grief reactions.

The treatment outcome literature for childhood PTSD shows that a variety of CBT approaches can be effective in helping traumatized young people. Treatments have been appropriately modified according to the nature of the trauma, and the age of the affected children. The available literature is small relative to the adult treatment outcome literature, and further replication and extension is required, especially in the form of randomized controlled trials. In the context of findings on broad effects of exposure to traumatic events, it is notable that most treatment outcome evaluations report on broad outcomes, including but not restricted to PTSD. Whether or not broad-spectrum problems are explicitly targeted, improvement across multiple domains is the norm.

Having noted the welcome increase in the number of studies of the treatment of PTSD in children and adolescents, it has to be acknowledged that the low level of investment in child treatment research means that it is difficult to make definitive conclusions and generalizations. As noted, many of the studies deal with children traumatized by sexual abuse so it is unclear how far findings from such studies generalize to those where children are subject to other physical abuse or interpersonal violence or road traffic accidents, let alone to war or natural disasters. In a recent review, Silverman *et al.* (2008) note the high quality of the studies they considered and concluded that in future there should be attention paid to developing a core set of measures of PTSD as well as depression and conduct problems. There is a need for larger studies with more adequate power to detect moderate effects sizes and longer follow-up is essential. It is premature to talk of dismantling studies before good replications have been completed. As noted earlier, many more studies of very young children are overdue. Finally, studies should incorporate broader measures of predictor, moderator, and mediator variables so that the healing processes can be better understood and enhanced.

Summary

Exposure to traumatic events is common in young people, especially among older adolescents. Although some traumatic events may be seen as chance "acts of fate," others are more or less predictable to the extent that a range of risk factors for exposure have been consistently identified across different studies. Following exposure to trauma, only a minority of young people develop persistent PTSD, most of whom will recover spontaneously within a few months. Over and above trauma-related factors (such as the number, type, and severity of exposure), a range of demographic and personal vulnerability factors can help to explain why some young people develop persistent PTSD. Factors derived from cognitive models, such as memory functioning, appraisal process, and unhelpful coping, are especially important because they account for a large proportion of the variance in outcome.

Exposure to trauma has broad effects in that rates of general psychopathology, particularly other anxiety disorders and depression, as well as externalizing problems and substance abuse, are raised among trauma-exposed young people. Substantial comorbidity of other disorders with PTSD is clearly the norm. The growing treatment outcome literature has focused on PTSD, but explicitly addresses these broad outcomes, and results for a variety of CBT approaches are generally favorable. Further research will help to detail more clearly the complex relationships between traumatic events and a range of psychological difficulties, and it is hoped that this will lead to the further development and dissemination of effective treatments for young people.

References

Aerni, A., Traber, R., Hock, C., Roozendaal, B., Schelling, G., Papassotiropoulos, A., *et al.* (2004). Low dose cortisol for symptoms of posttraumatic stress disorder. *American Journal of Psychiatry,* **161**, 1488–1490.

American Psychiatric Association (1980). *Diagnostic and Statistical Manual of Mental Disorders,* 3rd edn. Washington, DC: American Psychiatric Association.

American Psychiatric Association (1987). *Diagnostic and Statistical Manual of Mental Disorders*, 3rd edn revised. Washington, DC: American Psychiatric Association.

American Psychiatric Association (1994). *Diagnostic and Statistical Manual of Mental Disorders*, 4th edn. Washington, DC: American Psychiatric Association.

American Psychiatric Association (2000). *Diagnostic and Statistical Manual of Mental Disorders*, 4th edn, text revision. Washington, DC: American Psychiatric Association.

Arroyo, W. & **Eth, S.** (1985). Children traumatized in Central American warfare. In: **S. Eth** & **R. Pynoos** (eds.) *Post Traumatic Stress Disorder in Children*, pp. 101–120. Washington, DC: American Psychiatric Press.

Bayer, C., Klasen, F., & **Adam, H.** (2007). Association of trauma and PTSD symptoms with openness to reconciliation and feelings of revenge among former Ugandan and Congolese child soldiers. *Journal of the American Medical Association*, **298**, 555–559.

Bolton, D. & **Hill, J.** (1996). *Mind, Meaning, and Mental Disorder: The Nature of Causal Explanation in Psychology and Psychiatry*. New York: Oxford University Press.

Bolton, D., O'Ryan, D., Udwin, O., Boyle, S., & **Yule, W.** (2000). The long-term psychological effects of a disaster experienced in adolescence. II: General psychopathology. *Journal of Child Psychology and Psychiatry*, **41**, 513–523.

Bolton, P. (2001). Local perceptions of the mental health effects of the Rwandan genocide. *Journal of Nervous and Mental Disease*, **189**, 243–248.

Boney-McCoy, S. & **Finkelhor, D.** (1995). Psychological sequelae of violent victimization in a national sample of youth. *Journal of Consulting and Clinical Psychology*, **63**, 726–736.

Breslau, N. & **Kessler, R.** (2001). The stressor criterion in DSM-IV post traumatic stress disorder: an empirical investigation. *Biological Psychiatry*, **50**, 699–704.

Breslau, N., Davis, G., Peterson, E., & **Schultz, L.** (2000). A second look at comorbidity in victims of trauma: the posttraumatic stress disorder–major depression connection. *Biological Psychiatry*, **48**, 902–909.

Breslau, N., Kessler, R., Chilcoat, H., Schultz, L., Davis, G., & **Andreski, P.** (1998). Trauma and posttraumatic stress disorder in the community: the 1996 Detroit Area Survey of Trauma. *Archives of General Psychiatry*, **55**, 626–632.

Breslau, N., Lucia, V., & **Alvarado, G.** (2006). Intelligence and other predisposing factors in exposure to trauma and posttraumatic stress disorder. *Archives of General Psychiatry*, **63**, 238–245.

Brewin, C. R., Andrews, B., & **Valentine, J. D.** (2000). Meta-analysis of risk factors for posttraumatic stress disorder in trauma-exposed adults. *Journal of Consulting and Clinical Psychology*, **68**, 747–766.

Brewin, C. R., Hunter, E., Carroll, F., & **Tata, P.** (1996). Intrusive memories in depression: an index of schema activation? *Psychological Medicine*, **26**, 1271–1276.

Brown, G. & **Harris, T.** (1978). *The Social Origins of Depression: A Study of Psychiatric Disorder in Women*. London: Tavistock Press.

Bryant, R. A., Salmon, K., Sinclair, E., & **Davidson, P.** (2007). A prospective study of appraisals in childhood posttraumatic stress disorder. *Behaviour Research and Therapy*, **45**, 2502–2507.

Carrion, V. G., Weems, C. F., Ray, R. D., Glaser, B. H., Hessl, D., & **Reiss, A. L.** (2002). Diurnal salivary cortisol in pediatric posttraumatic stress disorder. *Biological Psychiatry*, **51**, 575–582.

Cohen, J. A., Deblinger, E., Mannarino, A. P., & **Steer, R. A.** (2004). A multisite randomized controlled trial for children with sexual abuse-related PTSD symptoms. *Journal of the American Academy of Child and Adolescent Psychiatry*, **43**, 393–402.

Cohen, J. A., Mannarino, A. P., & **Deblinger, E.** (2006). *Treating Trauma and Traumatic Grief in Children and Adolescents*. New York: Guilford Press.

Cohen, J., Mannarino, A., Greenberg, T., Padlo, S., & Shipley, C. (2002). Childhood traumatic grief: concepts and controversies. *Trauma, Violence, and Abuse*, **3**, 307–327.

Cohen, J., Mannarino, A., & Knudsen, K. (2005). Treating sexually abused children: 1 year follow-up of a randomized controlled trial. *Child Abuse and Neglect*, **29**, 135–145.

Cohen, J., Mannarino, A., & Staron, V. (2006). A pilot study of modified cognitive behavioral therapy for childhood traumatic grief (CBT-CTG). *Journal of the American Academy of Child and Adolescent Psychiatry*, **45**, 1465–1473.

Cohen, J. A., Perel, J. M., DeBellis, M., Friedman, M., & Putnam, F. W. (2002). Treating traumatized children: clinical implications of the psychobiology of posttraumatic stress disorder. *Trauma, Violence, and Abuse*, **3**, 91–108.

Copeland, W. E., Keeler, G., Angold, A., & Costello, E. J. (2007). Traumatic events and posttraumatic stress in childhood. *Archives of General Psychiatry*, **64**, 577–584.

Costello, E. J., Erkanli, A., Fairbank, J., & Angold, A. (2002). The prevalence of potentially traumatic events in childhood and adolescence. *Journal of Traumatic Stress*, **15**, 99–112.

Dalgleish, T. (2004). Cognitive approaches to posttraumatic stress disorder: the evolution of multirepresentational theorizing. *Psychological Bulletin*, **130**, 228–260.

Dalgleish, T. & Power, M. (2004). Emotion-specific and emotion-non-specific components of posttraumatic stress disorder (PTSD): implications for a taxonomy of related psychopathology. *Behaviour Research and Therapy*, **42**, 1069–1088.

Dalgleish, T., Meiser-Stedman, R., Kassam-Adams, N., Ehlers, A., Winston, F., Smith, P., et al. (2008). Predictive value of acute stress disorder in children and adolescents. *British Journal of Psychiatry*, **192**, 392–393.

Dalgleish, T., Meiser-Stedman, R., & Smith, P. (2005). Cognitive aspects of posttraumatic stress reactions and their treatment in children and adolescents: an empirical review and some recommendations. *Behavioural and Cognitive Psychotherapy*, **33**, 459–486.

DeBellis, M. (2001). Developmental traumatology: the psychobiological development of maltreated children and its implications for research, treatment, and policy. *Development and Psychopathology*, **13**, 539–564.

DeBellis, M. D., Baum, A. S., Birmaher, B., Keshavan, M. S., Eccard, C. H., Boring, A. M., et al. (1999). Developmental traumatology. I. Biological stress systems. *Biological Psychiatry*, **45**, 1259–1270.

DeBellis, M. D., Chrousos, G. P., Dorn, L. D., Burke, L., Helmers, K., Kling, M. A., et al. (1994). Hypothalamic–pituitary–adrenal axis dysregulation in sexually abused girls. *Journal of Clinical Endocrinology and Metabolism*, **78**, 249–255.

DeBellis, M. D., Keshavan, M. S, Clark, D. B., Casey, B. J, Giedd, J. N., Boring, A. M., et al. (1999). Developmental traumatology. II Brain development. *Biological Psychiatry*, **45**, 1271–1284.

Deblinger, E., Steer, R. A., & Lippmann, J. (1999). Two-year follow-up study of cognitive behavioral therapy for sexually abused children suffering post-traumatic stress symptoms. *Child Abuse and Neglect*, **23**, 1371–1378.

Dyregrov, A. (2008). *Grief in Children: A Handbook for Adults*, 2nd edn. London: Jessica Kingsley.

Dyregrov, A., Kuterovac, G., & Barath, A. (1996). Factor analysis of the Impact of Event Scale with children in war. *Scandinavian Journal of Psychology*, **37**, 339–350.

Ehlers, A. & Clark, D. M. (2000). A cognitive model of posttraumatic stress disorder. *Behaviour Research and Therapy*, **38**, 319–345.

Ehlers, A., Clark, D.M., Hackmann, A., McManus, F., & Fennell, M. (2005). Cognitive therapy for PTSD: development and evaluation. *Behaviour Research and Therapy*, **43**, 413–431.

Ehlers, A., Mayou, R. A., & Bryant, B. (2003). Cognitive predictors of posttraumatic stress disorder in children: results of a prospective longitudinal study. *Behaviour Research and Therapy*, **41**, 1–10.

Eley, T. & **Stevenson, J.** (2000). Specific life events and chronic experiences differentially associated with depression and anxiety in young twins. *Journal of Abnormal Child Psychology*, **28**, 383–394.

Elkit, A. (2002). Victimization and PTSD in a Danish national youth probability sample. *Journal of the American Academy of Child and Adolescent Psychiatry*, **41**, 174–181.

Feeny, N. C., Foa, E. B., Treadwell, K. R., & **March, J.** (2004). Posttraumatic stress disorder in youth: a critical review of the cognitive and behavioral treatment outcome literature. *Professional Psychology: Research and Practice*, **35**, 466–476.

Foa, E. B. & **Kozak, M. J.** (1986). Emotional processing of fear: exposure to corrective information. *Psychological Bulletin*, **99**, 20–35.

Foa, E. B., Steketee, G., & **Olasov-Rothbaum, B.** (1989). Behavioral/cognitive conceptualizations of post-traumatic stress disorder. *Behavior Therapy*, **20**, 155–176.

Giaconia, R. M., Reinherz, H. Z., Silverman, A. B., Pakiz, B., Frost, A. K., & **Cohen, E.** (1995). Traumas and posttraumatic stress disorder in a community population of older adolescents. *Journal of the American Academy of Child and Adolescent Psychiatry*, **34**, 1369–1380.

Giannopoulou, I., Dikaiakou, A., & **Yule, W.** (2006). Cognitive-behavioral group intervention for PTSD symptoms in children following the Athens 1999 earthquake: a pilot study. *Clinical Child Psychology and Psychiatry*, **11**, 543–553.

Giannopoulou, I., Strouthos, M., Smith, P., Dikaiakou, A., Galanopoulou, V., & **Yule, W.** (2006). Post-traumatic stress reactions of children and adolescents exposed to the Athens 1999 earthquake. *European Psychiatry*, **21**, 160–166.

Goenjian, A., Walling, D., Steinberg, A., Karayan, I., Najarian, L., & **Pynoos, R.** (2005). A prospective study of posttraumatic stress and depressive reactions among treated and untreated adolescents 5 years after a catastrophic disaster. *American Journal of Psychiatry*, **162**, 2302–2308.

Goenjian, A. K., Yehuda, R., Pynoos, R. S. Steinberg, A. M., Tashian, M., Yaug, R., *et al.* (1996). Basal cortisol, dexamethasone suppression of cortisol, and MHPG in adolescents after the 1988 earthquake in Armenia. *American Journal of Psychiatry*, **153**, 929–934.

Goodyer, I. M., Herbert, J., Tamplin, A., & **Altham, P.** (2000). Recent life events, cortisol, dehydroepiandrosterone and the onset of major depression in high risk adolescents. *British Journal of Psychiatry*, **177**, 499–504.

Green, B. L., Korol, M., Grace, M. C., Vary, M. G., Leonard, A. C., Glesser, G. C., *et al.* (1991). Children and disaster: age, gender, and parental effects on PTSD symptoms. *Journal of the American Academy of Child and Adolescent Psychiatry*, **30**, 945–951.

Ippen, C., Briscoe-Smith, A., & **Lieberman, A.** (2004). PTSD symptomatology in young children. Paper presented at the 20th Annual Meeting of the International Society for Traumatic Stress Studies. New Orleans, LA.

Janoff-Bulman, R. (1985). The aftermath of victimization: rebuilding shattered assumptions. In: **C. R. Figley** (ed.) *Trauma and its Wake*, pp. 15–35. New York: Brunner/Mazel.

Kassam-Adams, N. & **Winston, F. K.** (2004). Predicting child PTSD: the relationship between acute stress disorder and PTSD in injured children. *Journal of the American Academy of Child and Adolescent Psychiatry*, **43**, 403–411.

Kaufman, J., Birmaher, B., Perel, J., Dahl, R. E., Moreci, P., Nelson, B., *et al.* (1997). The corticotropin-releasing hormone challenge in depressed abused, depressed non-abused, and normal control children. *Biological Psychiatry*, **42**, 669–679.

Kessler, R. C., Sonnega, A., Bromet, E., Hughes, M., & **Nelson, C. B.** (1995). Posttraumatic stress disorder in the National Comorbidity Survey. *Archives of General Psychiatry*, **52**, 1048–1060.

Kilpatrick, D., Ruggiero, K., Acierno, R., Saunders, B., Resnick, H., & **Best, C.** (2003). Violence and risk of PTSD, major depression, substance abuse/dependence, and comorbidity: results from the National Survey of Adolescents. *Journal of Consulting and Clinical Psychology*, **71**, 692–700.

Kuyken, W., Watkins, E., Holden, E., & Cook, W. (2006). Rumination in adolescents at risk for depression. *Journal of Affective Disorders*, **96**, 39–47.

La Greca, A. M., Silverman, W. K., & Wasserstein, S. B. (1998). Children's predisaster functioning as a predictor of posttraumatic stress following Hurricane Andrew. *Journal of Consulting and Clinical Psychology*, **66**, 883–892.

Laor, N., Wolmer, L., & Cohen, D. (2001). Mothers' functioning and children's symptoms 5 years after a SCUD missile attack. *American Journal of Psychiatry*, **158**, 1020–1026.

Layne, C., Pynoos, R., Saltzman, W., Arslanagic, B., Black, M., Savjak, N., *et al.* (2001). Trauma/grief-focused group psychotherapy: school-based postwar intervention with traumatized Bosnian adolescents. *Group Dynamics: Theory, Research, and Practice*, **5**, 277–290.

Layne, C., Saltzman, W., Poppleton, L., Burlingame, G., Pasalic, A., Durakovic, E., *et al.* (2008). Effectiveness of a school-based group psychotherapy program for war-exposed adolescents: a randomized controlled trial. *Journal of the American Academy of Child and Adolescent Psychiatry*, **47**, 1048–1062.

Lengua, L., Long, A., & Meltzoff, A. (2006). Pre-attack stress-load, appraisals, and coping in children's responses to the 9/11 terrorist attacks. *Journal of Child Psychology and Psychiatry*, **47**, 1219–1227.

Lengua, L., Long, A., Smith, K., & Meltzoff, A. (2005) Pre-attack symptomatology and temperament as predictors of children's responses to the September 11 terrorist attacks. *Journal of Child Psychology and Psychiatry*, **46**, 631–645.

McFarlane, A. C. (1987). Family functioning and overprotection following a natural disaster: the longitudinal effects of post traumatic morbidity. *Australia and New Zealand Journal of Psychiatry*, **21**, 210–218.

Masinda, M. & Muhesi, M. (2004). Children and adolescents' exposure to traumatic war stressors in the Democratic Republic of Congo. *Journal of Child and Adolescent Mental Health*, **16**, 25–30.

Meiser-Stedman, R. (2002). Towards a cognitive-behavioural model of PTSD in children and adolescents. *Clinical Child and Family Psychology Review*, **5**, 217–232.

Meiser-Stedman, R., Dalgleish, T., Smith, P., Yule, W., & Glucksman, E. (2007). Diagnostic, demographic, memory quality, and cognitive variables associated with acute stress disorder in children and adolescents. *Journal of Abnormal Psychology*, **116**, 65–79.

Meiser-Stedman, R., Smith, P., Bryant, R., Salmon, K., Yule, W., Dalgleish, T., *et al.* (2009). Development and validation of the child post traumatic cognitions inventory (CPTCI). *Journal of Child Psychology and Psychiatry*, **50**, 432–440.

Meiser-Stedman, R., Smith, P., Glucksman, E., Yule, W., & Dalgleish, T. (2008). The post-traumatic stress disorder (PTSD) diagnosis in pre-school and elementary school-aged children exposed to motor vehicle accidents. *American Journal of Psychiatry*, **165**, 1326–1337.

Meiser-Stedman, R., Yule, W., Dalgleish, T., Smith P., & Glucksman E. (2006). The role of the family in child and adolescent posttraumatic stress following attendance at an emergency department. *Journal of Pediatric Psychology*, **31**, 397–402.

Meiser-Stedman, R., Yule, W., Smith, P., Glucksman, E., & Dalgleish, T. (2005). Acute stress disorder and posttraumatic stress disorder in children and adolescents involved in assaults or motor vehicle accidents. *American Journal of Psychiatry*, **162**, 1381–1383.

Meltzer, H., Gatward, R., Goodman, R., & Ford, T. (2003). Mental health of children and adolescents in Great Britain. *International Review of Psychiatry*, **15**, 185–187.

Morgan, L., Scourfield, J., Williams, D., Jasper, A., & Lewis, G. (2003). The Aberfan disaster: 33-year follow-up of survivors. *British Journal of Psychiatry*, **182**, 532–536.

National Institute for Clinical Excellence (2005). *Post-Traumatic Stress Disorder: The Management of PTSD in Adults and Children in Primary and Secondary Care*, Clinical Guideline No. 26. London: British Psychological Society.

Neuner, F., Schauer, E., Catani, C., Ruf, M., & Elbert, T. (2006). Post-tsunami stress: a study of posttraumatic stress disorder in children living in three severely affected regions in Sri Lanka. *Journal of Traumatic Stress*, **19**, 339–347.

Nolen-Hoeksema, S. (2000). The role of rumination in depressive disorders and mixed anxiety/depressive symptoms. *Journal of Abnormal Psychology*, **109**, 504–511.

Ohmi, H., Kojima, S., Awai, Y., Kamata, S., Sasaki, K., Tanaka, Y., *et al.* (2002). Post-traumatic stress disorder in pre-school aged children after a gas explosion. *European Journal of Pediatrics*, **161**, 643–648.

Ozer, E. J., Best, S., Lipsey, T., & Weiss, D. (2003). Predictors of posttraumatic stress disorder and symptoms in adults: a meta-analysis. *Psychological Bulletin*, **129**, 52–73.

Perrin, S., Smith, P., & Yule, W. (2000). Practitioner review: the assessment and treatment of post-traumatic stress disorder in children and adolescents. *Journal of Child Psychology and Psychiatry*, **41**, 277–289.

Perry, B. D. (1994) Neurobiological sequelae of childhood trauma: post-traumatic stress disorder in children. In: M. M. Murburg (ed.) *Catecholamine Function in Posttraumatic Stress Disorder: Emerging Concepts*, pp. 233–255. Washington, DC: American Psychiatric Press.

Pfefferbaum, B., DeVoe, E., Stuber, J., Schiff, M., Klein, T., & Fairbrother, G. (2004). Psychological impact of terrorism on children and families in the United States. *Journal of Aggression, Maltreatment, and Trauma*, **9**, 305–317.

Pine, D. S. (2003). Developmental psychobiology and response to threats: relevance to trauma in children and adolescents. *Biological Psychiatry*, **53**, 796–808.

Pine, D. S. & Cohen, J. (2002). Trauma in children and adolescents: risk and treatment of psychiatric sequelae. *Biological Psychiatry*, **51**, 519 – 531.

Pynoos, R., Fairbank, J., Steinberg, A., Amaya-Jackson, L., Gerrity, E., Mount, M., *et al.* (2008). The National Child Traumatic Stress Network: collaborating to improve the standard of care. *Professional Psychology: Research and Practice*, **39**, 389–395.

Pynoos, R. S., Goenjian, A., Karakashian, M., Tashjian, M., Manjikian, R., Manoukian, G., *et al.* (1993). Posttraumatic stress reactions in children after the 1988 Armenian earthquake. *British Journal of Psychiatry*, **163**, 239–247.

Rachman, S. (1980). Emotional processing. *Behaviour Research and Therapy*, **18**, 51–60.

Ramchandani, P. & Jones, D. P. H. (2003). Treating psychological symptoms in sexually abused children: from research findings to service provision. *British Journal of Psychiatry*, **183**, 484–490.

Resnick, H., Kilpatrick, D., Dansky, B., Saunders, B., & Best, C. (1993). Prevalence of civilian trauma and posttraumatic stress disorder in a representative national sample of women. *Journal of Consulting and Clinical Psychology*, **61**, 984–991.

Sack, W., Him, C., & Dickason, D. (1999). Twelve-year follow-up study of Khmer youths who suffered massive war trauma as children. *Journal of the American Academy of Child and Adolescent Psychiatry*, **38**, 1173–1179.

Sack, W., Seeley, J., & Clarke, G. (1997). Does PTSD transcend cultural barriers? A study from the Khmer Adolescent Refugee Project. *Journal of the American Academy of Child and Adolescent Psychiatry*, **36**, 49–54.

Sack, W., Seeley, J., Him, C., & Clarke, G. (1998). Psychometric properties of the Impact of Events Scale in traumatized Cambodian refugee youth. *Personality and Individual Differences*, **25**, 57–67.

Salmon K. & Bryant, R. A. (2002). Posttraumatic stress disorder in children: the influence of developmental factors. *Clinical Psychology Review*, **22**, 163–188.

Salmon, K., Sinclair, E., & Bryant, R. A. (2007). The role of maladaptive appraisals in child acute stress reactions. *British Journal of Clinical Psychology*, **46**, 203–210.

Sandberg, S. & Rutter, M. (2008). Acute life stresses. In: M. Rutter, D. Bishop, D. Pine, S. Scott, J. Stevenson, E. Taylor, *et al.* (eds.) *Rutter's Child and Adolescent Psychiatry*, 5th edn, pp. 392–406, London: Blackwell.

Scheeringa, M. S., Peebles, C. D., Cook, C. A., & Zeanah, C. H. (2001). Toward establishing procedural, criterion, and discriminant validity for PTSD in early childhood. *Journal of the American Academy of Child and Adolescent Psychiatry*, **40**, 52–60.

Scheeringa, M., Salloum, A., Arnberger, R., Weems, C., Amaya-Jackson, L., & Cohen, J. (2007). Feasibility and effectiveness of cognitive-behavioral therapy for posttraumatic stress disorder in preschool children: two case reports. *Journal of Traumatic Stress*, **20**, 631–636.

Scheeringa, M., Wright, M., Hunt, J. P., & Zeanah, C. H. (2006). Factors affecting the diagnosis and prediction of PTSD symptomatology in children and adolescents. *American Journal of Psychiatry*, **163**, 644–651.

Scheeringa, M. S., Zeanah, C. H., Drell, M. J., & Larrieu, J. A. (1995). Two approaches to diagnosing posttraumatic stress disorder in infancy and early childhood. *Journal of the American Academy of Child and Adolescent Psychiatry*, **34**, 191–200.

Scheeringa, M., Zeanah, C. H., Myers, L. & Putnam, F. (2003). New findings on alternative criteria for PTSD in preschool children. *Journal of the American Academy of Child and Adolescent Psychiatry*, **42**, 561 – 570.

Scheeringa, M. S., Zeanah, C. H., Myers, L., & Putnam, F. (2004). Heart period and variability findings in preschool children with posttraumatic stress symptoms. *Biological Psychiatry*, **55**, 685–691.

Schwab-Stone, M. E., Ayers, T. S., Kasprow, W., Voyce, C., Barone, C., Shriver, T., *et al.* (1995). No safe haven: a study of violence exposure in an urban community. *Journal of the American Academy of Child and Adolescent Psychiatry*, **34**, 1343–1352.

Shaw, J. A., Applegate, B., Tanner, S., Perez, D., Rothe, E., Campo-Bowen, A. E., *et al.* (1995). Pychological effects of Hurricane Andrew on an elementary school population. *Journal of the American Academy of Child and Adolescent Psychiatry*, **39**, 1185–1192.

Silverman, W. K., Ortiz, C. D., Viswesvaran, C., Burns, B. J., Kolko., D. J., Putnam, F. W. *et al.* (2008). Evidence-based psychosocial treatments for children and adolescents exposed to traumatic events. *Journal of Clinical Child and Adolescent Psychology*, **37**, 156–183.

Smith, P., Perrin, S., Dyregov, A., & Yule W. (2003). Principal components analysis of the Impact of Event Scale with children in war. *Personality and Individual Differences*, **34**, 315–322.

Smith, P., Perrin, S., Yule, W., & Clark, D. M. (2010). *Post Traumatic Stress Disorder: Cognitive Therapy with Children and Young People*. London: Routledge.

Smith, P., Perrin, S. G., Yule, W., Hacam, B., & Stuvland, R. (2002). War exposure among children from Bosnia-Hercegovina: psychological adjustment in a community sample. *Journal of Traumatic Stress*, **15**, 147–156.

Smith, P., Perrin, S., Yule, W., & Rabe-Hesketh, S. (2001). War-exposure and maternal reactions in the psychological adjustment of children from Bosnia-Hercegovina. *Journal of Child Psychology and Psychiatry*, **42**, 395–404.

Smith, P., Yule, W., Perrin, S., Tranah, T., Dalgleish, T., & Clark, D. M. (2007). Cognitive-behavioral therapy for PTSD in children and adolescents: a preliminary randomized controlled trial. *Journal of the American Academy of Child and Adolescent Psychiatry*, **46**, 1051–1061.

Stallard, P. (2003). A retrospective analysis to explore the applicability of the Ehlers and Clark (2000) cognitive model to explain PTSD in children. *Behavioural and Cognitive Psychotherapy*, **31**, 337–345.

Stallard, P. (2006). Psychological interventions for post traumatic stress reactions in children and young people: a review of randomised controlled trials. *Clinical Psychology Review*, **26**, 895–911.

Stallard, P. & Smith, E. (2007). Appraisals and cognitive coping styles associated with chronic post-traumatic symptoms in child road traffic accident survivors. *Journal of Child Psychology and Psychiatry*, **48**, 194–201.

Stallard, P., Salter, E., & Velleman, R. (2004). Posttraumatic stress disorder following road traffic accidents: a second prospective study. *European Child and Adolescent Psychiatry*, **13**, 172–178.

Stein, B. D., Jaycox, L. H., Kataoka, S. H., Wong, M., Tu, W., Elliott, M. N., *et al.* (2003). A mental health intervention for schoolchildren exposed to violence: a randomized controlled trial. *Journal of the American Medical Association*, **290**, 603–611.

Storr, C. L., Ialongo, N. S., Anthony, J., & Breslau, N. (2007). Childhood antecedents of exposure to traumatic events and post traumatic stress disorder. *American Journal of Psychiatry*, **164**, 119–125.

Thabet, A., Karim, K., & Vostanis, P. (2006). Trauma exposure in pre-school children in a war zone. *British Journal of Psychiatry*, **188**, 154–158.

Udwin, O., Boyle, S., Yule, W., Bolton, D., & O'Ryan, D. (2000). Risk factors for long-term psychological effects of a disaster experienced in adolescence: predictors of posttraumatic stress disorder. *Journal of Child Psychology and Psychiatry*, **41**, 969–979.

Vernberg, E. M., La Greca, A., Silverman, W. K., & Prinstein, M. J. (1996). Prediction of post-traumatic stress symptoms in children after hurricane Andrew. *Journal of Abnormal Psychology*, **105**, 237–248.

Weems, C. F., Pina, A. A., Costa, N. M., Watts, S. E., Taylor, L. K., & Cannon, M. F. (2007). Predisaster trait anxiety and negative affect predict posttraumatic stress in youth after Hurricane Katrina. *Journal of Consulting and Clinical Psychology*, **75**, 154–159.

World Health Organization (1991). *International Classification of Diseases*, 10th edn (ICD-10). Geneva: World Health Organization.

Yule, W., Bolton, D., Udwin, O., Boyle, S., O'Ryan, D., & Nurrish, J. (2000). The long-term psychological effects of a disaster experienced in adolescence. I. The incidence and course of post traumatic stress disorder. *Journal of Child Psychology and Psychiatry*, **41**, 503–511.

13

Child–parent relations: attachment and anxiety disorders

Katharina Manassis

Attachment theory provides an intriguing perspective on possible mechanisms for the development and maintenance of childhood anxiety disorders. It is a well-researched paradigm of parent–child relationships, providing the opportunity to test these mechanisms empirically. Attachment theory postulates that to promote survival infants tend to behave in ways that enhance proximity to their caregivers, and caregivers tend to behave reciprocally (Bowlby, 1973). As a result of these tendencies, an interactive system focused on a specific caregiver (usually the infant's mother) develops during the first year of life. When the infant has adequate proximity or contact with the caregiver for a given situation, attachment behaviors subside. When proximity or contact is inadequate, attachment behaviors escalate and compete with other behavioral systems, for example, the exploratory system (Bowlby, 1973).

Attachment theory and measurement

As described in more detail below, suboptimal attachment has been linked to anxiety at various stages of development (reviewed in Manassis, Bradley, Goldberg, Hood, & Swinson, 1994). This is thought to occur because a suboptimal parent–infant attachment relationship (called "insecure attachment") is not a time-limited risk factor, but rather serves as a template for the developing child's expectations of future relationships (Main, Kaplan, & Cassidy, 1985). Thus, expectations borne of an insecure parent–infant attachment are thought to continue to place the child at risk of anxiety disorders throughout development.

Using an experimental procedure involving two brief separations and reunions between parents and their 1-year-old infants (termed the "Strange Situation Procedure"), Ainsworth, Blehar, Waters, and Wall (1978) were able to classify infant attachments as "secure" (B classification) or "insecure." Secure infants were distressed when separated from their caregiver and responded positively when reunited with him or her. Insecure infants showed either minimal distress on separation and ignored the caregiver on reunion (termed "insecure–avoidant" attachment, A classification) or high distress on separation and anger towards the caregiver on reunion (termed "insecure–ambivalent/resistant" attachment, C classification). A later study identified one further group, termed "insecure–disorganized" (D classification), which showed a variety of unusual responses to the strange situation procedure (Main & Solomon, 1986). Caregivers of secure infants were found to respond sensitively and predictably to their infants' expressions of distress, while caregivers of

Anxiety Disorders in Children and Adolescents, 2nd edn, ed. W. K. Silverman and A. P. Field. Published by Cambridge University Press. © Cambridge University Press 2011.

insecure infants did not (Ainsworth *et al.*, 1978). Caregivers of avoidant, ambivalent/ resistant, and disorganized infants showed rejection or unavailability towards their infants, inconsistent or intrusive caregiving, and parenting affected by personal trauma or loss respectively (Ainsworth *et al.*, 1978).

According to attachment theory, infants of different attachment types are thought to develop different cognitions pertaining to interpersonal relationships and different ways of regulating affect. The cognitions are thought to be organized as "internal working models" (Main *et al.*, 1985), defined as mental representations of the self, intimate others, and the world that guide appraisals of experience and guide interpersonal behavior. Once organized, internal working models are thought to function outside conscious experience and therefore are difficult to change.

The nature of these models has been explored in adults using the Adult Attachment Interview (Main & Goldwyn, 1991), which examines how a discussion of one's attachment relationships affects the ability to maintain a coherent conversation. Using this interview, the following adult attachment types (with the corresponding infant–parent types in parentheses) have been elucidated: autonomous (secure), dismissive (avoidant), preoccupied (ambivalent/resistant), and unresolved (disorganized). In attachment theory, such models are thought to account for the intergenerational transmission of anxiety in that insecure adult internal working models are predictive of insecure infant attachment classification (Main & Goldwyn, 1991), and thus presumably the development of insecure internal working models in these children which predispose to anxiety.

Given the caregiving styles associated with different adult attachment types, the content of the corresponding internal working models children develop has been inferred (Main & Goldwyn, 1991). According to attachment theory, secure children see themselves as worthy and capable of eliciting needed care when distressed; they see others as trustworthy and protective, and the world as generally safe. Insecure–avoidant children see themselves as unworthy and incapable of eliciting needed care when distressed, others as uncaring or indifferent, and the world as generally unsafe. By implication, self-reliance is very important in ensuring safety when threatened. Insecure–ambivalent/resistant children see themselves as worthy and capable of eliciting needed care only under certain circumstances (largely dependent on the whims of the inconsistent caregiver), the caregiver as capable of giving love but frequently withholding it, and the world as unpredictable. By implication, the ability to maintain the caregiver's involvement is important for ensuring safety when threatened. Disorganized children struggle to find ways of coping with emotionally wounded caregivers, typically by exhibiting caregiving or controlling behaviors towards them (Main & Solomon, 1986).

Infants of different attachment types have been found to differ in their preferred means of regulating affect (reviewed in Goldberg, MacKay-Soroka, & Rochester, 1994). Secure infants express all affects genuinely in response to situations, confident of others' caring responses. Insecure–avoidant infants restrict expressions of distress, having experienced rejection in response to these in the past. Insecure–ambivalent/resistant infants exaggerate expressions of distress, having learned that expressing distress persistently eventually pays off. Disorganized infants do not have a coherent strategy for regulating affect.

Optimal means of measuring attachment have been the subject of debate, as measures are not well validated for all stages of development, and the measures considered ideal are often difficult to administer in non-academic settings. In addition to the Strange Situation Procedure for parent–infant attachment and the Adult Attachment Interview, attachment measures involving separation and reunion between parents and children have been validated for preschoolers (Moss, Bureau, Cyr, Mongeau, & St-Laurent, 2004). Adolescents can often complete the Adult Attachment Interview. Attachment measures for children in middle childhood (approximately ages 7 to 12), however, are still being evaluated (Bureau, Easlerbrooks, & Lyons-Ruth, 2009; Shmueli-Goetz, Target, Fonagy, & Datta, 2008).

Although the Adult Attachment Interview and the Strange Situation Procedure are still considered "gold standards" for measuring attachment in adulthood and infancy, respectively, they require intensive training, are time-consuming, and can be difficult to administer outside academic settings. A number of newer attachment measures have been developed for intermediate age groups and for various research populations (see Bifulco, 2002), but they may not all categorize children in exactly the same manner. For example, if children with avoidant attachment styles typically minimize expressions of affect, they may under-report emotionally distressing interactions with their parents on questionnaires, making them difficult to distinguish from secure children on questionnaire measures. Similarly, they may under-report anxiety despite high physiological arousal (Goldberg *et al.*, 1994), affecting questionnaire-based anxiety measures.

In addition, several authors have suggested that attachment measures may be biased by Western values (Rothbaum, Rosen, Ujiie, & Uchida, 2002; Rothbaum, Weisz, Pott, Miyake, & Morelli, 2000). The measures emphasize autonomy, individuation, and exploration as childhood goals, but these goals may not be congruent with cultural expectations in some Asian countries. In Japan, for example, an extremely close mother–child relationship is valued and would not be considered suboptimal (Rothbaum *et al.*, 2002). Racial bias effects also have been cited as problematic in child welfare assessments of attachment (Surbeck, 2003), where biased assessments could have serious consequences for child placements. White caseworkers were found to assess White mothers more positively than African American mothers in this study, although the same was not true of African American caseworkers.

Attachment and other risk factors

Attachment must be understood in the context of other constitutional and environmental risks. Therefore, before detailing possible links between attachment and childhood anxiety disorders, relationships between attachment and other risk factors are described; the concepts of behavioral inhibition, prone-to-distress temperament, temperament–attachment interaction, and the heritability of anxiety disorders are relevant to this discussion.

As discussed in detail in Lonigan, Phillips, Wilson, and Allan (Chapter 10, this volume) about 10% of toddlers (21 months of age or more) can be described as "behaviorally inhibited," defined as "tending to withdraw, to seek a parent, and to inhibit play and vocalization following encounter with unfamiliar people and events" (Kagan, Reznick, & Snidman, 1990). Inhibition is demonstrated by measuring the toddler or child's responses to novel stimuli and new situations. Many behaviorally inhibited toddlers become less inhibited over time. As a group, however, they develop anxiety disorders at higher rates than children who are not inhibited (Biederman, Rosenbaum, & Hirshfeld, 1990), and may be at particularly high risk for social anxiety (Schwartz, Snidman, & Kagan, 1999). The high levels of sympathetic arousal evident in inhibited toddlers (Kagan, Reznick, & Snidman, 1987) and high rates of inhibition among children of anxious parents (Manassis,

Bradley, Goldberg, Hood, & Swinson, 1995) suggest a temperamental basis for behavioral inhibition. A genetic basis for behavioral inhibition has been proposed by Suomi (1987) who selectively bred non-human primates who were either highly inhibited or highly uninhibited. He demonstrated behavioral and physiological differences between the two groups of offspring, consistent with their inhibited or uninhibited parentage.

Inhibited children and toddlers often have histories of high levels of motor activity and high levels of crying in infancy (Arcus, 1991). These behaviors, termed "prone-to-distress temperament," may affect attachment classification (reviewed in Goldberg, 1991). For example, an infant highly prone to distress at all times may appear very distressed during the Strange Situation Procedure, which (according to the scoring system for this procedure) increases the likelihood of either an insecure–ambivalent classification, or one of the subtypes of secure classification associated with high distress. However, the infant could still be scored as either secure or insecure based on other aspects of his or her behavior during the Strange Situation Procedure. Thus, temperament per se does not appear to significantly predict security. There is no significant association between parental reports of temperament and security of attachment (Sroufe, 1985). Also, security of attachment to the mother is reasonably independent of security of attachment to the father in most studies (Belsky & Rovine, 1987; Fox, Kimmerly, & Schafer, 1991), suggesting that temperament is not critical in predicting attachment security.

In the development of anxiety, temperamental risk factors could thus operate independently of the predisposition to anxiety associated with insecure attachment. The heritability of anxiety disorders, however, must also be considered (see Gregory & Eley, Chapter 8, this volume). Given the tendency for anxiety disorders to run in families, many infants with temperamental risk factors for anxiety are raised by caregivers who are anxious themselves (see Creswell, Murray, Stacey, & Cooper, Chapter 14, this volume). Mothers with anxiety disorders have been found to have high rates of insecure adult attachment, and the attachment relationships with their infants are also largely insecure (Manassis et al., 1994). Thus, among infants temperamentally vulnerable to anxiety, a greater than average number would be expected to have the additional risk factor of insecure attachment.

Shamir-Essakow, Ungerer, and Rapee (2005) examined the concurrent associations between attachment security, behavioral inhibition, maternal anxiety, and child anxiety in an at-risk sample of 104 children aged 3 to 4 years. Insecure attachment and behavioral inhibition were independently associated with child anxiety, even after controlling for the effect of maternal anxiety. However, maternal anxiety was also independently associated with child anxiety. Thus, maximal risk for child anxiety was conferred by the combination of insecure attachment, behavioral inhibition, and maternal anxiety. In a smaller sample of preschool children of anxious mothers, Manassis et al. (1995) also found that behavioral inhibition and insecure attachment independently increased child anxiety risk. Longitudinal studies are needed to further elucidate the manner in which these effects influence children's developmental trajectories, ultimately resulting in anxiety in young people when occurring in combination with other risk factors.

Attachment in relation to other anxiety risks

Caregivers with few social supports (Jacobson & Frye, 1991) and high levels of life stress (Vaughn, Egeland, Sroufe, & Waters, 1979) have an increased risk of developing insecure attachments with their infants. Maternal depression has also been associated with an increased risk of insecure mother–child attachment (Kochanska, 1991). Thus, one would predict an increased incidence of childhood anxiety disorders in the presence of these factors. In addition, depressed mothers show less facilitation of their children's attempts to approach unfamiliar situations (Kochanska, 1991), thus reducing opportunities for desensitization in temperamentally vulnerable children.

The role of the marital relationship has received little attention in studies of childhood anxiety disorders, but the presence of two parents has been found to reduce the risk of separation anxiety disorder (Last, Perrin, & Hersen, 1992). Spouses may ameliorate the effects of a child's insecure attachment with the primary caregiver (Fox *et al.*, 1991), provided the marital relationship is supportive.

Familial openness to outside influences, perhaps related to parental attachment status, can affect the development of children's anxiety (Schneewind, 1989). For example, the opportunity to interact with peers enhances social skills (Rubin, 1982) and may thus protect children from social phobia. Given their diminished ability to trust others, parents with insecure adult attachments would be less likely to encourage their children to interact with peers than parents with secure adult attachments.

Attachment status may also moderate the effect of life events or other stresses on anxiety risk. Dallaire and Weinraub (2007) studied a large and diverse sample of children from the National Institute of Child Health and Human Development Study of Early Child Care and Youth Development. They evaluated attachment security at 15 months and examined symptoms of anxiety at 4.5 years of age. Children who were insecurely attached and experienced many stressful life events exhibited more anxiety symptoms than children classified as securely attached who experienced similar events. This finding suggests that attachment security may protect some children from the potential anxiety-provoking effects of negative life events.

Similarly, Bifulco, Kwon, Jacobs, Moran, Bunn, and Beer (2006) examined 154 "high-risk" adult women, many of whom had experienced childhood neglect or abuse. New onset of anxiety or depression in the 5-year follow-up period was predicted by markedly or moderately insecure attachment style as determined by the Attachment Style Interview at baseline. Two styles, termed Fearful and Angry–Dismissive, partially mediated the relationship between childhood adversity and depression or anxiety. In an interesting study of 140 adolescents, Irons and Gilbert (2005) found that adolescents' concerns about their social rank in a peer group related to anxiety or depression symptoms in the presence of insecure attachment, but not in the presence of secure attachment. The authors suggest that insecure attachment sensitizes adolescents to become focused on the competitive dynamics of groups, and the power of others to shame, hurt, or reject while secure attachment may protect teens from this focus. Consistent with this idea, Brown and Wright (2003) found that adolescents with ambivalent attachment patterns (a form of insecurity) reported significantly more interpersonal difficulties and symptoms of psychopathology than adolescents with secure attachment patterns.

Attachment and various aspects of child anxiety

Within the framework of attachment theory, links to behavioral, cognitive, and emotional aspects of anxiety will now be described. It is important to distinguish three terms used in the literature: anxious attachment, anxiety, and anxiety disorder. Anxiety is an excessively fearful reaction relative to the degree of danger (Kaplan & Sadock, 1988). All people have such reactions occasionally, so they are not necessarily considered pathological. They become pathological, and are termed anxiety disorders, when they persist for long periods of time and interfere with the individual's day-to-day functioning (American Psychiatric Association, 1994). Anxious attachment, by contrast, is synonymous with insecure attachment. It is considered within the norm and not pathological.

Behaviorally, secure infants are freer to explore their environment than insecure infants (Bowlby, 1973). Confident in their caregivers' availability, secure infants' attachment systems are only activated in truly dangerous situations. In non-dangerous situations, their attachment systems are deactivated and the infants are free to explore, using their caregivers as a "secure base." Because insecure infants lack confidence in their caregiver's availability, their attachment systems are chronically activated, even in situations with little danger, and exploration is curtailed. Such overly cautious behavior is characteristic of anxious individuals, and resembles the "behavioral inhibition" linked to anxiety disorders by temperament theorists (discussed above and by Lonigan *et al.*, Chapter 10, this volume). Avoidance of new situations related to extreme caution also perpetuates anxiety, as it prevents the desensitization necessary to overcoming anxiety (reviewed in Compton, March, Brent, Albano, Weersing, & Curry, 2004).

Cognitively, the separation distress experienced repeatedly by insecure infants is considered one of the earliest forms of anxiety (Sroufe, 1996). When children internalize this distress, the internal working models described above may develop, which can result in distorted cognitions that predispose to further anxiety For example, children who are repeatedly unable to elicit caregiver attention when distressed may interpret this inability to get help from their caregivers as a sign of overall personal helplessness, predisposing to anxiety. The internal working models arising in insecurely attached children share common cognitive distortions: views of (1) the self as unworthy or incapable of eliciting needed care; (2) the world as unsafe or unpredictable; and (3) others as untrustworthy (Main & Goldwyn, 1991). These cognitive distortions are also found with greater frequency among anxious individuals than among non-anxious individuals (Beck, Brown, Steer, Eidelson, & Riskind, 1987). Of course, such distortions may also relate to other developmental factors apart from attachment.

Chronic reliance on internal models based on insecure attachment may also contribute to the selective encoding of threatening information discovered among anxious adults (Macleod, 1991) and anxious children and adolescents (Manassis, Tannock, & Masellis, 1996; Vasey, el-Hag, & Daleiden, 1996). Interestingly, a study that examined adults' attachment in relation to selective processing of threatening information (Zeijlmans van Emmichoven, van IJzendoorn, de Ruiter, & Brosschot, 2003) found that securely attached, anxiety disordered adults recalled *more* threatening words than adults who were insecurely attached. The authors explained this counter-intuitive result by proposing that adults' security allows for open communication about and processing of threatening information, leading to less defensive exclusion of negative material and better recall of threatening information. Thus, according to attachment theory, secure attachment might facilitate processing of threatening cognitions so the individual can examine them and evaluate their veracity. Implicit, unexamined cognitions associated with insecurity might be more deleterious, as these cognitions might result in individuals behaving towards others as if their internal models were accurate. For example, an internal model based on avoidant attachment could result in a perception of others as uncaring or indifferent. Therefore, an avoidant individual might manifest suspicious or emotionally distant responses to others when distressed. Such behavior could in turn elicit indifference or hostility from others, confirming the perception of others as uncaring or indifferent. In this way, the threat-focused cognitive models associated with insecurity may become self-perpetuating and thus maintain childhood anxiety.

Security of attachment has also been linked to affect regulation in infants and children. Confident of maternal care, secure infants appear to be open to appropriate negative feeling without being overly expressive (Shouldice & Stevenson-Hinde, 1992). Mothers of secure infants respond sensitively to both positive and negative affect (Goldberg *et al.*, 1994). Attachment theorists have linked these behaviors to the finding that secure children aged 3 to 6 years show a better understanding of emotion than insecure children of the same age (de Rosnay & Harris, 2002). Similarly, they have found that secure adults are able to discuss emotions about intimate others freely without either restricting emotional content or losing track of the conversation, as their insecure counterparts do (Main & Goldwyn, 1991).

Several studies now suggest that maternal responses that are sensitively attuned to their infants' needs (termed "maternal sensitivity") may mediate the relationship between secure attachment and affect regulation in children. Oyen, Landy, and Hillburn-Cobb (2000) studied 30 socially disadvantaged mother–child dyads, and found that autonomously attached mothers displayed the highest maternal sensitivity in videotaped interactions with their children, and preoccupied mothers displayed the lowest. Warren and Simmens (2005) followed over 1200 infants, and found that those displaying signs of difficult temperament who were raised by highly sensitive mothers (as rated by trained observers) showed fewer anxiety and depressive symptoms at 2 and 3 years of age than those who received less sensitive maternal care. Dallaire and Weinraub (2005) studied a sample of mother–child dyads from infancy to age 6, and found that the effect of mothers' separation anxiety on children's separation anxiety was mediated by maternal sensitivity. That is, high maternal sensitivity appeared to be protective in reducing the intergenerational transmission of separation anxiety. Mothers in secure dyads were more likely to show this high sensitivity than those in insecure dyads. Finally, mothers of 3- and 4-year-old insecure, behaviorally inhibited children were found to be less likely than mothers of secure inhibited children to validate their children's emotional experiences and more likely to show boundary violations and defense against negative affect (Shamir-Essakow, Ungerer, Rapee, & Safier, 2004), which the authors considered signs of maternal insensitivity.

Regarding the types of infant insecurity, mothers of insecure–avoidant infants respond preferentially to infants' positive emotions, while those of insecure–ambivalent/resistant infants respond preferentially to infants' negative emotions (Goldberg *et al.*, 1994), due to differences in their maternal perceptions of emotional distress (Zeanah, Benoit, Barton, Regan, Hirshberg, & Lipsitt, 1993). Therefore, attachment theorists postulate that to ensure receiving care when distressed avoidant infants minimize their displays of distress while ambivalent/resistant infants maximize them. In frightening situations, ambivalent/resistant infants thus show an exaggerated fear response, constituting overt anxiety. Avoidant infants do not display such overt anxiety, but do show elevated heart rates in frightening situations (Spangler & Grossman, 1993) indicating a high physiological fear response. Both strategies are considered suboptimal for regulating affect (Goldberg *et al.*, 1994).

A further link between physiological arousal and security of attachment has been postulated by Kramer (1992), who reviewed evidence that secure attachment may influence neurotransmitter levels. Since then, security has been found to enhance the function of serotonin systems (Kramer, 1992) and oxytocin systems (Tops, van Peer, Korf, Wijers, & Tucker, 2007), and decrease the cortisol response to acute stress (Quirin, Pruessner, & Kuhl, 2008). Dysregulation of serotonin or oxytocin systems, and heightened cortisol response to stress have all been linked to anxiety disorders (Kramer, 1992). Quirin *et al.* (2008) have related these findings to the effect of early life experiences, including attachment experiences, in programming the hypothalamus–pituitary–adrenal axis that regulates multiple stress response systems. This early programming is thought to establish a trajectory of physiological responsiveness throughout life, and thus form the basis of ongoing vulnerability to anxiety.

In summary, the nature of infants' attachment relationships can influence infants' behavioral, cognitive, emotional, and even physiological responses to frightening or distressing situations, thus increasing or decreasing their risk of developing anxiety disorders. Proposed links between attachment and anxiety disorders are now described.

Evidence for attachment–anxiety disorder links

Security of attachment has consistently been linked with favorable developmental outcomes, and insecurity of attachment has consistently been linked with unfavorable developmental outcomes (reviewed in Bakermans-Kranenburg & van IJzendoorn, 2007; Main, 1996), but only a subset of studies specifically examined anxiety or anxiety disorders in children.

Three studies have examined the link between insecure attachment and anxiety disorders in youth and several studies have examined the link between insecure attachment and subclinical levels of anxiety in youth. These studies will now be described, including the specific age group examined in each study.

Manassis *et al.* (1994) examined adult attachment and mother–child attachment in 20 mother–child dyads (children ages 18 to 59 months) in which the mothers suffered from anxiety disorders. The mothers all had insecure adult attachments, and 80% also had insecure attachments with their children. Among the insecurely attached children, three of 16 met DSM-III diagnostic criteria for anxiety disorders while none of the secure children did. Two had separation anxiety disorder (one with disorganized attachment, one with avoidant attachment) and one had avoidant disorder (with disorganized attachment). Insecure children also had higher internalizing scores on the Child Behavior Checklist (Achenbach & Edelbrock, 1983) than secure children (Manassis *et al.*, 1995).

Disorganized attachment predominated for both adult and mother–child attachment, indicating that many mothers' attachments were affected by unresolved trauma or loss (Manassis *et al.*, 1994). When dyads classified as disorganized and mothers classified as unresolved were assigned their best alternate category and combined with the remaining three categories, a higher than expected rate of ambivalent/resistant attachment and a lower than expected rate of secure attachment were found (see Table 13.1). Small sample size and difficulties associated with measuring attachment in children of varying ages (i.e., from 18 months to 59 months) are potential limitations of this study. Nevertheless, it represents an important first step in examining childhood anxiety disorders, maternal attachment, and child attachment together in a high-risk sample.

Warren, Huston, Egeland, and Sroufe (1997) studied 172 adolescents aged 17.5 years who had participated in assessments of mother–child attachment at 12 months of age. Twenty-six met diagnostic criteria for anxiety disorders. More children with anxiety disorders

Table 13.1 Attachment distributions (%) in anxious versus normal samples

Sample	Attachment classification[a]		
	A	B	C
Manassis *et al.* (1994)			
(1) Children of anxious mothers, $n = 20$	25	36	24
(2) Anxious adults (female), $n = 18$	17	39	44
Warren *et al.* (1997)			
Anxious adolescents, $n = 26$	23	42	35
Ainsworth *et al.* (1978)			
Normative sample	22	66	12

[a]Attachment classifications: A, insecure–avoidant; B, secure; C, insecure–ambivalent/resistant.

were, as infants, classified as anxious/resistant and more children with other disorders were classified as avoidant. Anxious/resistant attachment doubled the risk of subsequently developing an anxiety disorder, and was a better predictor of adolescent anxiety disorders than either maternal anxiety or child temperament. The interaction between anxious/resistant attachment and one aspect of temperament (slow habituation to stimuli) further increased the risk of a subsequent anxiety disorder. Nevertheless, secure, insecure–avoidant, and insecure–resistant attachment were all represented among the adolescents with anxiety disorders (see Table 13.1). The insecure–disorganized classification was not yet available at the time of the attachment assessments.

Asking questions based on attachment theory, Cassidy (1995) found that adolescents and adults with generalized anxiety disorder reported more memories of caregiver unresponsiveness and role-reversal/enmeshment, and more past and current feelings of anger toward their mothers than did controls. Although these reports closely resemble the descriptions of parents commonly provided by individuals with preoccupied adult attachment, formal assessments of adult attachment would be required to confirm high rates of preoccupation.

Studies linking attachment and subclinical anxiety in children are also reviewed now, as subclinical anxiety can impact child development. For example, subclinical levels of anxiety have been associated with concurrent functional impairment in adults and school-aged children (Ialongo, Edelsohn, Werthamer-Larsson, Crockett, & Kellam, 1995; Roy-Byrne, Katon, Broadhead, Lepine, & Richards, 1994), and have been associated with subsequent development of anxiety disorders when occurring in preschool children (Biederman *et al.*, 1990). As mentioned above, Shamir-Essakow *et al.* (2005) found anxiety levels increased in preschoolers who were insecurely attached. Two studies have linked high self-reported worry to self-reported ambivalent attachment style in school-aged children (Brown & Whiteside, 2008; Muris, Meesters, Merckelbach, & Hülsenbeck, 2000), and Brumariu and Kerns (2008) linked high self-reported social anxiety symptoms in 5th grade students to insecure ambivalent attachment. The lack of well-validated measures of attachment in school-aged children is a limitation of these studies.

Crowell, O'Connor, Wollmers, and Sprafkin (1991) found that behaviorally disturbed school-aged children whose mothers were classified as secure on the Adult Attachment Interview showed less self-rated anxiety and depression than children whose mothers were insecure–dismissing. Cassidy and Berlin (1994) reported increased fearfulness across several studies of insecure–ambivalent/resistant children.

Longitudinal studies have demonstrated that insecure attachment can precede the development of child anxiety disorders. Bar-Haim, Dan, Eshel, and Sagi-Schwartz (2007) followed 136 children assessed using Ainsworth's Strange Situation Procedure at 12 months to age 11 years. Compared to children who were securely attached, children who had insecure–ambivalent attachment at 12 months had higher levels of self- and maternal-report school phobia on questionnaires at 11 years. Boys who were ambivalently attached also had higher levels of social phobia on questionnaires at 11 years than those who were securely attached. Nevertheless, the anxiety levels reported for the insecure–ambivalent children were generally subclinical.

Another longitudinal study (Dallaire & Weinraub, 2005) followed 99 mother–child dyads assessed for attachment security in infancy to age 6. They found that previously insecurely attached children reported more separation anxiety at age 6 than previously securely attached children, regardless of type of insecurity or of the presence of maternal separation anxiety. Calkins and Fox (1992) found insecure–ambivalent/resistant attachment at 14 months to be predictive of inhibited behavior at 24 months.

Belsky and Rovine (1987) have suggested that the link between anxiety and attachment is best understood when the secure, ambivalent/resistant, and avoidant attachment categories are placed on a spectrum from those associated with the most overt distress (ambivalent/resistant) to those associated with the least overt distress (avoidant). Secures are in the middle of the spectrum, with some exhibiting relatively high distress and some exhibiting relatively low distress. Consistent with this suggestion, Stevenson-Hinde and Shouldice (1990) found that 2.5-year-old children who were either insecure–ambivalent/resistant or secure with relatively high distress showed higher indices of fear and separation distress than young children in other attachment classifications. Bar Haim *et al.*'s (2007) findings (see above) are also consistent with Belsky and Rovine's (1987) idea.

In summary, insecure attachment at various ages has been linked consistently with both clinical and subclinical anxiety. Insecure–disorganized attachment and insecure–ambivalent/resistant attachment have been associated with anxiety disorders by Manassis *et al.* (1994) and Warren *et al.* (1997), respectively. When insecure–disorganized subjects were assigned their best alternate classification (commonly done to further interpret attachment in disorganized subjects), both of these studies (Manassis *et al.*, 1994; Warren *et al.*, 1997) found increased rates of ambivalent/resistant attachment and decreased rates of secure attachment among anxious participants relative to a normative sample (see Table 13.1). However, all attachment types were represented in the anxious groups, consistent with the idea that other risk factors besides attachment must be considered in understanding the etiology of childhood anxiety. Insecure–ambivalent/resistant attachment was also associated with subclinical levels of anxiety in several studies. Thus, insecure attachment (especially ambivalent/resistant attachment) appears to be a risk factor in the development of elevated anxiety levels and anxiety disorders, and secure attachment may be protective.

Possible mechanisms for the development and maintenance of childhood anxiety disorders

Descriptions of specific anxiety disorders do not imply any particular etiology, with the exception of post-traumatic stress disorder where a traumatic etiology is implied (American Psychiatric Association, 1994). The high comorbidity among anxiety disorders (Last,

Hersen, Kazdin, Finkelstein, & Strauss, 1987) and the presence of similar physiological characteristics among individuals with various disorders has led some theorists to propose a common temperamental etiology (see Lonigan *et al.*, Chapter 10, this volume for a review). Temperament theories, however, do not account for the varied manifestations of anxiety in children and adults.

Attachment theory proposes that anxiety originates in the infant's uncertainty about caregiver availability, but responses to that uncertainty vary. These varied responses could partly account for the varied manifestations of childhood anxiety. However, because not all insecurely attached infants develop anxiety disorders, other risk factors must also play a role. For this discussion, it is assumed that insecure attachment contributes to at least some childhood anxiety disorders.

Within the framework of attachment theory, hypothetical links between different types of insecure attachment and different manifestations of anxiety can be made. In this framework, securely attached children could only develop anxiety disorders in the presence of high temperamental vulnerability (for example, severe, persistent behavioral inhibition resulting in social avoidance and eventually social phobia) or traumatic life events (for example, a specific phobia of dogs after a dog bite, or post-traumatic stress disorder after a serious accident). Anxiety would be unlikely to persist, however, because securely attached children engage in more exploratory behavior than insecure children (Ainsworth *et al.*, 1978) allowing for desensitization, and are more likely to make appropriate requests for help than insecure children (Cassidy, 1995), creating opportunities to learn strategies for coping with anxiety.

Ambivalent/resistant attachment has been associated most consistently with childhood anxiety. A hypothetical pathway from this type of attachment to anxiety can be inferred. In this case, intermittent availability of the parent strongly reinforces attachment behavior in the infant or child (Main *et al.*, 1985). A temperamentally vulnerable infant or child would thus become preoccupied with obtaining the parent's comfort, reducing exploratory behavior (Ainsworth *et al.*, 1978). This process would reduce exposure to new situations that would otherwise desensitize the child to some forms of anxiety. Further, parents of such children may express frustration at the child's clinging (Manassis, 2008), thus increasing the child's sense of insecurity. In addition, the parent's selective attention to negative affect in ambivalent/resistant attachment (Goldberg *et al.*, 1994) would reinforce it rather than reassuring the child.

An escalating cycle of anxiety could thus develop between parent and child, with the child attempting to alleviate anxiety by being near the parent, but then experiencing parental hostility resulting in increased anxiety. Separation anxiety is a possible outcome. Anxiety could be maintained through preoccupation with obtaining parental comfort (reducing the opportunity to learn coping strategies and engage in desensitization) and exaggerated, overly dramatic displays of negative affect that fail to elicit reassurance from others.

One can also hypothesize greater anxiety in children with avoidant and disorganized attachment, as these styles have been linked to suboptimal affect regulation compared to secure attachment. A hypothetical pathway from avoidant attachment to anxiety would start with the child's perception of being rejected by the parent when emotionally demonstrative, resulting in the child restricting displays of emotional distress (Main *et al.*, 1985). In the presence of temperamental vulnerability, the need to disavow or restrict overt expressions of emotional distress could result in anxiety-related physical symptoms (e.g., stomach aches, headaches) or other somatic manifestations. Difficulty asking for help, or fear of rejection, could maintain these symptoms. In disorganized attachment, the child's caregiver has been psychologically affected by unresolved trauma or loss, and therefore does not provide a predictable response to child distress (Main & Solomon, 1986). The children sometimes respond by denying their distress to look after the emotionally unstable parent (Main & Solomon, 1986). This response could certainly contribute to anxiety. For example, the need to look after a physically or mentally ill parent at home has been cited as a frequent contributing factor to children's school avoidance (Manassis, 1995).

Several adult studies have examined attachment styles in relation to various types of anxiety or anxiety-related conditions. Unfortunately, different studies use different terminology and measures for the various attachment styles. "Fearful" attachment (which appears similar to "preoccupied") was linked to depression and social phobia in 154 "high-risk" women, most of whom had histories of childhood neglect or abuse by Bifulco *et al.* (2006). The same study linked generalized anxiety disorder to Angry–Dismissive attachment style. By contrast, Marazziti, Dell'osso, Dell'Osso, Consoli, Del Debbio, Mungai, *et al.* (2007) found that preoccupied attachment prevailed among 126 adults with mood and anxiety disorders, but was not linked to any specific disorder. Troisi, Di Lorenzo, Alcini, Nanni, Di Pasquale, and Siracusano (2006) linked preoccupied attachment with a history of self-reported separation anxiety symptoms and with high body dissatisfaction in 65 women with eating disorders. Finally, Eng, Heimberg, Hart, Schneier, and Liebowitz (2001) studied 118 adults with social anxiety disorder, and found both secure and "anxious" (similar to "preoccupied") attachment styles. Anxious attachment was associated with more severe social anxiety, greater depression, and greater impairment than secure attachment. No child-focused studies have linked specific child attachment styles to specific child anxiety disorders.

The nature of the stresses that commonly trigger anxiety disorders may also differ depending on attachment type. As noted, avoidant children tend to use self-reliance to allay anxiety when threatened. Such children would be expected to develop anxiety symptoms in response to events involving personal vulnerability or failure. On the other hand, ambivalent/resistant children tend to use the ability to maintain emotional involvement with the caregiver to allay anxiety. Therefore, such children would be expected to be more stressed by events involving caregiver vulnerability or absence.

Differing parental attachment types may contribute to the maintenance of childhood anxiety. For example, an insecure–dismissive parent may consider a child's anxiety "silly" or "manipulative" while an insecure–preoccupied parent may see the same child as emotionally fragile, but difficult to manage (Manassis, 2008). If two parents have these different insecure attachment types, disagreements about how to respond to the child's anxiety can result in marital conflict that is anxiety-provoking to the child or in inconsistent management of the child's anxiety-related behaviors, resulting in treatment failure (Manassis, 2008).

Clinical and research implications

Attachment theory has implications for the prevention, assessment, and treatment of childhood anxiety disorders. Intervening with parents and infants to reduce insecurity offers the hope of preventing some anxiety disorders. Lieberman, Weston, and Pawl (1991) used infant–parent psychotherapy to improve the quality of attachment and social–emotional functioning in mothers and infants with insecure attachments and low socioeconomic status. At post-treatment, treated dyads were indistinguishable from secure controls. Erickson, Korfmacher, and Egeland (1993) used an attachment-based preventive intervention with children of poor, young, or poorly educated mothers. The treated mothers developed a better understanding of their babies' needs and showed less depression and anxiety than a control group. Similar interventions could be targeted to populations at risk for anxiety disorders (for example, behaviorally inhibited children with insecure attachments, or children of parents with anxiety disorders).

When intervening to prevent anxiety, the concept of sensitivity is important. Reliable, sensitive responses to infants' signals of distress foster the development of secure infant–parent attachments (Bowlby, 1973). Warren and Simmens (2005) also found that maternal sensitivity was a significant predictor of decreased anxiety/depressive symptoms for temperamentally difficult boys. In children predisposed to anxiety, this approach may seem to contradict the need to desensitize the child to frightening or distressing stimuli. In fact, overattentive parenting appears to perpetuate behavioral inhibition (Arcus, 1991). Sensitivity, however, does not imply extreme parental vigilance for any signal of infant upset or discomfort. Instead, the sensitive parent learns to "read" his or her infant's signals accurately and intervenes only when the infant is significantly distressed. Thus, the infant learns to take minor upsets and discomforts in its stride without parental help, but is confident of the parent's availability when he or she is genuinely distressed.

In the assessment of children with anxiety disorders, knowledge of how attachment can contribute to the development and maintenance of children's anxiety is helpful. Questions about the child's early temperament, parental response to it, and parents' own ways of coping with anxiety (often reflective of adult attachments) may elucidate the mechanisms predisposing a child to an anxiety disorder. Asking about attachment-related, anxiety-provoking events may reveal triggers for the onset of the disorder. Observing parent–child interactions and considering possible attachment-related mechanisms that may perpetuate anxiety may provide clues about likely obstacles to treatment success. Recall, however, that what is considered optimal closeness or distance in the parent–child relationship can vary from one culture to another (Rothbaum *et al.*, 2002).

In treating childhood anxiety disorders, attachment theory highlights the importance of parental involvement. Secure parent–child relationships may facilitate treatment, as the securely attached child is able to learn new coping strategies and engage in necessary desensitization confident of parental support. With minimal psycho-education, secure parents can often coach their children in ways of better managing their anxiety, reducing the need for lengthy clinical interventions (Manassis, 2008). When longer therapeutic involvement is needed, treatment is more likely to succeed if the therapist can act as a secure base for the anxious child (Warren *et al.*, 1997).

The high rate of ambivalent/resistant attachment in anxious samples suggests a need to identify and address familial frustration with the anxious child. Parents with this attachment style may also be so focused on negative interactions with their child that they have difficulty identifying his or her strengths. Helping the parent see the anxious child's abilities may allow him or her to encourage the child to participate in exposure tasks. The potentially anxiety-provoking effects of disorganized attachment suggest a need to identify and address unresolved parental losses or traumas. Dismissive parents may benefit from learning empathic responses to the child's anxiety, as these are likely to be reassuring. Identifying spousal differences in attachment style may further their understanding of one another's parenting style, and allow caregivers to develop a more consistent and effective approach to their anxious child.

Awareness of how insecure attachment can perpetuate anxiety may allow therapists to focus treatment on anxious children's coping styles (related to their internal working models), rather than just working towards symptom relief. Changing coping styles may ameliorate the recurrent exacerbations of anxiety symptoms that are common among anxious children (Bernstein, Borchardt, & Perwien, 1996), thus reducing long-term morbidity. Parental involvement in treatment of anxious children has been shown to contribute to the children's development of more adaptive coping styles (Mendlowitz, Manassis, Bradley, Scapillato, Miezitis, & Shaw, 1999).

Attachment theory should not be used to assign blame to parents or other individuals in the anxious child's life. As a careful review of the evidence reveals, insecure attachment is only one of several risk factors for childhood anxiety disorders, and it frequently contributes to these disorders as a result of interactions with child temperament or other factors. Even if insecure attachment is thought to play a role in a particular child's anxiety, the processes that perpetuate maladaptive attachment-related behaviors and cognitions are largely outside the child's and parent's awareness. Finally, given the tendency of parents of children with emotional problems to blame themselves, it is more helpful to focus on what they can do to help the child, rather than blaming them further. When parents are encouraged to show empathy to their anxious child's distress but express confidence in his or her ability to face what is feared (an attitude characteristic of secure attachment relationships), they can facilitate their child's ability to overcome anxiety (Manassis, 2008).

Research is needed to examine links between specific attachment types and specific childhood anxiety disorders to clarify their developmental trajectories. The role of individuals outside the caregiver–child dyad (e.g., other family members, peers) in the development of anxiety disorders must be clarified. Furthermore, all of these factors clearly interact with stressful life events and developmental changes, affecting the risk of anxiety disorders at various ages. Given all of the above, more longitudinal studies are needed to accurately describe the development of various childhood anxiety disorders.

Further studies that investigate behavioral, cognitive, and affective mechanisms that may mediate the relationship between attachment and childhood anxiety have also been advocated (Bogels & Brechman-Toussaint, 2006). Understanding these mechanisms is likely to suggest additional avenues for intervention.

The effectiveness of attachment-based preventive interventions in samples at risk for childhood anxiety disorders should also be examined. Their potential for reducing parental anxiety (Erickson *et al.*, 1993) suggests that they may be especially beneficial for children of anxious parents. Outcomes for anxious children receiving attachment-based treatments (i.e., those with high parental involvement and emphasis on changing coping styles) also require further study.

Practice guidelines

Key practice guidelines that can be derived from the above include:

- Consider preventive intervention to improve parental sensitivity in populations at high risk for child anxiety (for example, children with high temperamental vulnerability; children of anxiety-disordered parents).

During assessment

- Ask about parental attempts to modify the anxious child's temperament. Are they providing empathic encouragement to help the child face anxious situations?
- Observe parental attempts to soothe the child's anxiety or distress (for example, if a brief separation between parent and child occurs as you interview one alone), as this may provide clues about insecure attachment patterns.
- Be aware of cultural differences in what is considered optimal closeness or distance in the parent–child relationship, to avoid mistakenly assuming that culturally determined behaviors represent insecure attachment.
- Ask the anxious child's parents about their own ways of coping with anxiety to reveal: (a) the forms of affect regulation they model for the child; and (b) parental tendencies to dismiss or dwell on negative affect (typical of dismissive and preoccupied insecure attachment styles respectively).
- Enquire about separations, losses, and traumas in the history of the anxious child or the parents. For the child, these attachment-related threats may trigger anxiety; for the parents, these attachment-related threats may predispose to disorganized attachment if not addressed. The latter may require separate therapy for the parent.

In therapy

- Try to serve as a "secure base," offering consistent emotional availability and empathy, but expressing encouraging confidence in the child's ability to master anxious states.
- Avoid blaming parents for anxious children's difficulties.
- Involve parents in treatment to (a) allow them to contribute to the child's progress; and (b) foster more secure parent–child interactions.
- Help frustrated, preoccupied parents identify the negative interaction patterns they engage in with their child, step back from these patterns, and think about more effective parenting strategies. Also, help them see their anxious child's strengths.
- Help dismissive parents develop empathy for their child's distress so they can reassure him or her more effectively.
- Help spouses identify disparate styles of affect regulation and develop a consistent approach to managing their anxious child's behavior.

References

Achenbach, T. M. & Edelbrock, C. (1983). *Manual for the Child Behavior Checklist and Revised Child Behavior Profile*. Burlington, VT: University of Vermont Department of Psychiatry.

Ainsworth, M. D. S., Blehar, M. C., Waters, E. L., & Wall, E. (1978). *Patterns of Attachment: A Psychological Study of the Strange Situation*. Hillsdale, NJ: Erlbaum.

American Psychiatric Association (1994). *Diagnostic and Statistical Manual of Mental Disorders*, 4th edn. Washington, DC: American Psychiatric Association.

Arcus, D. (1991). The experiential modification of temperamental bias in inhibited and uninhibited children. Unpublished Ph.D. dissertation, Harvard University, Boston, MA.

Bakermans-Kranenburg, M. J. & van IJzendoorn, M. H. (2007). Research review: genetic vulnerability or differential susceptibility in child development: the case of attachment. *Journal of Child Psychology and Psychiatry*, **48**, 1160–1173.

Bar-Haim, Y., Dan, O., Eshel, Y., & Sagi-Schwartz, A. (2007). Predicting children's anxiety from early attachment relationships. *Journal of Anxiety Disorders*, **21**, 1061–1068.

Beck, A. T., Brown, G., Steer, R. A., Eidelson, J. I., & Riskind, J. H. (1987). Differentiating anxiety and depression: a test of the cognitive content-specificity hypothesis. *Journal of Abnormal Psychology*, **96**, 179–183.

Belsky, J. & Rovine, M. (1987). Temperament and attachment security in the strange situation: an empirical rapprochement. *Child Development*, **58**, 787–795.

Bernstein, G. A., Borchardt, C. M., & Perwien, A. R. (1996). Anxiety disorders in children and adolescents: a review of the past 10 years. *Journal of the American Academy of Child and Adolescent Psychiatry*, **35**, 1110–1119.

Biederman, J., Rosenbaum, J. F., & Hirshfeld, D. R. (1990). Psychiatric correlates of behavioral inhibition in young children of parents with and without psychiatric disorders. *Archives of General Psychiatry*, **47**, 21–26.

Bifulco, A. (2002). Attachment style measurement: a clinical and epidemiological perspective. *Attachment and Human Development*, **4**, 180–188.

Bifulco, A., Kwon, J., Jacobs, C., Moran, P. M., Bunn, A., & Beer, N. (2006). Adult attachment style as mediator between childhood neglect/abuse and adult depression and anxiety. *Social Psychiatry and Psychiatric Epidemiology*, **41**, 796–805.

Bogels, S. M. & Brechman-Toussaint, M. L. (2006). Family issues in child anxiety: attachment, family functioning, parental rearing and beliefs. *Clinical Psychology Review*, **26**, 834–856.

Bowlby, J. (1973). *Attachment and Loss: Attachment.* New York: Basic Books.

Brown, A. M. & Whiteside, S. P. (2008). Relations among perceived parental rearing behaviours, attachment style, and worry in anxious children. *Journal of Anxiety Disorders*, **22**, 263–272.

Brown, L. S. & Wright, J. (2003). The relationship between attachment strategies and psychopathology in adolescence. *Psychology and Psychotherapy*, **76**, 351–367.

Brumariu, L. E. & Kerns, K. A. (2008). Mother–child attachment and social anxiety symptoms in middle childhood. *Journal of Applied Developmental Psychology*, **29**, 393–402.

Bureau, J. F., Easterbrooks, M. A., & Lyons-Ruth, K. (2009). Attachment disorganization and controlling behavior in middle childhood: maternal and child precursors and correlates. *Attachment and Human Development*, **11**, 265–284.

Calkins, S. D. & Fox, N. A. (1992). The relations among infant temperament, security of attachment, and behavioral inhibition at twenty-four months. *Child Development*, **63**, 1456–1472.

Cassidy, J. (1995). Attachment and generalized anxiety disorder. In: D. Cicchetti & S. Toth (eds.) *Emotion, Cognition, and Representation: Rochester Symposium on Developmental Psychopathology VI*, pp. 343–370. Rochester, NY: University of Rochester Press.

Cassidy, J. & Berlin, L. J. (1994). The insecure/ambivalent pattern of attachment: theory and research. *Child Development*, **65**, 971–991.

Compton, S. N., March, J. S., Brent, D., Albano, A. M., Weersing, V. R., & Curry, J. (2004). Cognitive–behavioral psychotherapy for anxiety and depressive disorders in children and adolescents: an evidence-based medicine review. *Journal of the American Academy of Child and Adolescent Psychiatry*, **43**, 930–959.

Crowell, J. A., O'Connor, E., Wollmers, G., Sprafkin, J., & Rao, U. (1991). Mothers' conceptualizations of parent–child relationships: relation to mother–child interaction and child behavior problems. *Development and Psychopathology*, **3**, 431–444.

Dallaire, D. H. & Weinraub, M. (2005). Predicting children's separation anxiety at age 6: the contributions of infant–mother attachment security, maternal sensitivity, and maternal separation anxiety. *Attachment and Human Development*, **7**, 393–408.

Dallaire, D. H. & Weinraub, M. (2007). Infant–mother attachment security and children's anxiety and aggression at first grade. *Journal of Applied Developmental Psychology*, **28**, 477–492.

de Rosnay, M. & Harris, P. L. (2002). Individual differences in children's understanding of emotion: the roles of attachment and language. *Attachment and Human Development*, **4**, 39–54.

Eng, W., Heimberg, R. G., Hart, T. A., Schneier, F. R., & Liebowitz, M. R. (2001). Attachment in individuals with social anxiety disorder: the relationship among adult attachment styles, social anxiety, and depression. *Emotion*, **1**, 365–380.

Erickson, M. F., Korfmacher, J., & Egeland, B. R. (1993). Attachments past and present: implications for therapeutic intervention with mother–infant dyads. *Annual Progress in Child Psychiatry and Child Development*, pp. 459–476.

Fox, N., Kimmerly, N. L., & Schafer, W. D. (1991). Attachment to mother/attachment to father: a meta-analysis. *Child Development*, **62**, 210–225.

Goldberg, S. (1991). Recent developments in attachment theory and research. *Canadian Journal of Psychiatry*, **36**, 393–400.

Goldberg, S., MacKay-Soroka, S., & Rochester, M. (1994). Affect, attachment, and maternal responsiveness. *Infant Behavior and Development*, **17**, 335–340.

Ialongo, N., Edelsohn, G., Werthamer-Larsson, L., Crockett, L., & Kellam, S. (1995). The significance of self-reported anxious symptoms in first grade children: prediction to anxious symptoms and adaptive functioning in fifth grade. *Journal of Child Psychology and Psychiatry*, **36**, 427–437.

Irons, C. & Gilbert, P. (2005). Evolved mechanisms in adolescent anxiety and depression symptoms: the role of the attachment and social rank systems. *Journal of Adolescence*, **28**, 325–341.

Jacobson, S. W. & Frye, K. F. (1991). Effect of maternal social support on attachment: experimental evidence. *Child Development*, **62**, 572–582.

Kagan, J., Reznick, J. S., & Snidman, N. (1987). The physiology and psychology of behavioral inhibition in children. *Child Development*, **58**, 1459–1473.

Kagan, J., Reznick, J. S., & Snidman, N. (1990). Origins of panic disorder. In: J. C. Ballenger (ed.) *Neurobiology of Panic Disorder*, pp. 71–87. New York: Alan R. Liss.

Kaplan, H. I. & Sadock, B. J. (1988). *Synopsis of Psychiatry*, 5th edn. Baltimore, MD: Williams & Wilkins.

Kochanska, G. (1991). Patterns of inhibition to the unfamiliar in children of normal and affectively ill mothers. *Child Development*, **62**, 250–263.

Kramer, G. W. (1992). A psychobiological theory of attachment. *Behavioral and Brain Sciences*, **15**, 493–541.

Last, C. G., Hersen, M., Kazdin, A. E., Finkelstein, R., & Strauss, C. C. (1987). Comparison of DSM-III separation anxiety and overanxious disorders: demographic characteristics and patterns of comorbidity. *Journal of the American Academy of Child and Adolescent Psychiatry*, **26**, 527–531.

Last, C. G., Perrin, S., & Hersen, M. (1992). DSM-III-R anxiety disorders in children: sociodemographic and clinical characteristics. *Journal of the American Academy of Child and Adolescent Psychiatry*, **31**, 1070–1076.

Lieberman, A. F., Weston, D. R., & Pawl, J. H. (1991). Preventive intervention and outcome with anxiously attached dyads. *Child Development*, **62**, 199–209.

Macleod, C. (1991). Clinical anxiety and the selective encoding of threatening information. *International Review of Psychiatry*, **3**, 279–292.

Main, M. (1996). Introduction to the special section on attachment and psychopathology: overview of the field of attachment. *Journal of Consulting and Clinical Psychology*, **64**, 237–243.

Main, M. & Goldwyn, R. (1991). Adult attachment classification system. In: M. Main (ed.) *Behavior and the Development of Representational Models of Attachment: Five Methods of Assessment*. Cambridge, UK: Cambridge University Press.

Main, M. & Solomon, J. (1986). Discovery of an insecure-disorganized/disoriented attachment pattern. In *Affective Development in Infancy*, ed. T. B. Brazelton & M. Yogman. Norwood, NJ: Ablex.

Main, M., Kaplan, N., & Cassidy, J. (1985). Security in infancy, childhood and adulthood: a move to the level of representation. *Monographs of the Society for Research in Child Development*, **50**, 66–104.

Manassis, K. (1995). School refusal: how to address the underlying factors. *Canadian Journal of Diagnosis*, **12**, 55–68.

Manassis, K. (2008). *Keys to Parenting Your Anxious Child*, 2nd edn. New York: Barron's Educational.

Manassis, K., Bradley, S., Goldberg S., Hood, J., & Swinson, R. P. (1994). Attachment in mothers with anxiety disorders and their children. *Journal of the American Academy of Child and Adolescent Psychiatry*, **33**, 1106–1113.

Manassis, K., Bradley, S., Goldberg, S., Hood, J., & Swinson, R. P. (1995). Behavioral inhibition, attachment and anxiety in children of mothers with anxiety disorders. *Canadian Journal of Psychiatry*, **40**, 87–92.

Manassis, K., Hudson, J., Webb, A., & Albano, A. M. (2004). Development of childhood anxiety disorders: beyond behavioral inhibition. *Cognitive and Behavioral Practice*, **11**, 3–12.

Manassis, K., Tannock, R., & Masellis, M. (1996). Cognitive differences between anxious, normal, and ADHD children on a dichotic listening task. *Anxiety*, **2**, 279–285.

Marazziti, D., Dell'osso, B., Dell'Osso, M. C., Consoli, G., Del Debbio, A., Mungai, F., *et al.* (2007). Romantic attachment in patients with mood and anxiety disorders. *CNS Spectrum*, **12**, 751–756.

Mendlowitz, S., Manassis, K., Bradley, S., Scapillato, D., Miezitis, S., & Shaw, B. (1999). Cognitive behavioral group treatments in childhood anxiety disorders: the role of parental involvement. *Journal of the American Academy of Child and Adolescent Psychiatry*, **38**, 1223–1229.

Moss, E., Bureau, J. F., Cyr, C., Mongeau, C., & St-Laurent, D. (2004). Correlates of attachment at age 3: construct validity of the preschool attachment classification system. *Developmental Psychology*, **40**, 323–334.

Muris, P., Meesters, C., Merckelbach, H., & Hülsenbeck, P. (2000). Worry in children is related to perceived parental rearing and attachment. *Behaviour Research and Therapy*, **38**, 487–497.

Oyen, A. S., Landy, S., & Hillburn-Cobb, C. (2000). Maternal attachment and sensitivity in an at-risk sample. *Attachment and Human Development*, **2**, 203–217.

Quirin, M., Pruessner, J. C., & Kuhl, J. (2008). HPA system regulation and adult attachment anxiety: individual differences in reactive and awakening cortisol. *Psychoneuroendocrinology*, **33**, 581–590.

Rothbaum, F., Rosen, K., Ujiie, T., & Uchida, N. (2002). Family systems theory, attachment theory, and culture. *Family Process*, **41**, 328–350.

Rothbaum, F., Weisz, J., Pott, M., Miyake, K., & Morelli, G. (2000). Attachment and culture: security in the United States and Japan. *American Psychologist*, **55**, 1093–1104.

Roy-Byrne, P., Katon, W., Broadhead, W. E., Lepine, J. P., & Richards, J. (1994). Subsyndromal ("mixed") anxiety–depression in primary care. *Journal of General Internal Medicine*, **9**, 507–512.

Rubin, K. H. (1982). Social and social–cognitive developmental characteristics of young isolate, normal and sociable children. In: K. H. Rubin & H. S. Ross (eds.) *Peer Relationships and Social Skills in Childhood*, pp. 353–374. New York: Springer.

Schneewind, K. A. (1989). Contextual approaches to family systems research: the macro-micro puzzle. In: K. Kreppner & R. M. Lerner (eds.) *Family Systems and Life Span Development*, pp. 197–221. Hillsdale, NJ: Erlbaum.

Schwartz, C. E., Snidman, N., & Kagan, J. (1999). Adolescent social anxiety as an outcome of inhibited temperament in childhood. *Journal of the American Academy of Child and Adolescent Psychiatry*, **38**, 1008–1015.

Shamir-Essakow, G., Ungerer, J. A., & Rapee, R. M. (2005). Attachment, behavioral inhibition, and anxiety in preschool children. *Journal of Abnormal Child Psychology*, **33**, 131–143.

Shamir-Essakow, G., Ungerer, J. A., Rapee, R. M., & Safier, R. (2004). Caregiving representations of mothers of behaviorally inhibited and uninhibited preschool children. *Development and Psychopathology*, **40**, 899–910.

Shmueli-Goetz, Y., Target, M., Fonagy, P., & Datta, A. (2008). The Child Attachment Interview: a psychometric study of reliability and discriminant validity. *Developmental Psychology*, **44**, 939–956.

Shouldice, A. & Stevenson-Hinde, J. (1992). Coping with security distress: The Separation Anxiety Test and attachment classification at 4.5 years. *Journal of Child Psychology and Psychiatry*, **33**, 331–348.

Spangler, G. & Grossman, K. E. (1993). Biobehavioral organization in securely and insecurely attached infants. *Child Development*, **64**, 1439–1450.

Sroufe, L. A. (1985). Attachment classification from the perspective of infant–caregiver relationships and infant temperament. *Child Development*, **56**, 1–14.

Sroufe, L. A. (1996). *Emotional Development*. New York: Cambridge University Press.

Stevenson-Hinde, J. & Shouldice, A. (1990). Fear and attachment in 2.5-year-olds. *British Journal of Developmental Psychology*, **8**, 319–333.

Suomi, S. J. (1987). Genetic and maternal contributions to individual differences in rhesus monkey biobehavioral development. In: N. A. Kresnegor (ed.) *Perinatal Development: A Psychobiological Perspective*, pp. 397–417. Orlando, FL: Academic Press.

Surbeck, B. C. (2003). An investigation of racial partiality in child welfare assessments of attachment. *American Journal of Orthopsychiatry*, **73**, 13–23.

Tops, M., van Peer, J. M., Korf, J., Wijers, A. A., & Tucker, D. M. (2007). Anxiety, cortisol, and attachment predict plasma oxytocin. *Psychophysiology*, **44**, 444–449.

Troisi, A., Di Lorenzo, G., Alcini, S., Nanni, R. C., Di Pasquale, C., & Siracusano, A. (2006). Body dissatisfaction in women with eating disorders: relationship to early separation anxiety and insecure attachment. *Psychosomatic Medicine*, **68**, 449–453.

Vasey, M. W., el-Hag, N., & Daleiden, E. L. (1996). Anxiety and processing of emotionally threatening stimuli: distinctive patterns of selective attention among high- and low-test-anxious children. *Child Development*, **67**, 1173–1185.

Vaughn, B., Egeland, B., Sroufe, L. A., & Waters, E. (1979). Individual differences in infant–mother attachment at 12 and 18 months: stability and change in families under stress. *Child Development*, **50**, 971–975.

Warren, S. L. & Simmens, S. J. (2005). Predicting toddler anxiety/depressive symptoms: effects of caregiver sensitivity on temperamentally vulnerable children. *Infant Mental Health Journal*, **26**, 40–55.

Warren, S. L., Huston, L., Egeland, B., & Sroufe, L. A. (1997). Child and adolescent anxiety disorders and early attachment. *Journal of the American Academy of Child and Adolescent Psychiatry*, **36**, 637–644.

Zeanah, C., Benoit, D., Barton, M., Regan, C., Hirshberg, L. M., & Lipsitt, L. P. (1993). Representations of attachment in mothers and their one-year-old infants. *Journal of the American Academy of Child and Adolescent Psychiatry*, **32**, 278–286.

Zeijlmans van Emmichoven, I. A., van IJzendoorn, M. H., de Ruiter, C., & Brosschot, J. F. (2003). Selective processing of threatening information: effects of attachment representation and anxiety disorder on attention and memory. *Development and Psychopathology*, **15**, 219–237.

14

Parenting and child anxiety

Cathy Creswell, Lynne Murray, James Stacey, and Peter Cooper

Parenting and child and adolescent anxiety disorders

Intergenerational studies have shown that anxiety disorders commonly run in families (e.g., Noyes, Clarkson, Crowe, Yates, & McChesney, 1987), yet genetic research consistently points to a strong environmental component in the etiology of childhood anxiety disorders (e.g., Gregory & Eley, 2007). As such, research attention is increasingly looking to the role of parenting to help explain the intergenerational transmission of anxiety. The aim of this chapter is to review recent evidence and present a model of the influence of parental cognitions, expressed affect, and behavior in the development of anxiety disorders in children and adolescents.

A cautionary note

A large number of studies conducted over the past two decades have found associations between parenting and youth anxiety; however, in many the associations have been of modest magnitude. McLeod, Wood, and Weisz (2007) reported that parenting (as a general construct incorporating rejection and control) accounted for only 4% of the variance in childhood anxiety. For this reason it is important to consider parental factors as one potential risk or maintenance pathway amongst others. The exact contribution that parental factors make remains unclear for several reasons.

First, some parenting factors are likely to be of greater significance to anxiety than others; this review will consider the strength of evidence for the prime candidates that have been subjected to empirical evaluation. Second, methodological factors account for much variation in the degree of association between parenting and youth anxiety reported: high-quality, observational assessments of parenting, for example, are typically associated with stronger effects than parent or child reports, and stronger associations are found when anxiety diagnoses are established as opposed to when anxiety is assessed by questionnaire (e.g., McLeod *et al.*, 2007). Third, studies vary in both the parenting dimensions assessed, the operational definitions used (e.g., see sections on parental control/involvement and negativity), and whether assessments are made of specific behaviors or more general "parenting styles" (which may incorporate a collection of parental behaviors and cognitions). Effect sizes may also be influenced by the diagnostic composition of the anxiety-disordered participant groups, because specificity issues may be masked through the lumping together of disparate anxiety disorders. (For example, it is plausible that certain parental factors may be particularly pertinent in the case of separation anxiety disorder, e.g., Wood, 2006.)

Anxiety Disorders in Children and Adolescents, 2nd edn, ed. W. K. Silverman and A. P. Field. Published by Cambridge University Press. © Cambridge University Press 2011.

Fourth, parental factors are likely to vary in their importance at different stages in children's development and studies vary considerably in the age ranges of participants. Throughout this chapter, to identify participant groups we will use the terms infant (for under 2 years), children (for 2–11 years), adolescents (for 12–18 years), and youth (for studies including both children and adolescents).

Finally, recent studies have emphasized the importance of interactive effects on the development of childhood anxiety disorder. It is now clear that a particular style of parenting may have a specific impact on one child, and have no such impact on another (e.g., a sibling; see Hudson & Rapee, 2002), and this is likely to be due to interactions between parenting and a range of other variables, including biological vulnerability and life events/lifestyle factors (e.g., Murray, Creswell, & Cooper, 2009). It is also essential to note that the great majority of studies include a single parent (most commonly the mother); and it is not clear, therefore, whether effects found are true for parents or caregivers in general, or are specific to parents of a particular sex or in a particular childcare role. Three questions that are of particular importance here relate to whether mothers and fathers tend to parent in similar ways, whether the impact of particular parental behaviors is the same whether it comes from mother or father, and whether there are distinctive features of mothers' and fathers' parental interactions that make a specific contribution to the development of child anxiety (e.g., Bögels & Phares, 2008). The current evidence base is limited but we have considered each of these issues further below.

The intergenerational transmission of anxiety disorders

The familiality of anxiety disorders has been well documented from studies of mixed generations (e.g., Noyes *et al.*, 1987) including those focused on parent–child associations. For example, "top–down" studies have consistently demonstrated that offspring of adults with anxiety disorders have an increased risk of anxiety disorder themselves (e.g., Beidel & Turner, 1997; Biederman, Rosenbaum, Bolduc, Faraone, & Hirshfeld, 1991; Silverman, Cerny, & Nelles, 1988; Turner, Beidel, & Costello, 1987; Warner, Mufson, & Weissman, 1995; Weissman, Leckman, Merikangas, Gammon, & Prusoff, 1984). Similarly, "bottom–up" studies have noted the increased prevalence of anxiety disorders amongst parents of children with an anxiety disorder (e.g., Cooper, Fearn, Willetts, Seabrook, & Parkinson, 2006; Last, Hersen, Kazdin, Francis, & Grubb, 1987; Last, Hersen, Kazdin, Orvaschel, & Perrin, 1991). Cooper *et al.* (2006) conducted diagnostic interviews with 85 parents of children aged 7–12 years presenting at a child anxiety disorders clinic and 45 community controls. They found that mothers of children with anxiety disorders were almost three times more likely to meet criteria for a current anxiety disorder than mothers of the non-anxious control group children. Although only 60% of fathers were assessed in this study, fathers did not demonstrate an increased prevalence of current anxiety disorders in comparison to community controls, although they did show a raised prevalence of lifetime anxiety disorders.

The development of anxiety in children

It is important that models of the development of anxiety in youth are able to account for the increased prevalence of anxiety disorders amongst children with anxious parents (particularly mothers). They must also, however, be able to explain the occurrence of anxiety disorders in the absence of high parental anxiety. An example of such a model is presented by Murray *et al.* (2009) who distinguish between pathways to child anxiety that are accounted for by parental anxiety (i.e., biological/genetic vulnerability) and pathways that may occur in the absence of parental anxiety, yet may be *more likely* to occur where parents are also anxious. These pathways are (1) lifestyle and socialization factors that increase the youth's perception of increased threat and reduced control in relation to the environment, and (2) parental responses, such as anxiogenic modeling and information transfer. Murray *et al.* (2009) also proposed that when youths exhibit signs of anxiety these may be reinforced or maintained by particular parental responses (increased involvement and reduced encouragement). These responses may be particularly likely to occur when parents are themselves anxious. In this chapter we focus on the parental aspects of this model, and expand it to incorporate the potential mediating role of parental cognitions in the association between parental anxiety and behaviors, thus highlighting potential targets for prevention and treatment to enhance the efficacy of interventions for anxiety in youth.

Parenting and child anxiety

Observational studies of parent–youth interactions have identified associations (of varying strengths) between youth anxiety and (1) vicarious learning, (2) information transfer, (3) parental involvement (vs. autonomy granting), and (4) negativity (vs. warmth). Although many studies have reported cross-sectional associations (e.g. Gar & Hudson, 2008; Hudson & Rapee, 2001; Moore, Whaley, & Sigman, 2004), experimental and longitudinal designs are increasingly being used to address the issue of the direction of effects (e.g., De Rosnay, Cooper, Tsigaras, & Murray, 2006; Gerull & Rapee, 2002; Murray, DeRosnay, *et al.*, 2008). This is an essential development in the field if independent parental *risk* factors are to be identified, in contrast to what may potentially be parental responses to child anxiety, or bidirectional influences (e.g., Silverman, Kurtines, Pina, & Jaccard, 2009). Thus, the following discussion pays particular attention to the extent to which conclusions can be drawn regarding the anxiogenic nature of particular parental behaviors.

Vicarious learning

Clinical accounts have long ascribed a role to observational learning in the development of children's fears (for a review see Askew & Field, 2008). For example, accounts of World War II experiences evidence the extent to which children expressed fears during air raids was closely related to the level of maternal expressed fear (Lewis, 1942). However, although observational studies have the advantage of high levels of ecological validity, they commonly lack sufficient control of other potentially contributing variables. The challenge for researchers is to develop tightly controlled methods to examine the direction of effects between parenting and child anxiety, while retaining high levels of ecological validity. The studies of Mineka, Cook, and colleagues (e.g., Cook & Mineka, 1987, 1989, 1990; Mineka & Cook, 1986, 1993), and recent experimental extensions of this work with human populations (e.g., De Rosnay *et al.*, 2006; Gerull & Rapee, 2002), have successfully met this challenge, providing support for a causal effect of modeling on the development of anxiety in children. Mineka, Davidson, Cook, and Keir (1984) demonstrated that (non-snake-fearful) laboratory-reared rhesus monkeys developed persistent fears of snakes and snake-like objects after observing their wild-reared parents' fearful responses to snakes. Further studies demonstrated that these effects were enhanced in relation to stimuli where fear may be of an evolutionary advantage (e.g., snakes, but not flowers: Cook & Mineka, 1989, 1990).

To extend these findings to human populations, experimental methods have recently been applied. These experiments build on "social referencing" research with non-clinical populations, which has demonstrated that children's responses to potentially fear-provoking stimuli are influenced by observed adult behavior (see review by Feinman, Roberts, Hsieh, Sawyer, & Swanson, 1992). Gerull and Rapee (2002), for example, trained mothers to either express fear and disgust to potentially fear-provoking toys or display neutral expressions, when in the presence of their toddler (aged 15–20 months) offspring. They found that, in comparison to the benign/neutral control condition, maternal fear expression led to an increase in their offspring's expressed fear and avoidance of the toys. This effect has been found to extend beyond "prepared" fear-relevant stimuli. Dubi, Rapee, Emerton, and Schneiring (2008) found that, following negative maternal expression, toddlers were similarly fearful of fear-irrelevant stimuli (toy mushroom and flower) and fear-relevant ones (spider and snake). De Rosnay *et al.* (2006) adapted this paradigm to assess the transmission of social fear in infancy (12–14 months). Non-clinical mothers were trained to express either social anxiety (i.e., behaviors based on clinical and empirical descriptions of social phobia) or respond in their usual (non-anxious) way when interacting with a stranger. Again, in comparison to the control condition, expression of maternal anxiety was associated with increased infant fearfulness, avoidance, and reduced positive emotional tone when the infant was approached by the stranger. In this study, a significant interaction was reported with infant temperamental fearfulness (assessed using the Infant Behavior Questionnaire, a parent-report measure of infant activity level, smiling and laughter, fear, distress to limitations, soothability, and orienting: Rothbart, 1981, 1986): infants who were rated by their mothers as generally more fearful showed a heightened response to maternal expressed anxiety with the stranger.

Although such experimental designs (e.g., De Rosnay *et al.*, 2006; Gerull & Rapee, 2002) provide support for a causal effect of maternal modeling, one important limitation arises from the fact that a comparison is being made between how non-anxious mothers usually respond and their trained, anxious, response. In other words, infants might simply be responding with increased wariness to their mother reacting in an *unexpected* manner within the experimental paradigm. To overcome this limitation, it is essential to extend these findings to naturalistic studies. With regards to maternal modeling of anxiety, consistent results have been obtained in a recent prospective longitudinal study (Murray, De Rosnay, *et al.*, 2008). A sample of women diagnosed with social phobia and a non-anxious control group were recruited in pregnancy. The women and their children were then serially assessed. When the children were 10 and 14 months of age, mothers conversed with a stranger in the presence of their infant and the infant's subsequent responses to the stranger were rated. Maternal expressed anxiety at 10 months postpartum (which was, as expected, higher in the social phobia group than the control group) predicted increased infant avoidance of a stranger 4 months later. Again, infant temperament moderated the association: specifically, where infants of mothers with social phobia were behaviorally inhibited (classified on the basis of behavioral observations: Kagan, Reznick, & Snidman, 1987; see also Lonigan, Phillips, Wilson, & Allan, Chapter 10, this volume), they were particularly likely to show increased avoidance of the stranger. Boys appeared more vulnerable than girls to the effects of the mother's disorder. Further longitudinal follow-up of the children participating in this longitudinal study will be important to ascertain whether these factors constitute risk for the development of an anxiety disorder in later life. Nonetheless, the current findings provide strong support for the hypothesis that observed maternal anxiety influences the development of childhood anxiety, particularly in the context of pre-existing vulnerability (i.e., high behavioral inhibition).

Information transfer

A large body of research with non-clinical samples has demonstrated that children's anxious beliefs and behaviors are influenced by verbal information – for example, through tuition, spontaneous conversations, and recollections of past event, as well as plans for the future (Denham, Zoller, & Couchard, 1994; Fivush, 1991; Nelson, 1993). In a series of studies with non-clinical samples, Field and colleagues have shown that children's avoidant behaviors and fear beliefs are influenced by the information they are given (e.g., Field, Hamilton, Knowles, & Plews, 2003; Field & Lawson, 2003; Field, Lawson, & Banerjee, 2008; Lawson, Banerjee, & Field, 2007; and see Field & Purkis, Chapter 11, this volume).

Parents are likely to be an important source of fear-relevant information. Observational studies of children with anxiety disorders in conversation with their parents support the view that parental narratives can be an important influence on the development of children's anxiety. For example, Barrett, Rapee, Dadds, and Ryan (1996) instructed parents to discuss ambiguous scenarios with their 7–14-year-old offspring to help their child generate a plan for how they would respond to the scenarios. Following discussion with their parents, anxious youth were increasingly likely to propose an avoidant plan. In contrast, oppositional youth were more likely to propose an aggressive plan; and non-clinical control children were more likely to propose a proactive plan. Barrett *et al.* (1996) labeled this the "FEAR" effect: Family Enhancement of Aggressive or Avoidant Responses. In an accompanying paper, Dadds and Barrett (1996) described the process by which parents of anxious children appeared to support child avoidant responses, specifically by showing enthusiasm for avoidant plans and providing avoidant responses themselves. Similar results were reported by Chorpita, Albano, and Barlow (1996) who showed that child trait anxiety correlated positively and significantly with threat interpretations and avoidant plans, and that this was enhanced following family discussions. A limitation of these studies is that it is unclear whether parents of anxious children are encouraging their child to adopt a more anxious approach, or are instead encouraging their child (who may try to downplay his or her anxiety) to accurately represent how they would really respond to the scenarios presented. In other words, did parents reinforce anxiety, or did they simply encourage their child to give more accurate responses? To address this difficulty, Murray, Creswell, and Fearon (unpublished data) trained non-anxious mothers of 30 non-anxious children aged 7 to 8 years to act in a manner consistent with the FEAR effect, or in a contrasting manner ("Non-FEAR," i.e., showing enthusiasm for and reciprocating non-threatening interpretations and non-avoidant plans). Following the training period, the children and their mothers discussed two ambiguous scenarios. The children were then assessed on their interpretation of the scenarios that had been discussed, as well as of a novel set of ambiguous scenarios to assess whether the effects of the discussion generalized. Although the non-FEAR group exhibited a reduction in threat interpretation to both the discussed and novel scenarios, the FEAR group exhibited no change in threat interpretation. In other words, family discussions that reinforced children's adaptive (non-FEAR) interpretations led children to adopt and generalize a more adaptive style, whereas discussions that reinforced anxious interpretations maintained this processing style. The combination of findings from the quasi-experimental study of Barrett and colleagues and the experimental study of Murray and colleagues suggests that the discursive style of parents may, indeed, have an influential effect on children's developing fear beliefs.

Future research would benefit from extending these findings to investigate whether these effects lead to changes in observed anxiety when children subsequently enter relevant potentially anxiety-provoking situations. Preliminary evidence from a longitudinal study of adjustment to school in children of mothers with social phobia suggests this might be the case (Murray, Pella, *et al.*, 2008).

Parental control

Theories of the development of anxiety have commonly implicated parental control, in contrast to autonomy granting, as having an important causative role. Specifically, a parent's excessive regulation of the child's behaviors and discouragement of independence is likely to (a) give the child a message that the world is a dangerous and uncontrollable place (e.g., Hudson & Rapee, 2004), and (b) militate against the child's developing a sense of competence and mastery, reinforcing the avoidance of challenge (Chorpita & Barlow, 1998; Parker, 1983). Studies have differed in the specific nature of parental control assessed; some focus on parental over-involvement (where nurturance and support is given to the child when it is not needed, e.g., Hudson & Rapee, 2001); others on intrusive control (where the parent takes over or strongly directs the child, e.g., Wood, 2006); and others on lack of autonomy granting (where a parent fails to encourage the child to face challenges, e.g., Moore *et al.*, 2004). In a meta-analytic review, McLeod *et al.* (2007) reported overall effect sizes for the general construct of "control" and for over-involvement and autonomy granting specifically. Although the overall effect size for control was only $r = 0.25$ (i.e., accounting for 6% of the variance), this rose to 0.42 for autonomy granting (vs. 0.23 for over-involvement). The authors emphasize the need for the traditional parenting dimensions (such as "rejection" and "control") to be dissected into specific components that may represent more specific correlates with child anxiety. Notably, effects were strongest where direct observations of parenting were made (rather than child or parent report), and when child anxiety disorder was examined rather than trait anxiety or anxiety symptom scores.

An important question in relation to parental control is whether it arises in response to child anxiety, or plays an initiating role. Two recent experimental studies have attempted to address this issue. De Wilde and Rapee (2008) instructed 26 mothers of non-clinical children aged 7–13 years to act in either an overly controlling or minimally controlling manner while working with their child on the preparation of a practice speech. Children were subsequently asked to prepare and give a second speech independently of the parent. When children had to do the task alone, those whose mothers had acted in a controlling manner were rated as showing greater anxiety than those whose mothers had acted in a minimally controlling manner. A limitation of this study was that the instructions to mothers included the suggestion that they give the child a sense of how likely they were to succeed in the task, so it was unclear to what extent the effects found did arise from differences in maternal control, or from information transfer (see above), or other potentially overlapping parenting behaviors (e.g., negativity).

Support for the influence of parental control on child anxiety was found in a second experimental study. Thirlwall and Creswell (2010) adopted a repeated measures design in which 24 mothers, from a community population, were trained, using verbal instruction and a DVD presentation, to act in (1) a controlling, and (2) a child-led manner (counterbalanced across participants) while they worked with their 4–5-year-old children to prepare to speak to a videocamera. When mothers were more controlling, children predicted that they would be less able to perform well when it came to doing the task; most important, these differences were not accounted for by observed maternal negativity. Furthermore, for children rated as having high trait anxiety, observed child anxiety was significantly higher while delivering the speech when mothers had been controlling (vs. child-led). Whether a similar pattern of results will be obtained with children of other ages requires exploration; however, these preliminary studies suggest that higher levels of maternal control can lead to increases in child anxiety, particularly for children predisposed to being fearful. These conclusions are consistent with those drawn from a longitudinal, naturalistic study in which children who were inhibited at 2 years of age were only found to be socially reticent at 4 years of age if their mothers had shown intrusive control or were derisive towards the child at the initial assessment (Rubin, Burgess, & Hastings, 2002). Taken together, these studies support the hypothesis that parental control influences the development of childhood anxiety, and that this effect is exaggerated in the context of vulnerability factors such as high temperamental fearfulness.

As noted above, parental control has been implicated in the development of anxiety through its influence on children's cognitions about threat and control (e.g., Chorpita & Barlow, 1998; Hudson & Rapee, 2004). A recent study by Perez-Olivas, Stevenson, and Hadwin (2008) provided preliminary support for the hypothesis that the association between parental control and separation anxiety is mediated by how children process threat information. In this study, 129 non-clinical children (aged 6–14 years) completed a visual search task to assess attentional bias to angry faces, and mothers provided a Five-Minute Speech Sample (FMSS). The FMSS involves asking mothers to speak about their child (with minimal prompting) for 5 minutes; and ratings are then made on the basis of the content and tone of the narratives. The results provided evidence, consistent with a partially mediated pathway, that the child's vigilance for angry faces, which was associated with maternal over-involvement, in turn augmented the degree of separation anxiety in the child. Further studies are now required that are able to examine the temporal nature of these associations. Age was not taken in to account in this analysis; however, it is notable that anxiety-related differences in hypervigilance for angry faces were only present among children 10 years of age and older, highlighting the need for consideration of processes occurring within narrow age bands.

In another study, which addresses the cognitive mechanisms by which parental control might influence youth anxiety, Chorpita, Brown, and Barlow (1998) reported that, in a sample of 93 clinic and non-clinic children aged 6–15 years, children's perceived control mediated the association between a measure of control in the family environment and child negative affect (anxiety and depression). Similarly, an observational study by Gordon, Nowicki, and Wichern (1981) provides support for an association between parental over-involvement and children's cognitive style. These researchers administered a difficult puzzle task to 7–8-year-old children who were accompanied by their mothers, and found that offspring of mothers who tended to help more, give more directions, and generally interfere more, had a more external locus of control than offspring of less "controlling" mothers.

It is important to note, that none of the studies presented thus far provides any information on the impact of child anxiety on parenting behavior, or potential bidirectional associations. Although we can conclude that there is support for the hypothesis that controlling parenting can influence child anxiety, this does not rule out the possibility of a bidirectional relationship. As noted by Silverman *et al.* (2009), bidirectional influences have rarely been considered in relation to youth anxiety; however, the possibility that parents' behavior may change towards their child in response, for example, to a child's improvement from treatment, is highly plausible. Consistent with this hypothesis, Rubin, Nelson, Hastings, and Asendorpf (1999) reported that parents' perceptions of their child's shyness when aged 2 years significantly predicted observed maternal overprotection when children were 4 years of age (however, in the absence of an assessment of parenting at 2 years, it is unclear whether these results reflect changes over time or a continuity in overprotection).

Another approach to disentangling the relative contributions of child and parental influences is to assess parents' responses to multiple offspring with varying levels of anxiety. Hudson and Rapee (2002) and Barrett, Fox, and Farrell (2005) both used sibling controls and found no significant difference between non-anxious mothers' behavior with their anxious child and with the child's sibling; but these two sets of maternal interactions did differ from those of mothers of non-anxious control children. In other words, mothers with an anxious child differed in their parenting to mothers with non-anxious children, and their parenting was similar with both their anxious child and that child's sibling. The authors infer from these findings that the distinctive characteristics of the mothers of anxious children, namely, over-involvement (Hudson & Rapee, 2002), and overcontrol and lack of autonomy granting (Barrett *et al.*, 2005), arise primarily as a function of maternal rather than child characteristics.

Although this interpretation is consistent with their findings, it should be noted that, in Hudson and Rapee (2002) 13% of anxious children's siblings met criteria for a DSM-IV anxiety or behavior disorder and 30% experienced subclinical levels of anxiety. In the study by Barrett and colleagues, siblings who met criteria for a clinical-level anxiety disorder were excluded from analyses; however, the frequency of subclinical levels of anxiety is not reported and, notably, anxious children and their siblings did not differ in their behavior within the observed family discussion task. Caution should, therefore, be applied before rejecting the hypothesis that parental behaviors are a response to child anxiety. These studies also highlight the importance of examining interaction effects to explain the development of anxiety in youth, as despite both anxiety-disordered children and their siblings experiencing higher levels of parental control, in most cases only one sibling in the pair developed an anxiety disorder. As noted above, parental behaviors are likely to have a differential impact depending on child age and developmental stage. These studies both included children from wide age ranges (7 to 16 years: Hudson & Rapee, 2002; 6 to 16 years: Barrett *et al.*, 2005) and included same and mixed-sex sibling pairs; however, age and sex effects will be an important consideration in future research and neither study was sufficiently powered to look at these variables ($n = 57$ Hudson & Rapee, 2002; $n = 47$ Barrett *et al.*, 2005).

A recent study has applied a novel design to further investigate child and maternal contributions to maternal behavior. Mothers of a sample of 7–14-year-old children with anxiety disorders and mothers of non-clinical children were observed interacting with an unrelated child from the same diagnostic group as their own child, and an unrelated child from a different diagnostic group (i.e., anxious or not anxious) (Hudson, Doyle, & Gar, 2009). The anxious and non-anxious children did not differ on mean age or sex. In this study mothers were instructed to help the children prepare to give a speech. All mothers were more involved with clinically anxious children in comparison to non-clinical children, with no significant effects of maternal group, suggesting that the children's anxious behaviors influenced maternal involvement.

In summary, recent experimental studies suggest that increased parental control can *lead to* increased anxiety (in particular among children prone to high anxiety). In addition, observations of parents of clinically anxious children interacting with unrelated children suggest that parents may become more controlling or involved *in response to* high levels of child anxiety. No studies to date have been conducted with suitable methodology to elucidate fully the directionality of parental control in relation to anxiety in youth. This is clearly an essential direction for future research.

Parental negativity, or lack of warmth, has been implicated in the development of anxiety as it is suggested that it may lead the child to believe that the environment is fundamentally hostile and threatening, that outcomes will be negative, and to a sense of low self-worth and competence (Bögels & Tarrier, 2004; Parker, 1983). Although some have suggested that parental negativity may be associated with youth anxiety through their mutual association with low mood (e.g., Rapee, 1997), others have suggested that the experience of parental negativity may create a vulnerability for developing fear through other pathways. Price-Evans and Field (2008) reported that, among a sample of 6–10-year-old children, increased child perceptions of mothers as neglectful mediated the effect that verbal threat information (see above and Field & Purkis, Chapter 11, this volume) had on fear of novel animals. In this study there were no significant effects of child perceptions of punitive maternal style, maternal warmth, overprotection or monitoring, or perceptions about paternal rearing. Again, this finding highlights the importance of looking at specific parenting constructs rather than global indices of, for example, "negativity." Indeed, the precise definition of parental negativity has differed across studies, and has included withdrawal or a lack of positive affect, but also lack of acceptance, and actively aversive parenting or rejection.

Reviews based on both the broader definition and more specific subtypes of parental negativity have concluded that evidence for parental lack of warmth being associated with child anxiety is weak and inconsistent (DiBartolo & Helt, 2007; McLeod *et al.*, 2007; Wood, McLeod, Sigman, Hwang, & Chu, 2003). For example, on the basis of their meta-analysis, Mcleod and colleagues reported a small mean effect size of $r = 0.20$ for the general construct of "rejection," and, more specifically, mean effect sizes of $r = 0.06$ for warmth, 0.22 for withdrawal, and 0.23 for aversiveness. In addition, where associations have been found, studies have not been equipped to address issues of directionality. A recent exception is the study of Silverman *et al.* (2009). They studied a sample of 7–16-year-old clinically anxious youth before and after cognitive–behavioral therapy (CBT) treatment, with or without active parental involvement. They assessed their patients' perceptions of parental positive and negative behaviors, and conflict in the parent–youth relationship. From this study, evidence was strongest for the hypothesis that youth anxiety affects parenting; specifically, changes in youth anxiety from pre- to post-treatment were associated with reductions in parental negative behaviors at the post-treatment assessment. As this study relied on child reports of parenting variables it is unclear whether the results reflect changes in child perceptions of parenting, rather than actual parenting; however, it is notable that a similar pattern of findings existed for self-reported parental anxiety, i.e., a reduction in parent self-reported anxiety from pre- to post-treatment regardless of whether parents had been actively involved in treatment.

Hudson *et al.* (2009) also observed maternal negativity in their study of mothers of clinically anxious and non-anxious children. Mothers of clinically anxious children (in comparison to mothers of non-anxious children) were less negative in their interactions with non-clinical children compared to their interactions with their clinically anxious children. Although caution must be maintained, because the number of negative behaviors expressed was relatively low, the authors suggest that the fact that mothers of non-anxious children are less used to dealing with severely anxious behavior may enable them to be more warm and positive in their interactions. Once again, the results of both these studies provide a clear impetus in the field to seriously consider child to parent effects, and bidirectional associations.

Wider parenting practices

Although research interest in parenting outlined above has largely focused on observed parent–child interactions and the assessment of proximal parenting processes, it is important to note that wider parenting practices are also likely to be implicated in the development of child anxiety. Thus, parents' decisions concerning, for example, the use of day care, and family socialization and recreational activities, all stand to enhance or limit child exposure to potential challenges beyond the home, and thereby the opportunity for the child to develop coping skills. Research on these parenting dimensions in the context of youth anxiety is scant (although see Bögels & Brechman-Toussaint, 2006; Chorpita & Barlow, 1998). Nevertheless, there are grounds for suggesting that this is an important area for investigation, particularly in the preschool and early school years. For example, in non-clinical samples, where parents actively foster preschool social experiences, children show less anxious behavior and fewer absences from kindergarten in comparison to children whose parents were less active in fostering social experiences (Ladd & Hart, 1992; Ladd, Le Sieur, Profilet, & Duck, 1993; Ladd & Price, 1987).

Parental anxiety and parenting behaviors

If parental behaviors constitute a pathway to intergenerational transmission of anxiety then it is reasonable to expect a greater frequency of those parental behaviors that appear to reinforce child anxiety among parents who themselves experience high levels of anxiety than among low-anxious parents. To date there has been only a small number of studies that address this hypothesis.

Vicarious learning

It seems plausible to assume that children of anxious parents will have increased opportunities for vicarious learning, due to more frequent expression of anxiety by their parents in comparison to children of non-anxious parents. This assumption has been corroborated by findings from Murray *et al.*'s longitudinal study of the intergenerational transmission of social anxiety (Murray, Cooper, Creswell, Schofield, & Sack, 2007). Mothers and infants were studied from three demographically comparable groups: where the mother had social phobia ($n = 96$), where the mother had generalized anxiety disorder (GAD) ($n = 52$), and where the mother had no anxiety disorder ($n = 54$). Mothers' behaviors with their 10-week-old infants were observed in a face-to-face interaction and in a social challenge (conversation with a stranger). Mothers with social phobia ($n = 84$) were no less sensitive than control mothers with no anxiety disorder ($n = 89$) during interactions with their infants; however, mothers with social phobia exhibited significantly more anxiety, engaged less with the stranger, and were less encouraging of their child's interaction with the stranger than the non-anxious mothers. These differences appeared to be specific to mothers with social phobia, as they were not found among mothers with GAD. Furthermore, as reported above, continuing maternal expressed social anxiety at 10 months predicted subsequent infant avoidance of a stranger. Whether these findings extend to parental anxieties in other (non-social) domains warrants empirical examination.

Information transfer

Few studies have investigated in detail the extent to which potentially anxiogenic information is conveyed by highly anxious parents to their offspring. In a preliminary investigation, Moore et al., (2004) observed mother–child interactions in three discussion tasks (an "ideal person task," a conflict conversation, and an anxiety conversation). The 68 mother–child (7–15 years) pairs formed four groups based on the presence or absence of maternal as well as child anxiety disorder. There was a main effect of maternal anxiety disorder on the extent to which mothers made catastrophic comments, as well as an interaction with child anxiety diagnosis: specifically, when mothers were anxious, catastrophizing was present in the majority of dyads; but when mothers were not anxious, catastrophizing was elevated in dyads only where the child had an anxiety disorder diagnosis. These findings suggest that, as well as being a response to high child anxiety, a catastrophic narrative style may also be a function of maternal anxiety. These conclusions must be regarded as preliminary as group comparisons were based on small cell sizes (for example, there were only eight dyads in the anxious mother–non-anxious child group) and, thus, may not be generalizable. In addition, the findings reflect cross-sectional associations and studies that can investigate the direction of effects are required. Recent findings from a follow-up of the prospective, longitudinal study conducted by Murray, De Rosnay, et al. (2008) do suggest that anxious (in this case socially phobic) mothers do express more anxious cognitions (e.g., threat attributions) during a naturalistic, picture book, narrative interaction with their 5-year-old children about a potential social challenge (starting school), independent of previously assessed child behavioral inhibition (Murray, Pella, et al., 2008).

Parental control/involvement and negativity

Although studies of parental behaviors associated with parental anxiety disorder have found increased negativity and reduced autonomy granting (Whaley, Pinto, & Sigman, 1999), others have not found consistent associations (Ginsburg, Grover, & Ialongo, 2004; Turner, Beidel, Roberson-Nay, & Tervo, 2003; Woodruff-Borden, Morrow, Bourland, & Cambron, 2002). Indeed, because of the family aggregation of anxiety, it remains possible that associations found between parental anxiety and parenting behaviors are, in fact, the result of a shared association with increased child anxiety. The importance of the effect of the child on their parent has been emphasized by the few studies that take into account both the child and parent anxiety diagnoses. One such study by Moore et al. (2004), suggested that mothers of anxious children, regardless of their own anxiety, were less warm and granted less autonomy in interaction with their child than mothers of non-anxious children. Unfortunately, as noted above, in this study cell sizes were small which limits generalizability of the findings. Nevertheless, Gar and Hudson (2008) conducted a larger study employing a similar design and reported findings consistent with those of Moore *et al.*'s general conclusions. In this study, 155 mothers and their 4–16-year-old children participated, again grouped according to the presence or absence of child and maternal diagnosis (with a minimum cell size of $n = 28$). Based on both observed parent–child interactions (in preparation of a speech) and the Five Minute Speech Sample (FMSS), across the two procedures there was a main effect of child anxiety status on maternal over-involvement, but not of maternal anxiety status. Mothers of anxious children were also rated as being more negative on the FMSS. In this study, which focused on maternal control and negativity dimensions, no significant main effects or interaction effects with maternal anxiety were found. It appears, therefore, that more involved or controlling behavior, and possibly negativity, is a common parental response to having an anxious child which (see above) might reinforce child anxiety (in particular, when it occurs in interaction with other vulnerability factors).

Whether parental anxiety increases the likelihood of over-involved or controlling parenting behavior, thereby promoting the *development* of child anxiety, cannot be ascertained from these studies of already anxious children: information is required on the processes that occur before the onset of the child anxiety disorder. In fact, the results of prospective longitudinal studies suggest that infant or child inhibition may provoke these parenting styles more readily among anxious, compared to non-anxious, parents. For example, Hirshfeld, Biederman, Brody, Faraone, and Rosenbaum (1997) found that maternal criticism of the child (assessed via the FMSS) was a function of a significant interaction between child behavioral inhibition and maternal anxiety disorder status; that is, within the group of anxious mothers 65% of those with inhibited children were critical compared to 18% of those with non-inhibited children. Among non-anxious mothers, by contrast, the prevalence of maternal criticism was similar in those with inhibited and uninhibited children. Similar findings were obtained by Murray, De Rosnay, *et al.* (2008): mothers with social phobia showed low levels of encouragement to their infants to engage with a stranger *only* if their infant was behaviorally inhibited.

Cognitive mechanisms may underly the association between high parental anxiety and an increased tendency to respond to child symptoms in potentially anxiogenic ways. For example, Rubin, Cheah, and Fox (2001) suggest that parental beliefs about child vulnerability may lead to parenting behaviors that strengthen the relationship between child temperamental risk factors and child anxiety. In other words, parents' beliefs (and the behavior that follows) may determine whether or not temperamentally fearful children develop an anxiety disorder (and see Creswell, Murray, & Cooper, 2010a). Indeed, anxious parents, who are more inclined to interpret the world in a threatening manner themselves, have been found to make similar interpretations in relation to situations involving their child (Lester, Field, Oliver, & Cartwright-Hatton, 2009), to predict that their child will feel threatened and be more easily distressed (Creswell & O'Connor, 2006), and to have lower expectations of their own parental control of their child's behavior (Wheatcroft & Creswell, 2007); and these effects hold true after accounting for the contribution of child anxiety. Furthermore, parental predictions of increased child vulnerability appear to lead to more involved parental behaviors. Thus, in a preliminary experimental study, Creswell, O'Connor, and Brewin (2008) allocated mothers of 52 non-anxious children aged 7–11 years to either a "positive" or "negative" expectations group prior to completing a difficult anagram task with their child, in which the parent was led to believe the child would be likely to enjoy, or else be upset by, the task. The results showed that parents who were given negative expectations displayed increased levels of involvement during the task, suggesting that parental expectations about children's vulnerability are associated with more involved parenting behaviors. In this study, the increase in parental involvement that following experimental manipulation was small and did not lead to a significant increase in observed child anxiety. Future studies are required that include a sample that is sufficiently large to detect differences in child anxiety and to examine interactions with child trait anxiety. Nonetheless, based on these studies, one can speculate that targeting parental cognitions may be of particular value in interventions which aim to improve child anxiety by changing parental behavior.

Wider parenting practices

As noted above family socialization and use of childcare are likely to influence the development of anxiety in children, and may be affected by the presence of parental anxiety. For example, highly anxious parents may find it challenging to support their child's exposure to potential stressors or may provide only limited naturalistic opportunities for their child to face fears and develop coping skills. Initial support for this hypothesis has come from our prospective study of mothers diagnosed with social phobia, in which infants of non-anxious mothers experienced greater frequency of non-maternal care between 4 and 24 months of age (Creswell, Murray, & Cooper, 2010b).

Further investigation of parental anxiety and wider socialization practices is clearly warranted.

Further issues in research on parenting and child anxiety

Specificity of effects

Few studies to date have addressed the issues of specificity of effects. Several issues arise. The first concerns the question of whether particular parenting characteristics are uniquely associated with child anxiety disorders, rather than with more general child psychopathology. Second, there is the question of whether there are parenting characteristics that are specifically related to subtypes of both parent and child anxiety disorder. The third question is whether difficulties associated with either parental or child disorders are only manifest in specific, disorder-relevant contexts, or are apparent across situations. With regard to the first issue, studies (e.g., Dumas & LaFreniere, 1993; Dumas, Serketich, & LaFreniere, 1995; Hudson & Rapee, 2001) that have used observational methods to compare the parenting of anxious children with that of children with other disorders have produced inconsistent findings. Thus, compared to mothers of aggressive children, those of anxious children have been observed to be both more negative and more controlling (Dumas & LaFreniere, 1993; Dumas *et al.*, 1995); but also to be indistinguishable in terms of negativity and control (Hudson & Rapee, 2001). The use of more precise definitions of subtypes of parental behaviors within these broad categories, and comparisons with groups experiencing disorders that are commonly comorbid with anxiety, are likely to lead to greater consistency between findings and a clearer understanding of specific risks for childhood anxiety. Both the Virginia Twin Study (Kendler, Myers, & Prescott, 2000) and the Great Smoky Mountains epidemiological study (Shanahan, Copeland, Costello, & Angold, 2008) are notable for having used multiple informants (youth and parent), and for having carefully controlled for comorbid anxiety, mood, and behavioral disorders. The former study showed each of cold, overprotective, and authoritarian parenting to contribute to offspring anxiety, over and above their impact on other child diagnoses; while the latter study showed some evidence for over-intrusive parenting being specifically associated with anxiety disorders rather than conduct disorder, oppositional defiant disorder, and depression.

The majority of the studies discussed above concerned associations between parenting factors and childhood anxiety in general, grouping together disparate anxiety disorders (most commonly social phobia, GAD, and separation anxiety disorder [SAD], but also, commonly, specific phobias and obsessive–compulsive disorder). The issue of the diagnostic specificity of parental risk factors has received scant attention, despite emerging supportive evidence. Of note are the studies reported above concerning vicarious learning. Gerull and Rapee (2002), for example, showed that maternal modeling of fear to potentially fear-provoking objects led to infant expression of fearful and avoidant responses to those specific stimuli, and not to other novel stimuli to which mothers had not expressed fear. Similarly, specific effects on children's social reticence have been observed after mothers expressed anxiety and displayed reduced encouragement in a social setting (De Rosnay *et al.*, 2006; Murray, De Rosnay, *et al.*, 2008). Notably, such parental behaviors have been found to be specifically associated with the presence of maternal social phobia and not GAD (Murray *et al.*, 2007), suggesting that issues of diagnostic specificity will be important to take into account when considering the risks associated with parental anxiety disorder, as well as the development of child anxiety. A preliminary study of 55 clinically anxious children and their mothers (also assessed for anxiety disorder diagnoses) highlighted a potential clinical implication of this issue (Cooper, Gallop, Willetts, & Creswell, 2008). Specifically, clinically anxious children (aged 7–12 years), with a range of anxiety disorders, whose mothers met criteria for GAD had equivalent treatment outcomes to children of non-anxious mothers, whereas children who had mothers with social phobia did significantly less well following treatment. One possible interpretation of these findings is that mothers with social phobia may engage in specific behaviors which militate against positive treatment outcome (e.g., reduced encouragement/autonomy granting, increased fear modeling).

Results from studies of information transfer conducted with non-clinical populations are consistent with the notion of diagnostically specific effects on fear acquisition. Thus, in the studies of Field and colleagues, children typically show increased fear responses to the specific animal about which they receive negative information, and this effect does not generalize to animals about which they receive no information (e.g., Field *et al.*, 2003, 2008).

Few studies have examined diagnostic specificity in relation to the constructs of parental negativity and control, a notable exception being one reported by Wood (2006). Wood argues that parental intrusiveness may be a specific risk for SAD amongst children prone to anxiety, because it promotes reliance on the caregiver, reduces opportunities to experience feelings of mastery, control and self-efficacy, and reinforces clingy behavior. In Wood's study, the extent of parental intrusiveness was established for 40 6–13-year-old clinically anxious children. Intrusiveness was assessed using a composite of observed intrusive physical contact (in the "belt-buckling task"), parent- and child-reported degree of parental help with daily routines, and parent perceptions of help required by the child with daily living skills. Parental intrusiveness was significantly associated with severity of SAD (clinician, child, and parent reports), but not with severity of social phobia and GAD.

Both the Smoky Mountains and the Virginia twin studies mentioned above examined the question of specificities in children's perceived parenting within the anxiety disorders. Harsh discipline was associated with GAD in the Smoky Mountains study, as was the similar dimension of authoritative parenting in the Virginia study; however, in the latter, overprotection was also a significant factor. In the Smoky Mountains study, no perceived parenting dimension had a significant unique association with social phobia or child SAD, over and above their association with other child disorders, whereas in the Virginia study, all three parenting dimensions assessed (i.e., harsh discipline, authoritative parenting, and overprotection) made significant contributions to phobias (including social phobia), independent of effects on other disorders.

The final issue in relation to specificity is that parents may show particular parenting behaviors only within specific contexts, for example contexts that either the parent or the child (or both) find stressful. Wood's (2006) findings, for example, might have been different if parental intrusiveness had been assessed within a specific social stress task. Murray et al.'s (2007) findings are consistent with this idea: mothers with social phobia, but not mothers with GAD, differed from controls in key parenting behaviors within social, but not non-social, tasks.

In summary, research findings to date concerning the association between parenting characteristics and child anxiety may have been distorted by a failure to consider issues of specificity – that is, whether parenting characteristics are specifically associated with child anxiety disorders in comparison to child psychopathology generally, whether specific child and parental anxiety disorders are associated with particular behaviors, and whether anxiogenic parenting behaviors are elicited within specific domains (e.g., within particular stressful contexts). It is essential that future research takes account of these issues in order to identify specific targets for prevention and therapeutic intervention for anxious youth.

Effects of parent sex

As previously noted, the majority of studies conducted to date have either restricted their samples to mothers, or have included too few fathers to be able to look at differential effects of parent sex. While evidence does not clearly show that fathers, unlike mothers, of anxious children have a raised rate of current anxiety disorder (e.g., Cooper et al., 2006), there is evidence that fathers have an increased lifetime history of anxiety disorder when compared to fathers of non-anxious children (Cooper et al., 2006; Martin, Cabrol, Bouvard, Lepine, & Mouren-Simeoni, 1999). This consideration is important because studies have shown that a past history of psychological distress can continue to have an effect on cognitions (e.g., Hollon, Kendall, & Lumry, 1986) and parenting behaviors, even when there is no current disturbance (Stein et al., 2001). In other words, both maternal and paternal behaviors could contribute to the intergenerational transmission of anxiety. The issue resolves to three central questions: (a) do mothers and fathers tend to parent in similar ways? (b) Is the impact of particular parental behaviors the same whether it comes from mothers or fathers? And (c) are there distinctive features of mothers' and fathers' parental interactions that make a specific contribution to the development of child anxiety?

In relation to the first issue, few studies have directly addressed associations between both mothers' and fathers' cognitions and/or behaviors and child anxiety disorder. A notable exception is Barrett et al. (1996) in which fathers' and mothers' responses to ambiguous scenarios involving their child were assessed. Results for fathers were consistent with those reported for mothers. In particular, fathers of anxious children expected their children to respond in a more avoidant manner than fathers of non-anxious children. As noted above, however, this study is limited in that it is unclear to what extent the parents were simply representing their child's actual response, rather than evidencing a parental cognitive distortion. In their detailed analysis of parent–child discussions in a subset of families in the above study, Dadds and Barrett (1996) reported that fathers, like mothers, of clinically anxious children (anxious and aggressive) responded to an avoidant communication from their child with their own avoidant communication. Studies that have assessed children's perceptions of parenting have also found consistent patterns based on ratings of maternal and paternal behavior. Siqueland, Kendall, and Steinberg (1996), for example, reported that 9–12-year-old children with anxiety disorders rated both their mothers and fathers as significantly less accepting than control children. Most important, in this study, children's ratings of parental acceptance were significantly associated with independent observers' ratings of parental warmth. Similarly, Gruner, Muris, and Merckelbach (1999), in a community sample of 9–12-year-old children, found that (child-reported) maternal and paternal rejection, control, and anxious rearing, were associated with self-reported child anxiety.

In relation to the second issue, there is evidence to suggest that the impact of certain parental behaviors may be similar for both mothers and fathers. For example, Dadds and Barrett (1996) found that an avoidant communication pattern between both mothers and fathers and their children was associated with the extent to which children adopted avoidant plans following family conversations. Rubin *et al.* (1999), who also reported few differences between mothers' and fathers' expressed parenting styles at assessments made when their children were 2 and 4 years of age, found equivalent associations for mothers and fathers between perceived child shyness at 2 years and parental encouragement of independence at 4 years.

Despite these indications of equivalence, others have suggested that fathers may also typically take on a different role to mothers, due to biological and socially reinforced characteristics. For example, fathers may be important agents for children to experience boisterous, stimulating, and emotionally arousing play that encourages risk-taking and facing challenges which may buffer against early separation, stranger, and novelty anxiety (Bögels & Phares, 2008). There is some evidence that the parenting behaviors that distinguish anxious and non-anxious children may be different in fathers and mothers, although studies have largely been limited to non-clinical, adolescent samples and rely on measures of perceived parenting. For example, Brakel, van Muris, Bögels, and Thomassen (2006) reported that 11–15-year-old adolescents' reports of paternal (but not maternal) anxious rearing behaviors were associated with anxiety symptoms. The possibility that there may be specific effects of parental sex depending on child sex has been supported by Bosco, Renk, Dinger, Epstein, and Phares (2003) who found that adolescent daughters' (but not sons') reports of fathers', but not mothers', lower acceptance and higher control contributed to increased adolescent anxiety (independent of the association with depression). Similarly, in a sample of older adolescent girls, more negative perceptions of fathers were associated with increased anxiety (Renk, McKinney, Klein, & Oliveros, 2006). Unfortunately, most studies have not been equipped to identify whether these effects are specific to anxiety, and where comorbid difficulties have been assessed results have suggested that fathers' controlling and rejecting parenting (but not mothers') were associated with child externalizing symptoms, and not child social anxiety (Bögels, van Oostern, Muris, & Smulders, 2001) or shy and anxious behavior (McCabe, Clark, & Barnett, 1999).

However, in an important longitudinal study which included observational and parent report measures of father and mother behavior with their first-born sons (Belsky, Hsieh, & Crinic, 1998), the extent to which fathers, but not mothers, displayed what are traditionally viewed as *positive* rearing behaviors (sensitive and non-intrusive) was associated with increased inhibition in vulnerable male toddlers (previously classified as inhibited). These findings are contrary to models of the development of anxiety that postulate that higher levels of intrusiveness will be associated with increased child anxiety. The authors consider the possibility that inhibited boys may benefit from fathers who push their child to face challenges (appearing less sensitive), rather than fathers who are more sensitive to their child's vulnerability (and accept and potentially reinforce children's fears and worries). As this study only involved parents and their sons, whether these findings represented a specific effect for boys remains an open question.

Another important consideration is the impact of concordance between maternal and paternal anxiety. The findings to date on this point are highly inconsistent. Merikangas, Avenevoli, Dierker, and Grillon (1999) found that when both parents had an anxiety disorder, their 7–17-year-old offspring were nearly twice as likely to have an anxiety disorder than if just one parent has an anxiety disorder. In contrast, Dierker, Merikangas, and Szatmari (1999) found that parental concordance for anxiety and affective disorders did not significantly increase rates of anxiety disorders, again in 7–17-year-old offspring, beyond that found in families in which only one parent was affected. Consistent with the latter study, Jorm, Dear, Rodgers, and Christensen (2003) reported that although both paternal and maternal affection (as rated by adult offspring) correlated with offspring's reported anxiety symptoms, if mothers' affection was low, offspring continued to report high anxiety even in the presence of high paternal affection, suggesting that paternal affection did not compensate for a lack of maternal affection. However, in a longitudinal study of divorced families, father–adolescent closeness predicted less adolescent anxiety, over and above maternal variables (Summers, Forehand, Armistead, & Tannenbaum, 1998).

In summary, evidence is mixed with regard to whether maternal and paternal factors differ in relation to their association with child anxiety, although it has been suggested that fathers may commonly serve a particular role in encouraging risk-taking behavior, whereas mothers are more commonly responsible for care (Bögels & Phares, 2008). Further research is clearly warranted in this area, in particular, systematic evaluations of the behaviors of mothers and fathers, with their daughters and sons, using rigorous observational methodologies.

Summary

Although many limitations remain in our understanding of parenting pathways to the development of childhood anxiety disorder, the evidence reviewed suggests an interplay between several parenting factors (Figure 14.1), which are likely to be exacerbated by the presence of parental anxiety. First, research on parenting suggests that child anxiety may be promoted by learning processes of modeling and information transfer. We also suggest that wider parenting practices, such as family socialization and childcare arrangements, may influence the development of child anxiety by supporting or limiting opportunities for exposure to potential stressors. Although these parental behaviors are likely to be exacerbated in the context of parental anxiety, it is important to note that they may occur independently of parental anxiety (e.g., provision of negative information or modeling by other influential sources). Furthermore, some parenting dimensions associated with child disorder appear to be provoked by particular child characteristics, like temperamental fearfulness or, indeed, child anxiety itself. These include behaviors such as over-involvement or overprotection, lack of encouragement, or autonomy-promotion. We suggest that these

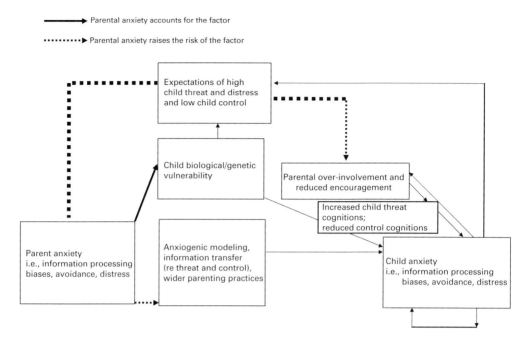

Figure 14.1 Parenting pathways to child anxiety. (Adapted from Murray *et al.* [2009] and Creswell *et al.* [2008].)

behaviors may relate to parental beliefs that the child is vulnerable in the face of a potentially dangerous world. Notably, such cognitions and behaviors are especially likely to arise in parents who are themselves prone to anxiety. These parenting styles initiated by the child's behavior also play a role in maintaining child inhibition and anxiety by reinforcing developing child cognitions that the world is threatening and that s/he is not capable of coping with or controlling this threat.

Clinical implications

The proposed model has potential implications for the prevention and clinical management of child anxiety disorders. While individual vulnerability factors may not be strong predictors of later anxiety disorder (see, e.g., McLeod *et al.*, 2007), identifying children who experience a combination of vulnerability factors (e.g., high temperamental fearfulness and "anxiogenic" parenting) may allow effective targeting of preventive interventions. Furthermore, the model identifies key parenting practices that are likely to require specific intervention (e.g., reduced encouragement and autonomy granting; see, e.g., Wood, Piacentini, Southam-Gerow, Chu, & Sigman, 2006) and associated parental cognitions, particularly in the context of high parental anxiety. Indeed, the presence of high levels of parental anxiety is likely to be a barrier to optimal child treatment outcome (e.g., Cobham, Spence, & Dadds, 1998; Creswell, Willetts, Murray, Singhal, & Cooper, 2008). Findings to date relating to improving outcomes for this group have been intriguing. Cobham *et al.* (1998), for example, reported a significant benefit to children whose anxious parents (in terms of the proportion of children who were diagnostic free post-treatment) received Parent Anxiety Management in addition to individual child cognitive–behavioral therapy

(CBT), although parents themselves did not appear to evidence a reduction in their own anxiety. It is possible that these parents responded to the intervention by becoming aware of their anxiogenic parenting and changing their parenting behaviors. The suggestion that parental behaviors, rather than parental anxiety per se, may be important in relation to treatment outcome is supported by findings of a preliminary study in which maternal modeling of anxiety during interactions with the child was a significant predictor of child treatment outcome (Creswell, Willetts, *et al.*, 2008). Future studies, which systematically address both parental anxiety and parental behaviors, will help determine whether it is necessary to address parental anxiety itself, or whether it is sufficient to deal only with the parenting consequences of that anxiety.

References

Askew, C. & Field, A. (2008). The vicarious learning pathway to fear 40 years on. *Clinical Psychology Review*, **28**, 1249–1265.

Barrett, P. M., Fox, T., & Farrell, L. (2005). Parent–child interactions with anxious children and their siblings: an observational study. *Behavior Change*, **22**, 220–235.

Barrett, P. M., Rapee, R. M., & Dadds, M. R. (1996). Family treatment of childhood anxiety: a controlled trial. *Journal of Consulting and Clinical Psychology*, **64**, 333–342.

Barrett, P. M., Rapee, R. M., Dadds, M. M., & Ryan, S. M. (1996). Family enhancement of cognitive style in anxious and aggressive children. *Journal of Abnormal Child Psychology*, **24**, 197–203.

Beidel, D. C. & Turner, S. M. (1997). At risk for anxiety. I. Psychopathology in the offspring of anxious parents. *Journal of the American Academy of Child and Adolescent Psychiatry*, **36**, 918–924.

Belsky, J., Hsieh, K., & Crnic, K. (1998). Mothering, fathering and infant negativity as antecedents of boys' externalizing problems and inhibition at age 3: differential susceptibility to rearing experiences? *Development and Psychopathology*, **10**, 301–319.

Biederman, J., Rosenbaum, J. F., Bolduc, E. A., Faraone, S. V., & Hirshfeld, D. R. (1991). A high risk study of young children of parents with panic disorder and agoraphobia with and without comorbid major depression. *Psychiatry Research*, **37**, 333–348.

Bögels, S. M. & Brechman-Toussaint, M. L. (2006). Family issues in child anxiety: attachment, family functioning, parental rearing and beliefs. *Clinical Psychology Review*, **26**, 834–856.

Bögels, S. M. & Phares, V. (2008). Fathers' role in the etiology, prevention and treatment of child anxiety: a review and new model. *Clinical Psychology Review*, **28**, 539–558.

Bögels, S. M. & Tarrier, N. (2004). Unexplored issues and future directions in social phobia research. *Clinical Psychology Review*, **24**, 731–736.

Bögels, S. M., van Oostern, A., Muris, P., & Smulders, D. (2001). Familial correlates of social anxiety in children and adolescents. *Behaviour Research and Therapy*, **39**, 273–287.

Bosco, G. L., Renk, K., Dinger, T. M., Epstein, M. K., & Phares, V. (2003). The connections between adolescents' perceptions of parents, parental psychological symptoms, and adolescent functioning. *Journal of Applied Developmental Psychology*, **24**, 179–200.

Brakel, A. M. L., van Muris, P., Bögels, S. M., & Thomassen, C. (2006). A multifactorial model for the aetiology of anxiety in non-clinical adolescents: main and interactive effects of behavioural inhibition, attachment, and parental rearing. *Journal of Child and Family Studies*, **15**, 568–578.

Chorpita B. F. & Barlow D. H. (1998). The development of anxiety: the role of control in the early environment. *Psychological Bulletin*, **124**, 3–21.

Chorpita, B. F., Albano, A. M., & Barlow, D. H. (1996). Cognitive processing in children: relationship to anxiety and family influences. *Journal of Clinical Child Psychology*, **25**, 170–176.

Chorpita, B. F., Brown, T. A., & Barlow, D. H. (1998). Perceived control as a mediator of family environment in etiological models of childhood anxiety. *Behavior Therapy*, **29**, 457–476.

Cobham, V. E., Spence, S. H., & Dadds, M. R. (1998). The role of parental anxiety in the treatment of childhood anxiety. *Journal of Consulting and Clinical Psychology*, **66**, 893–905.

Cook, M. & Mineka, S. (1987). Second-order conditioning and overshadowing in the observational conditioning of fear in monkeys. *Behaviour Research and Therapy*, **25**, 349–364.

Cook, M. & Mineka, S. (1989). Observational conditioning of fear to fear-relevant versus fear-irrelevant stimuli in rhesus monkeys. *Journal of Abnormal Psychology*, **98**, 448–459.

Cook, M. & Mineka, S. (1990). Selective associations in the observational conditioning of fear in rhesus monkeys. *Journal of Experimental Psychology – Animal Behaviour Processes*, **16**, 372–389.

Cooper, P. J., Fearn, V., Willetts, L, Seabrook, H., & Parkinson, M. (2006). Affective disorder in the parents of a clinic sample of children with anxiety disorders. *Journal of Affective Disorder*, **93**, 205–212.

Cooper, P. J., Gallop, C., Willetts, L., & Creswell, C. (2008). Treatment response in child anxiety is differentially related to the form of maternal anxiety disorder. *Behavioural and Cognitive Psychotherapy*, **36**, 41–48.

Creswell, C. & O'Connor, T. (2006). "Anxious cognitions" in children: an exploration of associations and mediators. *British Journal of Developmental Psychology*, **24**, 761–766.

Creswell, C., Murray, L. M., & Cooper, P. J. (2010a). Intergenerational transmission of anxious information processing bias. In: J. A. Hadwin & A. P. Field (eds.) *Information Processing Biases in Child and Adolescent Anxiety*, pp. 279–296. Chichester, UK: Wiley-Blackwell.

Creswell, C., Murray, L. M., & Cooper, P. J. (2010b). Use of non-maternal care amongst mothers with social phobia: comparisons with non-anxious mothers and associations with child outcomes. Paper presented at World Congress of Behavioural and Cognitive Therapies conference, June 26–29 2010, Boston University, Boston, MA.

Creswell, C., O'Connor, T., & Brewin, C. (2008). The impact of parents' expectations on parenting behaviour: an experimental investigation. *Behavioural and Cognitive Psychotherapy*, **36**, 483–490.

Creswell, C., Willetts, L., Murray, L., Singhal, M., & Cooper, P. (2008). Treatment of child anxiety: an exploratory study of the role of maternal anxiety and behaviours in treatment outcome. *Clinical Psychology and Psychotherapy*, **15**, 38–44.

Dadds, M. R. & Barrett, P. M. (1996). Family processes in child and adolescent anxiety and depression. *Behavior Change*, **13**, 231–239.

De Rosnay, M., Cooper, P. J., Tsigaras, N. & Murray, L. (2006). Transmission of social anxiety from mother to infant: an experimental study using a social referencing paradigm. *Behaviour Research and Therapy*, **44**, 1165–1175.

De Wilde, A. & Rapee, R. M. (2008). Do controlling maternal behaviours increase state anxiety in children's responses to a social threat? A pilot study. *Journal of Behavior Therapy and Experimental Psychiatry*, **39**, 526–537.

Denham, S., Zoller, D., & Couchard, E. (1994). Socialisation of pre-schoolers emotion understanding. *Developmental Psychology*, **30**, 928–936.

DiBartolo, P. M. & Helt, M. (2007). Theoretical models of affectionate versus affectionless control in anxious families: a critical examination based on observations of parent–child interactions. *Clinical Child and Family Psychology*, **10**, 253–274.

Dierker, L. C., Merikangas, K. R., & Szatmari, P. (1999). Influence of parental concordance for psychiatric disorders on psychopathology in offspring. *Journal of American Academy of Child and Adolescent Psychiatry*, **38**, 280–288.

Dubi, K., Rapee, R. M., Emerton, J. L., & Schneiring, C. A. (2008). Maternal modelling and the acquisition of fear and avoidance in toddlers: influence of stimulus preparedness and child temperament. *Journal of Abnormal Child Psychology*, **36**, 499–512.

Dumas, J. E. & LaFreniere, P. J. (1993). Mother–child relationships as sources of support or stress: a comparison of competent, average, aggressive, and anxious dyads. *Child Development*, **64**, 1732–1754.

Dumas, J. E., Serketich, W. J., & LaFreniere, P. J. (1995). "Balance of power": a transactional analysis of control in mother–child dyads involving socially competent, aggressive, and anxious children. *Journal of Abnormal Psychology*, **104**, 104–113.

Feinman, S., Roberts, D., Hsieh, K., Sawyer, D., & Swanson, D. (1992). A critical review of social referencing in infancy. In: S. Feinman (ed.) *Social Referencing and the Social Construction of Reality in Infancy*, pp. 15–54. New York: Plenum Press.

Field, A. P. & Lawson, J. (2003). Fear information and the development of fears during childhood: effects on implicit fear responses and behavioural avoidance. *Behaviour Research and Therapy*, **41**, 1277–1293.

Field, A. P., Hamilton, S. J., Knowles, K. A., & Plews, E. L. (2003). Fear information and social phobic beliefs in children: a prospective paradigm and preliminary results. *Behaviour Research and Therapy*, **41**, 113–123.

Field, A. P., Lawson, J., & Banerjee, R. (2008). The verbal threat information pathway to fear in children: the longitudinal effects on fear cognitions and the immediate effects on avoidance behavior. *Journal of Abnormal Psychology*, **117**, 214–224.

Fivush, R. (1991). The social construction of personal narratives. *Merrill-Palmer Quarterly*, **37**, 59–82.

Gar, N. S. & Hudson, J. L. (2008). An examination of the interactions between mothers and children with anxiety disorders. *Behaviour Research and Therapy*, **46**, 1266–1274.

Gerull, F. C. & Rapee, R. M. (2002). Mother knows best: effects of maternal modelling on the acquisition of fear and avoidance behaviour in toddlers. *Behaviour Research and Therapy*, **40**, 279–287.

Ginsburg, G. S., Grover, R. L., & Ialongo, N. (2004). Parenting behaviors among anxious and non-anxious mothers: relation with concurrent and long-term child outcomes. *Child and Family Behavior Therapy*, **26**, 23–41.

Gordon, D., Nowicki, S., Jr., & Wichern, F. (1981). Observed maternal and child behaviors in a dependency producing task as a function of children's locus of control orientation. *Merrill-Palmer Quarterly*, **27**, 43–52.

Gregory, A. M. & Eley, T. C. (2007). Genetic influences on anxiety in children: what we've learned and where we're heading. *Clinical Child and Family Psychology Review*, **10**, 199–212.

Gruner, K., Muris, P., & Merckelbach, H. (1999). The relationship between anxious rearing behaviours and anxiety disorders symptomatology in normal children. *Journal of Behavior Therapy and Experimental Psychiatry*, **30**, 27–35.

Hirshfeld, D. R., Biederman, J., Brody, L., Faraone, S. V., & Rosenbaum, J. F. (1997). Expressed emotion toward children with behavioral inhibition: associations with maternal anxiety disorder. *Journal of the American Academy of Child and Adolescent Psychiatry*, **36**, 910–917.

Hollon, S. D., Kendall, P. C., & Lumry, A. (1986). Specificity of depressotypic cognition in clinical depression. *Journal of Abnormal Psychology*, **95**, 52–59.

Hudson, J. L. & Rapee, R. M. (2001). Parent–child interactions and anxiety disorders: an observational study. *Behaviour Research and Therapy*, **39**, 1411–1427.

Hudson, J. L. & Rapee, R. M. (2002). Parent–child interactions in clinically anxious children and their siblings. *Journal of Clinical Child and Adolescent Psychology*, **31**, 548–555.

Hudson, J. L. & Rapee, R. M. (2004). From anxious temperament to disorder: an etiological model of generalized anxiety disorder. In: **R. G. Heimberg, C. L. Turk,** & **D. S. Mennin** (eds.) *Generalized Anxiety Disorder: Advances in Research and Practice*, pp. 51–74. New York: Guilford Press.

Hudson, J. L., Doyle, A. M., & Gar, N. (2009). Child and maternal influence on parenting behaviour in clinically anxious children. *Journal of Clinical Child and Adolescent Psychology*, **38**, 256–262.

Jorm, A. F., Dear, K. B. G., Rodgers, B., & Christensen, H. (2003). Interaction between mother's and father's affection as a risk factor for anxiety and depression symptoms. *Social Psychiatry and Psychiatric Epidemiology*, **38**, 173–179.

Kagan, J., Reznick, J., & Snidman, N. (1987). The physiology and psychology of behavioural inhibition in children. *Child Development*, **58**, 1459–1473.

Kendler, K. S., Myers, J., & Prescott, C. A. (2000). Parenting and adult mood, anxiety and substance disorders in female twins: an epidemiological, multi-informant, retrospective study. *Psychological Medicine*, **30**, 281–294.

Ladd, G. W. & Hart, C. H. (1992). Creating informal play opportunities: are parents' and preschoolers' initiations related to children's competence with peers? *Developmental Psychology*, **28**, 1179–1187.

Ladd, G. W. & Price, J. M. (1987). Predicting children's social and school adjustment following the transition from preschool to kindergarten. *Child Development*, **58**, 1168–1189.

Ladd, G. W., Le Sieur, K. D., Profilet, S. M., & Duck, S. (1993). Direct parental influences on young children's peer relationships. In: **S. Duck** (ed.) *Learning about relationships*, vol. 2, pp. 152–183. Thousand Oaks, CA: Sage Publications.

Last, C. G., Hersen, M., Kazdin, A. E., Francis, G., & Grubb, H. J. (1987) Psychiatric illness in the mothers of anxious children. *American Journal of Psychiatry*, **144**, 1580–1583.

Last, C. G., Hersen, M., Kazdin, A. E., Orvaschel, H., & Perrin, S. (1991). Anxiety disorders in children and their families. *Archives of General Psychiatry*, **48**, 928–939.

Lawson, J., Banerjee, R., & Field, A. P. (2007). The effects of verbal information on children's fear beliefs about social situations. *Behaviour Research and Therapy*, **45**, 21–37.

Lester, K. J., Field, A. P., Oliver, S., & Cartwright-Hatton, S. (2009). Do anxious parents interpretive biases towards threat extend into their child's environment? *Behaviour Research and Therapy*, **47**, 170–174.

Lewis, A. (1942). Incidence of neurosis in England under war conditions. *Lancet*, **2**, 175–183.

Martin, C., Cabrol, S., Bouvard, M. P., Lepine, J. P., & Mouren-Simeoni, M. P. (1999). Anxiety and depressive disorders in fathers and mothers of anxious school-refusing children. *Journal of the American Academy of Child and Adolescent Psychiatry*, **38**, 916–922.

McCabe, K. M., Clark, R., & Barnett, D. (1999). Family protective factors among urban African American youth. *Journal of Clinical Child Psychology*, **28**, 137–150.

McLeod, B. D., Wood, J. J., & Weisz, J. R. (2007). Examining the association between parenting and childhood anxiety: a meta-analysis. *Clinical Psychology Review*, **27**, 155–172.

Merikangas, K. R., Avenevoli, S., Dierker, L., & Grillon, C. (1999). Vulnerability factors among children at risk of anxiety disorders. *Biological Psychiatry*, **46**, 1523–1535.

Mineka, S. & Cook, M. (1986). Immunization against the observational conditioning of snake fear in rhesus monkeys. *Journal of Abnormal Psychology*, **95**, 307–318.

Mineka, S. & Cook, M. (1993). Mechanisms involved in the observational conditioning of fear. *Journal of Experimental Psychology*, **122**, 23–38.

Mineka, S., Davidson, M., Cook, M., & Keir, R. (1984). Observational conditioning of snake fear in rhesus monkeys. *Journal of Abnormal Psychology*, **93**, 355–372.

Moore, P. S., Whaley, S. E., & Sigman, M. (2004). Interactions between mothers and children: impacts of maternal and child anxiety. *Journal of Abnormal Psychology*, **113**, 471–476.

Murray, L., Cooper, P. J., Creswell, C., Schofield, E., & Sack, C. (2007). The effects of maternal social phobia on mother–infant interactions and infant social responsiveness. *Journal of Child Psychology and Psychiatry*, **48**, 45–52.

Murray, L. M., Creswell, C., & Cooper, P. J. (2009) Anxiety disorders in childhood. *Psychological Medicine*, **39**, 1413–1423.

Murray, L., De Rosnay, M., Pearson, J., Bergeron, C., Schofield, L., Royal-Lawson, M., *et al*. (2008). Intergenerational transmission of maternal social anxiety: the role of the social referencing process. *Child Development*, **79**, 1049–1064.

Murray, L. M., Pella, J., Schofield, E., Arteche, A., Royal-Lawson, M., Creswell, C., *et al*. (2008). Intergenerational factors in the development of child psychopathology. Presented at BPS Developmental Section Annual Conference, Sept 1–3, 2008, Oxford Brookes University, UK.

Nelson, K. (1993). The psychological and social origins of autobiographic memory. *Psychological Science*, **4**, 1–8.

Noyes, R., Clarkson, C., Crowe, R. R., Yates, W. R., & McChesney, C. M. (1987). A family study of generalized anxiety disorder. *American Journal of Psychiatry*, **144**, 1019–1024.

Parker, G. (1983). *Parental Overprotection: A Risk Factor in Psychosocial Development*. New York: Grune & Stratton.

Perez-Olivas, G., Stevenson, J., & Hadwin, J. (2008). Do anxiety-related attentional biases mediate the link between maternal over involvement and separation anxiety in children? *Cognition and Emotion*, **22**, 509–521.

Price-Evans, K. & Field, A. P. (2008). A neglectful parenting style moderates the effect of the verbal threat information pathway on children's heart rate responses to novel animals. *Behavioural and Cognitive Psychotherapy*, **36**, 473–482.

Rapee, R. M. (1997). Potential role of childrearing practices in the development of anxiety and depression. *Clinical Psychology Review*, **17**, 47–67.

Renk, K., McKinney, C., Klein, J., & Oliveros, A. (2006). Childhood discipline, perceptions of parents, and current functioning in female college students. *Journal of Adolescence*, **29**, 73–88.

Rothbart, M. K. (1981). Measurement of temperament in infancy. *Child Development*, **52**, 569–578.

Rothbart, M. K. (1986). Longitudinal observation of temperament. *Developmental Psychology*, **22**, 356–365.

Rubin, K. H., Burgess, K. B., & Hastings, P. D. (2002). Stability and social-behavioral consequences of toddlers' inhibited temperament and parenting behaviors. *Child Development*, **73**, 483–495.

Rubin, K. H., Cheah, C. S. L., & Fox, N. (2001). Emotion regulation, parenting and display of social reticence in preschoolers. *Early Education and Development*, **12**, 97–115.

Rubin, K. H., Nelson, L. J., Hastings, P. D., & Asendorpf, J. B. (1999). The transaction between parents' perceptions of their children's shyness and their parenting styles. *International Journal of Behavioral Development*, **23**, 937–957.

Shanahan, L., Copeland, W., Costello, E. J., & Angold, A. (2008). Specificity of putative psychosocial risk factors for psychiatric disorders in children and adolescents. *Journal of Child Psychology and Psychiatry*, **49**, 34–42.

Silverman, W. K., Cerny, J. A., & Nelles, W. B. (1988). The familial influence in anxiety disorders: studies of the offspring of patients with anxiety disorders. In: B. B. Lahey & A. Kazdin (eds.) *Advances in Clinical Child Psychology*, vol. 11, pp. 223–248. New York: Plenum Press.

Silverman, W. K., Kurtines, W. M., Pina, A. A., & Jaccard, J. (2009). Directionality of change in youth anxiety treatment involving parents: an initial examination. *Journal of Consulting and Clinical Psychology*, **77**, 474–485.

Siqueland, L., Kendall, P. C., & Steinberg, L. (1996). Anxiety in children: perceived family environments and observed family interaction. *Journal of Clinical Child Psychology*, **25**, 225–237.

Stein, A., Woolley, H., Murray, L., Cooper, P., Cooper, S., Noble, F., *et al.* (2001). Influence of psychiatric disorder on the controlling behaviour of mothers with 1-year-old infants: a study of women with maternal eating disorder, postnatal depression and a healthy comparison group. *British Journal of Psychiatry*, **179**, 157–162.

Summers, P., Forehand, R., Armistead, L., & Tannenbaum, L. (1998). Parental divorce during early adolescence in Caucasian families: the role of family process variables in predicting the long-term consequences for early adult psychosocial adjustment. *Journal of Consulting and Clinical Psychology*, **66**, 327–336.

Thirlwall, K. & Creswell, C. (2010). The impact of maternal control on children's anxious cognitions, behaviour and affect: an experimental study. *Behaviour Research and Therapy*, **48**, 1041–1046.

Turner, S. M., Beidel, D. C., & Costello, A. (1987). Psychopathology in the offspring of anxiety disordered patients. *Journal of Consulting and Clinical Psychology*, **55**, 229–235.

Turner, S. M., Beidel, D. C., Roberson-Nay, R., & Tervo, K. (2003). Parenting behaviours in parents with anxiety disorders. *Behaviour Research and Therapy*, **41**, 541–554.

Warner, V., Mufson, L., & Weissman, M. M. (1995). Offspring at low and high risk for depression and anxiety: mechanisms of psychiatric disorder. *Journal of the Academy of Child and Adolescent Psychiatry*, **34**, 786–797.

Weissman, M. M., Leckman, J. F., Merikangas, K. R., Gammon, G. D., & Prusoff, B. A. (1984). Depression and anxiety disorders in parents and children. *Archives of General Psychiatry*, **41**, 845–852.

Whaley, S. E., Pinto, A., & Sigman, M. (1999). Characterizing interactions between anxious mothers and their children. *Journal of Consulting and Clinical Psychology*, **67**, 826–836.

Wheatcroft, R. & Creswell, C. (2007). Parental cognitions and expectations of their preschool children: the contribution of parental anxiety and child anxiety. *British Journal of Developmental Psychology*, **25**, 435–441.

Wood, J. J. (2006). Parental intrusiveness and children's separation anxiety in a clinical sample. *Child Psychiatry and Human Development*, **37**, 73–87.

Wood, J. J., McLeod, B. D., Sigman, M., Hwang, W., & Chu, B. C. (2003). Parenting and childhood anxiety: theory, empirical findings, and future directions. *Journal of Child Psychology and Psychiatry*, **44**, 134–151.

Wood, J. J., Piacentini, J. C., Southam-Gerow, M., Chu, B. C., & Sigman, M. (2006). Family cognitive behavioral therapy for child anxiety disorders. *Journal of the American Academy of Child and Adolescent Psychiatry*, **45**, 314–321.

Woodruff-Borden, J., Morrow, C., Bourland, S., & Cambron, S. (2002). The behavior of anxious parents: examining mechanisms of transmission of anxiety from parent to child. *Journal of Clinical Child and Adolescent Psychology*, **31**, 364–374.

15

Peer influences

Annette M. La Greca and Ryan R. Landoll

Peer relationships play an important role in youngsters' social and emotional development. From early childhood on, children spend a considerable amount of time with peers, and by age 7, children spend most of their daytime hours in school or play settings with classmates and friends. This trend continues, and accelerates, through adolescence (La Greca & Prinstein, 1999).

Successful peer relationships contribute to youngsters' emotional health, facilitating the development of social skills and fostering feelings of personal competence that are essential for adult interpersonal functioning (Hartup, 1996). Supportive friendships also serve a protective function, such as by moderating the adverse effects of parental conflict (Wasserstein & La Greca, 1996).

At the same time, problematic peer relations represent a significant stressor. Abundant evidence suggests that children who experience interpersonal difficulties with peers during the elementary school years are at substantial risk for later emotional problems (Kupersmidt & Coie, 1990). Among adolescents, problems in the peer arena have been identified as strong predictors of internalizing problems (Hawker & Boulton, 2000; Prinstein, Boergers, & Vernberg, 2001), including social anxiety (La Greca & Harrison, 2005; Siegel, La Greca, & Harrison, 2009).

This chapter focuses on peer processes that contribute to the etiology or maintenance of anxiety in youth. As discussed in other chapters, the etiology and maintenance of anxiety disorders is complex, with multiple factors contributing. It is surprising, however, that little attention has been given to *interpersonal* processes as a contributing factor. Current conceptualizations of anxiety disorders, as reflected in DSM-IV (American Psychiatric Association, 2000) or ICD-10 (World Health Organization, 2009) make almost no mention of interpersonal processes contributing to anxiety. The only exceptions are social phobia (which implicate peer processes) and separation anxiety disorder (which implicate family interactions). Thus, the bulk of the research examining peer processes in anxiety disorders has focused specifically on social anxiety or social phobia. Almost no research has examined peer processes involved in the development of general anxiety, and the few exceptions are reviewed in this chapter.

Among youth with various anxiety disorders, social-anxiety-related symptoms, social dysfunction, or both are likely to be part of the clinical picture. This is because many youth with anxiety disorders have multiple psychological problems. Epidemiological studies show that most children with one anxiety disorder also have other phobic and/or anxiety

Anxiety Disorders in Children and Adolescents, 2nd edn, ed. W. K. Silverman and A. P. Field. Published by Cambridge University Press. © Cambridge University Press 2011.

disorders. It is not unusual for children screened in community studies to meet criteria for three or more anxiety disorders (Ollendick & Seligman, 2006); rates of comorbidity are even higher among children in clinic samples (Ollendick, King, & Muris, 2002) (see Costello, Egger, Copeland, Erkanli, & Angold, Chapter 3, this volume). Given high rates of comorbidity, youth who are seen for the treatment of an anxiety disorder, even one that does not have obvious interpersonal components, may have comorbid social phobia or subclinical levels of social anxiety. This suggests that attention to peer processes in the assessment and treatment of youth with anxiety disorders is important.

Another issue worth noting is that the current state of research often makes it difficult to disentangle peer influences on social anxiety, specifically, versus anxiety, more generally, as well as depression, more generally. Interpersonal processes are important to the development and maintenance of both anxiety and depression (Davila, La Greca, Starr, & Landoll, 2010; La Greca, Davila, & Siegel, 2008). Research on peer influences has focused on "internalizing problems" that include both anxiety and depression, which are often comorbid. Wherever possible in this chapter, we highlight research that allows for a more precise differentiation between peer processes linked to anxiety versus depression.

This chapter is organized into several main sections. The first reviews key aspects of peer relationships in youth, with attention to developmental, gender, and cultural issues. Next, we describe theoretical formulations that may underlie contributions of peer relationships to anxiety in youth, and then we review existing empirical data in support of such connections. This sets the stage for a brief description of methods used for assessing peer relationships. Finally, we briefly review psychological interventions for anxiety in youth that incorporate peer processes, and highlight potential avenues for addressing peer issues in treatment. Within each section, we first review evidence pertaining to school-aged children and then adolescents.

Developmental aspects of peer relationships

During elementary school, children spend most of the day in self-contained classrooms with a specific group of classmates, some of whom may also be friends. Children also have friends in their neighborhood, friends who participate in shared extracurricular activities (e.g., scouts, sports), or both. As children enter middle school and high school, peer networks expand considerably and are likely to include best friends, other close friends, larger friendship groups or cliques, peer crowds, and even romantic relationships (La Greca & Prinstein, 1999).

Peer acceptance

Youths' social status – or degree of *acceptance from the peer group* – is a critical aspect of peer relationships. Peer acceptance provides children and adolescents with a sense of belonging and inclusion (La Greca & Prinstein, 1999).

For children, social status often has been identified by classmates' nominations of acceptance (or "liking") and rejection (or "disliking"). Peer nominations have been used to identify *popular* youth (high on liking and low on disliking) as well as *rejected* youth (low on liking and high on disliking) (Coie, Dodge, & Kupersmidt, 1990). Popular children often have good social and academic skills (Estell, Jones, Pearl, Van Acker, Farmer, & Rodkin, 2008), whereas rejected children may display interpersonal, emotional, and academic difficulties, such as aggressive, disruptive behaviors (Hartup, 1996) and internalizing problems, such as social anxiety (La Greca & Stone, 1993).

For adolescents, affiliating with a peer crowd is a way of gaining peer acceptance and social status (La Greca & Prinstein, 1999). Peer crowds are distinct from smaller friendship groups in that they are much larger, and members may not be friends with one another (Brown, 1990). Typical peer crowds include: *Jocks, Populars, Brains, Burnouts, Alternatives, Loners*, although alternative names exist for each of these groups (Brown, 1990; La Greca, Prinstein, & Fetter, 2001). Peer crowds provide opportunities for social activities, friendships, and romantic relationships, as well as a sense of acceptance, belonging, and identity. Peer crowds' importance peaks in mid-adolescence and then declines in late adolescence when close friends and romantic relationships become more prominent (Brown, 1990).

The Jocks, Populars, Brains, and Burnouts, or their equivalents, are the most consistently observed peer crowds (Brown, Herman, Haamm, & Heck, 2008; Sussman, Pokhrel, Ashmore, & Brown, 2007). There is remarkable consistency in the types, roles, and functions of adolescent peer crowds across diverse contexts, including rural, suburban, and urban schools; across youth from different ethnic/cultural backgrounds; and even across multiple countries (Brown *et al.*, 2008; Kinney, 1993; La Greca & Prinstein, 1999).

Ethnicity is a salient aspect of peer crowd affiliation for many minority youth (e.g., African-Americans affiliate with other African-Americans, Asians with other Asians). However, recent findings indicate that adolescents from minority ethnic backgrounds are *more* likely to affiliate with the "traditional" peer crowds described above (e.g., Jocks, Brains), than with crowds that are defined by ethnic background (Brown *et al.*, 2008). In terms of sex differences, girls are more likely to affiliate with the Popular, Brain, Alternative, and Average peer crowds than boys, and boys are more likely to affiliate with the Jocks and Burnouts than girls (Brown, Mounts, Lamborn, & Steinberg, 1993; La Greca *et al.*, 2001; Strouse, 1999).

Close friendships

Children and adolescents place high value on *close friendships*, which provide intimacy and companionship, and enhance self-esteem (La Greca & Prinstein, 1999). Children's close friendships occur almost exclusively between same-sex peers until adolescence, when other-sex close friendships become common and set the stage for romantic relationships (Kuttler, La Greca, & Prinstein, 1999). At all ages, girls are more likely to have a "best friend" than boys and to have more close friends (Parker & Asher, 1993).

Common qualities of close friendships for children and adolescents include companionship, affection, receiving help, trust, and sharing. Intimacy (i.e., sharing private thoughts and feelings, knowing intimate details about friends) and emotional support also are evident in children's friendships and increase during adolescence (La Greca & Prinstein, 1999). In fact, during adolescence, close friends may surpass parents as the primary source of social support (Furman, McDunn, & Young, 2008).

Friendships also have negative aspects, such as conflict, pressure, and betrayal, although youth report more positive than negative qualities in their close friendships (Kuttler & La Greca, 2004; La Greca & Harrison, 2005; La Greca & Mackey, 2007). Girls report more positive and fewer negative qualities in their close friendships than boys (La Greca & Harrison, 2005; La Greca & Mackey, 2007). Across development, youth with better-quality friendships (more positive and fewer negative interactions) have fewer behavioral and emotional problems, and display greater social competence (La Greca & Prinstein, 1999).

Romantic relationships

Romantic relationships represent an important but relatively understudied aspect of adolescent peer relations, even though, by age 16, most adolescents have had a romantic relationship (Carver, Joyner, & Udry, 2003). Such relationships may have mental health benefits, such as the provision of social support, the enhancement of self-esteem, preparation for adult relationships, and the development of intimacy (Collins, 2003; Connolly & Goldberg, 1999).

Developmentally, early adolescence is marked by the emergence of mixed-sex peer groups, while romantically involved couples become prominent in later adolescence (Connolly & Goldberg, 1999). Adolescent girls are more likely to be romantically involved than are boys (Glickman & La Greca, 2004; La Greca & Harrison, 2005; La Greca & Mackey, 2007). Sex differences in the qualities of adolescents' romantic relationships have been less consistent. When sex differences are apparent, girls report more positive (La Greca & Mackey, 2007) and fewer negative qualities than boys (La Greca & Harrison, 2005).

Although adolescent romantic relationships are a normative aspect of development and may be beneficial to emotional functioning, such relationships can represent significant stressors. Romantic relationships explain 25–34% of the strong emotions that high school students' experience, and about 42% of these strong emotions are negative feelings, such as anxiety, anger, jealousy, and depression (Larson, Clore, & Wood, 1999). Involvement in romantic relationships during adolescence, particularly if frequent or steady, is associated with internalizing and depressive symptoms, particularly for girls (Davila, Steinberg, Kachadourian, Cobb, & Fincham, 2004).

Data from the National Longitudinal Study of Adolescent Health (Carver *et al.*, 2003; O'Sullivan, Cheng, Harris, & Brooks-Gunn, 2007), suggest that the occurrence and progression of adolescents' romantic relationships is substantially similar across different US ethnic groups (White, Black, Asian, Hispanic, and Mixed Ethnicity). One exception is that Asian adolescents are less likely to report having a romantic relationship than adolescents from other major ethnic groups (O'Sullivan *et al.*, 2007). Asian and Hispanic adolescents who are involved in romantic relationships are also less likely to report engaging in sexual events (e.g., touching partner under clothing, sexual intercourse) than White or Black adolescents (O'Sullivan *et al.*, 2007).

Peer victimization

A final aspect of peer influences to consider is that of peer victimization. Initially, peer victimization was examined among school-aged children in the context of understanding peer aggression and its impact (Crick, 1996). Two types of peer aggression/victimization experiences were identified: overt victimization (e.g., hitting, pushing, and other forms of physical violence) and relational victimization (e.g., social exclusion, isolation, and manipulation of friendships). Among school-aged children, girls report more relational and less overt victimization than boys and both forms of victimization predict adjustment difficulties (Crick & Bigbee, 1998)

In adolescence, peer victimization is a relatively common experience, with 20–30% of adolescents reporting victimization on a regular basis (i.e., weekly) (Dinkes, Cataldi, & Lin-Kelly, 2007; La Greca & Harrison, 2005; Storch, Brassard, & Masia-Warner, 2003). *Relational* peer victimization appears to be particularly distressing for adolescents, perhaps because the aggressor is likely to be a friend rather than an acquaintance. Relational victimization is associated with internalizing problems in adolescents beyond the contributions of other types of peer victimization (La Greca & Harrison, 2005; Siegel *et al.*, 2009).

In terms of sex differences, adolescent boys report more overt victimization than girls (De Los Reyes & Prinstein, 2004; La Greca & Harrison, 2005). However, boys also report higher levels of relational victimization than girls in some studies (La Greca & Harrison, 2005) but not others (Coyne, Archer, & Eslea, 2006; De Los Reyes & Prinstein, 2004; Prinstein *et al.*, 2001; Siegel *et al.*, 2009).

Studies have begun to examine "cyber-victimization" which occurs through new technologies such as social networking sites, instant messaging, or text messages (Landoll & La Greca, 2009; Slonje & Smith, 2008; Williams & Guerra, 2007). Evidence links cyber-victimization with high levels of social anxiety in adolescents and young adults (Landoll & La Greca, 2009). Although research on cyber-victimization is in its early stages, evidence suggests it may be a unique and particularly salient form of peer victimization for adolescents (Slonje & Smith, 2008; Williams & Guerra, 2007).

At this point there is little evidence for cultural/ethnic differences in peer victimization. Studies that included ethnically diverse samples have not found significant ethnic differences (La Greca & Harrison, 2005; Prinstein *et al.*, 2001; Siegel *et al.*, 2009).

Peer relations and anxiety: theoretical perspectives

Several theoretical perspectives are consistent with the notion that youths' peer relationships play a causal role in the development and maintenance of anxiety symptoms and disorders. Relevant to this discussion are the concepts of multifinality (that a particular risk factor may lead to multiple psychological outcomes) and equifinality (that any given psychological outcome may have multiple pathways that contribute to its development) (Hinshaw, 2008). In this framework, problematic peer relationships are viewed as a causal risk factor that is associated with multiple problematic outcomes, including anxiety in youth (especially social anxiety). In addition, problematic peer relationships may be one among a host of other causal factors, such as genetic make-up and parenting, which contribute to the development and maintenance of anxiety disorders, as discussed in other chapters.

Problematic peer relationships as significant interpersonal stressors

Perhaps the broadest way to conceptualize how peer relationships contribute to symptoms of anxiety and anxiety disorder in youth is to view problematic peer relationships, especially peer rejection and victimization, as significant interpersonal stressors that lead to feelings of anxiety and distress. Once anxious feelings develop, these feelings may exacerbate interpersonal problems. For example, anxious youth may appear nervous or uncomfortable with peers, may worry about peers' reactions to them, and may avoid peer-oriented social situations altogether (La Greca, 2001). Once socially anxious feelings and behavior patterns develop, they may interfere with interpersonal functioning. Youth who avoid peers miss out on important socialization experiences that are necessary for normal development (Coie *et al.*, 1990); and youth who are uncomfortable around peers may be less desirable companions, making them targets for exclusion from peer activities (Blote & Westenberg, 2007).

Although some degree of social anxiety is normative (La Greca, 1999), when socially anxious feelings and behaviors are sufficiently extreme, persist over time, and interfere with functioning, they may be consistent with the diagnosis of social phobia or social anxiety disorder (American Psychiatric Association, 2000). Evidence suggests that anxiety disorders, including social phobia or social anxiety disorder, are a potential gateway to psychological disorders such as depression (Essau, 2003; Grant, Beck, Farrow, & Davila, 2007). In fact, social anxiety disorder shares a high degree of comorbidity with depression (Costello, Egger, & Angold, 2005). Interpersonal aspects of socially anxious behaviors, especially social avoidance, have been prospectively associated with subsequent feelings of depression (see Grant *et al.*, 2007).

Aversive peer experiences as traumatic events

Traumatic experiences have long been viewed as a causal pathway to the development of anxiety disorders in youth (Silverman, Ortiz, *et al.*, 2008), potentially contributing to the development of specific phobias, generalized anxiety disorder, and post-traumatic stress disorder. In this context, extreme forms of peer rejection or victimization – especially overt and relational victimization, as well as chronic bullying (i.e., frequent and repeated victimization without provocation) – may represent traumatic events that contribute to the development and maintenance of anxiety symptoms and disorders in youth. As discussed later, peer victimization can lead to symptoms of social anxiety and social anxiety disorder in youth (La Greca & Harrison, 2005; Siegel *et al.*, 2009). High levels of peer victimization also are associated with symptoms of post-traumatic stress (Mynard, Joseph, & Alexander, 2000; Storch & Esposito, 2003).

Peer selection and socialization processes

Homophily (Kandel, 1978a, 1978b) is another theoretical perspective that provides a useful framework for understanding the role of peer relationships in the development of anxiety disorders and related symptoms. Homophily comprises the processes of "selection" (peers with similar interests and characteristics cluster together and seek one another out) and "socialization" (peers reward and reinforce similar attitudes and behaviors among group members or friends).

Consistent with the selection process, children choose friends based on having similar characteristics, such as age, sex, race, and preference for certain activities (La Greca & Prinstein, 1999). By adolescence, friendship choices are based on subtle and less observable factors, such as personality, attitudes, and self-esteem (Aboud & Mendelson, 1998). Friends also "socialize" each other by supporting and reinforcing each others' behaviors and feelings (Prinstein, 2007).

Selection and socialization processes have been studied predominantly with regard to externalizing behavior problems (Bukowski, Brendgen, & Vitaro, 2006), but these processes also play a role in youths' internalizing problems. Specifically, adolescents seek friends with similar levels of internalizing problems; adolescents also display increases in internalizing symptoms over time when their close friends are high on internalizing symptoms (Deater-Deckard, 2001; Hogue & Steinberg, 1995). As Prinstein (2007) illustrated in a recent 18-month longitudinal study of "peer contagion," adolescents whose close friends reported high levels of internalizing symptoms showed increases in their own internalizing symptoms over time.

Peer relations and anxiety: empirical data

Having described theoretical frameworks to explain how peer processes could contribute to the development of anxiety symptoms or disorders, we now review empirical support for such connections. Before proceeding, it is worth noting that evidence linking peer processes and anxiety comes mainly from community-based studies that examined anxiety from a dimensional rather than diagnostic or categorical perspective. The findings support important connections between peer processes and anxiety, but may not be specific to specific anxiety diagnostic categories. Wherever the research allows, we review prospective studies that may help to elucidate etiological pathways, as well as studies of peer relations among youth with specific anxiety disorders. Sometimes it was not possible to determine whether peer processes are antecedent or consequent to the development of anxiety disorders – an important issue that requires further research attention.

Peer rejection, peer victimization

Theory and research support the notion that anxiety, particularly social anxiety, may result from problematic peer relations, such as peer rejection, peer victimization, and social exclusion (Davila *et al.*, 2010; La Greca & Prinstein, 1999).

Peer rejection (low acceptance)

Community studies find that children who are rejected by peers have substantial interpersonal, emotional, and academic difficulties (La Greca & Prinstein, 1999). Rejected children often demonstrate aggressive, disruptive, or inattentive behaviors (Coie *et al.*, 1990), although peer-rejected children also display high levels of anxiety, especially social anxiety (La Greca, Dandes, Wick, Shaw, & Stone, 1988; La Greca & Stone, 1993). Children who are neglected by peers (i.e., neither liked nor disliked, but mostly unnoticed) also display high levels of social withdrawal and social anxiety (La Greca *et al.*, 1988; La Greca & Stone, 1993).

Studies of clinically diagnosed children also support associations between peer rejection and anxiety. Strauss and colleagues (Strauss, Frame, & Forehand, 1987; Strauss, Lahey, Frick, Frame, & Hynd, 1988) found that anxiety-disordered (AD) children received fewer positive peer nominations than non-anxiety-disordered (NAD) youth. Ginsburg, La Greca, and Silverman (1998) examined children (ages 6 to 11) with simple phobia; those with a comorbid diagnosis of social phobia reported significantly lower levels of peer acceptance and more negative peer interactions than those without comorbid social phobia. Finally, a recent study (Verduin & Kendall, 2008) found that AD children received significantly lower ratings of peer-liking than NAD children. Moreover, AD children with a diagnosis of social phobia were significantly less liked by peers than those without social phobia. Differences in peer-liking did not emerge for children with another anxiety disorder compared to NAD. Thus, evidence with children supports a linkage between peer rejection and anxiety, especially social anxiety, in both community and clinical samples.

Among adolescents, similar findings are apparent. In community samples, adolescents who are actively rejected by peers report significantly higher levels of social anxiety than those who are more accepted (Inderbitzen, Walters, & Bukowski, 1997; La Greca & Lopez, 1998). Rejected adolescents report both social evaluative concerns and high levels of social avoidance and distress (La Greca & Lopez, 1998). In addition, "submissive rejected" adolescents (who are unassertive and inhibited) report more social anxiety than "aggressive rejected" adolescents (Inderbitzen *et al.*, 1997), suggesting that peer rejection may elicit social anxiety in youth whose interpersonal style is more consistent with internalizing than externalizing behavior problems.

Community studies also have examined adolescents' peer crowd affiliations, which reflect social status in the larger peer group. Adolescents who identify with peer crowds, regardless of whether they are high status (e.g., Jocks, Populars) or low status (e.g., Burnouts, Alternatives), report less social anxiety than other adolescents (La Greca & Harrison, 2005). This pattern highlights the potential benefits of affiliating with a crowd (e.g., sense of belonging and acceptance; opportunities for companionship) that may protect against feelings of social anxiety, even if the crowd has a low social status. It further suggests that adolescents who do not affiliate with peer crowds may be more vulnerable to feeling socially anxious.

In summary, community studies demonstrate a linkage between peer rejection and adolescents' reports of social anxiety. However, studies have not specifically examined peer acceptance or rejection among adolescents with anxiety disorders.

Peer victimization

Peer victimization experiences also have a significant impact on anxiety. With respect to children, a meta-analysis (Hawker & Boulton, 2000), conducted before investigators began differentiating between different types of peer victimization (i.e., overt, relational), found moderate associations between peer victimization and anxiety (both general anxiety and social anxiety) across child-focused studies.

Recent investigations have evaluated specific types of peer victimization in children, finding that both overt and relational victimization are strongly associated with a variety of adjustment difficulties, including anxiety (Crick & Grotpeter, 1996; Schwartz, Gorman, Dodge, Pettit, & Bates, 2008). For example, Storch, Phil, Nock, Masia-Warner, and Barlas (2003) found that overt victimization was significantly and positively associated with children's social anxiety (fear of negative evaluation and social avoidance) as well as with symptoms of depression and loneliness. For relational victimization, associations with symptoms of social anxiety, depression, and loneliness were observed for girls, but not for boys (Storch *et al.*, 2003). These findings are consistent with other reports that girls display greater distress than boys in response to relational victimization (Crick & Nelson, 2002; Galen & Underwood, 1997).

Among clinical samples of children, the literature on peer victimization is sparse. One study examined the frequency of peer victimization among children with obsessive–compulsive disorder (OCD), comparing them to healthy controls and children with type 1 diabetes (Storch *et al.*, 2006). Greater rates of peer victimization were observed for the children with OCD, relative to controls. Additionally, in a separate sample of children and adolescents (ages 7–18 years) with OCD, peer victimization was related to OCD youths' perfectionism (Ye, Rice, & Storch, 2008). Based on these findings, the authors highlight the importance of addressing problematic peer relations when treating youth with OCD.

Among adolescents, community studies provide strong evidence that peer victimization is associated with social anxiety (La Greca & Harrison, 2005; Siegel *et al.*, 2009; Storch & Masia-Warner, 2004; Storch, Masia-Warner, Crisp, & Klein, 2005). Further, relational victimization is uniquely and strongly associated with social anxiety, even when controlling for other forms of peer victimization (La Greca & Harrison, 2005; Siegel *et al.*, 2009). Findings indicate *stronger* effect sizes for the association between peer victimization and social anxiety than between peer victimization and depression (La Greca & Harrison, 2005). Further, in a study of over 3000 adolescents (15 to 16 years), Ranta, Kaltiala-Heino, Pelkonen, and Marttunen (2009) demonstrated that peer victimization was significantly associated with adolescents' symptoms of social phobia (with and without comorbid depressive symptoms), but not with adolescents' depressive symptoms alone.

Prospective studies with adolescents also elucidate potential bidirectional pathways between peer victimization and anxiety in youth. Vernberg, Abwender, Ewell, and Beery (1992) evaluated adolescents at three time points during a school year (September, November, and May) assessing the quality of their peer relationships, occurrence of peer victimization experiences, and levels of social anxiety. Analyses examined peer experiences as predictors of subsequent social anxiety (controlling for initial social anxiety) and social anxiety as a predictor of subsequent peer experiences (controlling for initial peer experiences). Among the study findings, rejecting and exclusionary peer experiences that reflected relational victimization predicted increases in adolescents' social anxiety over a 2-month period and increases in social avoidance and distress over the school year. Other recent prospective work also points to relational victimization as leading to *increases* in adolescents' symptoms of social anxiety over time (Siegel *et al.*, 2009) and to increases in symptoms of social phobia (Storch *et al.*, 2005).

In contrast, these same prospective studies provide mixed evidence regarding the reverse pathway – that is, that social anxiety leads to *subsequent* peer victimization in adolescents. Two of the studies did not find that social anxiety led to increases in peer victimization over the school year (Storch *et al.*, 2005; Vernberg *et al.*, 1992). However, Siegel *et al.* (2009) did find that higher levels of social anxiety predicted increases in adolescents' relational victimization over a two-month period. Others have found evidence that socially anxious youth are treated more negatively by their classmates than youth who are not socially anxious (Blote & Westenberg, 2007).

It may be difficult to evaluate whether social anxiety leads to increased peer victimization because socially anxious youth who are victimized may learn to avoid social situations in order to limit their opportunities for further peer victimization. Over time, socially anxious adolescents may avoid social situations that could make them the targets of further peer victimization. Studies that examine the bidirectional influences of peer victimization and social anxiety, as well as mediating and moderating variables, are needed. For example, one important moderating variable may be the presence of a close friend in the school setting, as socially anxious adolescents with a close school friend may be less victimized by peers than those who are loners or have no close friends in school. These issues will be valuable to examine in future research.

Clinical samples of adolescents also provide evidence that peer victimization is associated with clinical levels of social anxiety. Ranta *et al.* (2009) found that adolescents (12 to 17 years) who met criteria for social phobia had substantially higher rates of peer victimization than those without social phobia.

Close friendships

Problems in close friendships represent an interpersonal stressor that could contribute to feelings of anxiety, and lead to avoidance or inhibition in close relationships. Such inhibition could interfere with the development of close, supportive ties (La Greca & Lopez, 1998). Among children, a recent review suggests that those who are socially withdrawn, a characteristic associated with both anxious and depressive symptoms, have more difficulty forming larger friendship groups, have friends who are more likely to display internalizing problems, and have lower-quality friendships (Rubin, Coplan, & Bowker, 2009). Additionally, children who report higher levels of social anxiety report more negative qualities within their best friendships (Greco & Morris, 2005).

Scant data are available on the close friendships of children with anxiety disorders. In a rare study (Schneider, 2009), clinically referred youth with high levels of social withdrawal and social anxiety were observed while interacting with friends. Compared to community controls, the withdrawn/anxious youth displayed more reticence in their social interactions and less positive affect. As noted earlier, Ginsburg *et al.* (1998) found that children with social phobia reported more negative peer interactions than other phobic children.

Among adolescents, community studies have found that impairments in close friendships are associated with social anxiety. Specifically, adolescent girls who had fewer best friends, felt less competent in friendships, and perceived that their friendships were less supportive, less intimate, and lower in companionship, reported higher levels of social anxiety than other adolescents (La Greca & Lopez, 1998). Social avoidance was the aspect of social anxiety most strongly associated with impairments in friendships.

La Greca and Harrison (2005) also examined adolescents' peer relationships as predictors of concurrent social anxiety. Even after controlling for other aspects of peer relations, such as peer crowd affiliations and peer victimization, adolescents who reported fewer positive interactions (e.g., companionship, support, intimacy) and more negative interactions (e.g., conflict, pressure) in their best friendships reported significantly higher levels of social anxiety. Only the negative qualities of adolescents' close friendships were related to depressive symptoms, suggesting some differentiation in the association between friendship qualities and adolescents' social anxiety versus depression. Subsequently, La Greca and Mackey (2007) evaluated connections between close relationships and dating anxiety (i.e., anxiety experienced in heterosocial situations), revealing that adolescents with fewer other-sex friends and those with fewer positive and more negative interactions with their best friends reported more dating anxiety than other teens.

A prospective study by Vernberg *et al.* (1992) provided support for bidirectional influences between social anxiety and close friendships among youth. Specifically high levels of social anxiety at the beginning of the school year predicted less intimacy and companionship in adolescents' close friendships months later, especially for girls. Moreover, as social anxiety increased over the school year, concomitant decreases were observed in adolescents' levels of intimacy and companionship in their close friendships.

These findings implicate problems in close friendships as contributing to social anxiety, especially for girls, and further suggest that feelings of social anxiety can interfere with adolescents' close friendships. Because girls emphasize intimacy and emotional support in their close friendships to a greater extent than boys (Buhrmester & Furman, 1987), girls may be more vulnerable than boys to experiencing social anxiety when they encounter friendship problems.

No studies could be found on the friendships of adolescents with anxiety disorders. It is likely, however, that impairments in close friendships would be apparent for youth with anxiety disorders, especially those with social anxiety disorder or social phobia, as such youth may be less likely to participate in friendship activities (e.g., going out with friends, going to parties). A survey of adults with social anxiety disorder revealed that about half of the respondents did not have any close friends at all (Anxiety Disorders Association of America, 2007).

Romantic relationships

Little research has addressed the contributions of romantic relationships to anxiety symptoms or disorder in adolescents. One complication is that adolescents who are socially anxious are significantly less likely to date or be involved in romantic relationships than their less socially anxious peers (Glickman & La Greca, 2004; La Greca & Harrison, 2005), possibly because they avoid or are uncomfortable in romantic situations. Similarly, among adults, those with high levels of social anxiety are less likely to have romantic relationships or to marry (Wittchen, Fuetsch, Sonntag, Mueller, & Liebowitz, 2000).

Among adolescents involved in romantic relationships (and thus less socially anxious in general), high levels of social and dating anxiety have been associated with low levels of positive interactions (e.g., support, intimacy) and high levels of negative interactions (e.g., conflict, pressure) with romantic partners (La Greca & Harrison, 2005; La Greca & Mackey, 2007). La Greca and Mackey (2007) also found that adolescents with high levels of dating anxiety were more likely than others to report that they never had a romantic relationship, did not have a current romantic partner, and, if involved in a romantic relationship, had less positive and more negative interactions with their partner.

It is not surprising that negative interactions with a romantic partner might contribute to social or dating anxiety. A critical aspect of romantic relationships is to make one feel accepted and loved. Adolescents, in particular, have a heightened sensitivity to rejection from romantic partners (Downey, Bonica, & Rincon, 1999). Thus, when conflict, exclusion, or other negative interactions emerge in a romantic relationship, these interactions may foster considerable anxiety and distress.

It is also not surprising that fewer positive interactions with romantic partners were associated with higher levels of social or dating anxiety; this suggests that socially anxious and dating anxious adolescents are "less engaged" in their romantic relationships. Socially anxious adolescents might be more inhibited and display fewer positive interactions with their partners. Alternatively, low levels of positive interactions with a partner may elicit concerns about the quality of the relationship, and thus contribute to feelings of social or dating anxiety.

Understanding the psychological impact of romantic relationships is important because troubled romantic relationships in adolescence foreshadow difficulties in adult romantic relationships (Downey *et al.*, 1999). Continued research, and especially prospective studies on the interplay of romantic relationships and anxiety in adolescents over time, will be important.

Assessing peer relationships

Peer relationships can be challenging to evaluate, as they may be temporary and dynamic (Brown, 2004). The utility of peer relationship measures also vary with the developmental level or age of the child and with the purpose of assessment (La Greca & Lemanek, 1996). Peer, self-, parent, and teacher reports have been used to evaluate various aspects of children's peer relations (La Greca & Prinstein, 1999). Self-ratings are widely used to assess the qualities of children's friendships, as well as perceptions of social acceptance, social support, and peer victimization. Peer nominations are useful for evaluating peer acceptance/rejection and for identifying mutual close friendships; ratings by classroom teachers are also useful for evaluating children's peer acceptance/rejection. Parents may be useful informants for children's peer status and social skills. However the overall utility of teacher and parent reports declines during adolescence (La Greca & Lemanek, 1996).

For adolescents, self-reports are the most common method of assessment. Peer nominations are impractical or challenging, as adolescents have large, extensive peer networks that extend across multiple classes and grade levels; thus school-based peer nominations for social acceptance or mutual friendships may be difficult to obtain. Teachers also are poor informants for adolescents' peer relations as they may have little direct contact with adolescents in social contexts. Although used infrequently, parents have served as informants for certain aspects of adolescents' peer relations, such as peer rejection, the number of close friends, and social skills (Bagwell, Molina, Pelham, & Hoza, 2001; Gresham & Elliot, 1990).

Table 15.1 lists several peer-relations constructs with examples of appropriate measures for children and adolescents. (Detailed discussions of measures can be found in La Greca & Prinstein, 1999 and LeBlanc, Sautter, & Dore, 2006.)

When evaluating anxious children and adolescents in clinical settings, it would be useful to develop a brief screening battery of peer relationship measures. For children, this might include their self-reports of: (a) social acceptance/rejection (e.g., the 6-item *Social Acceptance* subscale of the *Self-Perception Profile for Children*, (b) peer victimization (e.g., the 10 items from the *Social Experiences Questionnaire – Self-Report* which assesses overt and relational peer victimization), (c) close friendships (e.g., the close friends subscale of the *Social Support Scale for Children and Adolescents*), and (d) social anxiety (e.g., the *Social Anxiety Scale for Children – Revised*). For adolescents, the screen might include self-reports of: (a) social acceptance/rejection (e.g., the 6-item *Social Acceptance* subscale of the *Self-Perception Profile for Adolescents*), (b) peer victimization (e.g., items from the *Revised Peer Experiences Questionnaire*), (c) close friendships (e.g., 13-item short form of the *Network of Relationships – Revised*), and (d) social anxiety (e.g., the *Social Anxiety Scale for Adolescents*).

In addition to self-reports, parents and/or teachers could complete items from the *Child Behavior Checklist* (CBCL) or *Teacher Report Form* (TRF), respectively, that index peer rejection (e.g., "is not liked by other kids," "gets teased a lot," and "does not get along with other kids"). Similarly, relevant items from the *Social Competence* subscale of the CBCL or TRF could be used to index children's friendships (e.g., number of close friends). Children or adolescents who screen positive or show elevations on any of these brief measures might then complete additional measures of peer relations (see Table 15.1).

Interventions addressing peer processes

Cognitive–behavioral treatment (CBT) is the most common treatment modality for anxiety disorders in youth. It is an efficacious form of treatment and can be delivered in individual or group format, with or without parent involvement (Kendall, Furr, & Podell, 2010; Pahl & Barrett, 2010; Silverman, Pina, & Viswesvaran, 2008). Below, we briefly discuss CBT interventions for socially anxious youth and the role of peers in "general CBT" programs for child and adolescent anxiety.

Social anxiety disorder

Social Effectiveness Therapy for Children (SET-C) is a CBT intervention that focuses on children (8 to 12 years) with social phobia (Beidel, Turner, & Morris, 2000; Beidel, Turner, Sallee, Ammerman, Crosby, & Pathak, 2007; Beidel, Turner, Young, & Paulson, 2005). SET-C is unique in its approach to incorporating peer processes, as it has a strong focus on children's interpersonal skills and incorporates non-anxious peers as agents of change (Beidel *et al.*, 2000). During the intensive 12-week program, children attend two sessions per week, one in a peer-group format (60 to 90 minutes) and one individual session (60 minutes). SET-C focuses on developing children's social skills, using non-anxious peers as facilitators to help youth practice and generalize their social skills during "real-life"

Table 15.1 Commonly used assessments of youths' peer relations and representative reference sources

Peer process/construct	Informant	Children	Adolescents	Description
Peer acceptance/rejection	Self-report	Self-Perception Profile for Children (Harter, 1988)	Self-Perception Profile for Adolescents (Harter, 1988)	Brief 6-item *Social Acceptance* subscale
			Peer Crowd Questionnaire (La Greca et al., 2001)	Measures affiliation with peer crowds
	Peer report	Peer nomination (e.g., Coie et al., 1990)	Peer nomination (Prinstein & Aikins, 2004)	Asks peers to nominate most liked/most disliked youth
	Teacher report	Teacher nominations (Anthonysamy & Zimmer-Gembeck, 2007)		Teachers identify accepted and rejected youth
	Parent/teacher report	Child Behavior Checklist (Achenbach, 1991)		Items like "Is not liked by other kids." "Gets teased a lot."
Close relationships	Self-report	Friendship Quality Questionnaire (Parker & Asher, 1993)		40-item questionnaire on quality and satisfaction with best friendship
		Friendship Qualities Scale (Bukowski, Hoza, & Boivin, 1994)		Original scale contains 30 items based on five subscales (companionship, conflict, help, closeness, security)
		Friendship Qualities Measure (Grotpeter & Crick, 1996)		43-items; includes six subscales from *Friendship Quality Questionnaire*, one from *Friendship Qualities Scale*, and additional ones on negative interactions
		Self-Perception Profile for Children (Harter, 1988)		*Close Friendship* subscale
			Network of Relationships Inventory (Furman, 1998)	39-items; 13 subscales of both positive and negative relationship qualities, can be used for friends and romantic relationships; short form available
	Peer report	Peer nominations of best friends (Crick & Nelson, 2002)		Ask peers to nominate their best friends

(cont.)

Table 15.1 (*cont.*)

Peer process/ construct	Informant	Children	Adolescents	Description
	Parent report	*Child Behavior Checklist* (Achenbach, 1991)		Parent report from social competence items
Peer victimization	Self-report	*Friendship Qualities Measure* (Grotpeter & Crick, 1996)		*Relational Aggression* (4 items) and *Physical Aggression* (3 items) subscales
		Social Experiences Questionnaire (Crick & Bigbee, 1998)		15 items; 3 subscales (overt, relational victimization, and receipt of pro-social acts)
			Revised Peer Experiences Questionnaire (De Los Reyes & Prinstein, 2004)	18 items; measures relational, reputation, overt victimization, and pro-social behavior; parallel version for bullying
	Peer report	*Social Experiences Questionnaire* (Crick & Bigbee, 1998)		15 items; 3 subscales (overt, relational, and receipt of pro-social acts)
	Teacher report	*Social Experiences Questionnaire – Teacher Report* (Cullerton-Sen & Crick, 2005)		15 items; 3 subscales (overt, relational, and receipt of pro-social acts)
Social skills	Self-report	*Child and Adolescent Social Support Scale* (Malecki, Demaray, & Elliot, 2000)	*Child and Adolescent Social Support Scale* (Malecki et al., 2000)	48 items; measures social support from parents, teachers, classmates, and a close friend
		Social Support Scale for Children and Adolescents (Harter, 1985)	*Social Support Scale for Children and Adolescents* (Harter, 1985)	24 items; measures social support from parents, teachers, classmates, and a close friend
		Survey of Children's Social Support (Dubow & Ullman, 1989)		Measures frequency of support (38 items), appraisal of support (31 items), and size of support network
		Social Skills Rating System (Gresham & Elliot, 1990)	*Social Skills Rating System* (Gresham & Elliot, 1990)	30 items assessing cooperation, assertion, and empathy
	Teacher and parent report	*Social Skills Rating System* (Gresham & Elliot, 1990)	*Social Skills Rating System* (Gresham & Elliot, 1990)	30 items assessing cooperation, assertion, and empathy

group activities (e.g., pizza parties, bowling). These group activities approximate children's natural peer groups and social interactions. SET-C also uses in vivo exposure therapy for anxiety-provoking social situations (Beidel *et al.*, 2000).

SET-C has demonstrated promising results in several clinical trials. With 67 children, aged 8 to 12 years, Beidel *et al.* (2000) found that treated children reported higher social skills, less fear and anxiety, and more social interaction than children in the control condition. Furthermore, two-thirds of the youth who received SET-C no longer met criteria for social phobia at post-treatment, compared to 5% of youth in the credible control condition ("test busters" to reduce test anxiety). Additionally, most children who participated in follow-up remained diagnosis-free at 3 years (Beidel *et al.*, 2005) and 5 years post-treatment (Beidel, Turner, & Young, 2006).

SET-C has been extended to include adolescents (e.g., ages 7 to 17 years; also referred to as SET-A). Compared to pharmacological treatment (fluoxetine) for social phobia, Beidel *et al.* 2007 found SET-C to be as efficacious as fluoxetine treatment, but with the added benefits of enhancing youths' social skills and exerting longer-lasting effects. Garcia-Lopez, Olivares, Beidel, Albano, Turner, and Rosa (2006) also found that treatment effects were maintained at 5-year follow-up for socially anxious adolescents treated with SET-A (Spanish version).

Overall, the treatment outcome data for SET-C and SET-A are positive. The SET-C and SET-A programs address youths' interpersonal skills and behavioral inhibition in social situations, and demonstrate reductions in anxiety (and anxiety diagnoses) and in youths' reports of loneliness, as well as improvements in social skills (Beidel *et al.*, 2006). Unlike earlier CBT programs to address social anxiety disorder in youth (e.g., Albano, Marten, Holt, Heimberg, & Barlow, 1995; Spence, 2000) that revealed benefits relative to wait-list control conditions, SET-C and SET-A demonstrate treatment gains relative to active attention-control conditions. In fact, in reviewing treatments for anxiety disorders in youth, Silverman, Pina, *et al.* (2008) considered SET-C to be one of the few treatments that was "probably efficacious."

Another program developed for social anxiety disorder is Skills for Social and Academic Success (SSAS: Fisher, Masia-Warner, & Klein, 2004; Masia-Warner, Fisher, Shrout, Rathor, & Klein, 2007). SSAS is a school-based CBT intervention for socially anxious adolescents, who are rarely identified and referred for treatment (Masia, Klein, Storch, & Corda, 2001). Similar to SET-C, SSAS sessions emphasize social skills and exposures for anxiety-provoking social situations. In addition to 12 40-minute group sessions with peers, adolescents have two brief individual sessions, and four weekend social events with non-anxious peer facilitators. Additionally, parents attend group meetings that focus on psycho-educational issues, and teachers facilitate classroom exposures.

Preliminary evidence suggests that SSAS is effective. Following positive treatment effects in an open trial (Masia *et al.*, 2001), Masia-Warner *et al.* (2007) conducted a randomized controlled trial of SSAS with 36 socially anxious adolescents. They found that 59% of the adolescents receiving SSAS no longer met criteria for social anxiety disorder compared to 0% of the adolescents in the credible attention–control condition. Also encouraging was the fact that clinical improvements for adolescents treated with SSAS were maintained at 6 months post-treatment. The use of a school-based approach is appealing given that socially anxious adolescents experience distress in school (Masia-Warner *et al.*, 2007), although further study of SSAS with larger, more ethnically diverse samples would be desirable.

As reviewed by Silverman, Pina, *et al.* (2008), one other "probably efficacious" treatment for youth with social anxiety disorder is Group CBT for Social Phobia (GCBT for SOP). Studies by Spence, Donovan, and Brechman-Toussaint (2000) with 50 youth aged 7–14 years, and Hayward, Varady, Albano, Thienemann, Henderson, and Schatzberg (2000) with 35 adolescent girls (mean age = 15.8 years) provide support for GCBT for SOP relative to wait-list controls or no treatment. In the Hayward *et al.* study, significant post-treatment effects for GCBT did not hold up at 12-month follow-up; the authors suggested the possibility that girls' heterosocial anxiety (i.e., anxiety in dating and mixed-sex social situations), which was not a target of treatment, may have played a role.

In summary, SET-C, SET-A, and SSAS are important and valuable treatments for youth with social anxiety disorder. These treatments reduce social anxiety and anxiety disorder diagnoses, and improve aspects of interpersonal functioning, such as social skills.

At the same time, the impacts of these treatments on peer processes that contribute to social anxiety have not been examined. It is not known, for example, whether CBT interventions for social anxiety improve youths' friendships, romantic relationships, levels of peer support, or social acceptance. In the future, these peer processes might be evaluated as treatment outcomes or as mediators of treatment outcome. Efforts to target heterosocial anxiety, a strong correlate of social anxiety (Glickman & La Greca, 2004), in treatments for adolescent social anxiety also may be valuable.

Anxiety disorders in general

Individual CBT (ICBT) and GCBT have been used for a wide range of phobic and anxiety disorders in youth and represent "probably efficacious" treatments (Silverman, Pina, *et al.*, 2008). These treatments often include youth with a primary or secondary diagnosis of social anxiety disorder, who may evidence social impairments (Ginsburg *et al.*, 1998). Although it is beyond the scope of this chapter to review these treatment studies in detail, a few observations will be offered regarding the attention to peer processes in these interventions.

GCBT programs incorporate peers in treatment through the use of group-based treatment procedures (e.g., Barrett, 1998; Flannery-Schroeder & Kendall, 2000; Silverman, Kurtines, Ginsburg, Weems, Lumpkin, & Carmichael, 1999). However, it is not clear whether the inclusion of other anxious peers in GCBT is beneficial (e.g., provides social support and "real-life" peers for practicing exposures) or not (e.g., intensifies anxious feelings for socially avoidant youth).

Both GCBT and ICBT have been effective with anxious youth (Silverman, Pina, *et al.*, 2008). Although data are sparse, in some trials and among certain outcome measures, ICBT appeared to perform better than GCBT (Flannery-Schroeder & Kendall, 2000; Manassis *et al.*, 2002). In reflecting on this finding, Manassis *et al.* (2002) speculated that children with social evaluative concerns might be overwhelmed by the group format of GCBT at first. Thus, the mere inclusion of peers with similar difficulties may not automatically enhance treatment outcomes for certain anxious youth.

The issue of peer processes that contribute to anxiety (and especially social anxiety) in youth raises some intriguing possibilities for future intervention studies. For general ICBT and GCBT interventions, it may be worth examining whether high levels of social anxiety moderate treatment outcome. Understanding how these interventions affect important social outcomes for youth, such as the number and quality of their best friendships, or levels of social support, may also be instructive, and lead to future treatment targets to enhance effectiveness.

Even for treatments designed for social anxiety disorder, greater attention to peer variables that may moderate treatment outcome would be useful. For example, does youths' level of peer victimization moderate treatment outcome? It may not be sufficient to teach social skills and reduce social avoidance among youth who are actively victimized. Peer victimization can represent a "real threat" that must be dealt with in some manner. Consistent with a "personalized medicine" approach to treatment, if peer victimization levels moderate treatment outcome, CBT treatments may need to be adapted for such youth to incorporate strategies for effectively dealing with victimization experiences. It also may be useful to examine close friend support as a treatment moderator, as peer support can buffer the impact of interpersonal stressors. Other peer processes described in this chapter (e.g., presence and quality of close friendships or romantic relationships) could also be important moderators to examine, and may contribute to the next generation of treatment studies in this area (La Greca, Silverman, & Lochman, 2009).

Conclusions

This chapter highlighted peer processes associated with anxiety symptoms and disorders in youth. In the theoretical frameworks reviewed, aversive peer processes (peer victimization, peer rejection) were conceptualized as directly contributing to anxiety, especially social anxiety, and research supports this view. In some cases, the direction of causal pathways between interpersonal functioning with peers (e.g., qualities of close friendships and romantic relationships) and anxiety are less clear, although these associations are conceptualized as bidirectional. Future studies that directly examine causal pathways between anxiety and interpersonal functioning, and that evaluate the interpersonal functioning of youth with anxiety disorders would be instructive.

The chapter also briefly highlighted measures for assessing peer variables. These may be useful in clinical situations to characterize the interpersonal functioning of youth with anxiety disorders, or for examining peer processes that may mediate or moderate treatment outcome.

Finally, we considered the role of peer processes in CBT treatments for youth anxiety. A recent commentary on the future direction of the child and adolescent intervention literature (La Greca *et al.*, 2009) stressed the importance of evaluating mediators, moderators, and predictors of treatment outcome in psychological interventions for youth. Many of the peer processes reviewed in this chapter would be fruitful to consider in this context. This is a fertile area of investigation that holds promise for further refinement of interventions for youth with anxiety disorders.

References

Aboud, F. E. & Mendelson, M. J. (1998). Determinants of friendship selection and quality: developmental perspectives. In: W. M. Bukowski, A. F. Newcomb, & W. W. Hartup (eds.) *The Company They Keep: Friendships in Childhood and Adolescence*, pp. 87–112. New York: Cambridge University Press.

Albano, A., Marten, P. A., Holt, C. S., Heimberg, R. G., & Barlow, D. H. (1995). Cognitive–behavioral group treatment for social phobia in adolescents: a preliminary study. *Journal of Nervous and Mental Disease*, **183**, 649–656.

Achenbach, T. M. (1991). *Integrative Guide for the 1991 CBCL/4–18, YSR, and TRF Profiles.* Burlington, VT: University of Vermont Department of Psychiatry.

American Psychiatric Association (2000). *Diagnostic and Statistical Manual of Mental Disorders,* 4th edn, text revision. Washington, DC: American Psychiatric Association.

Anthonysamy, A. & **Zimmer-Gembeck, M. J.** (2007). Peer status and behaviors of maltreated children and their classmates in the early years of school. *Child Abuse and Neglect,* **31**, 971–991.

Anxiety Disorders Association of America (2007). ADAA survey results: friendships. Available at http://socialanxietydisorder.about.com/od/researchreports/p/adaafriends.htm.

Bagwell, C. L., Molina, B. S. G., Pelham, W. E., & **Hoza, B.** (2001). Attention-deficit hyperactivity disorder and problems in peer relations: predictions from childhood to adolescence. *Journal of the American Academy of Child and Adolescent Psychiatry,* **40**, 1285–1292.

Barrett, P. M. (1998). Evaluation of cognitive–behavioral group treatments for childhood anxiety disorders. *Journal of Clinical Child Psychology,* **27**, 459–468.

Beidel, D. C., Turner, S. M., & **Morris, T. L.** (2000). Behavioral treatment of childhood social phobia. *Journal of Consulting and Clinical Psychology,* **68**, 1072–1080.

Beidel, D. C., Turner, S. M., Sallee, F. R., Ammerman, R. T., Crosby, L. A., & **Pathak, S.** (2007). SET-C versus fluoxetine in the treatment of childhood social phobia. *Journal of the American Academy of Child and Adolescent Psychiatry,* **46**, 1622–1632.

Beidel, D. C., Turner, S. M., & **Young, B. J.** (2006). Social effectiveness therapy for children: five years later. *Behavior Therapy,* **37**, 416–425.

Beidel, D. C., Turner, S. M., Young, B., & **Paulson, A.** (2005). Social effectiveness therapy for children: three-year follow-up. *Journal of Consulting and Clinical Psychology,* **73**, 721–725.

Blöte, A. W. & **Westenberg, P. M.** (2007). Socially anxious adolescents' perception of treatment by classmates. *Behaviour Research and Therapy,* **45**, 189–198.

Brown, B. B. (1990). Peer groups and peer cultures. In: **S. S. Feldman** & **G. R. Elliot** (eds.) *At the Threshold: The Developing Adolescent,* pp. 171–196. Cambridge, MA: Harvard University Press.

Brown, B. B. (2004). Adolescents' relationship with peers. In: **R. M. Lerner** & **L. Steinberg** (eds.) *Handbook of Adolescent Psychology,* 2nd edn, pp. 363–394. Hoboken, NJ: Wiley & Sons.

Brown, B. B., Herman, M., Hamm, J. V., & **Heck, D. J.** (2008). Ethnicity and image: correlates of crowd affiliation among ethnic minority youth. *Child Development,* **79**, 529–546.

Brown, B. B., Mounts, N., Lamborn, S. D., & **Steinberg, L.** (1993). Parenting practices and peer group affiliation in adolescence. *Child Development,* **64**, 467–482.

Buhrmester, D. & **Furman, W.** (1987). The development of companionship and intimacy. *Child Development,* **58**, 1101–1113.

Bukowski, W. M., Brendgen, M., & **Vitaro. F.** (2006). Peers and socialization. In: **J. E. Grusec** & **P. D. Hastings** (eds.) *Handbook of Socialization Theory and Research,* pp. 355 – 381. New York: Guilford Press.

Bukowski, W. M., Hoza, B., & **Boivin, M.** (1994). Measuring friendship quality during pre- and early adolescence: the development and psychometric properties of the Friendship Qualities Scale. *Journal of Social and Personal Relationships,* **11**, 471–484.

Carver, K., Joyner K., & **Udry, J. R.** (2003). National estimates of adolescent romantic relationships. In: **P. Florsheim** (ed.) *Adolescent Romantic Relationships and Sexual Behavior: Theory, Research, and Practical Implications,* pp. 291–329. New York: Cambridge University Press.

Coie, J. D., Dodge, K. A., & **Kupersmidt, J. B.** (1990). Peer group behavior and social status. In: **S. R. Asher** & **J. D. Coie** (eds.) *Peer Rejection in Childhood,* pp. 17–59. New York: Cambridge University Press.

Collins, W. A. (2003). More than myth: the developmental significance of romantic relationships during adolescence. *Journal of Research on Adolescence,* **13**, 1–24.

Connolly, J. A. & **Goldberg, A.** (1999). Romantic relationships in adolescence: the role of friends and peers in their emergence and development. In: **W. Furman, B. B. Brown,** & **C. Feiring** (eds.) *The Development of Romantic Relationships in Adolescence*, pp. 266–290. New York: Cambridge University Press.

Costello, E. J., Egger, H. L., & **Angold, A.** (2005). The developmental epidemiology of anxiety disorders: phenomenology, prevalence, and comorbidity. *Child and Adolescent Psychiatric Clinics of North America*, **14**, 631–648.

Coyne, S. M., Archer, J., & **Eslea, M.** (2006). "We're not friends anymore! Unless . . . ": the frequency and harmfulness of indirect, relational and social aggression. *Aggressive Behavior*, **32**, 294–307.

Crick, N. R. (1996). The role of overt aggression, relational aggression and prosocial behavior in the prediction of children's future social adjustment. *Child Development*, **67**, 2317–2327.

Crick, N. R. & **Bigbee, M. A.** (1998). Relational and overt forms of peer victimization: a multi-informant approach. *Journal of Consulting and Clinical Psychology*, **66**, 337–347.

Crick, N. R. & **Grotpeter, J. K.** (1996). Children's treatment by peers: victims of relational and overt aggression. *Development and Psychopathology*, **8**, 367–380.

Crick, N. R. & **Nelson, D. A.** (2002). Relational and physical victimization within friendships: nobody told me there'd be friends like these. *Journal of Abnormal Child Psychology*, **30**, 599–607.

Cullerton-Sen, C. & **Crick, N. R.** (2005). Understanding the effects of physical and relational victimization: the utility of multiple perspectives in predicting social–emotional adjustment. *School Psychology Review*, **34**, 147–160.

Davila, J., La Greca, A. M., Starr, L. R., & **Landoll, R. R.** (2010). Anxiety disorders in adolescence. In: **J. G. Beck** (ed.) *Interpersonal Processes in the Anxiety Disorders: Implications for Understanding Psychopathology and Treatment*. Washington, DC: American Psychological Association.

Davila, J., Steinberg, S. J., Kachadourian, L., Cobb, R., & **Fincham, F.** (2004). Romantic involvement and depressive symptoms in early and late adolescence: the role of preoccupied relational style. *Personal Relationships*, **11**, 161–178.

Deater-Deckard, K. (2001). Annotation: recent research examining the role of peer relationships in the development of psychopathology. *Journal of Child Psychology and Psychiatry*, **42**, 565–579.

De Los Reyes, A. & **Prinstein, M. J.** (2004). Applying depression-distortion hypotheses to the assessment of peer victimization in adolescents. *Journal of Clinical Child and Adolescent Psychology*, **33**, 325–335.

Dinkes, R., Cataldi, E. F., & **Lin-Kelly, W.** (2007). *Indicators of School Crime and Safety: 2007*. Washington, DC: National Center for Education Statistics, Institute of Education Sciences, US Department of Education.

Downey, G., Bonica, C., & **Rincon, C.** (1999). Rejection sensitivity and adolescent romantic relationships. In: **W. Furman, B.B. Brown,** & **C. Feiring** (eds.) *The Development of Romantic Relationships in Adolescence*, pp. 148–174. New York: Cambridge University Press.

Dubow, E. F. & **Ullman, D. G.** (1989). Assessing social support in elementary school children: the Survey of Children's Social Support. *Journal of Clinical Child Psychology*, **18**, 52–64.

Essau, C. A. (2003). Comorbidity of anxiety disorders in adolescents. *Depression and Anxiety*, **18**, 1–6.

Estell, D. B., Jones, M. H., Pearl, R., Van Acker, R., Farmer, T. W., & **Rodkin, P. C.** (2008). Peer groups, popularity, and social preference: trajectories of social functioning among students with and without learning disabilities. *Journal of Learning Disabilities*, **41**, 5 – 14.

Fisher, P. H., Masia-Warner, C., & **Klein, R. G.** (2004). Skills for Social and Academic Success: a school-based intervention for social anxiety disorder in adolescents. *Clinical Child and Family Psychology Review*, **7**, 241–249.

Flannery-Schroeder, E. C. & Kendall, P. C. (2000). Group and individual cognitive–behavioral treatments for youth with anxiety disorders: a randomized clinical trial. *Cognitive Therapy and Research*, **24**, 251–278.

Furman, W. (1998). The measurement of friendship perceptions: conceptual and methodological issues. In: W. M. Bukowski, A. F. Newcomb, & W. W. Hartup (eds.) *The Company They Keep: Friendships in Childhood and Adolescence*, pp. 41–65. New York: Cambridge University Press.

Furman, W., McDunn, C., & Young, B. J. (2008). The role of peer and romantic relationships in adolescent affective development. In: N. Allen & L. Sheeber (eds.) *Adolescent Emotional Development and the Emergence of Depressive Disorders*, pp. 299–317. New York: Cambridge University Press.

Galen, B. R. & Underwood, M. K. (1997). A developmental investigation of social aggression among children. *Developmental Psychology*, **33**, 589–600.

Garcia-Lopez, L. J., Olivares, J., Beidel, D., Albano, A. M., Turner, S., & Rosa, A. I. (2006). Efficacy of three treatment protocols for adolescents with social anxiety disorder: a 5-year follow-up assessment. *Journal of Anxiety Disorders*, **20**, 175–191.

Ginsburg, G. S., La Greca, A. M., & Silverman, W. K. (1998). Social anxiety in children with anxiety disorders: relation with social and emotional functioning. *Journal of Abnormal Child Psychology*, **26**, 175–185.

Glickman, A. R. & La Greca, A. M. (2004). The Dating Anxiety Scale for Adolescents: scale development and associations with adolescent functioning. *Journal of Clinical Child and Adolescent Psychology*, **33**, 566–578.

Grant, D. M., Beck, J. G., Farrow, S. M., & Davila, J. (2007). Do interpersonal features of social anxiety influence the development of depressive symptoms? *Cognition and Emotion*, **21**, 646–663.

Greco, L. A. & Morris, T. L. (2005). Factors influencing the link between social anxiety and peer acceptance: contributions of social skills and close friendships during middle childhood. *Behavior Therapy*, **36**, 197–205.

Gresham, F. M. & Elliot, S. N. (1990). *Social Skills Rating System Manual*. Circle Pines, MN: American Guidance Service.

Grotpeter, J. K. & Crick, N. R. (1996). Relational aggression, overt aggression, and friendship. *Child Development*, **67**, 2328–2338.

Harter, S. (1985). *The Social Support Scale for Children and Adolescents*. Denver, CO: University of Denver.

Harter, S. (1988). *Manual for the Self-Perception Profile for Children and Adolescents*. Denver, CO: Author.

Hartup, W. W. (1996). The company they keep: friendships and their developmental significance. *Child Development*, **67**, 1–13.

Hawker, D. S. J. & Boulton, M. J. (2000). Twenty years' research on peer victimization and psychosocial maladjustment: a meta-analytic review of cross-sectional studies. *Journal of Child Psychology and Psychiatry*, **41**, 441–455.

Hayward, C., Varady, S., Albano, A. M. Thienemann, M., Henderson, L., & Schatzberg, A. F. (2000). Cognitive–behavioral group therapy for social phobia in female adolescents: results of a pilot study. *Journal of the American Academy of Child and Adolescent Psychiatry*, **39**, 721–726.

Hinshaw, S. P. (2008). Developmental psychopathology as a scientific discipline: relevance to behavioral and emotional disorders of childhood and adolescence. In: T. P. Beauchaine & S. P. Hinshaw (eds.) *Child and Adolescent Psychopathology*, pp. 3–26. Hoboken, NJ: Wiley & Sons.

Hogue, A. & Steinberg, L. (1995). Homophily of internalized distress in adolescent peer groups. *Developmental Psychology*, **31**, 897–906.

Inderbitzen, H. M., Walters, K. S., & Bukowski, A. L. (1997). The role of social anxiety in adolescent peer relations: differences among sociometric status groups and rejected subgroups. *Journal of Clinical Child Psychology*, **26**, 338–348.

Kandel, D. B. (1978a). Homophily, selection, and socialization in adolescent friendships. *American Journal of Sociology*, **84**, 427–436.

Kandel, D. B. (1978b). Similarity in real-life adolescent friendship pairs. *Journal of Personality and Social Psychology*, **36**, 306–312.

Kendall, P. C., Furr, J. M., & Podell, J. L. (2010). Child-focused treatment of anxiety. In: J. R. Weisz & A. E. Kazdin (eds.) *Evidence-Based Psychotherapies for Children and Adolescents*, 2nd edn, pp. 45–60. New York: Guilford Press.

Kinney, D. A. (1993). From nerds to normals: the recovery of identify among adolescents from middle school to high school. *Sociology of Education*, **66**, 21–40.

Kupersmidt, J. B. & Coie, J. D. (1990). Preadolescent peer status, aggression, and school adjustment as predictors of externalizing problems in adolescence. *Child Development*, **61**, 1350–1362.

Kuttler, A. F. & La Greca, A. M. (2004). Adolescents' romantic relationships: do they help or hinder close friendships? *Journal of Adolescence*, **27**, 395–414.

Kuttler, A. F., La Greca, A. M., & Prinstein. M. J. (1999). Adolescents' close friendships: same- versus cross-sex friends. *Journal of Research in Adolescence*, **9**, 339–366.

La Greca, A. M. (1999). The Social Anxiety Scales for Children and Adolescents. *The Behavior Therapist*, **22**, 133–136.

La Greca, A. M. (2001). Friends or foes? Peer influences on anxiety among children and adolescents. In: W. K. Silverman & P. D. A. Treffers (eds.) *Anxiety Disorders in Children and Adolescents: Research, Assessment, and Intervention*, pp. 159–186. New York: Cambridge University Press.

La Greca, A. M. & Harrison, H. W. (2005). Adolescent peer relations, friendships and romantic relationships: do they predict social anxiety and depression? *Journal of Clinical Child and Adolescent Psychology*, **34**, 49–61.

La Greca, A. M. & Lemanek, K. L. (1996). Assessment as a process in pediatric psychology. *Journal of Pediatric Psychology*, **21**, 137–151.

La Greca, A. M. & Lopez, N. (1998). Social anxiety among adolescents: linkages with peer relations and friendships. *Journal of Abnormal Child Psychology*, **26**, 83–94.

La Greca, A. M. & Mackey, E. R. (2007). Adolescents' anxiety in dating situations: do friends and romantic partners contribute? *Journal of Clinical Child and Adolescent Psychology*, **34**, 522–533.

La Greca, A. M. & Prinstein, M. J. (1999). Peer group. In: W. K. Silverman & T. H. Ollendick (eds.) *Developmental Issues in the Clinical Treatment of Children*, pp. 171–198. Needham Heights, MA: Allyn & Bacon.

La Greca, A. M. & Stone, W. L. (1993). The Social Anxiety Scale for Children – Revised: factor structure and concurrent validity. *Journal of Clinical Child Psychology*, **22**, 17–27.

La Greca, A. M., Dandes, S. K., Wick, P., Shaw, K., & Stone, W. L. (1988). Development of the Social Anxiety Scale for Children: reliability and concurrent validity. *Journal of Clinical Child Psychology*, **17**, 84–91.

La Greca, A. M., Davila, J., & Siegel, R. (2008). Friendships, romantic relationships, and depression. In: N. Allen & L. Sheeber (eds.) *Adolescent Emotional Development and the Emergence of Depressive Disorders*, pp. 318–336. New York: Cambridge University Press.

La Greca, A. M., Prinstein, M. J., & Fetter, M. (2001). Adolescent peer crowd affiliation: linkages with health-risk behaviors and close friendships. *Journal of Pediatric Psychology*, **26**, 131–143.

La Greca, A. M., Silverman, W. K., & Lochman, J. E. (2009). Moving beyond efficacy and effectiveness in child and adolescent intervention research. *Journal of Consulting and Clinical Psychology*, **77**, 373–382.

Landoll, R. R. & La Greca, A. M. (2009). Peer victimization in a new generation: understanding victimization via social networking sites. In: **A. M. La Greca** & **J. Davila** (Chairs) *Interpersonal Processes Contributing to Adolescents' Internalizing Symptoms: Implications for Research and Intervention*. New York: Association for Behavioral and Cognitive Therapies.

Larson, R. W., Clore, G. L., & Wood, G. A. (1999). The emotions of romantic relationships: do they wreck havoc on adolescents? In **W. Furman, B. B. Brown,** & **C. Feiring** (eds.) *The Development of Romantic Relationships in Adolescence*, pp. 19–49. New York: Cambridge University Press.

LeBlanc, L. A., Sautter, R. A., & Dore, D. J. (2006). Peer relationship problems. In: **M. Hersen** (ed.) *Clinician's Handbook of Child Behavioral Assessment*, pp. 377–399. San Diego, CA: Academic Press.

Malecki, C. K., Demaray, M. K., & Elliot, S. N. (2000). *The Child and Adolescent Social Support Scale*. DeKalb, IL: Northern Illinois University.

Manassis, K., Mendlowitz, S. L., Scapillato, D., Avery, D., Fiksenbaum, L., Freire, M., et al. (2002). Group and individual cognitive–behavioral therapy for childhood anxiety disorders: a randomized trial. *Journal of the American Academy of Child and Adolescent Psychiatry*, **41**, 1423–1430.

Masia, C. L., Klein, R. G., Storch, E. A., & Corda, B. (2001). School-based behavioral treatment for social anxiety disorder in adolescents: results of a pilot study. *Journal of the American Academy of Child and Adolescent Psychiatry*, **40**, 780–786.

Masia-Warner, C., Fisher, P. H., Shrout, P. E., Rathor, S., & Klein, R. G. (2007). Treating adolescents with social anxiety disorder in school: an attention control trial. *Journal of Child Psychology and Psychiatry*, **48**, 676–686.

Mynard, H., Joseph, S., & Alexander, J. (2000). Peer-victimization and post-traumatic stress in adolescents. *Personality and Individual Differences*, **28**, 815–821.

Ollendick, T. H. & Seligman, L. D. (2006). Anxiety disorders in children and adolescents. In: **C. Gillberg, R. Harrington,** & **H. Steinhausen** (eds.) *Clinician's Desk Book of Child and Adolescent Psychiatry*, pp. 144–187. Cambridge: Cambridge University Press.

Ollendick, T. H., King, N. J., & Muris, P. (2002). Fears and phobias in children: phenomenology, epidemiology, and etiology. *Child and Adolescent Mental Health*, **7**, 98–106.

O'Sullivan, L. F., Cheng, M. M., Harris, K. M., & Brooks-Gunn, J. (2007). I wanna hold your hand: the progression of social, romantic and sexual events in adolescent relationships. *Perspectives on Sexual and Reproductive Health*, **39**, 100–107.

Pahl, K. M. & Barrett, P. M. (2010). Interventions for anxiety disorders in children using group cognitive–behavioral therapy with family involvement. In: **J. R. Weisz** & **A. E. Kazdin** (eds.) *Evidence-Based Psychotherapies for Children and Adolescents*, 2nd edn, pp. 61–79. New York: Guilford Press.

Parker, J. G. & Asher, S. R. (1993). Friendship and friendship quality in middle childhood: links with peer group acceptance and feelings of loneliness and social dissatisfaction. *Developmental Psychology*, **29**, 611–621.

Prinstein, M. J. (2007). Moderators of peer contagion: a longitudinal examination of depression socialization between adolescents and their best friends. *Journal of Clinical Child and Adolescent Psychology*, **36**, 159–170.

Prinstein, M. J. & Aikins, J. W. (2004). Cognitive moderators of the longitudinal association between peer rejection and adolescent depressive symptoms. *Journal of Abnormal Child Psychology*, **32**, 147–158.

Prinstein, M. J., Boergers, J., & Vernberg, E. M. (2001). Overt and relational aggression in adolescents: social–psychological functioning of aggressors and victims. *Journal of Clinical Child Psychology*, **30**, 447–489.

Ranta, K., Kaltiala-Heino, R., Pelkonen, M., & Marttunen, M. (2009). Associations between peer victimization, self-reported depression and social phobia among adolescents: the role of comorbidity. *Journal of Adolescence*, **32**, 77–93.

Rubin, K. H., Coplan, R. J., & Bowker, J. C. (2009). Social withdrawal in childhood. *Annual Review of Psychology*, **60**, 141–171.

Schneider, B. H. (2009). An observational study of the interactions of socially withdrawn/anxious early adolescents and their friends. *Journal of Child Psychology and Psychiatry*, **50**, 799–806.

Schwartz, D., Gorman, A. H., Dodge, K. A., Pettit, G. S. & Bates, J. E. (2008). Friendships with peers who are low or high in aggression as moderators of the link between peer victimization and declines in academic functioning. *Journal of Abnormal Child Psychology*, **36**, 719–730.

Siegel, R. S., La Greca, A. M., & Harrison, H. M. (2009). Peer victimization and social anxiety in adolescents: prospective and reciprocal relationships. *Journal of Youth and Adolescence*, **38**, 1096–1109.

Silverman, W. K., Kurtines, W. M., Ginsburg, G. S., Weems, C. F., Lumpkin, P. W., & Carmichael, D. H. (1999). Treating anxiety disorders in children with group cognitive–behavioral therapy: a randomized clinical trial. *Journal of Consulting and Clinical Psychology*, **67**, 995–1003.

Silverman, W. K., Ortiz, C. D., Viswesvaran, C., Kolko, D. J., Amaya-Jackson, L., Putnam, F. W., *et al.* (2008). Evidence-based psychosocial treatments for children and adolescents exposed to traumatic events. *Journal of Clinical Child and Adolescent Psychology*, **37**, 156–183.

Silverman, W. K., Pina, A., & Viswesvaran, C. (2008). Evidence-based psychosocial treatments for phobic and anxiety disorders in children and adolescents. *Journal of Clinical Child and Adolescent Psychology*, **37**, 105–130.

Slonje, R. & Smith, P. K. (2008). Cyberbullying: another main type of bullying? *Scandinavian Journal of Psychology*, **49**, 147–154.

Spence, S. H. (2000). *Social Skills Training: Enhancing Social Competence with Children and Adolescents*. Windsor, UK: NRER-Nelson.

Spence, S. H., Donovan, C., & Brechman-Toussaint, M. (2000). The treatment of childhood social phobia: the effectiveness of a social skills training-based, cognitive–behavioral intervention, with and without parental involvement. *Journal of Child Psychology and Psychiatry*, **41**, 713–726.

Storch, E. A. & Esposito, L. E. (2003). Peer victimization and post-traumatic stress among children. *Child Study Journal*, **33**, 91–98.

Storch, E. A. & Masia-Warner, C. (2004). The relationship of peer victimization to social anxiety and loneliness in adolescent females. *Journal of Adolescence*, **27**, 351–362.

Storch, E. A., Brassard, M. R., & Masia-Warner, C. L. (2003). The relationship of peer victimization to social anxiety and loneliness in adolescence. *Child Study Journal*, **33**, 1–18.

Storch, E. A., Ledley, D. R., Lewin, A. B., Murphy, T. K., Johns, N. B., Goodman, W. K., *et al.* (2006). Peer victimization in children with obsessive–compulsive disorder: relations with symptoms of psychopathology. *Journal of Clinical Child and Adolescent Psychology*, **35**, 446–455.

Storch, E. A., Masia-Warner, C., Crisp, H., & Klein, R. G. (2005). Peer victimization and social anxiety in adolescence: a prospective study. *Aggressive Behavior*, **31**, 437–452.

Storch, E. A., Phil, M., Nock, M. K., Masia-Warner, C., & Barlas, M. E. (2003). Peer victimization and social–psychological adjustment in Hispanic and African-American children. *Journal of Child and Family Studies*, **12**, 439–452.

Strauss, C. C., Frame, C. L., & Forehand, R. (1987). Psychosocial impairment associated with anxiety in children. *Journal of Clinical Child Psychology*, **16**, 235–239.

Strauss, C. C., Lahey, B. B., Frick, P., Frame, C. L., & Hynd, G. W. (1988). Peer social status of children with anxiety disorders. *Journal of Consulting and Clinical Psychology*, **56**, 137–141.

Strouse, D. L. (1999). Adolescent crowd orientations: a social and temporal analysis. In: **J. A. McLellan** & **M. J. V. Pugh** (eds.) *The Role of Peer Groups in Adolescent Social Identity: Exploring the Importance of Stability and Change*, pp. 37–54. San Francisco, CA: Jossey-Bass.

Sussman, S., Pokhrel, P., Ashmore, R. D., & Brown, B. B. (2007). Adolescent peer group identification and characteristics: a review of the literature. *Addictive Behaviors*, **32**, 1602–1627.

Vernberg, E. M., Abwender, D. A., Ewell, K. K., & Beery, S. H. (1992). Social anxiety and peer relationships in early adolescence: a prospective analysis. *Journal of Clinical Child Psychology*, **21**, 189–196.

Verduin, T. L. & Kendall, P. C. (2008). Peer perceptions and liking of children with anxiety disorders. *Journal of Abnormal Child Psychology*, **36**, 459–469.

Wasserstein, S. B. & La Greca, A. M. (1996). Can peer support buffer against behavioral consequences of parental discord? *Journal of Clinical Child Psychology*, **25**, 177–182.

Williams, K. R. & Guerra, N. G. (2007). Prevalence and predictors of Internet bullying. *Journal of Adolescent Health*, **41**, S14–S21.

Wittchen, H.U., Fuetsch, M., Sonntag, H., Mueller, N., & Liebowitz, M. (2000). Disability and quality of life in pure and comorbid social phobia: Findings from a controlled study. *European Psychiatry*, **15**, 46–58.

World Health Organization (2009). *The International Statistical Classification of Diseases and Health Related Problems: ICD-10*, 2008 edn. Geneva: World Health Organization.

Ye, H. J., Rice, K. G., & Storch, E. A. (2008). Perfectionism and peer relations among children with obsessive-compulsive disorder. *Child Psychiatry and Human Development*, **39**, 415–426.

Prevention and treatment of child and adolescent anxiety

16

Prevention of child and adolescent anxiety disorders

Heidi J. Lyneham and Ron M. Rapee

Anxiety disorders are the most frequently reported mental health concern in child, adolescent, and adult populations (see Costello, Egger, Copeland, Erkanli, & Angold, Chapter 3, this volume) with lifetime prevalence reaching approximately 30% (Kessler, Berglund, Demler, Jin, Merikangas, & Walters, 2005). These disorders exceed the health costs and societal burden of most other physical and mental health problems (Begg, Vos, Barker, Stevenson, & Lopez, 2007; Kessler & Greenburg, 2002). At the individual level, anxiety disorders are associated with immediate distress and impairment (Ialongo, Edelsohn, Werthamer-Larsson, Crockett, & Kellam, 1996; Strauss, Frame, & Forehand, 1987), are a known risk factor in the development of suicidal ideation and of mood and substance use disorders (Hofstra, Van der Ende, & Verhulst, 2000, 2002; Last, Perrin, Hersen, & Kazdin, 1996; Sareen *et al.*, 2005), and are associated with poor long-term outcomes in social, academic, and career domains (Last, Hansen, & Franco, 1997; Weissman *et al.*, 1999). Age of onset for anxiety disorders is typically in childhood or early adolescence (Kessler *et al.*, 2005) and without treatment these disorders persist throughout a person's lifetime (Keller, Lavori, Wunder, Beardslee, Schwartz, & Roth, 1992). Set against this poor prognosis is research showing that the majority of people with anxiety disorders will not receive clinical intervention (Canino *et al.*, 2004; Farmer, Stangl, Burns, Costello, & Angold, 1999).

The costs associated with anxiety disorders coupled with the remarkably early onset suggests that a preventative approach during childhood or adolescence may be of value. Recent developments in the literature have certainly argued this point and several programs targeting anxiety prevention have been examined (e.g., Barrett, Lowry-Webster, & Turner, 2000; Dadds & Roth, 2008; Rapee, Kennedy, Ingram, Edwards, & Sweeney, 2005). The majority of these prevention programs have been conducted in schools, primarily due to the ease of access to large numbers of children that this environment allows (Neil & Christensen, 2009). A smaller number have been implemented in university or clinic settings (e.g., Ginsburg, 2009). A review of this research will be split into the three categories: universal, selective, and indicated prevention, categories proposed by the Institute of Medicines subcommittee on Prevention of Mental Disorders (Mrazek & Haggerty, 1994).

Within this structure, universal refers to application of a prevention program across an entire population (or subpopulation) regardless of individual risk. Selective interventions refer to those that target known risk factors for a given problem or disorder. Finally, indicated intervention refers to selection of individuals based on early indicators or symptoms of the relevant disorder. In the review below, only programs specifically targeting anxiety

Anxiety Disorders in Children and Adolescents, 2nd edn, ed. W. K. Silverman and A. P. Field. Published by Cambridge University Press. © Cambridge University Press 2011.

have been included. However, programs targeting other internalizing disorders such as depression and general resiliency have also been shown to have some impact on anxiety (for review see Neil & Christensen, 2009).

In addition to the three levels of prevention highlighted above, a concept that is rarely discussed is that of "treatment-based" prevention (Rapee, 2008). There are many circumstances where traditional treatment at one point in development might provide prevention at a later developmental stage. This is particularly true of child anxiety where treatment for children who have an anxiety disorder has been shown to be highly efficacious (Cartwright-Hatton, Roberts, Chitsabesan, Fothergill, & Harrington, 2004; Silverman, Pina, & Viswesvaran, 2008). Given that anxiety in childhood and adolescence is a risk factor for a variety of later disorders (Woodward & Ferguson, 2001), it is possible that successful treatment of the anxiety disorder in childhood may provide prevention of issues such as adolescent depression, early adult substance abuse, and adult anxiety (Flannery-Schroeder, 2006). The blur between prevention and treatment also exists between prevention and early intervention. As will be seen in the review of prevention programs below, the majority of the children who report high anxiety symptoms (which is interpreted as an early indicator of a potential anxiety disorder) already meet criteria for an anxiety disorder when subjected to a diagnostic interview. The prevention programs that these children complete arguably become a form of early intervention.

Universal interventions

The majority of research on universal interventions that target child anxiety have been studies of the FRIENDS program (e.g., Barrett *et al.*, 2000). This program has separate versions for primary and high school students, with 10 in-school sessions for the child/adolescent, two booster sessions, and nil to four parent sessions (dependent on the study), and involves homework between sessions for the children. The content of the program is based on traditional cognitive–behavioral treatment for child anxiety incorporating psycho-education, relaxation, positive self-talk, graduated exposure, problem-solving, and rewards (Barrett & Turner, 2001). For example, children learn to face their fears in a graduated manner and to manage anxiety through relaxation and positive self-talk. Each of the FRIENDS studies has examined a different aspect of implementation regarding the preventative intervention.

Barrett and Turner (2001) implemented FRIENDS with 489 6th grade children, comparing psychologist-led and teacher-led programs with usual care (i.e., standard curriculum). Children in the two intervention conditions reported significant improvement in self-reported anxiety and the usual care children showed no significant change. Further there was a non-significant trend for the intervention groups to be more likely to move from at-risk to healthy range scores of anxiety self-report questionnaires, if they had been in the clinical range pre-intervention. Insufficient statistical power prevented conclusions regarding differences between psychologist- and teacher-led prevention.

A second study (Lowry-Webster, Barrett, & Dadds, 2001; Lowry-Webster, Barrett, & Lock, 2003) examined teacher-led FRIENDS against a no-intervention control in 594 10–13-year-old children (allocated via classes). Although all children showed improvement, significantly greater symptom reduction was seen in the prevention group and a larger proportion of the prevention group were no longer "at-risk" (based on clinical level scores on both anxiety and depression measures) when compared to the control group.

After 12 months these group differences were maintained. In addition, children who were previously identified as "at risk" completed a diagnostic interview (child report only). In the prevention group 85% of children previously "at risk" were disorder-free compared to 31% of the control group.

A third study examined outcomes up to 3 years post-prevention in two age groups compared with a monitoring-only control (Barrett, Farrell, Ollendick, & Dadds, 2006; Lock & Barrett, 2003). Children in Year 6 ($n = 336/334$ at allocation and 12 months) and Year 9 ($n = 401/335$ at allocation and 12 months) were participants in the studies (representing a 77–79% response rate for the whole grades). Relatively substantial attrition was seen at the 2-year (34%) and 3-year (47%) follow-up points, with greater attrition in the control group. Outcomes were measured using child self-report of anxiety and depression using questionnaire measures. Short-term outcomes showed general reductions across time for all groups but significantly greater reductions in the intervention group. Younger children showed a greater response, particularly younger female children. At the 3-year follow-up, significantly more control children were considered high risk (a finding not present at the 2-year mark). Patterns over time specifically on the anxiety measure showed that Year 6 intervention children scored significantly lower over time than the Year 6 controls whereas no group differences were identified for the Year 9 groups. The studies also highlighted that girls tend to be at higher risk and initially respond more to intervention; however, this was not a durable effect.

A fourth study (Barrett, Lock, & Farrell, 2005), similar to the one above, compared Year 6 and Year 9 prevention with monitoring. The results showed that anxiety dropped in all groups over time, but a greater drop was reported by the prevention groups at the 12-month mark.

Several studies by other, independent research groups have shown more equivocal results. In the only study reporting a comparison of FRIENDS with an attention control group (who were read *Harry Potter*) findings indicated few significant effects. The trial involved 253 4th grade to 6th grade children in Canada, and no significant differences between the intervention and control groups were demonstrated on reported anxiety symptoms, even for those whose anxiety was elevated or at clinical levels prior to intervention (Laye–Gindhu *et al.*, 2005, cited in Miller, 2008). In an uncontrolled study in the United Kingdom where trained school nurses implemented the FRIENDS program with 106 9- and 10-year-old children, assessments were conducted 6 months prior to the program, immediately before the program, and 3 and 12 months after the program (Stallard, Simpson, Anderson, & Goddard, 2008; Stallard, Simpson, Anderson, Hibbert, & Osborn, 2007). Reductions in child-reported anxiety and increases in self-esteem were found at the 3-month and 12-month follow-up when compared to the initial assessment but not when compared to anxiety symptoms and self-esteem immediately before treatment. Examination of the high-risk children found that 67% moved from high to low risk and no child moved from low to high risk. Of course the changes over time often noted in children with no intervention (e.g., Barrett *et al.*, 2006) makes these small changes especially surprising. It is unclear why these two independent studies seem to have demonstrated somewhat smaller effects than the studies by Barrett's group. Perhaps more experience and/or more allegiance among the originators of the program, as well as other such factors, may lead to stronger effects. If this is true, it might suggest that programs such as FRIENDS need to be implemented by highly trained and experienced staff (compared with for example, school nurses in the work by Stallard's group).

In a recent study utilizing a different program small but positive effects of universal intervention were demonstrated (Aune & Stiles, 2009). Children from 6th to 9th grade were offered three 45-minute sessions providing information and strategies to manage social anxiety. Teachers, parents, and mental health professionals were also offered supportive information and were encouraged to support the young people to implement strategies. A total of 1439 children participated and returned follow-up data (67% of the total population) and assessments were conducted around 12 months apart. Compared with a wait-list group, those in the intervention showed significantly greater reductions in general anxiety symptoms (effect size = 0.21) and symptoms of social anxiety (effect size = 0.20). There were no significant differences on general symptoms of distress or depression.

A final universal prevention program worth noting targeted preschool children in Australia (Dadds & Roth, 2008). The program consisted of six sessions for parents conducted at the child's preschool. The sessions targeted development of positive future expectations through self-talk, behavioral change, and problem-solving strategies, with an overarching emphasis on building preschoolers' strengths and competencies. Of the parents invited to participate in the study 45% consented with 355 children being allocated to intervention and 379 to a no-intervention comparison. Assessments occurred at baseline, pre- and post-intervention, and 7 months after intervention and were taken from both parent and teacher perspectives.

Of those participants invited to attend the intervention, 57.5% expressed an interest in coming and only 34% of these interested parents actually attended most sessions. By the follow-up, participation in assessments had reduced to 496 participants. Sampling biases made findings in this study difficult to interpret. In the beginning parents of emotionally healthier children tended not to be interested in attending the program while the most stressed parents self-selected into the program. In contrast, drop-out from assessment differed between groups: in the comparison condition those parents who were initially more stressed dropped out while in the intervention condition the less stressed parents were twice as likely to drop out.

The general pattern of results was that parents reported no change and teachers reported that all children were significantly better adjusted over time, with relatively greater improvement at post-treatment only for anxiety symptoms. When examining initial risk status a higher percentage of treated preschoolers moved from at-risk to low-risk than occurred for the comparison preschoolers despite the differential drop-out impacting on findings. In general, these results point to the marked difficulty that is common to many universal programs, of delivering intervention to those who need it. The results also do not provide strong optimism for the efficacy of universal delivery at this very early age. Nevertheless, future developments may result in stronger effects.

Although universal trials contain some promising results, it should be noted that effect sizes are commonly in the small to moderate range (−0.24 to 0.7 at follow-up) (Neil & Christensen, 2009). These findings are also tempered by several methodological limitations. The assessment methods used in the child and adolescent studies are based on child report alone. It is commonly accepted that adequate assessment of child anxiety should involve multiple methods and multiple informants (Schniering, Hudson, & Rapee, 2000; Silverman & Ollendick, 2005; see also Cartwright-Hatton, Reynolds, & Wilson, Chapter 7, this volume). Additionally, there is lack of methods other than questionnaire to assess outcomes. The addition of diagnostic interviews for all children (rather than a subset of high-risk children after intervention) would be valuable in understanding whether the results reflect true prevention. Given the strong similarities between these universal prevention programs and standard clinical interventions for anxious children, it is possible that any effects are due to treatment of already diagnostic children rather than to the prevention of anxiety disorders in non-diagnostic children.

The statistical methods used to determine outcomes within these studies also tend to be limited. For example, appropriate intent-to-treat analyses have not been conducted. This is particularly concerning given the high rates of attrition across follow-up points seen in most universal intervention studies. Failure to consider outcomes for children who do not participate in follow-up may result in conclusions that interventions have been successful, when at a population level, they may not be. Further, the clustered nature of the data collected (given that classes or schools are allocated to intervention or control) has not been controlled for in any of the data analyses. Baldwin, Murray, and Shadish (2005) illustrate the substantial increase in type 1 error rates when dependencies in data collected are not accounted for. In school settings clustering may have a particularly substantial impact given that the success of the program could easily be impacted by the level of support provided by school management and staff and the socioeconomic disparities that exist between schools. These statistical anomalies bring in to question existing positive findings and indicate a need for further research to determine the efficacy of universal prevention. A final limitation in all of the studies reviewed so far relates to participant informed consent (see discussion later in this chapter).

Selective interventions

Prevention programs that target children who demonstrate a specific risk factor for anxiety are rare. This can be partly attributed to the infancy of research into risk factors for anxiety and consequently insufficient time having passed for prevention programs to have been developed and tested. Three early developments in this arena include a program targeting children of parents with an anxiety disorder, a program targeting coping with stressful life events (specifically ongoing exposure to terrorism violence) and a program targeting preschool children who were high on behavioral inhibition/withdrawal.

The Child Anxiety Prevention Study (CAPS: Ginsburg, 2009) is a preventative intervention designed to reduce anxiety symptoms and prevent the onset of anxiety disorders among children of anxious parents, one of the strongest known risk factors. The CAPS program is conducted during six to eight individual family sessions with a psychologist and is maintained by three booster sessions. The program focuses on increasing child strengths and resilience (e.g., by teaching cognitive restructuring and problem-solving), reducing known risk factors (e.g., reducing parental overprotection by teaching appropriate contingency management), and increasing knowledge and communication about anxiety within the family (e.g., factual information on anxiety and communication skills).The program evaluation was conducted on 40 7–12-year-old children who had a parent with a primary diagnosis of an anxiety disorder. Each family volunteered to complete the program, which was conducted in a clinic setting. Children were excluded from the study if they met criteria for an anxiety disorder based on diagnostic interview, making it the only prevention study to only target children who were yet to develop a disorder.

The children were randomly assigned to either intervention or wait-list and both conditions were assessed pre- and post-intervention and at 6 and 12 months follow-up. At 12 months 30% of the wait-list children had developed an anxiety disorder compared to none of the intervention children. Although child report of anxiety did not show significant group differences, independent evaluator (estimated effect size $d = 1.99$ at 12 months) and parent report (estimated effect size $d = 0.82$ at 12 months) of symptoms showed significant decreases in level of anxiety for the intervention children when compared to those on wait-list. Program attendance (average of 7.47/8 sessions) and parent satisfaction ratings indicated positive engagement and a perception of having benefited from participation. Replication and expansion of this study is needed; however, its results show promise in providing evidence for an effective preventative program.

The second study to take a selected preventive approach was implemented by Berger and colleagues in a program targeting terror-related distress and anxiety in Israeli primary school children (Berger, Pat-Horenczyk, & Gelkopf, 2007). The program, presented by teachers, was completed during eight, 90-minute sessions during class time and two parent information sessions. The program included psycho-education, coping skill development, cognitive restructuring, and specific discussion of building a positive future outlook despite the ongoing distress associated with terror. Consent was obtained from 46% ($n = 142$) of Year 2 to 6 children to participate in the evaluation. More than 50% of the participating children had had personal exposure to a terror-related incident, with a further 25% having had near-misses. Assessments occurred 1 week before and 2 months after the intervention.

In a comparison of wait-list to intervention, significant reductions in post-traumatic stress syndrome (PTSD) symptoms, somatic complaints, generalized anxiety, and separation anxiety symptoms were found in the intervention group (estimated $ds = 0.55$ to 1.07), with greater effects noted for younger children. A significantly greater improvement in functional impairment for boys was also noted. Of children meeting PTSD criteria (based on child questionnaire responses) 6/6 no longer met criteria and no new cases were identified in the intervention group compared to 2/5 no longer meeting criteria with an additional 2/67 who newly met criteria in the comparison group. This study showed a promising option to assist children exposed to ongoing community-based stressors such as terrorism that may overcome the additional risk that this exposure adds.

In a study that targeted preschool children, Rapee and colleagues (Rapee *et al.*, 2005) identified through questionnaire and laboratory screening, 146 temperamentally and behaviorally inhibited (see Lonigan, Phillips, Wilson, & Allan, Chapter 10, this volume) children aged 3–5 years. These children were randomly allocated to either intervention or a no-intervention control (i.e., families were simply told that their child would be assessed on a yearly basis). The intervention consisted of six parent-group sessions where parents were trained in exposure tasks, confidence-building, reduced parental control, and appropriate modeling of managing anxiety. Outcomes were measured based on diagnostic interview (parent report), temperament questionnaires, and laboratory assessments of behavioral inhibition. Although the selection for the trial was based on the risk factor of behavioral inhibition at the pre-intervention over 90% of the children already met criteria for an anxiety disorder.

The intervention led to a significantly greater decrease in anxiety diagnoses at 12-month follow-up in comparison to the control group. No significant changes were evident, however, in measures of the risk factors inhibition or withdrawal. This study, while originally aimed at reduction of a significant risk factor, found that even at this early stage anxiety disorders are present and are amenable to brief format early intervention.

A later follow-up for this same cohort showed continued divergence between the intervention and no-intervention groups (Rapee, Kennedy, Ingram, Edwards, & Sweeney, 2010).

Three years after entry to the study, when the children were aged around 7 years, children whose parents had been in intervention continued to show significantly fewer anxiety disorders than children whose parents received no intervention. Further, at this later assessment point, the intervention group also showed lower levels of anxiety symptoms according to maternal, paternal, and child self-report. Interestingly, temperamental features of inhibition stilled failed to differ significantly between groups.

One possible reason that the initial study by Rapee *et al.* (2005) failed to show group differences on measures of temperament may have been the relatively low level of risk of the children included, possibly leading to marked changes over time in the no-intervention children. Therefore a later study selected 71 3–4-year-old children who scored extremely high (2 standard deviations above norm) on inhibition and who also had a parent with an anxiety disorder (Kennedy, Rapee, & Edwards, 2009). Commensurate with their high-risk status, all children in this study met criteria for an anxiety disorder at pre-intervention. Intervention was similar to that in the previous study, but was extended to nine sessions. At 6-months follow-up children whose parents engaged in the intervention had significantly fewer anxiety disorders, but also showed significantly less life interference from their anxiety and demonstrated lower behavioral inhibition according to both parent report and laboratory observation.

At this stage selective intervention for anxiety appears to show promise. However, the extent of research is still far behind that of universal programs. The few studies that have been done vary in terms of populations and risk factors targeted in addition to their outcomes. As for universal interventions it is also impossible to know how much of their effects can be described as true "prevention" given that only one study has excluded participants with pre-existing anxiety disorders.

Indicated interventions

Indicated interventions target individuals at risk for a disorder based on early indicators or low level symptoms of the disorder. One of the largest studies of prevention of anxiety disorders was conducted by Dadds and colleagues (Dadds, Holland, Laurens, Mullins, Barrett, & Spence, 1999; Dadds, Spence, Holland, Barrett, & Laurens, 1997). This program was conducted in schools with students aged 7–14 years and involved 10 child sessions and three parent sessions delivered by clinical psychologists. Participants were selected to participate if they had a high score on the Revised Children's Manifest Anxiety Scale (RCMAS: Reynolds & Richmond, 1978) or if they were identified as anxious by their teacher (but not identified as disruptive). Parents of identified children then completed a diagnostic interview to determine if their child had either subclinical anxiety or a mild clinical anxiety disorder, and would therefore be suitable for the preventative intervention. Subsequently 128 children were allocated (by virtue of school attended) to either intervention or usual care control, with assessments occurring post-treatment and every 6 months for 2 years.

No significant differences between groups were found immediately post-treatment. At the 6-month follow-up fewer diagnoses were evident in the intervention group; however, this difference disappeared at the 12-month follow-up. At the 2-year mark, parents of the intervention group children reported less avoidance (estimated $d = 0.56$) and children received lower global severity ratings (estimated $d = 0.72$) and lower rates of anxiety disorders than those children in the control group. Furthermore, those children who were more severe to start with had the greatest difference in anxiety disorder rates between intervention (<20%) and control conditions (∼50%). Specifically looking at the small group of children who were subclinical at the initial assessment (and therefore truly a prevention rather than early intervention target) at the 6-month assessment 54% of the control group versus 16% of the intervention had progressed to clinical disorders. However, by the 2-year assessment the difference in this subgroup was minimal, suggesting that the risk of subclinical anxious children progressing to clinical status in the long term is not high.

In a replication of the Dadds early intervention study, Bernstein, Layne, Egan, and Tennison (2005) used similar screening procedures and implemented the FRIENDS program using clinical psychologists in a school setting for children with subclinical and mild clinical anxiety disorders ($n = 61$). In addition to the replication, this study examined the efficacy of the addition of a comprehensive parent program to the standard child-focused FRIENDS sessions. The study compared the parent + child approach to child sessions alone and a no-treatment control. Findings demonstrated significant benefits according to parent, child, and therapist report in both intervention groups when compared to the no-treatment control group (effect size of $d = 0.58$). The child + parent intervention produced slightly stronger effects on clinical global impression. The particularly small sample size limits conclusions that can be drawn, especially on comparing active interventions.

A similar study was conducted by Mifsud and Rapee (2005) specifically focusing on children in low socioeconomic status schools. Following a process of child-report screening and teacher/school counselor nomination or exclusion similar to that used by Dadds *et al.* (1997), 91 high anxious 4th or 5th grade children were randomly allocated to wait-list or intervention. The intervention, "Cool Kids," was an eight-session in-school program for children supported by an additional two parent information evenings. The program was conducted in small groups by the school counselor and a community mental health worker. Symptom monitoring was completed by child, parent, and teacher. Symptoms of anxiety showed a significantly greater reduction in the intervention compared to the wait-list according to both child report (estimated $d = 0.58$) and teacher report (estimated $d = 0.57$) at post-intervention and 4-month follow-up. Data from parents showed a similar pattern of means but return rates were too poor to analyze the data.

In general, data from indicated programs show positive intervention effects and point to a moderate reduction in symptoms of anxiety. Once again actual prevention effects are difficult to determine since selection of children scoring high on anxiety symptoms is likely to include a large proportion of those with anxiety disorders. A notable exception is the study by Dadds *et al.* (1997, 1999), which did analyze data based on a subsample of children who did not meet criteria for disorder at the commencement of the research. Prevention effects for this subsample were inconsistent. Nevertheless, one advantage of this form of intervention is the delivery of treatment to children who otherwise are unlikely to access traditional services. For example, in the study by Mifsud and Rapee (2005), only two of their sample of 91 children had ever seen a mental health professional previously.

Moderators of prevention effects

In several of the studies described above gender and age effects were noted. In particular the literature suggests that younger children and girls (Barrett *et al.*, 2006; Berger *et al.*, 2007; Lock & Barrett, 2003) may benefit more from anxiety prevention programs than boys and older children. These studies have not indicated reasons for these discrepancies but it is very likely that both boys and older children are more difficult to engage in programs of this type. Most prevention programs at present are based on a traditional model of expert-delivered education and it is likely that more innovative means of training will need to be developed to engage adolescents and boys. Importantly, socioeconomic status does not seem to have an influence on outcome. Studies have been conducted across a variety of socioeconomic environments with good outcomes. The one study that specifically focused on disadvantaged students (Mifsud & Rapee, 2005) showed effects sizes consistent with other research. This study also highlighted another potentially important issue. It was indicated that some of the children in the sample had anxiety related to real social or environmental problems (such as domestic violence, inadequate housing, etc.). It is unlikely that these types of issues can be dealt with in an anxiety-focused intervention. Therefore the effects of prevention programs may be more consistent with more detailed and focused screening.

A further issue related to potential for differential outcome relates to the issue of culture. Several studies have implemented prevention programs with specific cultural groups. The FRIENDS program has been examined as a selective prevention approach in Chinese, former-Yugoslavian, and mixed non-English-speaking background migrant children and adolescents (Barrett, Sonderegger, & Sonderegger, 2001; Barrett, Sonderegger, & Xenos, 2003) and with inner-city African-American children (Cooley, Boyd, & Grades, 2004). Among the migrant populations who completed FRIENDS increases in self-esteem, decreases in anxiety, and improvement in future outlook amongst children, and decreases in anxiety, depression, anger, post-traumatic stress, and dissociation for adolescents were demonstrated. Wait-list comparison groups at both ages showed increase in anxiety, deterioration of outlook, and maintenance of other factors. Some evidence for differential effectiveness according to culture was also identified. For example the former-Yugoslavian group exhibited greater reductions in anxiety despite starting at a higher point pre-treatment. Interaction of the prevention program with adjustment to their new cultural environment (such as ease of affiliation) was highlighted as a possible explanation.

In an example of an indicated prevention program, inner-city African-American children living with high levels of community violence were chosen via child-reported anxiety, teacher nomination/exclusion, parent consent, and diagnostic interview to identify children with subclinical or low clinical anxiety. In this study, following a clinical psychologist led implementation of FRIENDS, self-reported anxiety dropped (based on the RCMAS) and a trend for improvement (effect size not given) in therapist-rated levels of clinical anxiety was noted. However, there were no significant group differences on anxiety symptoms according to the Multidimensional Anxiety Scale for Children (March, Parker, Sullivan, Stallings, & Conners, 1997) or symptoms of depression. The authors suggested that minor adaptations were needed to the manual to make it culturally relevant and respectful (e.g., incorporating multigenerational family structures rather than two-parent examples). Such changes, however, are unlikely to undermine the fundamental cognitive–behavioral concepts relevant to the treatment components and are an appropriate example of applying a manualized program with flexibility.

Hence, the preliminary evidence suggests that prevention programs do transport successfully across cultures. However, further work on culturally appropriate assessment and treatment of anxiety (and other mental health) issues is needed. This would ensure that services are both culturally sensitive and effective at identifying symptoms and experiences that may be defined and valued differently across cultures.

Barriers to implementation of prevention programs

There are many issues that present barriers to the implementation of prevention programs. These barriers impact on the conclusions that can be drawn from research at this stage, and undermine the implementation and sustainability of programs in the community. Barriers that particularly limit conclusions from research include issues of consent, engagement, and identification of participants. Sustainability is further impacted by limitations to the maintenance of gains, access, and sociopolitical pressures.

Consent and engagement

All universal and the majority of indicated prevention programs have been implemented in school or preschool settings. School-based settings provide the advantage of easy access to a population and allowing an entire subpopulation to be targeted with relatively few resources needing to be spent on accessing suitable targets. However, the research that results from these studies is plagued by highly variable and typically relatively low levels of consent either to participate in the intervention or to participate in appropriate evaluation. In the studies reviewed above consent from parents for their child to participate in a universal program or screening varied from 29% to 99%. The one study that attained a 99% consent rate used an "opt-out" procedure for screening rather than active consent (Stallard *et al.*, 2008). Such a procedure may improve screening rates and passive access to the program, but is unlikely to change active participation and engagement with programs. In cases where children are selected following screening as suitable for intervention, consent to participate in intensive screening (diagnostic interview) ranged from 30% to 62%. Thereafter, actual participation in the intervention program was lower again.

Engagement of parents, especially in school-based prevention programs, is particularly difficult (McLoone, Hudson, & Rapee, 2006). Given research implicating a key role for parents in the cause and maintenance of anxiety disorders (Hudson & Rapee, 2008; see Creswell, Murray, Stacey, & Cooper, Chapter 14, this volume) and evidence that parent participation may improve child outcomes for younger children from both prevention and treatment studies (Barrett, Dadds, & Rapee, 1996; Bernstein *et al.*, 2005), involvement of parents in anxiety prevention programs may be crucial to their long-term success, especially for younger children. Unfortunately, attendance of parents in offered programs is typically very poor. In the preschool setting for a universal intervention only 23% of all invited parents attended more than half of the program sessions (Dadds & Roth, 2008). In the school setting, attendance is repeatedly poor for universal programs, one study noting an average attendance of 10 parents per school (despite enrolment of 692 children from seven schools: Barrett *et al.*, 2005). Parent attendance for indicated programs has been approximately 30–58% (Dadds *et al.*, 1997; Mifsud & Rapee, 2005).

These poor engagement and consent rates raise two important issues. First, while the intervention or screening may be defined as universal, the reality is that small to large proportions of the population are not participating. As a result, the validity of any conclusions that can be drawn from the research is highly suspect. More importantly, the value of the programs becomes limited because they do not necessarily reach the populations they are designed to help. In fact, a common aspect of universal interventions is that they are least likely to be implemented by the very people who most need them (Offord, Chmura Kraemer, Kazdin, Jensen, & Harrington, 1998). Indeed, low attendance is a common phenomenon in prevention studies across disorders, especially in universal applications (Heinrichs, Bertram, Kuschel, & Hahlweg, 2005; Offord *et al.*, 1998). One of the strongest motivators for engagement with an intervention is current distress. Given that by definition prevention programs target populations who are suffering little or no current distress, engagement will always be one of the most difficult challenges. Clearly one of the key issues for future research will be to work on methods to increase attendance and engagement with prevention programs.

Identification of target children

A barrier specific to selected and indicated prevention programs is the accurate identification of target children. The standard for the assessment of anxiety is the use of multi-method, multi-informant approaches (Schniering *et al.*, 2000; Silverman & Ollendick, 2005; Cartwright-Hatton *et al.*, Chapter 7, this volume). This is however an expensive and time-consuming process. Screening via child report alone is likely to produce poor sensitivity and specificity. While children may have good knowledge of their internal state, they are often inaccurate in reporting on their actual behaviors (Comer & Kendall, 2004; DiBartolo, Albano, Barlow, & Heimberg, 1998; Herjanic & Reich, 1997) undermining the value of their report when used in isolation. The accuracy of teacher screening by nomination of "the most anxious children in your class" used in several indicated studies has not been investigated and may be highly reliant on the teacher's personal definition of anxiety and recognition of symptoms. In addition, teachers tend to have a better recognition of certain forms of anxiety than others (Lyneham, Street, Abbott, & Rapee, 2008), which makes their report of limited value to identify some forms of anxiety in children. Given the above issues, it is not surprising that agreement between teacher identification and child report of high anxiety in indicated studies has been as low as 2% (Dadds *et al.*, 1997). In addition, for identified children who go on to complete diagnostic interviews, rates of subclinical and clinical diagnoses have been approximately 75%. This rate may however be exaggerated as it does not account for the large number of children whose parents do not consent to diagnostic interview potentially because they do not believe their child to be anxious (McLoone, 2007).

Overall existing evidence suggests that accurate detection of at-risk children is likely to be best achieved through use of multiple informants and multiple methods. The costs associated with such increased accuracy however are high and need to be balanced against the gains made in targeting appropriately at-risk children. From an implementation perspective, public bodies are rarely interested in high-cost options. Research on the cost-effectiveness balance is needed to indicate the most appropriate screening battery for future prevention/early intervention programs.

Maintenance of gains, sustainability, access, and the sociopolitical imperative

Maintenance of early gains is difficult in any form of intervention. In prevention it is an especially crucial issue since the target for prevention is often at highest risk many years after the prevention program has been completed. The long-term evidence from current anxiety prevention studies is minimal but suggests that gains are inconsistent over time and may not maintain over the long term (e.g., Barrett *et al.*, 2006; Dadds *et al.*, 1999). If prevention programs are going to prevent onset of new cases, the reduction in risks needs to be maintained for many years. Strategies such as booster sessions, environmental prompts to implement skills learnt, programs that are presented across several school years with material adapted to the developmental level and challenges unique to each age, and incorporation of the prevention principles into the targeted subculture may all be ways of improving long-term maintenance of gains for anxiety prevention programs (Rapee, 2008).

A large number of prevention programs are developed and conducted within a research framework. In most cases, however, once the research is completed these programs disappear (Heady *et al.*, 2006). It is necessary for researchers to incorporate systems for the distribution and sustainability of their programs following evaluation. The best opportunity for sustainability and distribution is to incorporate programs into the daily workings of existing systems (Heady *et al.*, 2006). The implementation of the FRIENDS program at national and international levels is a good example of attempted ongoing sustainability. Significant enthusiasm for training in such programs is generated, often outstripping demand (Miller, 2008; Rapee, 2008). However when those trained in appropriate programs are followed up, the early enthusiasm and training rarely translates into continued implementation (McLoone *et al.*, 2006). The most common story is a lack of support from the system (e.g., lack of time, competing demands, lack of resources) that tempers any initial enthusiasm. Even national government supported implementations of broad-based mental health programs such as the Australian MindMatters program have had limited uptake and success. An estimated two-thirds of secondary schools implemented "in some way" (Ainley, Withers, Underwood, & Frigo, 2006) the MindMatters whole-school approach to mental health which incorporates promotion, prevention, and early intervention programs. However, fewer than one in five noted it as a key resource in determining the approach taken to students' mental health (Ainley *et al.*, 2006).

Selection of the most appropriate system to implement and maintain a prevention program needs to be not only informed by considerations of convenience but also by the ability of that system to conduct the intervention. Schools have become the vehicle of choice for the delivery of the vast majority of mental health prevention programs in children and adolescents. Yet whether schools are the most appropriate system to implement and maintain interventions has rarely been considered (McLoone *et al.*, 2006). The primary mandate of any educational system is education. Because many schools are stretched to the limit to deliver the level of education that is expected from increasingly sophisticated communities, expecting them also to deliver mental health interventions is potentially unrealistic. Indeed evidence from the MindMatters program suggests that insufficient curriculum space, the skill and appropriateness of teaching staff to be responsible for mental health, insufficient access to mental health specialists, lack of parent/community support for mental health interventions, and the mismatch between available resources and individual student needs are all barriers undermining implementation of prevention and early intervention in schools (Ainley *et al.*, 2006). Consequently, despite the fact that schools provide a convenient point of access to children, prevention programs may need to consider alternative systems such as programs delivered via the Internet, social networking websites, or other mass media to support their long-term sustainability and distribution.

A final challenge worth noting is that social and political needs frequently produce barriers to good, systematic science. It is often difficult to conduct the careful evaluation required to develop the most effective programs when society is applying pressure for instant success (Rapee, 2008). Miller's (2008) description of the enthusiasm and uptake of the FRIENDS program across British Columbia despite evidence for its efficacy being equivocal (Laye-Gindhu *et al.*, 2005, cited in Miller, 2008) and its long-term efficacy unknown, is a good example of perceived need overriding a lack of evidence. Juxtaposed to this are programs with proven efficacy that are not funded due to high resource costs. Funding of high-cost programs, particularly if the targeted issue is perceived as relatively trivial, may not be seen by the public and therefore in turn by the government, to be worthy of funding for implementation. Implementation of anxiety prevention is especially vulnerable to this issue since most communities perceive overt problems such as substance abuse, delinquency, and suicide as far more worthy of investment than anxiety, despite the high social burden of anxiety disorders across the lifespan. Sustainable prevention programs will require social advocacy in order to become a part of the political agenda.

Conclusions and future directions

Although in its infancy, research into the prevention of child and adolescent anxiety has a substantial base. The evidence for universal approaches is mixed, long-term stability of gains questionable, and effect sizes are small. However, as Miller (2008) highlights, these universal approaches may result in a greater understanding and awareness of anxiety disorders in children, schools allow easiest access to the population and the interventionists (i.e., teachers within schools) are keen to add these skills to their professional repertoire. More importantly, even small effects when applied across whole populations are extremely valuable. Consequently universal programs provide one component of clear value in the prevention of anxiety disorders. Evidence for the efficacy of selective programs, although in its infancy, shows a moderate to large preventative effect in the short term when children at high risk are targeted. Evidence for indicated prevention programs is also promising with moderate effects on anxiety symptoms and diagnoses. In addition to the direct evidence provided by indicated prevention studies it should also be considered that existing evidence from traditional treatment trials supports the long-term efficacy of these programs (Barrett, Duffy, Dadds, & Rapee, 2001; Kendall, Safford, Flannery-Schroeder, & Webb, 2004), in turn suggesting a possible preventative spin-off.

A substantial amount of research remains to be done in the field of the prevention of child and adolescent anxiety disorders. Studies of the cost-effectiveness of all programs that include the impact of prevention on comorbidity and service use in addition to standard change in anxiety symptoms and risk will be important to inform appropriate program and audience selection. A second avenue for investigation is a thorough understanding of etiology, risk, and protective factors that is needed to specifically inform appropriate targets for prevention programs (Ginsburg, 2004; Rapee, 2008). The CAPS approach of preventing anxiety in children at risk by virtue of an anxious parent shows the promise of understanding and successfully targeting proven risk factors. In addition identifying children at risk by virtue of presence or absence of multiple risk factors may be most effective. Ashford and colleagues (2008), for example, found that identification of multiple rather than single risk factors amongst preschool children increased the likelihood of high anxiety at age 11 from 15% to 48%. Targeting a child who is behaviorally inhibited, has an anxious parent, and who has an anxious cognitive style may be a better use of preventative resources than targeting children based on only one of these risk factors. Consistent with this suggestion, Kennedy *et al.* (2009) showed stronger prevention effects when targeting children who were both inhibited and had an anxious parent than was previously shown by Rapee *et al.* (2005) who selected children only on the basis of their inhibition. Other outstanding questions for future research include an understanding of moderators and mediators of prevention outcomes to better enable selection of targeted participants and improve program content.

Based on the evidence to date an interesting way forward may be consistent with the model proposed by Weisz, Sandler, Durlak, and Anton (2005). They argue that there is a level before universal prevention, that of health promotion/positive development strategies. Given that most currently identified risk factors are relevant to internalizing disorders in general rather than to any one specific disorder, it may be appropriate to use the evidence for current universal programs to encourage a mental health promotion approach that focuses on the development of coping strategies and builds on personal, community, and environmental strengths. Such health promotion could take advantage of school-based populations as well as various forms of media and community forums in order to reach the broad population. This may also lead to flow on benefits beyond the targeted children and adolescents to parents and the wider community. In turn, this broad, universal health promotion initiative could be backed up by more focused selective and indicated programs offered to particular subgroups of the community.

References

Ainley, J., Withers, G., Underwood, C., & Frigo, T. (2006). *National Survey of Health and Well-Being Promotion Policies and Practices in Secondary Schools.* Camberwell, VIC: Australian Council for Educational Research.

Ashford, J., Smit, F., van Lier, P. A., Cuijpers, P., Koot, H. M., Ashford, J., et al. (2008). Early risk indicators of internalizing problems in late childhood: a 9-year longitudinal study. *Journal of Child Psychology and Psychiatry and Allied Disciplines*, **49**, 774–780.

Aune, T. & Stiles, T. C. (2009). Universal-based prevention of syndromal and subsyndromal social anxiety: a randomized controlled study. *Journal of Consulting and Clinical Psychology*, **77**, 867–879.

Baldwin, S.A., Murray, D. M., & Shadish, W. R. (2005). Empirically supported treatments or type I errors? Problems with the analysis of data from group-administered treatments. *Journal of Consulting and Clinical Psychology*, **73**, 924–935.

Barrett, P. M. & Turner, C. (2001). Prevention of anxiety symptoms in primary school children: preliminary results from a universal school-based trial. *British Journal of Clinical Psychology*, **40**, 399–410.

Barrett, P. M., Dadds, M. R., & Rapee, R. M. (1996). Family treatment of childhood anxiety: a controlled trial. *Journal of Consulting and Clinical Psychology*, **64**, 333–342.

Barrett, P. M., Duffy, A. L., Dadds, M. R., & Rapee, R. M. (2001). Cognitive–behavioral treatment of anxiety disorders in children: long-term (6-year) follow-up. *Journal of Consulting and Clinical Psychology*, **69**, 135–141.

Barrett, P. M., Farrell, L. J., Ollendick, T. H., & Dadds, M. (2006). Long-term outcomes of an Australian universal prevention trial of anxiety and depression symptoms in children and youth: an evaluation of the FRIENDS program. *Journal of Clinical Child and Adolescent Psychology*, **35**, 403–411.

Barrett, P. M., Lock, S., & Farrell, L. J. (2005). Developmental differences in universal preventive intervention for child anxiety. *Clinical Child Psychology and Psychiatry*, **10**, 539–555.

Barrett, P. M., Lowry-Webster, H., & Turner, C. (2000). *FRIENDS Program for Children: Group Leaders' Manual.* Brisbane, QLD: Australian Academic Press.

Barrett, P. M., Sonderegger, R., & Sonderegger, N. L. (2001). Evaluation of an anxiety-prevention and positive-coping program (FRIENDS) for children and adolescents of non-English-speaking background. *Behaviour Change*, **18**, 78–91.

Barrett, P. M., Sonderegger, R., & Xenos, S. (2003). Using FRIENDS to combat anxiety and adjustment problems among young migrants to Australia: a national trial. *Clinical Child Psychology and Psychiatry*, **8**, 241–260.

Begg, S., Vos, T., Barker, B., Stevenson, C., & Lopez, A. D. (2007). *The Burden of Disease and Injury in Australia 2003*. Canberra, ACT: Australian Institute of Health and Welfare.

Berger, R., Pat-Horenczyk, R., & Gelkopf, M. (2007). School-based intervention for prevention and treatment of elementary-students' terror-related distress in Israel: a quasi-randomized controlled trial. *Journal of Traumatic Stress*, **20**, 541–551.

Bernstein, G. A., Layne, A. E., Egan, E. A., & Tennison, D. M. (2005). School-based interventions for anxious children. *Journal of the American Academy of Child and Adolescent Psychiatry*, **44**, 1118–1127.

Canino, G., Shrout, P. E., Rubio-Stipec, M., Bird, H. R., Bravo, M., Ramirez, R., et al. (2004). The DSM-IV rates of child and adolescent disorders in Puerto Rico. *Archives of General Psychiatry*, **61**, 85–93.

Cartwright-Hatton, S., Roberts, C., Chitsabesan, P., Fothergill, C., & Harrington, R. (2004). Systematic review of the efficacy of cognitive behaviour therapies for childhood and adolescent anxiety disorders. *British Journal of Clinical Psychology*, **43**, 421–436.

Comer, J. S. & Kendall, P. C. (2004). A symptom-level examination of parent–child agreement in the diagnosis of anxious youths. *Journal of the American Academy of Child and Adolescent Psychiatry*, **43**, 878–886.

Cooley, M. R., Boyd, R. C., & Grades, J. J. (2004). Feasibility of an anxiety preventive intervention for community violence exposed African-American children. *Journal of Primary Prevention*, **25**, 105–123.

Costello, E., Mustillo, S., Erkanli, A., Keeler, G., & Angold, A. (2003). Prevalence and development of psychiatric disorders in childhood and adolescence. *Archives of General Psychiatry*, **60**, 837–844.

Dadds, M. R. & Roth, J. H. (2008). Prevention of anxiety disorders: results of a universal trial with young children. *Journal of Child and Family Studies*, **17**, 320–335.

Dadds, M. R., Holland, D. E., Laurens, K. R., Mullins, M., Barrett, P. M., & Spence, S. H. (1999). Early intervention and prevention of anxiety disorders in children: results at 2-year follow-up. *Journal of Consulting and Clinical Psychology*, **67**, 145–150.

Dadds, M. R., Spence, S. H., Holland, D. E., Barrett, P. M., & Laurens, K. R. (1997). Prevention and early intervention for anxiety disorders: a controlled trial. *Journal of Consulting and Clinical Psychology*, **65**, 627–635.

DiBartolo, P. M., Albano, A. M., Barlow, D. H., & Heimberg, R. G. (1998). Cross-informant agreement in the assessment of social phobia in youth. *Journal of Abnormal Child Psychology*, **26**, 213–220.

Farmer, E. M., Stangl, D. K., Burns, B. J., Costello, E., & Angold, A. (1999). Use, persistence, and intensity: patterns of care for children's mental health across one year. *Community Mental Health Journal*, **35**, 31–46.

Flannery-Schroeder, E. C. (2006). Reducing anxiety to prevent depression. *American Journal of Preventive Medicine*, **31**(Suppl. 1), S136–S142.

Ginsburg, G. S. (2004). Anxiety prevention programs for youth: practical and theoretical considerations. *Clinical Psychology: Science and Practice*, **11**, 430–434.

Ginsburg, G. S. (2009). The Child Anxiety Prevention Study: intervention model and primary outcomes. *Journal of Consulting and Clinical Psychology*, **77**, 580–587.

Heady, A., Pirkis, J., Merner, B., VandenHeuvel, A., Mitchell, P., Robinson, J., *et al.* (2006). A review of 156 local projects funded under Australia's National Suicide Prevention Strategy: overview and lessons learned. *Australian e-Journal for the Advancement of Mental Health (AeJAMH)*, **5**(3), www.auseinet.com/journal/vol5iss3/headey.pdf.

Heinrichs, N., Bertram, H., Kuschel, A., & Hahlweg, K. (2005). Parent recruitment and retention in a universal prevention program for child behavior and emotional problems: barriers to research and program participation. *Prevention Science*, **6**, 275–286.

Herjanic, B. & Reich, W. (1997). Development of a structured psychiatric interview for children: agreement between child and parent on individual symptoms. *Journal of Abnormal Child Psychology*, **25**, 21–31.

Hofstra, M. B., Van der Ende, J., & Verhulst, F. C. (2000). Continuity and change of psychopathology from childhood into adulthood: a 14-year follow-up study. *Journal of the American Academy of Child and Adolescent Psychiatry*, **39**(7), 850–858.

Hofstra, M. B., Van der Ende, J., & Verhulst, F. C. (2002). Child and adolescent problems predict DSM-IV disorders in adulthood: a 14-year follow-up of a Dutch epidemiological sample. *Journal of the American Academy of Child and Adolescent Psychiatry*, **41**, 182–189.

Hudson, J. L. & Rapee, R. M. (2008). Familial and social environments in the etiology and maintenance of anxiety disorders. In: **M. M. Antony** & **M. B. Stein** (eds.) *Oxford Handbook of Anxiety and Related Disorders*, pp. 173–189. Oxford, UK: Oxford University Press.

Ialongo, N., Edelsohn, G., Werthamer-Larsson, L., Crockett, L., & Kellam, S. (1996). Social and cognitive impairment in first-grade children with anxious and depressive symptoms. *Journal of Clinical Child Psychology*, **25**, 15–24.

Keller, M. B., Lavori, P. W., Wunder, J., Beardslee, W. R., Schwartz, C. E., & Roth, J. (1992). Chronic course of anxiety disorders in children and adolescents. *Journal of the American Academy of Child and Adolescent Psychiatry*, **31**, 595–599.

Kendall, P. C., Safford, S., Flannery-Schroeder, E., & Webb, A. (2004). Child anxiety treatment: outcomes in adolescence and impact on substance use and depression at 7.4 year follow-up. *Journal of Consulting and Clinical Psychology*, **72**, 276–287.

Kennedy, S. J., Rapee, R. M., & Edwards, S. L. (2009). A selective intervention program for inhibited preschool-aged children of parents with an anxiety disorder: effects on current anxiety disorders and temperament. *Journal of the American Academy of Child and Adolescent Psychiatry*, **48**, 602–609.

Kessler, R. C. & Greenburg, P. E. (2002). The economic burden of anxiety and stress disorders. In: **K. L. Davis, D. Charney, J. T. Coyle**, & **C. Nemeroff** (eds.) *Neuropsychopharmacology: The Fifth Generation of Progress*, pp. 981–992. Philadelphia, PA: Lippincott Williams & Wilkins.

Kessler, R. C., Berglund, P., Demler, O., Jin, R., Merikangas, K., & Walters, E. (2005). Lifetime prevalence and age-of-onset distributions of DSM-IV disorders in the national comorbidity survey replication. *Archives of General Psychiatry*, **62**, 593–602.

Last, C. G., Hansen, C., & Franco, N. (1997). Anxious children in adulthood: a prospective study of adjustment. *Journal of the American Academy of Child and Adolescent Psychiatry*, **36**, 645–652.

Last, C. G., Perrin, S., Hersen, M., & Kazdin, A. E. (1996). A prospective study of childhood anxiety disorders. *Journal of the American Academy of Child and Adolescent Psychiatry*, **35**, 1502–1510.

Lock, S. & Barrett, P. M. (2003). A longitudinal study of developmental differences in universal preventative intervention for child anxiety. *Behaviour Change*, **20**, 183–199.

Lowry-Webster, H. M., Barrett, P. M., & Dadds, M. R. (2001). A universal prevention trial of anxiety and depressive symptomatology in childhood: preliminary data from an Australian study. *Behaviour Change*, **18**, 36–50.

Lowry-Webster, H. M., Barrett, P. M., & Lock, S. (2003). A universal prevention trial of anxiety and depressive symptomatology in childhood: results at one-year follow-up. *Behaviour Change*, **20**, 25–43.

Lyneham, H. J., Street, A., Abbott, M. J., & Rapee, R. M. (2008). Psychometric properties of the School Anxiety Scale – Teacher Report (SAS–TR). *Journal of Anxiety Disorders*, **22**, 292–300.

March, J. S., Parker, J. D. A., Sullivan, K., Stallings, P., & Conners, C. K. (1997). The Multidimensional Anxiety Scales for Children (MASC): factor structure, reliability, and validity. *Journal of the American Academy of Child and Adolescent Psychiatry*, **36**, 554–565.

McLoone, J. (2007). Companing the costs and effects of school-based and parent-run help for anxious children. Unpublished doctoral dissertation, Macquarie University, Sydney, NSW.

McLoone, J., Hudson, J. L., & Rapee, R. M. (2006). Treating anxiety disorders in a school setting. *Education and Treatment of Children*, **29**, 219–242.

Mifsud, C. & Rapee, R. M. (2005). Early intervention for childhood anxiety in a school setting: outcomes for a disadvantaged population. *Journal of the American Academy of Child and Adolescent Psychiatry*, **44**, 996–1004.

Miller, L. D. (2008). Facing fears: the feasibility of anxiety universal prevention efforts with children and adolescents. *Cognitive and Behavioral Practice*, **15**, 28–35.

Mrazek, P. J. & Haggerty, R. J. (1994). *Reducing Risks for Mental Disorders: Frontiers for Preventive Intervention Research*. Washington, DC: National Academy Press.

Neil, A. L. & Christensen, H. (2009). Efficacy and effectiveness of school-based prevention and early intervention programs for anxiety. *Clinical Psychology Review*, **29**, 208–215.

Offord, D. R., Chmura Kraemer, H., Kazdin, A. E., Jensen, P. S., & Harrington, R. (1998). Lowering the burden of suffering from child psychiatric disorder: trade-offs among clinical, targeted, and universal interventions. *Journal of the American Academy of Child and Adolescent Psychiatry*, **37**(7), 686–694.

Rapee, R. M. (2008). Prevention of mental disorders: promises, limitations, and barriers. *Cognitive and Behavioral Practice*, **15**, 47–52.

Rapee, R. M., Kennedy, S., Ingram, M., Edwards, S., & Sweeney, L. (2005). Prevention and early intervention of anxiety disorders in inhibited preschool children. *Journal of Consulting and Clinical Psychology*, **73**, 488–497.

Rapee, R. M., Kennedy, S., Ingram, M., Edwards, S. L., & Sweeney, L. (2010). Altering the trajectory of anxiety in at-risk young children. *American Journal of Psychiatry*, **167**, 1518–1525.

Reynolds, C. R. & Richmond, B. O. (1978). Factor structure and construct validity of "What I think and feel": The Revised Children's Manifest Anxiety Scale. *Journal of Personality Assessment*, **43**, 281–283.

Sareen, J., Cox, B. J., Afifi, T. O., de Graaf, R., Asmundson, G. J. G., ten Have, M., *et al.* (2005). Anxiety disorders and risk for suicidal ideation and suicide attempts. *Archives of General Anxiety*, **62**, 1249–1257.

Schniering, C. A., Hudson, J. L., & Rapee, R. M. (2000). Issues in the diagnosis and assessment of anxiety disorders in children and adolescents. *Clinical Psychology Review*, **20**(4), 453–478.

Silverman, W. K. & Ollendick, T. H. (2005) Evidence-based assessment of anxiety and its disorders in children and adolescents. *Journal of Clinical Child and Adolescent Psychology*, **34**, 380–411.

Silverman, W. K., Pina, A. A., & Viswesvaran, C. (2008). Evidence-based psychosocial treatments for phobic and anxiety disorders in children and adolescents. *Journal of Clinical Child and Adolescent Psychology*, **37**, 105–130.

Stallard, P., Simpson, N., Anderson, S., & Goddard, M. (2008). The FRIENDS emotional health prevention programme: 12 month follow-up of a universal UK school based trial. *European Child and Adolescent Psychiatry*, **17**, 283–289.

Stallard, P., Simpson, N., Anderson, S., Hibbert, S., & Osborn, C. (2007). The FRIENDS emotional health programme: initial findings from a school-based project. *Child and Adolescent Mental Health*, **12**, 32–37.

Strauss, C. C., Frame, C. L., & Forehand, R. (1987). Psychosocial impairment associated with anxiety in children. *Journal of Clinical Child Psychology*, **16**, 235–239.

Weissman, M. M., Wolk, S., Wickramaratne, P., Goldstein, R. B., Adams, P., Greenwald, S., *et al.* (1999). Children with prepubertal-onset major depressive disorder and anxiety grown up. *Archives of General Psychiatry*, **56**, 794–801.

Weisz, J. R., Sandler, I. N., Durlak, J. A., & Anton, B. S. (2005). Promoting and preventing youth mental health through evidence-based prevention and treatment. *American Psychologist*, **60**, 628–648.

Woodward, L. J. & Ferguson, D. M. (2001). Life course outcomes of young people with anxiety disorders in adolescence. *Journal of the American Academy of Child and Adolescent Psychiatry*, **40**, 1086–1093.

17

Pharmacological management of childhood and adolescent anxiety disorders

Laurel Pelligrino, Courtney Pierce, and John T. Walkup

Introduction

Psychotropic medications were first studied in anxious children and adolescents in the late 1950s. Early studies evaluated antipsychotic agents and minor tranquilizers, but did not find them to be more effective than placebo (for review, see Reinblatt & Walkup, 2005). However, in the early 1970s the efficacy of tricyclic antidepressants (TCAs) for panic disorder in adults and adult reports of anxiety onset in childhood led to the first demonstrated efficacy of medication – TCAs – in anxious children (Gittelman-Klein & Klein, 1971). For the next 20 years few pharmacological treatment studies of anxious children were conducted. However, in the early 1990s the arrival of the selective serotonin reuptake inhibitors (SSRIs) and safety concerns with the TCAs (Riddle, Geller, & Ryan, 1993) led to a number of studies of SSRIs in childhood obsessive–compulsive disorder (OCD)(Geller *et al.*, 2001, 2004; March *et al.*, 1998; Riddle *et al.*, 2001). Positive efficacy studies and a benign safety profile resulted in United States Food and Drug Administration (FDA) approval of fluoxetine, sertraline, and fluvoxamine for childhood OCD. With the success of the SSRIs in childhood OCD, studies focusing on the usefulness of SSRIs for separation, social, and generalized anxiety have been conducted subsequently (Birmaher *et al.*, 2003; RUPP, 2001). Although the SSRIs have demonstrated efficacy for these conditions, these studies have not led to FDA approval. Given a solid evidence base for the acute efficacy and safety of SSRIs for OCD and other anxiety disorders (Ipser, Stein, Hawkridge, & Hoppe, 2009), future studies will focus on four main issues: (1) the long-term durability and safety of medication treatment; (2) strategies for non-responders or partial responders, (3) identification of predictors and moderators of pharmacological and psychotherapeutic intervention to help determine which treatment is best for whom, and (4) how long to treat a child before he or she can safely discontinue medication with minimal risk for relapse. This chapter is a guide for prescribing anxiolytics for children and adolescents focusing on SSRIs. The current evidence base for treatment will be reviewed, and the processes of prescribing to terminating treatment will be discussed.

Basics of psychopharmacology

Rationale for treatment with medication

Normal anxiety is important to healthy child development (see Muris & Field, Chapter 4, this volume). Anxiety disorders, in contrast, plague children with excessive worry that lacks

Anxiety Disorders in Children and Adolescents, 2nd edn, ed. W. K. Silverman and A. P. Field. Published by Cambridge University Press. © Cambridge University Press 2011.

any normative purpose and interferes with development and functioning. For example, normal childhood rituals, such as ritualized closing a closet door at bedtime, are common and presumably a normative part of development. But unlike such transient rituals in childhood, obsessive–compulsive behaviors are maladaptive, have no developmental purpose, cause excessive distress, and are time-consuming (Leonard, Goldberger, Rapoport, Cheslow, & Swedo, 1990). In addition, although normal forms of anxiety can be understood dimensionally with a range of severity across individuals, from the perspective of pharmacological treatment, some forms of anxiety disorders are best considered as pathological categories with unique symptomatology and course, and discontinuous with normal anxiety. For example, a 9-year-old child with new-onset separation anxious symptoms is not consistent with developmentally normative separation worries and would be considered discontinuous with separation anxiety as seen in younger children. Or for example, fears of embarrassment in routine social interactions including using public toilets, ordering food at restaurants, or handing in homework for fear of scrutiny are not normative for a teenager who is prodromally an extrovert. Such symptoms are atypical for teen development, more commonly seen in disordered youth than in non-anxious youth, and potentially impairing (Labellarte, Ginsburg, Walkup, & Riddle, 1999). Similarly, OCD behaviors are differentiated from normal childhood superstitions based on their content (repetitive washing and grooming rituals versus superstitions involving good and bad luck), timing (normal childhood superstitions fade by age 8; OCD behaviors can present after age 7), and severity (Leonard *et al.*, 1990). Because anxiety disorders interfere with normal development and can increase the risk of developing anxiety and depressive disorders in adulthood, it is important to understand and use the evidence-based pharmacological tools that have been developed to treat them.

Neurotransmitter systems

Neurotransmitters are the chemicals that neurons (the basic cells of the brain) use to communicate with one another. Neurotransmitters are released into the spaces between neurons called synapses. The neuron that releases the neurotransmitter is called the presynaptic neuron and the one that responds to the neurotransmitter is called the postsynaptic neuron. After release, neurotransmitters are either degraded by enzymes in the synapse or reabsorbed by the presynaptic neuron and "recycled."

Six systems of neurotransmitters have been highlighted as critical to mood and anxiety disorders. The first two – the glutamatergic and GABAergic systems – are the major neurotransmitters of the central nervous system and have widespread effects on various neural systems. The glutamatergic system involves the neurotransmitter glutamate. The GABAergic system involves gamma-aminobutyric acid (GABA) as a neurotransmitter. The other four systems are clustered in specific areas of the nervous system and have more circumscribed effects. These are the cholinergic, dopaminergic, noradrenergic, and serotoninergic systems that involve the neurotransmitters acetylcholine, dopamine, norepinephrine, and serotonin, respectively. Each system has a host of functions in the brain. For example, the noradrenergic system is involved in regulating sleep cycles, appetite, mood, and cognition. The cholinergic system has been found to be involved in attention, novelty-seeking, memory, and sleep cycles.

Psychiatric disorders have been found to relate to disturbances in these neurotransmitter systems and the circuits and networks in which they function. Anxiety disorders, for example, have been linked to the malfunctioning of the serotoninergic system in the amygdala and the noradrenergic system in the locus ceruleus.

Psychotropic medications work by modulating these systems. Drugs that mimic the action of a given neurotransmitter are referred to as agonists and those that inhibit the action of a neurotransmitter are called antagonists. Benzodiazepines (BZs), for example, act as GABA agonists – that is, they bind to GABA receptors and mimic GABA's effects. Other anti-anxiety medications work by blocking the reuptake of neurotransmitters by presynaptic neurons, thus prolonging the effects of the neurotransmitter in the synapse. For example, SSRIs work this way, and result in increased synaptic serotonin.

Pharmacokinetics

Pharmacokinetics are the principles that explain how a particular dose of medicine results in a given concentration of the drug in the body. There are four processes that affect the concentration of medication in the body: absorption, distribution, metabolism, and excretion. Absorption and distribution generally determine the speed at which the drug makes its effects felt in the body. Metabolism and excretion generally determine the rate of termination of these effects.

The SSRIs are administered orally and after absorption in the gastrointestinal tract, pass through the liver where they undergo "first-pass" metabolism before entering the broader circulation. The "parent" drug is usually effective but for some of the SSRIs the metabolites from first pass through the liver can also be effective. The proportion of parent drug that reaches the systemic circulation after this first-pass metabolism is called bioavailability. With repeated dosing the concentration in the blood generally rises until the rate of absorption equals the rate of removal, the so-called "steady state." Thus, concentration in the blood reaches a steady state more quickly if the medication is metabolized and eliminated quickly; conversely, those medications that are metabolized slowly or eliminated slowly take longer to reach steady state.

The amount of time it takes for the concentration of a medicine in the blood to be reduced by half is called the half-life of the medication. Knowing the half-life allows one to predict the time to steady state (usually 5 × the half-life) and can be useful in determining dosing frequency – short half-life medications may require more frequent dosing than longer half-life medications.

For most psychotropic drugs doubling the dose effectively doubles the level of medication in the blood. This is referred to as linear pharmacokinetics. However, some of the SSRIs inhibit their own metabolic pathway, so with repeated dosing the amount of the drug in the blood increases disproportionally, so doubling the dose may result in a three- to four-fold increase in blood level (i.e., non-linear pharmacokinetics). For example, a single dose of paroxetine has a short half-life, but with repeated dosing paroxetine inhibits its own metabolism resulting in an increased half-life, which prolongs the period to steady state and the duration of time it takes to leave the body when the medication is discontinued.

Pharmacokinetics in children and adolescents

Children and adolescents have effective livers and kidneys so they have a faster metabolism in the liver and more efficient elimination by the kidneys than adults. With faster metabolism children can require adult doses of medication, but children also can be more sensitive to some medication side effects. For example, in SSRI trials average endpoint doses of medication in children are often similar to those in adult studies, yet children's side effect profile includes more activation and hyperactivity than adults. No general statements can be made about dose and side effects for medications in children so reviewing each medication's specific information is important for safe and effective prescribing. In clinical practice to maximize the opportunity to replicate finding from randomized controlled trials, it is useful to mimic the dosing and duration of acute treatment to prevent under-dosing or unnecessarily prolonged treatment trials.

Anti-anxiety agents

Antidepressants
Selective serotonin reuptake inhibitors

Selective serotonin reuptake inhibitors are the first-line pharmacological treatment for childhood anxiety disorders because of their demonstrated efficacy and safety profile. There are currently four SSRIs with FDA approval for children – fluoxetine for major depression and OCD for children down to age 7 years; sertraline for OCD down to age 6 years, fluvoxamine for OCD down to age 8, and escitalopram for major depression down to age 12. Despite the lack of FDA approval, other SSRIs antidepressants have demonstrated efficacy in children and adolescents including the SSRI paroxetine for OCD (Geller *et al.*, 2004) and social phobia (Wagner *et al.*, 2004), and the norepinephrine–serotonin reuptake inhibitor venlafaxine for social phobia (March, Entusah, Rynn, Albano, & Tourian, 2007).

It is important to note that the evidence base for antidepressant efficacy for anxiety disorders in children and FDA approval are not synonymous. A number of SSRIs have demonstrated efficacy for childhood anxiety (e.g., fluvoxamine, sertraline, and fluoxetine for separation, social, and generalized anxiety disorders and paroxetine and venlafaxine as noted above) but do not have FDA approval for a variety of reasons. Approval by the FDA requires a willing pharmaceutical manufacturer to prepare the data and pay for review by the FDA. Most of the SSRIs are no longer under patent so the relevant pharmaceutical companies no longer have a profit motive to pursue an indication. The FDA could initiate changes in the product information for the SSRIs for which there is evidence, but to date they have not done so. Although families and non-prescribers may express concern about "off-label" prescribing (using a medication for a purpose that is not FDA approved), evidence-based prescribing does not require using only FDA-approved medications. In actuality for child prescribers to practice evidence-based medicine they may be required to use medications "off label."

The SSRIs have fewer nuisance side effects (sedation, constipation, etc.) than TCAs and lack their cardiac side effects also. The SSRIs also lack the potentially severe drug–food interactions of an infrequently used class of antidepressants, the monoamine oxidase inhibitors (MAOIs). The SSRIs vary in their chemical structure, but they all selectively block the reuptake of serotonin by presynaptic neurons with little or no effect on adrenergic, cholinergic, or histaminic systems. While early-onset side effects appear to be related to this acute reuptake blockade of serotonin (i.e., transient serotonin excess in the synapse), it is believed that the longer-term effects on anxiety and depression are related to SSRI-induced changes in postsynaptic receptor density and sensitivity (Velosa & Riddle, 2000).

The greatest variation among SSRIs is in their metabolism, half-life, elimination, and potential for drug interactions. Fluoxetine, for example, has a long half-life and a potent active metabolite with an even longer half-life. Fluoxetine, therefore, takes a long time to reach steady state and remains in the body for a long time – weeks to months – after discontinuation. Sertraline and fluvoxamine, on the other hand, have a short half-life, so they reach steady state quickly and are also cleared from the body quickly – days to weeks (Chiu & Leonard, 2003; Labellarte *et al.*, 1999).

The SSRIs also affect the functioning of the metabolic enzymes in the liver. The major liver system responsible for metabolizing the SSRIs is the cytochrome P-450 system. Some of the enzymes are plentiful with nearly unlimited capacity (i.e., they cannot be saturated), However, others are less plentiful or are readily saturated, resulting in non-linear pharmacokinetics of the drug. Non-linear pharmacokinetics can lead to potentially unpredictable effects as clinicians and patients may assume that incremental dosing results in incremental effects, i.e. double the dose doubles the benefits, whereas drugs with non-linear pharmacokinetics have non-linear accumulation and effects – doubling the dose may result in a three- to four-fold increase in blood level and marked increased risk for side effects. In contrast to the SSRIs some medications can induce the creation of more enzymes (some anticonvulsants) resulting in increased metabolism, shorter half-life, drop in peak blood level, and perhaps loss of efficacy.

The SSRIs to a greater and less extent inhibit the cytochrome system, have non-linear accumulation (pharmacokinetics), and can impact the metabolism of drugs that are co-administered and metabolized by the same system (i.e., drug–drug interactions). Among the SSRIs those with the greatest risk for drug–drug interactions are fluoxetine, paroxetine, and, to a much lesser extent, sertraline. These three medications inhibit the cytochrome P-450 2D6 enzyme, which is an important enzyme for metabolism of other psychotropic medications. For example, combining SSRIs with TCAs may lead to increases in TCA blood levels. Without careful monitoring such combined use may increase a patient's risk for TCA cardiac side effects.

The SSRIs can also result in drug–drug interactions by interfering with another drug's distribution in the blood. A number of medications bind to proteins in the blood and become inactive as a result. If an SSRI disrupts the protein-binding process, a larger amount of the other drug becomes active in the blood, resulting in unpredictable benefit or side effects. For example, some SSRIs interfere with the protein-binding of the anti-clotting agent warfarin. Combined use of an SSRI and warfarin can be done, but may require a lowering of the warfarin dose and monitoring for an increased risk for bleeding.

Tricyclic antidepressants

Tricyclic antidepressants were synthesized in the 1940s and first used for adult depression and anxiety in the 1950s. The FDA has approved their use in children for OCD (clomipramine) and enuresis (imipramine), but not for the other anxiety disorders. Although there are data supporting their use for the non-OCD anxiety disorders (Bernstein *et al.*, 2000), their safety profile often makes them a second-line medication choice to be used when SSRIs are ineffective or not tolerated. Although SSRIs are the drug of choice, TCAs may have a particular advantage for children compared to SSRIs, as TCAs normalize sleep architecture, improve sleep onset (Armitage, 2000), increase appetite (some anxious children under-eat), and have fewer activation side effects than the SSRIs. The TCAs can also improve attention and concentration in attention deficit hyperactivity disorder (ADHD) (Spencer *et al.*, 2002).

The TCAs consist of a basic three-ring structure and they vary according to the attached amine group. All TCAs function by blocking the reuptake of norepinephrine and to a lesser extent serotonin at presynaptic reuptake sites. The TCAs also have antagonistic effects on muscarinic and histaminic receptors, which accounts for greater nuisance side effects as compared to the SSRIs.

Similar to the SSRIs, the TCAs cause downstream effects on the postsynaptic neuron including changes in receptor density and postsynaptic activity. These changes are not immediate but rather accumulate over time and it is hypothesized that changes in post-synaptic neuron activity is associated with clinical benefit and the resulting lag time in altering mood and anxiety. The TCAs are rapidly and completely absorbed by the body, and they are taken to the liver where they are metabolized and then excreted in the urine. Children metabolize TCAs more efficiently than adults, leading to more rapid clearance. The TCAs are highly protein-bound and highly soluble in fat (lipophilic), which means that they are widely distributed in the body and can cross the blood–brain barrier into the central nervous system.

The TCAs have more side effects than the SSRIs because they interact with a greater number of receptors. Most importantly, they increase autonomic nervous system tone, causing small increases in heart rate and blood pressure. There have also been reports of sudden death in children undergoing treatment with TCAs (Riddle *et al.*, 1993). Although the exact mechanism by which TCAs might increase some children's risk for sudden death is not known, screening children for periods of loss of consciousness due to cardiac arrhythmia (not due to seizure or vasovagal syncope i.e. common fainting), a family history of sudden cardiac death (not due to coronary artery disease), cardiac arrhythmias, and/or risk factors for these difficulties plus close monitoring with electrocardiograms is reasonable in the safe use of these medications (Wilens *et al.*, 1996). There is also a withdrawal syndrome associated with stopping TCAs, so patients should be slowly tapered off of TCAs as is done with most medication (Garner, Kelly, & Thompson, 1993).

Monoamine oxidase inhibitors

Monoamine oxidase inhibitors were used to treat depression before the advent of TCAs and SSRIs. The MAOIs function by inhibiting monoamine oxidase (MAO), an enzyme that breaks down neurotransmitters in the synapse and thus results in increased levels of neurotransmitters such as norepinephrine, serotonin, and dopamine. The MAOIs have short half-lives and need to be dosed daily, but their effects are enduring because they bind irreversibly to their enzyme targets. After being discontinued, MAOIs are cleared from the blood within 24 hours, but it can take up to 2 weeks for MAO enzyme to be regenerated. The MAOIs are primarily metabolized in the liver, but their metabolism is not well understood.

The MAOIs are used infrequently because of their potentially dangerous interactions with a large number of foods and drugs. For example, when combined with foods containing tyramine (such as aged meats and cheeses) or with medications with neurotransmitter agonist activity, they can lead to excessive neurotransmitter in the synapse and toxicity. Excessive norepinephrine in the synapse can cause hypertensive crises involve headaches, neck stiffness, chest discomfort, palpitations, confusion, and possibly even hemorrhage and stroke. Excessive serotonin activity is characterized by delirium, hyperthermia, autonomic instability, fever, neuromuscular excitability, and possibly coma and death. When switching from an MAOI to a serotoninergic drug such as an SSRI, it is important to wait 2 weeks for the MAO enzyme to be regenerated.

As such, MAOIs should be considered for use in childhood anxiety disorders only if several other medications and psychotherapy have failed. The child and family must understand the risks associated with the drug and agree to comply with the dietary and medication restrictions to avoid side effects.

Atypical or second-generation antidepressants

Trazodone is a triazolopyridine derivative that weakly inhibits serotonin reuptake and is indicated for adult depression. There are no studies evaluating the efficacy of trazodone in children with anxiety. Trazodone's metabolite *m*-chlorophenylpiperazine (mCPP) is a direct serotonin agonist, and works in combination with trazodone to increase levels of serotonin and exert its anxiolytic effects. It can also cause sustained erections (priapism) in males (Jayaram & Rao, 2005). Although there are very few reports of such problems in male children many clinicians are reluctant to use trazadone in any male patients. Due to its low antidepressant potency and substantial sedative side effects, trazodone is usually prescribed as a sleeping aid for those with primary insomnia or insomnia secondary to SSRI treatment, especially in females. However, combining trazodone with SSRIs may require special care as SSRIs that are inhibitors of CYP3A4 (Rotzinger, Fang, & Baker, 1998), such as fluvoxamine, may elevate serum levels of trazodone and mCPP (Rotzinger, Fang, Coutts, & Baker, 1998).

Nefazodone is a phenylpiperazine antidepressant, related to trazodone, that inhibits the reuptake of both norepinephrine and serotonin with an indication for adult depression. There are no studies supporting the use of nefazodone in the childhood anxiety disorders. In adults nefazodone is generally well tolerated. Common side effects include somnolence and increased appetite. The FDA has required a "black box" warning because nefazodone is associated with rare liver toxicity that may lead to death. Prior to the "black box" warning, nefazodone's sedative and anxiolytic properties as demonstrated in adults made it a clinically useful second-line agent for anxious children who did not tolerate the activating effects (including insomnia) of the SSRIs. Nefazodone also appears to have fewer sexual side effects than the SSRIs and may also be clinically useful in those anxious teens who experience such side effects with SSRI treatment. Nefazodone inhibits CYP3A4 so co-treatment with anti-anxiety agents such as the benzodiazepines, tiazolam, or alprazolam can significantly elevate their blood levels (Greene, Salazar, Dockens, Kroboth, & Barbhaiya, 1995).

Bupropion is an aminoketone that inhibits norepinephrine and dopamine reuptake with an indication for adult depression. Studies of bupropion are few in children and have focused on its potential utility in attentionally impaired children. Bupropion mechanism of action suggests that it might not be useful in the treatment of anxious adults or children. However, its efficacy for adult depression and presumably anxiety associated with depression may lead to its use as a second- or third-line medication for a group of anxious adults (Papakostas *et al.*, 2008) or children. Bupropion's unique mechanism of action is matched by its unique side-effect profile. Bupropion decreases appetite and has neutral or even positive effects of sexual function, which may lead to its use alone or in combination with SSRIs in those who experience increased appetite or sexual dysfunction on SSRIs. Other side effects reflect dopamine and norepinephrine excess and include behavioral effects, activation, insomnia, and stomach upset. The most serious adverse event is seizures, which may occur at high dosages or when doses of medication are not appropriately separated in time. For this reason, the first dose in adults or children should not exceed 150 mg and a second dose should not be taken before 8 hours have passed. Sustained release preparations of bupropion may mitigate this effect and allow for once a day dosing of greater than 150 mg. Bupropion is mainly used to treat children with depression and ADHD. Combining bupropion with SSRIs should be done with caution; combinations with MAOIs are contraindicated.

Mirtazapine, a member of the class of drugs called piperazinoazepines, blocks both serotonin and norepinephrine reuptake and is indicated for adult depression, but commonly used off label for a number of other conditions including anxiety disorders. It is also commonly used off label as a second drug in depressed adults with partial response to another antidepressant or to improve anxiety control or for insomnia. No studies have been completed in anxious children. It is provided in a pill form as well as a dissolving tablet. Adverse effects reported in adults include somnolence and increased appetite with weight gain, so risk factors for obesity should be considered before starting mirtazapine. Its sedative effects are greater at lower doses than at high doses, so when starting mirtazapine, clinicians should move more quickly to higher doses to avoid the prolonged period of sedation associated with lower doses (Preskorn, 2000); "starting low and going slow" as is done with other medications is not a useful strategy for mirtazapine. Regardless of age sedative effects are greater when used in conjunction with benzodiazepines and alcohol. Mirtazapine's efficacy across a number of conditions and unique side-effect profile may make it a good alternative for children with anxiety who cannot tolerate SSRIs. Its anti-anxiety properties can address daytime anxious symptoms as well as anxiety-associated insomnia. Its appetite-enhancing properties may also be useful in children who under-eat due to anxiety.

Venlafaxine, released in the USA in 1994, is a selective norepineprhine and serotonin reuptake inhibitor (NSRI). It blocks serotonin more effectively at low doses and norepinephrine more effectively at higher doses. Adverse events include nausea, drowsiness, insomnia, dizziness, headache, dry mouth, and elevations in blood pressure at high doses. For this reason, blood pressure should be monitored during treatment. Venlafaxine should not be taken in combination with MAOIs, but otherwise it shows few drug–drug interactions. Venlafaxine is currently used for treatment-refractory depression in adults but has been shown to be efficacious in youth with social anxiety disorder (March *et al.*, 2007).

Atomoxine is a selective norepinephrine reuptake inhibitor (NRI) FDA approved for the treatment of ADHD in children and adults. It is generally well tolerated. Atomoxine may have antidepressant and anti-anxiety properties so some clinicians may consider its use in attentionally impaired and anxious youth (Geller *et al.*, 2007). Side effects include anorexia, nausea, headache, insomnia, and rhinitis.

Reboxetine is a selective NRI released in Europe in 1997 for adult depression (Montgomery, 1998) and is not available in the USA. Reboxetine has been shown to be well tolerated in adults; reported adverse events include dry mouth, insomnia, tremor, hypertension, and somnolence. It may be useful in children with ADHD, depression, and anxiety (Arabgol, Panaghi, & Hebrani, 2009).

Benzodiazepines

Benzodiazepines are indicated for the treatment of anxiety in adults. Their only FDA approval for use in children is for pre-anesthesia. The first BZ entered the market in 1960 and today there are 10 available in the USA. BZs bind to GABA receptors, increasing GABA's effect on these receptors. As GABA is the primary inhibitory neurotransmitter of the central nervous system, BZs have widespread neurodepressive effects. Benzodiazepines do not have the risk in overdose that the barbiturates have but can be lethal when combined with alcohol or other central nervous system depressants, which is particularly relevant for adolescent patients.

Benzodiazepines are completely absorbed from the gastrointestinal tract and metabolized in the liver. They are readily soluble in fat, which allows them to cross the blood–brain barrier into the central nervous system. All BZs have similar pharmacodynamic properties, but they vary in their pharmacokinetic properties. Those BZs with longer half-lives are better for anxiety symptoms because they have more prolonged and consistent effects, but they may also cause daytime drowsiness.

The most common side effect of BZs is sedation. In children they may also cause problems with learning and memory when used long term. Patients can also develop tolerance to BZs after taking them chronically for 3–4 months. For these reasons, they should only be used short term for acute symptoms of anxiety or during known acute stressors (Barnett & Riddle, 2003).

Evidence base in children

A variety of medications are effective in treating anxiety disorders in children and adolescents. In a recent meta-analysis of 22 short-term randomized controlled trials ($n = 2519$), 11 of the 19 placebo controlled trials showed a significantly greater response with treatment for both OCD and non-OCD anxiety disorders (number needed to treat [NNT] = 4) (Ipser *et al.*, 2009). The greatest number of trials involved SSRIs, which are the first-line treatment for childhood anxiety disorders. No controlled evidence was found for the use of BZs, even though they are prescribed for the pediatric population. Maintenance studies suggested that long-term treatment with SSRIs may be required for sustained benefit and to avoid relapse (Cook *et al.*, 2001; RUPP, 2002).

Obsessive–compulsive disorder

The evidence base supporting the efficacy of pharmacological treatment of OCD is greater than pharmacological evidence for all of the other anxiety disorders. Both SSRIs and TCAs are effective in treating childhood OCD. Clomipramine has more side effects than the SSRIs and is generally considered second line. However, clomipramine is an important alternative to the SSRIs because it is more sedating than the SSRIs, less commonly activating, normalizes sleep architecture, enhances appetite, and may be useful for more severe or treatment-resistant cases of OCD because it has a broad spectrum of receptor activity.

Tricyclic antidepressants

The most significant trial showing clomipramine to be an effective treatment for childhood OCD was an 8-week, multicenter, double-blind, randomized controlled trial of clomipramine in doses up to 200 mg in children aged 10–17 (DeVeaugh-Geiss *et al.*, 1992). On the Children's Yale-Brown Obsessive Compulsive Scale (CY-BOCS) (Scahill *et al.*, 1997), 37% of children in the treatment group showed a reduction in symptoms as compared to 8% in the placebo group. Clomipramine was generally well tolerated; the most commonly reported adverse events were dry mouth, somnolence, and dizziness. Additionally, mild pulse-rate elevations, drops in systolic blood pressure, and weight gain were noted in the treatment group; but no clinically significant electrocardiogram changes were found. Efficacy was maintained over a 1-year, open-label extension trial.

Selective serotonin reuptake inhibitors

Fluvoxamine was shown to be effective in doses up to 200 mg/day in a 10-week, multicenter, double-blind, randomized controlled trial ($n = 120$) of children aged 8–17 (Riddle *et al.*, 2001). On the CY-BOCS, 42% of participants in the treatment group showed improvement, as compared to only 26% of the placebo group. Fluvoxamine was generally well tolerated; adverse events that occurred in greater frequency in the treatment group were insomnia and asthenia.

Sertraline was first shown to be effective in children ages 6–17 ($n = 187$) up to 200 mg/day (March *et al.*, 1998). Using the Clinical Global Impressions (CGI)-Improvement Scale (Guy, 1976), 16% more participants in the treatment group than the placebo group were very much or much improved at study endpoint with an approximate 30% reduction in symptoms. Adverse events in the treatment group included insomnia, nausea, agitation, and tremor. A 1-year open-label extension trial was completed for all participants regardless of assigned treatment or response ($n = 132$) with sertraline up to 200 mg/day; 85% of responders to acute treatment remained responsive at the endpoint of the extension study; and 43% of non-responders responded by the endpoint of the extension study (Cook *et al.*, 2001). Sertraline was well tolerated. Adverse events were mild to moderate, occurred early in treatment, and tended to decrease throughout treatment.

In a subsequent trial patients were treated with sertraline alone, cognitive–behavioral therapy (CBT) alone, sertraline and CBT combined, or placebo for 12 weeks (POTS, 2004). Participants taking only sertraline received doses up to 200 mg/day and showed significant improvement (17.8% more patients showed clinical remission than the placebo group). The group assigned to both sertraline and CBT showed even greater improvement (50% more showed clinical remission than the placebo group). Adverse events included decreased appetite, diarrhea, enuresis, motor overactivity, nausea, and stomach ache.

Fluoxetine was shown to be effective in doses up to 60 mg daily in a 13-week, double-blind, randomized controlled trial of children aged 7–17 ($n = 103$) with OCD. On the CY-BOCS, 24% more children in the treatment group were responders than those in the placebo group. There were no statistically significant differences in adverse events reported between the two groups.

Paroxetine was shown to be effective up to 50 mg/day in a 10-week randomized controlled trial of patients aged 7–17 ($n = 203$) (Geller *et al.*, 2004). Based on the CY-BOCS, the paroxetine group showed a significant reduction in symptoms in favor of paroxetine (an adjusted mean difference of -3.45 (95% confidence interval $= -5.60$ to -1.29, $p = 0.002$). Adverse events were mild to moderate and included headache, abdominal pain, nausea, respiratory disorder, somnolence, hyperkinesia, and trauma. A double-blind discontinuation trial showed that patients were less likely to relapse with continued treatment with paroxetine (Geller *et al.*, 2003). After a 16-week open-label treatment with paroxetine, participants were randomized to continued treatment or placebo for 16 more weeks. The overall rate of relapse was 10% greater in the placebo group than the continued-treatment group. This difference was even greater for patients with comorbid disorders.

Separation anxiety disorder, generalized anxiety disorder, and social phobia

Tricyclic antidepressants

The evidence for TCAs in non-OCD anxiety disorders is not as compelling as the evidence for the SSRIs. The first report of efficacy came in 1971 in a 6-week study by Gittelman-Klein and Klein of imipramine up to 200 mg/day in children with school phobia (presumably due to an anxiety disorder); school attendance improved in 34% more children in the imipramine group than the placebo group (Gittelman-Klein & Klein, 1971). This study was small, however, and subsequent studies failed to show statistically significant improvement (Klein, Koplewicz, & Kanner, 1992). In another study imipramine was found to be effective for school-refusing adolescents with anxiety and depression when combined with CBT (37.5% more patients on imipramine group than placebo met remission criteria of 75% school attendance) (Bernstein *et al.*, 2000).

Selective serotonin reuptake inhibitors

The SSRIs have replaced TCAs as the first-line treatment for anxiety disorders in children and adolescents, and their evidence base is much stronger. Fluvoxamine was shown to be effective in doses up to 300 mg in a large, multisite, double-blind, randomized controlled trial done by the Research Units of Pediatric Psychopharmacology (RUPP) Anxiety Study Group (RUPP, 2001). Children between the ages of 6 and 17 ($n = 128$) who did not respond to 3 weeks of psycho-education were randomized to fluvoxamine or placebo, and after 8 weeks the fluvoxamine group showed significantly greater improvement (76%) on the CGI-Improvement Scale than the placebo group (29%). The medication was generally well tolerated; side effects included gastrointestinal symptoms and behavioral activation. In a 6-month, open-label extension of this trial, 94% of patients who responded to acute treatment showed a continued remission of anxiety symptoms (RUPP, 2002). In addition, when fluvoxamine was not effective in acute treatment, a switch to fluoxetine improved symptoms over the next 6 months (71% of non-responders to fluvoxamine improved when switched to fluoxetine).

Fluoxetine was found to be effective up to 20 mg/day in a 12-week randomized controlled trial of children aged 7 to 17 (26% more patients in the fluoxetine group showed improvement than those of the placebo group). However, the doses (Birmaher *et al.*, 2003) may not have been high enough to maximize response rates. Side effects were mild and were limited to transient headaches and gastrointestinal symptoms. Fluoxetine was also found to be effective up to 40 mg in a randomized controlled trial comparing fluoxetine and psycho-education for social phobia in youths aged 7–17. Participants taking fluoxetine showed improvement on the CGI-Improvement Scale (30.1% more than placebo). Side effects were mild to moderate, the most common being nausea. Participants assigned to Social Effectiveness Therapy for Children (SET-C) showed even greater improvement (72.7% more than placebo) (Beidel, Turner, Sallee, Ammerman, Crosby, & Pathak, 2007).

Paroxetine was found to be effective in doses up to 50 mg in a large ($n = 322$), multicenter, double-blind, randomized controlled trial of children aged 8–17 with social anxiety disorder (Wagner, *et al.*, 2004). Participants taking paroxetine improved on the CGI-Improvement Scale (77.6%) more than the placebo group (38.3%). Adverse events were mild to moderate and included insomnia, decreased appetite, and vomiting.

Extended-release venlafaxine was found to be an effective short-term treatment for generalized anxiety disorder in doses up to 225 mg in children aged 6–17 in two double-blind randomized controlled trials (Rynn, Riddle, Yeung, & Kunz, 2007). Pooled data from the two studies showed a 21% greater improvement in the venlafaxine group than the placebo group on the CGI-Improvement Scale. Treatment was generally well tolerated; adverse events included asthenia, pain, anorexia, and somnolence.

Extended-release venlafaxine was also found to be effective in treating social phobia in doses up to 225 mg in a double-blind, randomized controlled trial of children aged 8–17 (March *et al.*, 2007). Participants in the treatment group showed a 19% greater response than the placebo group. Adverse events were mild to moderate, the most common being nausea and anorexia; the treatment group experienced a clinically significant weight loss. Three of the participants in the treatment group developed suicidal ideation as compared to none in the placebo group.

In the largest trial in children with separation, social or generalized anxiety disorders the Child Adolescent Anxiety Multimodal Study compared the efficacy of sertraline or CBT with their combination and pill placebo in 488 children and adolescents aged 7–17 (Walkup *et al.*, 2008). On a variety of categorical and dimensional outcome measures combination treatment was better than both of the monotherapies and pill placebo. The two monotherapies were similar in outcome and were superior to pill placebo. Sertraline was found to be safe with few medication-related drop-outs and few side effects of meaningful severity were present more often in the sertraline group as compared to placebo. There was no apparent risk for suicidal behavior in the sertraline group.

Benzodiazepines

Studies of benzodiazepines in children and adolescents with anxiety disorders have not shown significant benefit. A small, 8-week, double-blind, randomized controlled trial of alprazolam up to 0.03 mg/kg daily versus imipramine and placebo in children aged 7–18 ($n = 24$) with school refusal showed alprazolam to be the most effective treatment arm (Bernstein, Garfinkel, & Borchardt, 1990). However, when the data were analyzed taking baseline scores into account, no significant differences were found. Side effects were described as mild and did not interfere with functioning. In a small, 4-week, double-blind, randomized controlled trial of alprazolam up to 0.04 mg/kg daily in children aged 8–16 ($n = 30$) with overanxious or avoidant disorder, alprazolam showed slightly more improvement than placebo, but the difference was not statistically significant (Simeon & Ferguson, 1987). Another small, 4-week, double-blind, randomized controlled trial of clonazepam up to 2 mg/day in children aged 7–13 with mixed anxiety disorders (predominantly separation anxiety disorder) failed to show a significant difference between treatment and placebo (Graae, Milner, Rizzotto, & Klein, 1994).

Specific phobia

There is limited evidence for the treatment of specific phobia with anxiolytics. A small, open-label pilot study of six children and adolescents with specific phobia showed that fluoxetine was effective up to 80 mg/day; five of the six patients were improved or much improved on the CGI-Improvement Scale (Fairbanks *et al.*, 1997). Side effects were mild and transient. Another small, double-blind, randomized controlled trial of 11 children with specific phobia showed paroxetine to be effective up to 20 mg/day. Three out of five patients responded on paroxetine compared to only one of six on placebo (Benjamin, Costello, & Warren, 1990).

Post-traumatic stress disorder

Although there are no randomized controlled trials for treatment of post-traumatic stress disorder (PTSD) with medication in children and adolescents, there are some indications that medication can be an effective treatment (Donnelly, 2003). A small, open-label study of a clonidine patch in seven preschool children aged 3–6 indicated improvement in all seven patients (Harmon & Riggs, 1996). Another small, 4-week, open-label study of propranolol up to 2.5 mg/day in 11 children with PTSD showed a reduction in symptoms (Famularo, Kinscherff, & Fenton, 1988). Risperidone was also helpful in a small, uncontrolled trial of 18 boys with PTSD (Horrigan & Barnhill, 1999); 15 of the 18 boys showed significant improvement. Carbamazepine was useful based on an uncontrolled case series of 28 children and adolescents between the ages of 8 and 17 who received 300–1200 mg/day. All showed significant improvement and 15 became asymptomatic (Looff, Grimley, Kuller, Martin, & Shonfield, 1995).

Antidepressants may also be useful in PTSD. Citalopram up to 40 mg/day was helpful in a small, 8-week, open-label trial of 24 children and adolescents (Seedat *et al.*, 2002); 16 of the participants (67%) were responders on the CGI-Improvement Scale. Imipramine up to 100 mg/day was helpful in a small, prospective, randomized trial of pediatric burn patients (aged 2–19) with acute stress disorder (Robert, Blakeney, Villarreal, Rosenberg, & Meyer, 1999); 10 of 12 children given imipramine were considered responders.

Adverse events

Antidepressants

Selective serotonin reuptake inhibitors

Although SSRIs are generally well tolerated, treatment can be associated with changes in physical functioning and behavior. It is important to discuss potential problems in treatment with the patient and family before starting medications. Adverse events that are unexpected, late in onset, or manifest themselves in changes in behavior are the most challenging to assess and treat.

Common physical side effects of SSRIs include nausea, upset stomach, and possibly reflux symptoms. They are usually short-lived and can be reduced by taking the medication with meals or lowering the dose. Other physical side effects include decreased appetite, weight loss, headaches, insomnia or hypersomnia, drowsiness, constipation, and fatigue. Sexual dysfunction is a side effect frequently reported in the adult population, but is rarely reported in placebo-controlled trials of SSRIs in children (Scharko, 2004). Management of sexual dysfunction in teens is likely addressed similarly to adults (Martin-Du & Baumann, 2008), but there is limited evidence to guide clinicians in which approaches are best and for whom.

The most commonly reported behavioral adverse event on SSRIs is activation or increased motor activity (Hammad, Laughren, & Racoosin, 2006). In an analysis of pooled data from four large, placebo-controlled clinical trials that separated their adverse event findings by age group, activation was more commonly reported in children than in adolescents (7.3% more children on treatment reported activation than those in the placebo group compared to only 0.2% more adolescents) (Safer & Zito, 2006). Children with minimal brain dysfunction, such as pervasive developmental disorder, mental retardation, or autism, are more likely to experience activation as an adverse event to SSRI treatment. Activation is most often seen early in treatment. In an analysis of activation adverse events in the RUPP fluvoxamine for childhood anxiety study 45% of the treatment group experienced activation with most before week 4 (Reinblatt, dosReis, Walkup, & Riddle, 2009). Activation is easily managed by reducing or discontinuing the medication.

It is important to differentiate activation, which does not involve any real change in mood, from bipolar switching, which is characterized by a change in mood, behavior, and impulse control. Bipolar switching can also be associated with SSRIs, but it generally occurs later in treatment and, unlike activation, does not go away with dose reduction, and may require treatment with a mood stabilizer (Walkup & Labellarte, 2001). It is critical to differentiate activation from a manic reaction. Activation is commonly caused by a number of medications and may not have any prognostic significance, whereas a manic reaction is less common and may reflect an individual's risk for future bipolar disorder. For children with anxiety disorders mislabeling activation as mania may result in unnecessarily stopping antidepressant treatment and may leave children untreated and vulnerable to accumulated morbidity from ineffective mood stabilizer treatment.

Apathy is another possible complication of SSRI treatment. It has been well documented in adults (Hoehn-Saric, Harris, Pearlson, Cox, Machlin, & Camargo, 1991), but there is more limited evidence of its occurrence in the pediatric population. Five cases of apathy in children and adolescents were described that were similar in profile to that seen in adults (Garland & Baerg, 2001). Symptoms were often undetected for some period of time before being identified weeks or months after onset. Although apathy is a subtle symptom, it can interfere with social interactions, school work, and sports involvement. Symptoms are readily reversible with dose reduction. Whether apathy is medication-induced or anhedonia due to loss of antidepressant efficacy is an important distinction. Careful questioning can help the clinician differentiate the two as patients can often differentiate their depressive symptoms or sedative side effects from apathy. For those cases where it is difficult to differentiate, reducing the dose of medication will often alleviate apathy, but it may also result in a return of anxiety or depression. Reducing the dose in a patient with previous suicidal behavior will require close monitoring. An alternative approach is to increase the dose and see if the apathy remains or worsens; worsening would indicate that apathy is indeed a side effect of the medication, which should then be reduced or discontinued. If the dose increase results in an improvement in mood or anxiety, then the medication simply wasn't working to its full potential. Adding a stimulant or a dopaminergic agent such as bupropion may be useful in those patients who cannot come off their antidepressant (Walkup & Labellarte, 2001).

Once a child's anxiety is reduced with SSRI treatment, he or she may behave in ways that their parents have not seen before. Sometimes children are so happy that their anxiety is relieved and they can go to school again, go to their friend's house, or not worry about tests or feel so self-conscious. Sometime parents have never seen their children function without apprehension and wonder whether their child's energy and enthusiasm is hypomania or mania. Sometimes when a child gets better they are also more assertive, want to do things they haven't done before, and may actually become demanding or oppositional. If the parents are not made aware of such changes ahead of time they may not be prepared to deal appropriately with these changes and respond with relevant parenting strategies (Walkup & Labellarte, 2001).

Concern regarding treatment of emergent suicidality with SSRIs led the FDA to put a "black box" warning on SSRIs in 2004. The data from the FDA that supported the "black box" suggested a 1–2% risk difference between drug and placebo and a relative risk just above 1 (Hammad, 2004). A recent meta-analysis of 27 SSRI trials in children and adolescents identified a slight increase in suicidal ideation (0.7% more on the drug than placebo) that was not statistically significant (Bridge *et al.*, 2007). Among those studies that focused on anxiety disorders, the risk of suicidality was less with OCD and non-OCD anxiety disorders than depression. Data from high-quality depression studies and from OCD and non-OCD anxiety studies suggest a number needed to treat in the 3–5 range with a number needed to harm for suicidality in the 140–200 range making the overall benefit–risk ratio favorable for SSRIs in childhood anxiety and depression. This reassessment of the benefit–risk ratio for suicidal behavior on SSRIs is especially critical given the increased rate of suicide subsequent to the "black box" warning (Gibbons, Hur, Bhaumik, & Mann, 2005).

Tricyclic antidepressants

Tricyclic antidepressants have a host of side effects because, in addition to altering levels of serotonin, they also block cholinergic, histaminic, and adrenergic receptors. A common anticholinergic effect is dry mouth. Other side effects include sedation, hypotension, hypertension, increased heart rate, and subtle changes in electrocardiographic readings. Since patients can gain weight while taking TCAs, it is advised that they stick to a healthy diet and exercise, and do not consume high-calorie fluids to alleviate the dry mouth. Although overdose of SSRIs is not usually lethal, overdose with TCAs can be, presumably due to fatal arrhythmias.

Benzodiazepines

Benzodiazepines are generally well tolerated. The most common side effects are sedation, decreased concentration, and poor coordination, but in a few patients they may actually cause activation or disinhibition (Riddle, Bernstein, Cook, Leonard, March, & Swanson, 1999). Drowsiness and sedation are generally related to dosage, and often times resolve with time as patients develop tolerance. Other possible side effects include diplopia, tremor, and decreased mental acuity. In a report of two adolescents clonazepam had to be discontinued due to disinhibition and anger outbursts (Reiter & Kutcher, 1991). Alprazolam at a low dose (0.03 mg/kg) in a trial for childhood anxiety caused mild side effects including blurred vision, constipation, dizziness, dry mouth, and nausea (Bernstein *et al.*, 1990). Clonazepam titrated up to 2 mg/day in another children's trial caused drowsiness, irritability, and oppositional behavior, causing two of eight children to drop out (Graae *et al.*, 1994).

When overdosed and combined with other sedative drugs like alcohol, they can cause extreme drowsiness, coma, seizures, and possibly even death. When patients take benzodiazepines for extended periods of time they can develop tolerance and dependence. Withdrawal symptoms include anxiety, malaise, irritability, headache, sweating, gastrointestinal symptoms, and muscle tension (Riddle *et al.*, 1999). Withdrawal symptoms can be reduced with gradual tapering. Tapering off of 0.03 mg/kg alprazolam per day across 1–2 weeks did not result in any withdrawal symptoms (Bernstein *et al.*, 1990).

How to do it well

Preliminary work-up

The American Academy of Child and Adolescent Psychiatry has outlined several important principles that should be followed when prescribing psychiatric medication to children and adolescents.[1] Some of these principles are described here. First, a comprehensive psychiatric evaluation is crucial to determining which symptoms need to be treated with medication and which can be treated with psychosocial interventions. The evaluation should include interviews with both the child and their parents (or guardian). A clinician should also review records to see which interventions did or did not work in the past. This is important to determining the next logical step in the patient's treatment.

It is also advised that the prescriber communicate with other medical, mental health, and education professionals involved in the child's care to coordinate their treatment and reduce misunderstandings. Obtaining information from multiple informants helps to develop a more complete picture of the child's disorder. For example, a child with anxiety may be more aware of his or her inner discomfort, but parents and teachers may be more able to explain how the child's functioning is impaired in school and development (AACAP, 2009). There are multiple self-assessment tools for children for diagnosing anxiety disorders, such as the Multidimensional Anxiety Scale for Children (MASC) (March, Parker, Sullivan, Stallings, & Conners, 1997) and the Screen for Child Anxiety Related Emotional Disorders (SCARED) (Birmaher, Brent, Chiappetta, Bridge, Monga, & Baugher, 1999). There are also diagnostic interviews such as the Anxiety Disorders Interview Schedule (Silverman & Albano, 1994), Kiddie-Schedule for Affective Disorder and Schizophrenia (Kaufman *et al.*, 1997), and Diagnostic Interview Schedule for Children (Shaffer, Fisher, Dulcan, & Davies, 1996).

A complete medical history should be taken to rule out the possibility that a medical problem like hypothyroidism is causing psychiatric symptoms. The medical history is also important in determining whether the child is healthy enough to receive a psychiatric medication. For example, the patient may have a history of a cardiac arrhythmia that might influence medication choice. A physical examination by the pediatrician while not specifically required can be useful to allow the pediatrician to see and evaluate the patient before the start of a medication trial. Such an approach is an inclusive one and guarantees that the pediatrician is "in the loop" regarding the medication trial.

Specific medical testing may be appropriate, depending on the medical history, physical examination findings, or the known risks of the specific medication. Before prescribing TCAs, for example, a baseline electrocardiogram may be obtained to identify any rare condition that might increase the risks of these medications. A conservative laboratory work-up prior to initiating medication provides a baseline assessment for comparison later in the course of treatment should a medical problem develop. Also a "clean bill of health" can put both parents and clinicians at ease. By the end of the work-up, the clinician should have a diagnostic formulation that logically explains the various aspects and etiologies of the child's condition, including biological, social, and psychological factors; a treatment plan that encompass both pharmacological and psychosocial treatments for the patient's various symptoms; and a plan in place for monitoring the progress and side effects of the treatment (AACAP, 2009).

Obtaining informed consent

The first step to obtaining informed consent is to provide psycho-education to the patient and family regarding the assessment and treatment plan. The clinician should explain the

---

[1] Substantial portions of this section are based on the AACAP "Practice parameter on the use of psychotropic medication in children and adolescents" written by John Walkup and the Practice Parameter Work Group (AACAP, 2009).

child's disorder, its course, its symptoms, and the long-term prognosis. The clinician should also provide the name of the medication, the starting and estimated ending doses and timing of dose changes, possible side effects and strategies for monitoring and managing them, assessment strategies for monitoring the child's progress, and alternative treatment plans if the medication is unsuccessful. The clinician also explains how the treatment plan fits in with the current evidence base and standard of care, and displays an understanding of any recent controversies surrounding the medication.

It is also important to determine the family's attitude toward medication and directly address any negative feelings to ensure that treatment is properly maintained. A study of parents seeking treatment for children with anxiety disorders ($n = 71$) (Brown, Deacon, Abramowitz, Dammann, & Whiteside, 2007) showed that parents generally prefer CBT to pharmacological interventions and believe that CBT is more effective. Also, parents of children with no past medical treatment perceived pharmacological treatment less favorably than parents of children with a record of past treatment with medication, so these parents may need even more psycho-education.

Following psycho-education of the patient and family, the clinician should document the consent of the patient and family in the patient's medical records. Any subsequent changes to the treatment plan should be explained to the patient and family and consent should again be documented.

Starting the medication

Treatment with medication is considered to have three phases – an acute phase, a maintenance phase, and a discontinuation phase (AACAP, 2009). During the acute phase, medication is started and adjusted upward to a dose that achieves maximum benefit with minimum side effects. During the maintenance phase, recovery occurs, and during the discontinuation phase, medication is tapered without relapse.

Dosing

An adequate medication trial requires the proper dose of medication and the correct duration of treatment. Based on the above SSRIs trials benefit can be observed in the first 3–6 weeks of treatment but extended treatment of 12–16 weeks will be required to identify maximum benefit. Once maximum benefit is achieved children may build on their treatment gains over subsequent months. Maintaining the treatment dose may be required to maintain treatment gains. Any reduction in dose during the maintenance phase of treatment should be followed closely as dose reduction may undermine gains. There are no specific guidelines for dosing children and adolescents with anxiety disorders, but it is recommended that clinicians begin with a low dose and increase based on the patient's response to medication and side effects. Following dosing and maintenance schedules from randomized controlled trials can be useful to avoid using too low a dose or too long a treatment trial, both of which may lead to less than optimal treatment outcome.

During the acute phase of treatment, visits need to be frequent enough for the clinician to monitor the patient for the development of side effects and assess outcome. More frequent visits may be needed for medications that require multiple dose adjustment. Additionally, the clinician should provide psychosocial support for known stressors and address any problems with adherence.

Management of partial or non-response

If a patient does not respond or only partially responds to treatment, the clinician needs to determine the exact reason for this failure – whether the original assessment was inaccurate, the medication trial was not adequate, or the patient adhered poorly to the treatment. Common causes of unexpectedly poor outcome include erroneous assessment, poorly planned and monitored treatment, and inattention to psychosocial factors that impact illness presentation or adherence. Explicitly reviewing critical portions of the assessment, dosing plan, and adherence may be helpful. Consultation may be useful at any point when treatment does not appear to be progressing as expected.

Strategies to improve partial response

There is some evidence that switching SSRIs can be effective in treating non-responders (RUPP, 2002). Also adding CBT to treatment with an SSRI may also increase the chances of symptom reduction (POTS, 2004; Walkup *et al.*, 2008). Evidence for augmenting treatment with another medication is scant, but it is commonly done by prescribers. There are several reasons to use a combination of medications. One is to treat two comorbid disorders. Another is to treat the side effects of one medication with another medication. A third reason is that a combination of two medications may work particularly well for a certain disorder. For example the addition of an antipsychotic to an SSRI may be useful in those with OCD and a tic disorder (McDougle, Epperson, Pelton, Wasylink, & Price, 2000).

Maintenance treatment

During the maintenance phase of treatment, responders should be consolidating their gains and recovering from their disorder. Patients do not need to be seen as frequently during this time. For children who have responded well and adhered well to treatment, visits may be as infrequent as two to four times per year. Children with more stressors in their life or difficulty adhering to the treatment plan may need to be seen more frequently (AACAP, 2009).

Discontinuing medication

Medication should be discontinued if the patient is recovered and no longer requires treatment, if the medication is no longer working, or if the side effects are too severe. Given the lack of randomized controlled trials on discontinuation, recommendations for discontinuing treatment are based on a limited number of maintenance studies (Pine, 2002). For SSRIs, studies have shown that medication treatment up to 1 year is safe and effective. For this reason, a duration of treatment of at least a year could be considered reasonable before discontinuing treatment. Choosing an appropriate time with limited stressors for the discontinuation may minimize the potential for relapse. For example, it might not be helpful to take a child with separation anxiety off medication in the weeks before starting school or during a holiday break. All anti-anxiety medications should be slowly tapered to minimize symptoms of withdrawal. The patient needs to be monitored closely during the period of discontinuation for the return of symptoms, and if symptoms return, re-initiation of medication should be promptly reviewed. Following patients for a period of time after they are off medication insures that patients don't have a recurrence of symptoms and if they do that there is good access to treatment.

Future directions

Optimizing treatment

The majority of randomized controlled trials of anxiolytic medications in children and adolescents investigate only acute treatment over 1–3 months. While medications have proven useful in reducing symptoms, at the end of these trials a substantial number of children have residual symptoms which may be impairing or put them at risk for relapse. Very few studies have focused on how best to address the treatment needs of those who do not respond optimally. Strategies for augmenting treatment with other medication or psychological treatment are needed.

How long to treat

Medication treatments can be extremely helpful but there are limited data on how long to treat. A handful of open-label maintenance studies suggest that longer treatment (up to 1 year) may be useful to maintain medication treatment gains (Cook *et al.*, 2001; RUPP, 2002). Studies to identify those who can discontinue medication without loss of benefit and those who may need even longer treatment to maintain maximal gains are needed.

How early to treat

Analysis of studies following children over two decades showed that mood and anxiety disorders during childhood increase the risk for mood and anxiety disorders later in life (Pine, 2002), suggesting that the early anxiety may lead to poor outcomes later in life. Although it appears reasonable to assume, it is unknown whether early identification and treatment of childhood anxiety improves outcomes in the teen and adult years. More data are also needed to determine the effects of untreated anxiety disorders on the brain versus the effects of medications on the brain's development. Studies in rats showed that fluoxetine admininistered during development had long-lasting effects on both the frontal cortex (Wegerer, Moll, Bagli, Rothenberger, Ruther, & Huether, 1999) and hippocampal dendritic spines (Norrholm & Ouimet, 2001). Other studies have shown that stress during early development (like that experienced in anxiety disorders) also causes changes in brain development in rats (Levine, 1967; Levine & Mullins, 1966).

Personalized treatment

More data are also needed to determine the correct type and sequence of treatment for each patient. For example, for a given patient, what treatment should a clinician start with? How long should CBT be tried before moving onto medication? Which medication is best for whom? If ineffective, should medications be discontinued, changed, or augmented? What are the differences in efficacies between medications within classes? What are possible moderators of treatment outcome? One way to answer some of these questions will be through trials that assess dynamic treatment regimes (Lavori & Dawson, 2004). These trials evaluate the decision-making rules that optimize and individualize treatment for each patient.

Summary

The treatment of childhood anxiety disorders with medication has a long history. There is a convergence of evidence suggesting an important role of serotonin reuptake medications that have a positive benefit-to-risk ratio and are the medication treatment of choice for these conditions. Much more research is needed to personalized treatment with these agents to assure optimal outcome.

References

American Academy of Child and Adolescent Psychiatry (2009). Practice parameter on the use of psychotropic medication in children and adolescents. *Journal of the American Academy of Child and Adolescent Psychiatry*, **48**, 961–973. doi: 10.1097/CHI.0b013e3181ae0a08 00004583–200909000-00017 [pii]

Arabgol, F., Panaghi, L., & Hebrani, P. (2009). Reboxetine versus methylphenidate in treatment of children and adolescents with attention deficit-hyperactivity disorder. *European Child and Adolescent Psychiatry*, **18**, 53–59. doi: 10.1007/s00787–008-0705–9

Armitage, R. (2000). The effects of antidepressants on sleep in patients with depression. *Canadian Journal of Psychiatry*, **45**, 803–809.

Barnett, S. & Riddle, M. A. (2003). Anxiolytics: benzodiazepines, buspirone, and others. In: **A. Martin, L. Scahill, D. S. Charney, & J. F. Leckman** (eds.) *Pediatric Psychopharmacology: Principles and Practice*, pp. 341–351. New York: Oxford University Press.

Beidel, D. C., Turner, S. M., Sallee, F. R., Ammerman, R. T., Crosby, L. A., & Pathak, S. (2007). SET-C versus fluoxetine in the treatment of childhood social phobia. *Journal of American Academy of Child and Adolescent Psychiatry*, **46**, 1622–1632.

Benjamin, R. S., Costello, E. J., & Warren, M. (1990). Anxiety disorders in a pediatric sample. *Journal of Anxiety Disorders*, **4**, 293–316.

Bernstein, G. A., Borchardt, C. M., Perwien, A. R., Crosby, R. D., Kushner, M. G., Thuras, P. D., *et al.* (2000). Imipramine plus cognitive-behavioral therapy in the treatment of school refusal. *Journal of the American Academy of Child and Adolescent Psychiatry*, **39**, 276–283.

Bernstein, G. A., Garfinkel, B. D., & Borchardt, C. M. (1990). Comparative studies of pharmacotherapy for school refusal. *Journal of the American Academy of Child and Adolescent Psychiatry*, **29**, 773–781.

Birmaher, B., Axelson, D. A., Monk, K., Kalas, C., Clark, D. B., Ehmann, M., *et al.* (2003). Fluoxetine for the treatment of childhood anxiety disorders. *Journal of the American Academy of Child and Adolescent Psychiatry*, **42**, 415–423.

Birmaher, B., Brent, D. A., Chiappetta, L., Bridge, J., Monga, S., & Baugher, M. (1999). Psychometric properties of the Screen for Child Anxiety Related Emotional Disorders (SCARED): a replication study. *Journal of the American Academy of Child and Adolescent Psychiatry*, **38**, 1230–1236.

Bridge, J. A., Iyengar, S., Salary, C. B., Barbe, R. P., Birmaher, B., Pincus, H. A., *et al.* (2007). Clinical response and risk for reported suicidal ideation and suicide attempts in pediatric antidepressant treatment: a meta-analysis of randomized controlled trials. *Journal of the American Medical Association*, **297**, 1683–1696.

Brown, A. M., Deacon, B. J., Abramowitz, J. S., Dammann, J., & Whiteside, S. P. (2007). Parents' perceptions of pharmacological and cognitive-behavioral treatments for childhood anxiety disorders. *Behaviour Research and Therapy*, **45**, 819–828. doi: S0005–7967(06)00101-X [pii] 10.1016/j.brat.2006.04.010

Chiu, S. & Leonard, H. (2003). Antidepressant 1: selective serotonin reuptake inhibitors. In: **A. Martin, L. Scahill, D. S. Charney, & J. F. Leckman** (eds.) *Pediatric Psychopharmacology: Principles and Practice*, pp. 274–283. New York: Oxford University Press.

Cook, E. H., Wagner, K. D., March, J. S., Biederman, J., Landau, P., Wolkow, R., *et al.* (2001). Long-term sertraline treatment of children and adolescents with obsessive-compulsive disorder. *Journal of the American Academy of Child and Adolescent Psychiatry*, **40**, 1175–1181.

DeVeaugh-Geiss, J., Moroz, G., Biederman, J., Cantwell, D., Fontaine, R., Greist, J. H., *et al.* (1992). Clomipramine hydrochloride in childhood and adolescent obsessive-compulsive disorder: a multicenter trial. *Journal of the American Academy of Child and Adolescent Psychiatry*, **31**, 45–49.

Donnelly, C. L. (2003). Pharmacologic treatment approaches for children and adolescents with posttraumatic stress disorder. *Child and Adolescent Psychiatric Clinics of North America*, **12**, 251–269.

Fairbanks, J. M., Pine, D. S., Tancer, N. K., Dummit, E. S., III, Kentgen, L. M., Martin, J., *et al.* (1997). Open fluoxetine treatment of mixed anxiety disorders in children and adolescents. *Journal of Child and Adolescent Psychopharmacology*, **7**, 17–29.

Famularo, R., Kinscherff, R., & Fenton, T. (1988). Propranolol treatment for childhood posttraumatic stress disorder, acute type: a pilot study. *American Journal of Diseases of Children*, **142**, 1244–1247.

Garland, E. J., & Baerg, E. A. (2001). Amotivational syndrome associated with selective serotonin reuptake inhibitors in children and adolescents. *Journal of Child and Adolescent Psychopharmacology*, **11**, 181–186.

Garner, E. M., Kelly, M. W., & Thompson, D. F. (1993). Tricyclic antidepressant withdrawal syndrome. *Annals of Pharmacotherapy*, **27**, 1068–1072.

Geller, D. A., Biederman, J., Stewart, S. E., Mullin, B., Farrell, C., Wagner, K. D., *et al.* (2003). Impact of comorbidity on treatment response to paroxetine in pediatric obsessive-compulsive disorder: is the use of exclusion criteria empirically supported in randomized clinical trials? *Journal of Child and Adolescent Psychopharmacology*, **13**(Suppl. 1), S19–S29. doi: 10.1089/104454603322126313

Geller, D., Donnelly, C., Lopez, F., Rubin, R., Newcorn, J., Sutton, V., *et al.* (2007). Atomoxetine treatment for pediatric patients with attention-deficit/hyperactivity disorder with comorbid anxiety disorder. *Journal of the American Academy of Child and Adolescent Psychiatry*, **46**, 1119–1127. doi: 10.1097/chi.0b013e3180ca8385 S0890–8567(09)61930–4 [pii]

Geller, D. A., Hoog, S. L., Heiligenstein, J. H., Ricardi, R. K., Tamura, R., Kluszynski, S., *et al.* (2001). Fluoxetine treatment for obsessive-compulsive disorder in children and adolescents: a placebo-controlled clinical trial. *Journal of the American Academy of Child and Adolescent Psychiatry*, **40**, 773–779.

Geller, D. A., Wagner, K. D., Emslie, G., Murphy, T., Carpenter, D. J., Wetherhold, E., *et al.* (2004). Paroxetine treatment in children and adolescents with obsessive-compulsive disorder: a randomized, multicenter, double-blind, placebo-controlled trial. *Journal of the American Academy of Child and Adolescent Psychiatry*, **43**, 1387–1396.

Gibbons, R. D., Hur, K., Bhaumik, D. K., & Mann, J. J. (2005). The relationship between antidepressant medication use and rate of suicide. *Archives of General Psychiatry*, **62**, 165–172.

Gittelman-Klein, R. & Klein, D. (1971). Controlled imipramine treatment of school phobia. *Archives of General Psychiatry*, **25**, 204.

Graae, F., Milner, J., Rizzotto, L., & Klein, R. G. (1994). Clonazepam in childhood anxiety disorders. *Journal of the American Academy of Child and Adolescent Psychiatry*, **33**, 372–376.

Greene, D. S., Salazar, D. E., Dockens, R. C., Kroboth, P., & Barbhaiya, R. H. (1995). Coadministration of nefazodone and benzodiazepines. III. A pharmacokinetic interaction study with alprazolam. *Journal of Clinical Psychopharmacology*, **15**, 399–408.

Guy, W. (1976). The clinical global impression scale. In: *The ECDEU Assessment Manual for Psychopharmacology – Revised*, Vol. DHEW Publ. No. ADM 76–338, pp. 218–222. Rockville, MD: US Department of Health, Education, and Welfare Public Health Service, Alcohol, Drug Abuse, Mental Health Administration, NIMH Psychopharmacology Research Branch, Division of Extramural Research.

Hammad, T. (2004). Review and evaluation of clinical data: relationship between psychotropic drugs and pediatric suicidality. Available at www.fda.gov/ohrms/dockets/ac/04/briefing/2004–4065b1–10-TAB08-Hammads-Review.pdf.

Hammad, T. A., Laughren, T., & Racoosin, J. (2006). Suicidality in pediatric patients treated with antidepressant drugs. *Archives of General Psychiatry*, **63**, 332–339.

Harmon, R. J. & Riggs, P. D. (1996). Clonidine for posttraumatic stress disorder in preschool children. *Journal of the American Academy of Child and Adolescent Psychiatry*, **35**, 1247–1249. doi: S0890–8567(09)63499–7 [pii] 10.1097/00004583–199609000-00022

Hoehn-Saric, R., Harris, G. J., Pearlson, G. D., Cox, C. S., Machlin, S. R., & Camargo, E. E. (1991). A fluoxetine-induced frontal lobe syndrome in an obsessive compulsive patient. *Journal of Clinical Psychiatry*, **52**, 131–133.

Horrigan, J. P. & Barnhill, L. J. (1999). Risperidone and PTSD in boys. *Journal of Neuropsychiatry and Clinical Neurosciences*, **11**, 126–127.

Ipser, J. C., Stein, D. J., Hawkridge, S., & Hoppe, L. (2009). Pharmacotherapy for anxiety disorders in children and adolescents. *Cochrane Database of Systematic Reviews*, **3**, CD005170. doi: 10.1002/14651858.CD005170.pub2

Jayaram, G. & Rao, P. (2005). Safety of trazodone as a sleep agent for inpatients. *Psychosomatics*, **46**, 367–369. doi: 46/4/367 [pii] 10.1176/appi.psy.46.4.367

Kaufman, J., Birmaher, B., Brent, D., Rao, U., Flynn, C., Moreci, P., *et al.* (1997). Schedule for Affective Disorders and Schizophrenia for School-Age Children-Present and Lifetime Version (K-SADS-PL): initial reliability and validity data. *Journal of the American Academy of Child and Adolescent Psychiatry*, **36**, 980–988.

Klein, R. G., Koplewicz, H. S., & Kanner, A. (1992). Imipramine treatment of children with separation anxiety disorder. *Journal of the American Academy of Child and Adolescent Psychiatry*, **31**, 21–28.

Labellarte, M. J., Ginsburg, G. S., Walkup, J. T., & Riddle, M. A. (1999). The treatment of anxiety disorders in children and adolescents. *Biological Psychiatry*, **46**, 1567–1578. doi: S0006–3223(99)00248–6 [pii]

Lavori, P. W. & Dawson, R. (2004). Dynamic treatment regimes: practical design considerations. *Clinical Trials*, **1**, 9–20.

Leonard, H. L., Goldberger, E. L., Rapoport, J. L., Cheslow, D. L., & Swedo, S. E. (1990). Childhood rituals: normal development or obsessive-compulsive symptoms? *Journal of the American Academy of Child and Adolescent Psychiatry*, **29**, 17–23. doi: S0890–8567(09)65104–2 [pii] 10.1097/00004583–199001000-00004

Levine, S. (1967). Maternal and environmental influences on the adrenocortical response to stress in weanling rats. *Science*, **156**, 258–260.

Levine, S., & Mullins, R. F., Jr. (1966). Hormonal influences on brain organization in infant rats. *Science*, **152**, 1585–1592.

Looff, D., Grimley, P., Kuller, F., Martin, A., & Shonfield, L. (1995). Carbamazepine for PTSD. *Journal of the American Academy of Child and Adolescent Psychiatry*, **34**, 703–704. doi: S0890–8567(09)63566–8 [pii] 10.1097/00004583–199506000-00008

March, J. S., Biederman, J., Wolkow, R., Safferman, A., Mardekian, J., Cook, E. H., *et al.* (1998). Sertraline in children and adolescents with obsessive-compulsive disorder: a multicenter randomized controlled trial. *Journal of the American Medical Association*, **280**, 1752–1756.

March, J. S., Entusah, A. R., Rynn, M., Albano, A. M., & Tourian, K. A. (2007). A randomized controlled trial of venlafaxine ER versus placebo in pediatric social anxiety disorder. *Biological Psychiatry*, **62**, 1149–1154.

March, J. S., Parker, J. D., Sullivan, K., Stallings, P., & Conners, C. K. (1997). The Multidimensional Anxiety Scale for Children (MASC): factor structure, reliability, and validity. *Journal of the American Academy of Child and Adolescent Psychiatry*, **36**, 554–565.

Martin-Du, P. R. & Baumann, P. (2008). [Sexual dysfunctions induced by antidepressants and antipsychotics.] *Revue Medicale Suisse*, **4**, 758–762.

McDougle, C. J., Epperson, C. N., Pelton, G. H., Wasylink, S., & Price, L. H. (2000). A double-blind, placebo-controlled study of risperidone addition in serotonin reuptake inhibitor-refractory obsessive-compulsive disorder. *Archives of General Psychiatry*, **57**, 794–801.

Montgomery, S. A. (1998). Chairman's overview: The place of reboxetine in antidepressant therapy. *Journal of Clinical Psychiatry*, **59**(Suppl. 14), 26–29.

Norrholm, S. D. & Ouimet, C. C. (2001). Altered dendritic spine density in animal models of depression and in response to antidepressant treatment. *Synapse*, **42**, 151–163.

Papakostas, G. I., Stahl, S. M., Krishen, A., Seifert, C. A., Tucker, V. L., Goodale, E. P., *et al.* (2008). Efficacy of bupropion and the selective serotonin reuptake inhibitors in the treatment of major depressive disorder with high levels of anxiety (anxious depression): a pooled analysis of 10 studies. *Journal of Clinical Psychiatry*, **69**, 1287–1292. doi: ej07m03773 [pii]

Pine, D. S. (2002). Treating children and adolescents with selective serotonin reuptake inhibitors: how long is appropriate? *Journal of Child and Adolescent Psychopharmacology*, **12**, 189–203.

Pediatric OCD Treatment Study (2004). Cognitive–behavior therapy, sertraline, and their combination for children and adolescents with obsessive-compulsive disorder: the Pediatric OCD Treatment Study (POTS) randomized controlled trial. *Journal of the American Medical Association*, **292**, 1969–1976.

Preskorn, S. H. (2000). Imipramine, mirtazapine, and nefazodone: multiple targets. *Journal of Practical Psychiatry and Behavioral Health*, March, 97–102.

Reinblatt, S. P., dosReis, S., Walkup, J. T., & Riddle, M. A. (2009). Activation adverse events induced by the selective serotonin reuptake inhibitor fluvoxamine in children and adolescents. *Journal of Child and Adolescent Psychopharmacology*, **19**, 119–126. doi: 10.1089/cap.2008.040

Reinblatt, S. P. & Walkup, J. T. (2005). Psychopharmacologic treatment of pediatric anxiety disorders. *Child and Adolescent Psychiatric Clinics of North America*, **14**, 877–908.

Reiter, S. & Kutcher, S. P. (1991). Disinhibition and anger outbursts in adolescents treated with clonazepam. *Journal of Clinical Psychopharmacology*, **11**, 268.

Riddle, M. A., Bernstein, G. A., Cook, E. H., Leonard, H. L., March, J. S., & Swanson, J. M. (1999). Anxiolytics, adrenergic agents, and naltrexone. *Journal of the American Academy of Child and Adolescent Psychiatry*, **38**, 546–556.

Riddle, M. A., Geller, B., & Ryan, N. (1993). Another sudden death in a child treated with desipramine. *Journal of the American Academy of Child and Adolescent Psychiatry*, **32**, 792–797.

Riddle, M. A., Reeve, E. A., Yaryura-Tobias, J. A., Yang, H. M., Claghorn, J. L., Gaffney, G., *et al.* (2001). Fluvoxamine for children and adolescents with obsessive-compulsive disorder: a randomized, controlled, multicenter trial. *Journal of the American Academy of Child and Adolescent Psychiatry*, **40**, 222–229.

Robert, R., Blakeney, P. E., Villarreal, C., Rosenberg, L., & Meyer, W. J., III (1999). Imipramine treatment in pediatric burn patients with symptoms of acute stress disorder: a pilot study. *Journal of the American Academy of Child and Adolescent Psychiatry*, **38**, 873–882. doi: S0890–8567(09)66537–0 [pii] 10.1097/00004583–199907000-00018

Rotzinger, S., Fang, J., & Baker, G. B. (1998). Trazodone is metabolized to m-chlorophenylpiperazine by CYP3A4 from human sources. *Drug Metabolism and Disposition*, **26**, 572–575.

Rotzinger, S., Fang, J., Coutts, R. T., & Baker, G. B. (1998). Human CYP2D6 and metabolism of m-chlorophenylpiperazine. *Biological Psychiatry*, **44**, 1185–1191. doi: S0006–3223(97)00483–6 [pii]

Research Unit on Pediatric Psychopharmacology (2001). Fluvoxamine for the treatment of anxiety disorders in children and adolescents: the Research Unit on Pediatric Psychopharmacology Anxiety Study Group. *New England Journal of Medicine*, **344**, 1279–1285.

Research Unit on Pediatric Psychopharmacology (RUPP) (2002). Treatment of pediatric anxiety disorders: an open-label extension of the research units on pediatric psychopharmacology anxiety study. *Journal of Child and Adolescent Psychopharmacology*, **12**, 175–188.

Rynn, M. A., Riddle, M. A., Yeung, P. P., & Kunz, N. R. (2007). Efficacy and safety of extended-release venlafaxine in the treatment of generalized anxiety disorder in children and adolescents: two placebo-controlled trials. *American Journal of Psychiatry*, **164**, 290–300.

Safer, D. J. & Zito, J. M. (2006). Treatment-emergent adverse events from selective serotonin reuptake inhibitors by age group: children versus adolescents. *Journal of Child and Adolescent Psychopharmacology*, **16**, 159–169. doi: 10.1089/cap.2006.16.159

Scahill, L., Riddle, M. A., McSwiggin-Hardin, M., Ort, S. I., King, R. A., Goodman, W. K., et al. (1997). Children's Yale-Brown Obsessive Compulsive Scale: reliability and validity. *Journal of the American Academy of Child and Adolescent Psychiatry*, **36**, 844–852.

Scharko, A. M. (2004). Selective serotonin reuptake inhibitor-induced sexual dysfunction in adolescents: a review. *Journal of the American Academy of Child and Adolescent Psychiatry*, **43**, 1071–1079. doi: S0890–8567(09)61441–6 [pii] 10.1097/01.chi.0000131135.70992.58

Seedat, S., Stein, D. J., Ziervogel, C., Middleton, T., Kaminer, D., Emsley, R. A., et al. (2002). Comparison of response to a selective serotonin reuptake inhibitor in children, adolescents, and adults with posttraumatic stress disorder. *Journal of Child and Adolescent Psychopharmacology*, **12**, 37–46.

Shaffer, D., Fisher, P., Dulcan, M. K., & Davies, M. (1996). The NIMH Diagnostic Interview Schedule for Children Version 2.3 (DISC-2.3): description, acceptability, prevalence rates, and performance in the MECA study. *Journal of the American Academy of Child and Adolescent Psychiatry*, **35**, 865–877.

Silverman, W. K. & Albano, A. M. (1994). *The Anxiety Disorders Interview Schedule for DSM-IV: Research and Lifetime Version for Children and Parents (ADIS-RLV)*. New York: Columbia University.

Simeon, J. G. & Ferguson, H. B. (1987). Alprazolam effects in children with anxiety disorders. *Canadian Journal of Psychiatry*, **32**, 570–574.

Spencer, T., Biederman, J., Coffey, B., Geller, D., Crawford, M., Bearman, S. K., et al. (2002). A double-blind comparison of desipramine and placebo in children and adolescents with chronic tic disorder and comorbid attention-deficit/hyperactivity disorder. *Archives of General Psychiatry*, **59**, 649–656.

Velosa, J. F. & Riddle, M. A. (2000). Pharmacologic treatment of anxiety disorders in children and adolescents. *Child and Adolescent Psychiatric Clinics of North America*, **9**, 119–133.

Wagner, K. D., Berard, R., Stein, M. B., Wetherhold, E., Carpenter, D. J., Perera, P., et al. (2004). A multicenter, randomized, double-blind, placebo-controlled trial of paroxetine in children and adolescents with social anxiety disorder. *Archives of General Psychiatry*, **61**, 1153–1162.

Walkup, J. & Labellarte, M. (2001). Complications of SSRI treatment. *Journal of Child and Adolescent Psychopharmacology*, **11**, 1–4.

Walkup, J. T., Albano, A. M., Piacentini, J., Birmaher, B., Compton, S. N., Sherrill, J. T., et al. (2008). Cognitive behavioral therapy, sertraline, or a combination in childhood anxiety. *New England Journal of Medicine*, **359**, 2753–2766.

Wegerer, V., Moll, G. H., Bagli, M., Rothenberger, A., Ruther, E., & Huether, G. (1999). Persistently increased density of serotonin transporters in the frontal cortex of rats treated with fluoxetine during early juvenile life. *Journal of Child and Adolescent Psychopharmacology*, **9**, 13–24; discussion 25–26.

Wilens, T. E., Biederman, J., Baldessarini, R. J., Geller, B., Schleifer, D., Spencer, T. J., *et al.* (1996). Cardiovascular effects of therapeutic doses of tricyclic antidepressants in children and adolescents. *Journal of the American Academy of Child and Adolescent Psychiatry*, **35**, 1491–1501.

18

Treatment: an update and recommendations

Wendy K. Silverman and Luci M. Motoca

Introduction

In the psychosocial treatment chapter included in the previous edition of this volume, Silverman and Berman (2001) reviewed results of 10 randomized clinical trials. Each of these trials had evaluated cognitive–behavioral treatment (CBT) procedures to reduce anxiety disorders in children and adolescents (hereafter referred to as youth). Most of the trials compared CBT to a wait-list control condition (WLC). Several additional trials evaluated the efficacy of CBT using an individual treatment approach, either with or without (or minimal) parent involvement (Barrett, Dadds, & Rapee, 1996; Kendall, 1994; Kendall, Flannery-Schroeder, Panichelli-Mindel, Southam-Gerow, Henin, & Warman, 1997; King *et al.*, 1998). Several evaluated the efficacy of CBT using a group treatment approach, again, either with or without (or minimal) parent involvement (Barrett, 1998; Flannery-Schroeder & Kendall, 2000; Mendlowitz, Manassis, Bradley, Scapillato, Miezitis, & Shaw, 1999; Silverman, Kurtines, Ginsburg, Weems, Lumpkin, & Carmichael, 1999). From their review, Silverman and Berman (2001) concluded that these randomized clinical trials produced strong and consistent evidence that CBT, using either an individual or group approach, was more efficacious than WLCs in reducing anxiety disorders in youth. Silverman and Berman (2001) further concluded that the efficacy of CBT might be enhanced by involving parents in the treatment process; however, they noted the need for more research on this issue.

Silverman and Berman (2001) also summarized the results of two studies that went beyond WLCs. Each compared CBT to an active and credible comparison control condition – education support (Last, Hansen, & Franco, 1998; Silverman *et al.*, 1999a). Last *et al.* (1998) used a sample of youth with school refusal behavior. Silverman, Kurtines, Ginsburg, Weems, Rabian, & Serafini (1999) used a sample of youth with phobic disorders and compared two variants of CBT (self-control and contingency management) to education support. Both Last *et al.* (1998) and Silverman, Kurtines, Ginsburg, Weems, Rabian, *et al.* (1999) found significant gains were produced in the CBT and education support conditions, with no significant differences between conditions on most of the main outcome measures. In light of these findings, Silverman and Berman (2001) called for more randomized clinical trials that used active and credible comparison control conditions to help determine the robustness and generalizability of the Last *et al.* (1998) and Silverman, Kurtines, Ginsburg, Weems, Rabian, *et al.* (1999) findings.

Silverman and Berman (2001) also noted that research is needed to determine whether the positive findings obtained in university-based clinics would generalize to community-based clinics. Additionally, Silverman and Berman (2001) noted a dearth of research evaluating potential predictors, mediators, and moderators of positive child treatment outcome. They called for further research in these areas as well.

Because other evaluative reviews have appeared since publication of Silverman and Berman (2001), we refer the reader directly to these reviews for summaries of these subsequent randomized clinical trials (Barmish & Kendall, 2005; Cartwright-Hatton, Roberts, Chitsabesan, Fothergill, & Harrington, 2004; Creswell & Cartwright-Hatton, 2007; In-Albon & Schneider, 2007; James, Soler, & Weatherall, 2005; Nevo & Manassis, 2009; Pahl & Barrett, 2010; Rapee, Schniering, & Hudson, 2009; Silverman, Pina, & Viswesvaran, 2008). Our aim in this chapter is to provide a summary of clinical trials that were *not* covered in these evaluative reviews. In a few instances however we refer back to a few earlier trials because they serve as backdrops for subsequent follow-up studies, which are summarized in this chapter.

Thus, in this chapter, we summarize comparative treatment research studies that focused on the relative efficacy of (1) CBT compared to active and credible comparison control conditions; (2) individual CBT (ICBT) to group CBT (GCBT); and (3) CBT to pharmacological treatment (see Pelligrino, Pierce, & Walkup, Chapter 17, this volume for more detailed coverage of this last topic). Because several of these studies contained a treatment condition that included parent or family involvement (Bodden *et al.*, 2008; Kendall, Hudson, Gosch, Flannery-Schroeder, & Suveg, 2008; Silverman, Kurtines, Jaccard, & Pina, 2009; Wood, McLeod, Piacentini, & Sigman, 2009; Wood, Piacentini, Southam-Gerow, Chu, & Sigman, 2006), we also take another look at whether parent or family involvement enhances treatment effects compared to no (or minimal) parent or family involvement. We also update the work that has been conducted on evaluating potential predictors, mediators, and moderator of treatment outcome. We also include a summary of recent, innovative approaches for CBT delivery (i.e., Internet-based and computer-assisted).

As will be apparent from reading this chapter, a great deal of progress has been made since Silverman and Berman (2001). Nevertheless, more work is needed on several fronts. We highlight these fronts throughout the chapter. We now begin below with a brief overview of the main characteristics of the youth anxiety treatment research studies.

Main characteristics of youth anxiety treatment research

All the youth anxiety randomized trials used manualized CBT protocols and most often targeted the most prevalent anxiety disorders of childhood and adolescence: separation anxiety disorder (SAD), social phobia (SOP), generalized anxiety disorder (GAD), and specific phobias (SP). A few studies targeted a specific disorder, usually SOP or SP. Youth participants varied in age, within and across studies, with the age range usually from 6 to 17 years. The majority of participants were European Americans though a few studies contained high proportions of minority populations (e.g., Pina, Silverman, Fuentes, Kurtines, & Weems, 2003; see Silverman *et al.*, 2008 for review). These studies support the efficacy of CBT with these minority populations as well. Doctoral students, psychologists, or psychiatrists typically served as therapists, all of whom were carefully trained in using CBT. Treatment sessions most often ranged from 10 to 16 sessions and were 60 to 120 minutes in length.

The main components of the CBT protocols were: (1) having the child engage in graded exposures (in vivo or imaginary) and (2) assisting the child in developing coping and cognitive self-control strategies. When delivered in a group format, CBT programs emphasized social skills and assertiveness training. Studies with active parent involvement are referred to in this chapter as CBT/P, even though investigators might have referred to them as "family" CBT. Studies varied regarding whether the mother or both parents were involved in CBT/P. We identified only one study that involved the entire family, which we refer to as CBT/F (Bodden *et al.*, 2008); siblings attended three sessions along with the targeted child and parents. As summarized by Barmish and Kendall (2005), CBT/P and CBT/F most often emphasized at least one or more of the following: (1) teaching parents to remove their reinforcement of the child's anxious or avoidant behaviors, (2) reducing parent–child conflict, and (3) training parents to manage their own anxiety.

The most common outcomes across studies were diagnostic recovery rates (i.e., present/absent) assessed most often using the Anxiety Disorders Interview Schedule for DSM-IV: Child and Parent Versions (ADIS-C/P: Silverman & Albano, 1996) (see Fonseca & Perrin, Chapter 2, this volume). Common clinician outcomes were symptom severity ratings assessed using global ratings of impairment such as the clinician severity ratings (CSRs) on the ADIS-C/P, Children's Global Assessment Scale (C-GAS: Bird, Shaffer, Fisher, Gould, Staghezza, & Chen, 1993), and Clinician Global Impression – Improvement Scale (CGI-I: Guy & Bonato, 1970). Less commonly used were the Clinician Global Impression – Severity Scale (CGI-S: Guy & Bonato, 1970) and the Pediatric Anxiety Rating Scale (PARS: RUPP Anxiety Study Group, 2002).

Youth anxiety symptoms assessed using youth self-rating scales were other common primary outcomes. The Revised Children's Manifest Anxiety Scale (RCMAS: Reynolds & Richmond, 1978) and more recently, the Multidimensional Anxiety Scale for Children (MASC: March, Parker, Sullivan, Stallings, & Conners, 1997) have been most widely used. The Spence Children's Anxiety Scale (SCAS: Spence, 1998) has been widely used in the Australian studies.

Youths' symptoms from the parents' perspective also have been assessed most with the Child Behavior Checklist (CBCL) Internalizing broad-band scale, the Anxiety–Depression (A/D) narrow-band scale, or both (Achenbach, 1991). The parallel subscales on the Teacher Report Form (TRF: Achenbach & Edelbrock, 1986) have been used to assess teachers' perspectives. Several studies used other youth and/or parent rating scales, including the Strengths and Difficulties Questionnaire – Emotional Symptoms scale (SDQ-E: Goodman, 1997), State Trait Anxiety Inventory for Children (STAIC: Spielberger, 1973), Screen for Child Anxiety Related Emotional Disorders (SCARED: Birmaher *et al.*, 1997), and Social Phobia and Anxiety Inventory (SPAI: Beidel, Turner, & Morris, 1995).

Youth anxiety assessed using direct observation procedures, social evaluative tasks, behavioral approach tasks (BATs), and parent–youth interaction tasks, were additional outcomes in several trials (Barrett *et al.*, 1996; Beidel, Turner, & Morris, 2000; Beidel, Turner, Sallee, Ammerman, Crosby, & Pathak, 2007; Kendall, 1994; Ollendick, Öst, Reuter-skiöld, Costa, Cederlund, & Sirbu, 2009; Öst, Svensson, Hellström, & Lindwall, 2001). With regard to social evaluative tasks (Beidel *et al.*, 2000; Beidel *et al.*, 2007; Kendall, 1994), youth are asked to make a verbal presentation in front of a small audience and/or engage in a role-play scene with same-age peers. With regard to BATs (Ollendick *et al.*, 2009; Öst *et al.*, 2001), phobic youth are asked to approach or confront the feared stimulus in the clinic setting. With regard to the parent–youth interaction tasks (Barrett *et al.*, 1996), parents and their children engage in problem-solving situations. The reader is referred to Silverman and Ollendick (2005) for further details regarding direct observation procedures used with youth with phobic and anxiety disorders.

The most common secondary outcomes in the clinical trials were youth self-ratings of other emotional problems, including depression using the Children's Depression Inventory (CDI: Kovacs, 1992) and fear using the Fear Survey Schedule for Children – Revised (FSSC-R: Ollendick, 1983). Measures relating to children's coping also have been administered in a number of studies (e.g., child and parent versions of the Coping Questionnaire, CQ-C, CQ-P: P. C. Kendall & A. Marrs-Garcia, unpublished data; Children's Automatic Thoughts Scale (CATS: Schniering & Rapee, 2002). We now proceed with narrative summaries of the treatment research studies.

Comparative research outcomes studies

CBT compared to active, credible comparison control conditions
Parent-child GCBT versus parent-child group active control

Hudson, Rapee, Deveney, Schniering, Lyneham, and Bovopoulous (2009) randomized 112 youth (7 to 16 years) to either GCBT ($n = 60$) or an active, credible comparison control condition, Group Support and Attention (GSA: $n = 52$). GSA emphasized a supportive environment, activities to help youth express and understand emotions, and building relationships between and within participating families.

No statistically significant differences were found between GCBT and GSA in diagnostic recovery rates of the primary anxiety disorder at post-treatment: GCBT's recovery rate was 45.1% and GSA's was 29.6%. There also were no statistically significant differences between GCBT and GSA on youth-rated SCAS and SDQ-E at post-treatment and 3-month follow-up. However, statistically significant differences in diagnostic recovery rates of the primary anxiety disorder were found at 3-month follow-up (68.7% GCBT; 45.5% GSA), which the authors noted suggest a strengthening of GCBT's treatment effects on primary diagnostic recovery rates over time.

When it came to all anxiety disorders (not just primary), statistically significant differences in diagnostic recovery rates were found between GCBT and GSA at post-treatment (33.3% GCBT; 15.9% GSA), as well as 3-month follow-up (49.0% GCBT; 29.6% GSA). GCBT also showed significant improvement relative to GSA at post-treatment on CSRs and mother-rated SCAS and SDQ-E, though these differences were no longer significant at 3-month follow-up.

The overall pattern of findings in Hudson *et al.* (2009), using a group format, was thus similar to those of Last *et al.* (1998) and Silverman, Kurtines, Ginsburg, Weems, Rabian, *et al.* (1999), both of which used an individual format: an active comparison control condition resulted in positive treatment response. However, Hudson *et al.* (2009) showed this to be the case with youth diagnosed with a broader range of anxiety disorders including SAD, SOP, GAD, panic disorder, and SP. (Recall Last *et al.* showed this with school refusers; Silverman *et al.* showed this with phobics.) Further, except for diagnostic recovery rates of all anxiety disorders, the differences that were found between GCBT and GSA disappeared at 3-month follow-up. These findings highlight the same point made by Silverman and Berman (2001): there is need for additional research using credible active control conditions, as evidence for CBT dampens when CBT has been compared to such controls relative to WLCs.

One-session CBT versus active comparison control condition for specific phobia

In a multisite study conducted in the USA and Sweden, Ollendick *et al.* (2009) randomized 196 youth (7 to 16 years) with a primary diagnosis of SP to a single session of behavioral exposure treatment, referred to as One-Session Treatment (OST: $n = 85$), a single session of Education Support Treatment (EST: $n = 70$), or WLC ($n = 41$). Findings revealed that youth in OST and EST displayed significantly greater improvements than youth in the WLC on diagnostic recovery rates and CSRs from pre- to post-treatment. Other than these couple of positive effects, however, there was no superiority shown by OST over either EST or WLC on any of the other study measures (i.e., youth FSSC-R, MASC, and CDI ratings; parent CBCL-A/D and CBCL-I ratings; youth self-ratings of anxiety prior to the BATs and percentage of steps completed on the BATs).

With respect to significant pre- to post-treatment differences between OST and EST, OST outperformed EST on diagnostic recovery rates, CSRs, youth ratings of anxiety prior to the BATs, and youth and parent ratings of treatment satisfaction. However, no significant differences were found between OST and EST on any youth and parent rating scale, as well as on the percentage of steps completed on the BATs. Treatment gains were maintained at 6-month follow-up, with OST now outperforming EST only on diagnostic recovery rates and CSRs.

Ollendick *et al.* (2009) suggest that the overall lack of superior outcomes of OST relative to EST and WLC at both post-treatment and 6-month follow-up on the youth and parent rating scales may be explained in part by floor effects on these measures (i.e., the measures' pre-treatment means were all in the normative ranges, making change less likely). The failure of Ollendick *et al.* to find superiority of the two active conditions to the WLC on the majority of measures is an inconsistency when compared to past studies. These findings serve to highlight the importance of not just conducting more research using active credible comparison controls, but also conducting more research that examines participants' utilization of specific treatment strategies. Such research will help to discern what exactly participants are doing when they are randomized to particular arms of randomized trials, including WLCs. Also important is to ensure that comparison control conditions do not contain the hypothesized key change producing procedures of CBT (e.g., exposure), a concern noted earlier by Silverman, Kurtines, Ginsburg, Weems, Rabian, *et al.* (1999).

CBT with parent/family involvement compared to CBT with no (or minimal) parent/family involvement

CBT/P versus ICBT

Two studies compared CBT with parent involvement (CBT/P) to CBT with no (or minimal) parental involvement (ICBT) (Silverman *et al.*, 2009; Wood *et al.*, 2006). Wood *et al.* (2006) randomized 40 youth (ages 6 to 13) to either CBT/P ($n = 20$) or ICBT ($n = 20$). There were no statistically significant differences between the two treatments on diagnostic recovery rates of all anxiety disorders (78.9% CBT/P; 52.6% ICBT). However, significant pre- to post-treatment improvements were found for both treatments on the youth- and parent-rated MASC, as well as clinician-rated CSRs and CGI-I, with CBT/P significantly outperforming ICBT on all measures except the youth MASC.

In a 12-month follow-up, Wood *et al.* (2009) reported data for 35 (92%) of the treatment completers. A similar pattern of findings was obtained. There were no statistically significant differences between the two treatments on diagnostic recovery rates of all anxiety disorders. Again, however, CBT/P was superior to ICBT on the same measures as in Wood *et al.* (2006).

These were parent but not youth-rated MASC, and clinician rated CSRs and CGI-I. Overall then, involving parents in their child's treatment resulted in enhanced post-treatment and follow-up effects on clinician and parent ratings, but not diagnostic recovery rates and not youth ratings.

To help explain the lack of differential treatment effects on the youth self-ratings at post-treatment and 12-month follow-up, Wood *et al.* (2009) suggest these findings may partly reflect limitations of youth self-report data. However, the reason why youth ratings often have yielded positive effects coupled with the lack of statistically significant differences between CBT/P and ICBT in other past CBT trials makes this point somewhat ambiguous. Wood *et al.* (2009) further suggest that although clinician ratings were informed by both youth and parent interviews, parents in CBT/P likely influenced clinician ratings more, resulting in lower CSRs and higher CGI-I ratings in CBT/P than ICBT. This point highlights the importance of carefully training independent evaluators when conducting post-treatment and follow-up assessments in an effort to minimize potential biases in respondents' reports.

Further, we concur with Wood *et al.* (2009) for the need for improved measurement, as extant measures are certainly not sensitive enough in detecting the diverse skills that are being targeted in treatment programs. Further, there now are available advanced statistics to evaluate more fully the degree of systematic source and error effects in assessing child and adolescent anxiety outcomes, which ought to be more often utilized. There also is need to move beyond evaluating treatment outcome based on diagnoses and symptoms, towards also evaluating whether the treatment had meaningful impact on adaptive functioning (Silverman & Hinshaw, 2008).

In another randomized trial, Silverman *et al.* (2009) compared CBT/P ($n = 59$) to ICBT ($n = 60$) in youth 7 to 16 years of age. This study moved beyond the investigation of efficacy to examine preliminarily the directionality of change between youth anxiety and parent variables from pre- and post-treatment to 12-month follow-up. In this section, we summarize the efficacy results.

Overall, there were no statistically significant differences between CBT/P and ICBT: 78.4% of youth across both treatments were free of their primary anxiety diagnosis at post-treatment, and 91% at 12-month follow-up. Also across both treatments, 83% and 77% of youth fell below the clinical cut-off scores on the C-GAS and mother-rated CBCL-A/D. Pre- to post-treatment improvements also were observed on youth and parent RCMAS and parent CBCL-A/D, with no significant differences between conditions. Treatment gains were maintained at 12-month follow-up on all measures. The pattern of findings of Silverman *et al.* (2009) was therefore different from Wood *et al.* (2006) and Wood *et al.* (2009): in Silverman *et al.* (2009) involving parents in the child's treatment did not lead to any enhanced treatment effects.

CBT/P versus ICBT versus active comparison control condition

Kendall *et al.* (2008) compared the relative efficacy of CBT/P ($n = 56$), ICBT ($n = 55$), and an active comparison control condition, Education, Support, and Attention with Parents, or ESA/P ($n = 50$) in reducing youth anxiety (7 to 14 years). Significant pre- to post-treatment improvements were found in all three conditions on diagnostic recovery rates, CSRs, youth ratings on the MASC and CQ-C, mother and father ratings on the CBCL-I, CBCL-Anxiety (an anxiety scale derived by Kendall *et al.*, 2008), and CQ-P, and teacher ratings on the TRF-I and TRF-Anxiety (also derived by Kendall *et al.*, 2008). Only on diagnostic recovery rates and CSRs did the two CBTs differ significantly from ESA/P pre- to post-treatment.

The two CBTs differed significantly from one another only on teacher ratings, with ICBT showing superior performance. Kendall *et al.* (2008) suggest this latter finding is due to ICBT leading to changes that are especially visible in the school environment, though why this would occur more in ICBT than CBT/P was not further explained. Further, in Kendall (1994), the TRF was the only measure in which statistically greater pre- to post-treatment improvement in ICBT relative to WLC was not observed. Certainly, more research using teacher ratings is needed, as they have not been used as much as youth and parent ratings.

In Kendall *et al.*'s (2008) 12-month follow-up, there continued to be no statistically significant differences between the two CBTs and ESA/P on youth, mother, and father ratings, as well as now on diagnostic recovery rates and CSRs. Also at 12-month follow-up, there no longer were differential effects between ICBT and CBT/P on teacher reports using the TRF. These findings therefore align with Silverman *et al.* (2009), but not Wood *et al.* (2006, 2009), in that the overall pattern was that involving parents in the child's treatment did not lead to enhanced treatment effects.

Just as importantly, similar to other studies using education support conditions (Hudson *et al.*, 2009; Khanna & Kendall, 2010; Last *et al.*, 1998; Silverman, Kurtines, Ginsburg, Weems, Rabian, *et al.*, 1999; Ollendick *et al.*, 2009), there were no statistically significant differences between the active comparison control condition and CBT on any measure of anxiety symptoms from any source at post-treatment and 12-month follow-up. A similar pattern of findings were obtained at 12-month follow-up with one exception: significantly greater gains from post-treatment to 12-month follow-up were found in CBT/P than ESA/P on the TRF.

In explaining their study's findings, Kendall *et al.* (2008) note that treatment integrity checks indicated that ESA/P consisted of 65% CBT. In other words, according to the authors, ESA/P was not necessarily delivered to participants in a way to make it fully distinguishable from CBT. Because ESA/P was administered by therapists trained in CBT, Kendall *et al.* (2008) suggest future studies use comparison control therapists who are naïve to CBT. The other points we made above under our discussion of Ollendick *et al.* (2009) apply here as well.

CBT/F versus ICBT

In a sample of 128 youth (8 to 17 years) referred to community mental health clinics, Bodden *et al.* (2008) examined the efficacy and partial effectiveness of CBT/F ($n = 64$) and ICBT ($n = 64$) Nineteen of these families were initially randomized to an 8–12-week WLC, and still had anxiety disorders after waiting. Bodden *et al.* refer to their study as a partial effectiveness trial because youth were non-recruited clinic referred and treatments were performed by representative practitioners from clinical care settings.

Both CBT/F and ICBT displayed significantly greater improvements than the WLC. ICBT displayed significantly greater improvements than CBT/F on recovery rates of the primary diagnoses (70% ICBT; 41% CBT/F) and all anxiety disorder diagnoses (53% ICBT; 28% CBT/F), CSRs, and recovery rates using clinical cut-off scores of youth-rated STAI (ICBT 97%; CBT/F 83%). On all the other study measures, however, there were no statistically significant differences between treatment conditions. These include youth-rated SCARED, STAI, and CATS and combined mother- and father-rated SCARED, STAI, and CBCL-I, and recovery rates using clinical cut-off scores on some of the youth and parent rating scales.

Fifty-two percent of youth across both conditions maintained treatment gains at 3-month follow-up assessment. However, at the follow-up, there were no longer any differences at all between the two CBTs. The only exception was clinically significant change using combined mother and father CBCL-I (ICBT 91%; CBT/F 75%). Overall, similar to Kendall *et al.* (2008) and Silverman *et al.* (2009) involving families in the child's treatment did not account for enhanced treatment effects. To the contrary, ICBT was superior to CBT/F, albeit on only a small number of measures.

CBT using individual or group treatment approaches
ICBT versus GCBT

Liber, Van Widenfelt, Utens, Ferdinand, Van Der Leeden, and Van Gastel (2008) randomized 127 children (8 to 12 years) to ICBT ($n = 62$) or GCBT ($n = 65$). Both treatments included parent psycho-education sessions. There were no statistically significant differences between ICBT and GCBT on diagnostic recovery rates of the primary anxiety disorder (ICBT 62%; GCBT 54%), all anxiety disorders (48% ICBT; 41% GCBT), youth-rated MASC, CDI, and mother- and father-rated CBCL-I. Follow-up data were not reported. Based on the findings, Liber, Van Widenfelt, Utens, *et al.* (2008) concluded that CBT is efficacious whether delivered using an individual and group approach; however, they acknowledged the absence of retest and inter-rater reliability of diagnoses, among others, as study limitations.

Liber and colleagues' (2008) findings are generally consistent with past studies' findings (Flannery-Schroeder & Kendall, 2000; Manassis *et al.*, 2002). However, the absence of follow-up data in Liber, Van Widenfelt, Utens, *et al.* (2008) and Manassis *et al.* (2002) indicates the need for further ICBT and GCBT comparative research to investigate maintenance of treatment gains over time.

CBT compared to pharmacological treatment
CBT versus sertraline versus combined treatment versus placebo therapy

Walkup *et al.* (2008) randomized 488 youth (7 to 17 years) to ICBT ($n = 139$), sertraline ($n = 133$), ICBT in combination with sertraline ($n = 140$), or a placebo pill control condition ($n = 76$), in the Child/Adolescent Anxiety Multimodal Treatment Study (CAMS). CAMS is the first multisite, randomized controlled clinical trial to integrate selective serotonin reuptake inhibitors (SSRIs) and placebo in the treatment of GAD, SAD, and SOP. Treatment conditions varied by number and length of sessions (not a trivial point when interpreting the results). ICBT consisted of 14 sessions, 60 minutes in length. Sertraline alone and placebo alone consisted of eight sessions, 30 to 60 minutes in length. The combined treatment consisted of 14 sessions of ICBT 60 minutes in length plus eight sessions of sertraline 30 to 60 minutes in length. The combined treatment sessions were administered as much as possible on the same day, but not always. This resulted in a greater number of participant study visits in the ICBT plus sertraline condition than in the other conditions.

All three active treatments were superior to the placebo condition on the reported outcomes: the CGI-I, CGI-S, C-GAS, and PARS. On the CGI-I, 59.7% of ICBT participants, 54.9% of sertraline participants, 80.7% of combined ICBT and sertraline participants, and 23.7% of placebo participants were rated by clinicians as "improved or very much improved." All three conditions were statistically superior to the placebo, with the combined treatment being significantly different from the three other conditions. The authors conclude:

Our findings indicate that as compared with placebo, the three active therapies – combination therapy with both cognitive behavioral therapy and sertraline, cognitive behavioral therapy alone, and sertraline alone – are effective short-term treatments for children with separation and generalized anxiety disorders and social phobia, with combination treatment having superior response rates. (Walkup *et al.*, 2008, p. 2764)

Despite the critical importance of CAMS to the field, it is worth noting the study's main limitations. From our perspective, a key limitation is that only youths and parents who received either sertraline or placebo were blinded to their condition. The potential for expectancy effects cannot be ruled out. The use of independent evaluators was intended to counteract the unblinded nature of these two treatments. However, the same independent evaluators conducted the pretreatment assessment, as well as "all future assessments (Compton *et al.*, 2010, p. 5). Overall, then, it is unclear to us whether the use of independent evaluators, especially the same evaluators across assessment points, adequately reduces the potential of unwanted expectancy effects – on the part of youth and parent participants as well as the evaluators.

CAMS also examined the safety of pharmacological treatment of anxiety disorders. The combined treatment condition was characterized by the most reports of adverse events. Sertraline alone had significantly more adverse events than ICBT, though not significantly more than placebo. Walkup *et al.* (2008) suggest the number of adverse events in the combined treatment condition could have been inflated by the number of study visits and increased reporting opportunities, both of which were statistically significant greater in this condition than the other three conditions.

Research is needed to determine, not only the short-term, but also the long-term comparative efficacy of the treatments. Additional analyses using other outcomes beyond the clinician ratings also are critically important. We assume such work is in preparation and we are excited about summarizing this work in the third edition of this book. A follow-up study to determine this issue is in progress by the CAMS investigative team and we look forward to these findings as well. In addition, research is needed to determine the optimal duration of pharmacotherapy, as well as the most efficacious sequencing of medication regimens and CBT, including their combination. Pelligrino, Pierce, and Walkup (Chapter 17, this volume) elaborate on these and other directions for future pharmacological treatment research.

Long-term follow-up studies of CBT

The number of long-term follow-up (LTFU) studies that have followed treated anxious youth into late adolescence is small. The reader is referred to reviews cited earlier in the chapter for summaries of the LTFU studies conducted by the following investigative teams: Barrett and colleagues (Barrett, Duffy, Dadds, & Rapee, 2001), Beidel and colleagues (Beidel, Turner, & Young, 2006; Beidel, Turner, Young, & Paulson, 2005), Kendall and colleagues (Kendall & Southam-Gerow, 1996; Kendall, Safford, Flannery-Schroeder, & Webb, 2004); and Manassis and colleagues (Manassis, Avery, Butalia, & Mendlowitz, 2004). Most notably, all these studies found that the short-term benefits of targeting anxiety disorders extended over time. Specifically, post-treatment diagnostic recovery rates were maintained, or even enhanced. Youth and parent questionnaire data also showed maintenance of post-treatment gains at LTFU. We focus here on the most recent LTFU studies (Cobham, Dadds, Spence, & McDermott, 2010; Saavedra, Silverman, Morgan-Lopez, & Kurtines, 2010).

Cobham *et al.* (2010) reported on 60 of the 67 participants in Cobham, Dadds, and Spence (1998), an average of 2.66 years post-treatment (ages 10 to 17 years). In Cobham *et al.* (1998), mother-and-father dyads were classified according to parental anxiety levels, using the adult State Trait Anxiety Inventory (Trait) (i.e., "anxious," $n = 35$, "non-anxious," $n = 32$). All youth (7 to 14 years) met DSM-IV criteria for an anxiety disorder based on a modified ADIS-C/P and were randomized either to GCBT (referred to by the authors as "child focused cognitive behavioral therapy," $n = 32$) or GCBT with Parental Anxiety Management (GCBT with PAM, $n = 35$) (referred to by the authors as "child focused cognitive behavioral therapy plus parental anxiety management"). Results indicated that for youth whose parents were classified as non-anxious, 82% in GCBT no longer met criteria for an anxiety disorder compared to 80% in GCBT with PAM, a non-significant difference. For youth whose parents were classified as anxious, however, 39% in GCBT no longer met criteria for an anxiety disorder compared to 77% in GCBT with PAM, a significant difference. As Cobham *et al.* (1998) note, this significant difference based on post-treatment diagnoses may reflect the diagnosticians' expectancies for improvement because diagnosticians were not blind to participants' assigned condition. Furthermore, GCBT and GCBT with PAM showed significant improvement on the RCMAS and STAIC-S/T, with no statistically significant differences between the two treatment conditions. At 6- and 12-month follow-up, all treatment gains were maintained, again with no significant differences between treatment conditions.

The LTFU assessment consisted of questionnaires and the administration of the ADIS-IV to the parent only (i.e., ADIS-IV: Silverman & Albano, 1996). There were more similarities than differences between the treatment conditions in maintenance of treatment gains. Treatment gains based on clinician global ratings of improvement, and youth and parent ratings were maintained from 12-month follow-up through LTFU, with no statistically significant differences between GCBT and GCBT plus PAM.

A different picture emerged when it came to diagnostic recovery rates of all anxiety disorders (69.69% GCBT; 92.59% GCBT plus PAM). Cobham *et al.* (2010) explain that these significantly different diagnostic recovery rates between the two conditions at LTFU, which did not appear in Cobham *et al.* (1998), perhaps reflect parents in GCBT plus PAM being better equipped to support their children's treatment gains through the LTFU given the parent training they received in this condition, unlike parents in GCBT. Given that Cobham *et al.* (2010) is the first study to find statistically significant differences in diagnostic recovery rates in CBT conditions with and without parent involvement at LTFU, further LTFU studies focusing on this issue are needed.

Saavedra *et al.* (2010) reported on 67 of the 106 participants in Silverman, Kurtines, Ginsburg, Weems, Rabian, *et al.* (1999) and Silverman, Kurtines, Ginsburg, Weems, Lumpkin, *et al.* (1999), an average of 9.83 years post-treatment (ages 16 and 26 years). The first of these studies randomized youth (6 to 16 years) with a diagnosis of a phobic disorder (majority with SP) to one of two imaginal/in-vivo exposure conditions: Exposures plus Self Control (SC: $n = 41$) or Exposures plus Contingency Management (CM: $n = 40$). The remaining youth were randomized to an Educational Support (ES) condition ($n = 23$); these youth were not included in the LTFU. A statistically significant difference was found between the conditions with respect to primary/targeted phobic disorder diagnostic recovery rates (88% SC; 56% CM; 75% ES), with SC outperforming CM. The significant difference in diagnostic recovery rates was in contrast to the absence of any other significant treatment differences for any of the youth and parent rating scales, though significant pre- to post-treatment improvements were found on these scales for all three conditions. This same pattern of results was found at the follow-up assessments (3, 6, and 12 months).

In Silverman, Kurtines, Ginsburg, Weems, Lumpkin, *et al.* (1999) 56 youth (6 to 16 years) were randomized to either GCBT ($n = 37$) or a WLC ($n = 19$). At post-treatment, 64% of youth in GCBT no longer met primary diagnosis compared to 12.5% in WLC. Statistically significant improvements were observed pre- to post-treatment for treated but not wait-listed youth on CSRs, youth ratings on the RCMAS, FSSC-R, and CDI, and parent ratings on the CBCL-I, with continued maintenance of treatment gains at the follow-up assessments (6 and 12 months).

In Saavedra *et al.* (2010) follow-up of the two Silverman and colleagues (1999) trials, primary outcome was the targeted anxiety disorder and targeted symptoms. Secondary outcomes were other disorders and symptoms not directly targeted in the treatments including (1) other anxiety disorders and symptoms, (2) depressive disorders and symptoms, and (3) substance use disorders and symptoms. Academic and occupational outcomes also were assessed.

In terms of long-term recovery, results indicated that 86.5% of participants did not meet criteria for any anxiety disorder, 91% did not meet criteria for major depression, 95.5% did not meet criteria for dysthymia, 80.5% did not meet criteria for substance use, and 82.1% did not meet criteria for any new DSM-IV psychiatric disorders. Additionally, treatment gains were maintained from 12-month follow-up through LTFU across all youth and parent ratings and these gains showed no statistically significant different across GCBT, SC, and CM. However, participants who received individual treatment that emphasized cognitive facilitative strategies (SC) showed significantly better results for depression and internalizing disorder symptoms than participants who received GCBT. These findings raise the possibility that the more individualized attention to essential treatment procedures seen in an ICBT approach that emphasizes cognitive work equips children with important skills for managing targeted anxiety disorders, as well as other symptoms and disorders. Another noteworthy finding was the low rates of substance use disorder and symptoms observed in each of the treatment approaches, as well as the overall positive academic and occupational outcomes.

Thus, in line with past LTFU studies, Cobham *et al.* (2010) and Saavedra *et al.* (2010) provide empirical evidence for the long-term efficacy of CBT, including GCBT. Nevertheless, a limitation of both studies, which characterizes all the LTFU studies, is the absence of a non-active comparison condition. These studies therefore do not rule out the possibility of spontaneous remission that may come with maturation. Additional follow-up studies designed from the outset to evaluate the effect of spontaneous remission are needed. Sample size restrictions in both studies place further limits on drawing full inferences on the long-term effects for specific anxiety disorders.

New delivery approaches: Internet-based and computer-assisted CBT

Two recent studies examined the efficacy of internet-based and computer-assisted CBT (Khanna & Kendall, 2010; March, Spence, & Donovan, 2008). March *et al.* (2008) randomized 73 children (ages 7 to 12 years) to an Internet-based CBT (minimal therapist contact via phone or e-mail) with parents (referred by the authors as NET; $n = 40$) or WLC ($n = 33$). NET involved 10 child treatment sessions and six parent treatment sessions. Treatment was followed by booster sessions at 1 and 3 months.

The findings were mixed with regard to support for NET. Statistically significant greater improvements were found in NET than WLC on clinician-rated CSRs and C-GAS, and parent-rated SCAS and CBCL-I. However, no significant improvements were found on child-rated SCAS and diagnostic recovery rates of the primary anxiety disorder (30% NET; 10.3% WLC).

Six-month follow-up data were obtained for a small number of youth ($n = 23$) in NET. (WLC youth received treatment, but these youth were not included in the follow-up.) At 6-month follow-up, the diagnostic recovery rate of the primary anxiety disorder for these 23 NET participants had now increased to 75%. Further, a greater number of measures were now showing significant differences within NET from pre-treatment to 6-month follow-up relative to the number of measures showing significance from pre- to post-treatment. Specifically, now all the measures showed gains through 6-month follow-up including the child-rated SCAS.

March *et al.* (2008) note that compliance rates may account for the modest post-treatment outcomes in NET. Children and parents completed the post-treatment assessment whether or not they completed all sessions. However, following the post-treatment assessment, children and parents were given the opportunity to complete any remaining sessions. Thus, while at post-treatment only 33.3% of children and 60% of parents had completed all sessions, by 6-month follow-up, 62% of children and 72.3% of parents had completed all sessions. Outcome at the 6-month follow-up consequently was better than at post-treatment. In addition to this uneven pattern of treatment compliance, March *et al.* (2008) acknowledge other study limitations including the use of a small sample size comprising primarily Australian-born participants, the lack of comparative control data at 6-month follow-up, and the lack of any 12-month follow-up data.

In another effort, Khanna and Kendall (2010) randomized 49 youth (7 to 13 years) to one of three treatment conditions: ICBT ($n = 17$), computer-assisted CBT (therapist guided, with contact), referred to as Camp Cope-A-Lot (CCAL; $n = 16$), or Computer-linked Education, Support, and Attention (ESA/C; $n = 16$). Youth in ICBT and CCAL displayed significantly greater improvements than youth in ESA/C on diagnostic recovery rates of the primary anxiety disorder (70% ICBT; 81% CCAL; 19% ESA/C) and clinician-rated CSRs and C-GAS ratings, with no differences between ICBT and CCAL. However, on youth-rated MASC and CDI, youth not only in ICBT and CCAL reported significant pre- to post-treatment improvements, but so did youth in ESA/C, with no significant differences among conditions. There were continued improvements on these youth and clinician measures at 3-month follow-up. There also continued to be an absence of significant differences between ICBT and CCAL on any of the outcomes at 3-month follow-up. Follow-up data were not available for youth in ESA/C who were offered either CBT or were referred to other agencies.

Aside from March *et al.* (2008) and Khanna and Kendall (2010), one other study (Spence, Holmes, March, & Lipp, 2006) examined the utility of computers in the delivery of CBT (see Silverman *et al.*, 2008). Taken together, these studies are promising in that they suggest that Internet-based and computer-assisted CBT may have utility in anxiety reduction for youth. However, we concur with the conclusion of Khanna and Kendall (2010) that there is room for improvement, not only for CCAL, but ICBT. This is because in both conditions C-GAS ratings were on average only a few points above the clinical cut-off. We also concur with Khanna and Kendall's (2010) acknowledgments regarding these studies' limits including the small samples comprising primarily Whites, the lack of parent-rated outcomes, and the limited follow-ups.

Effectiveness of CBT in community-based clinics

A critical question for the field is whether CBT produces better outcomes than the usual interventions employed with children and adolescents in community mental health clinics (CMHCs). This question has been addressed in only two studies (Barrington, Prior, Richardson, & Allen, 2005; Southam-Gerow, Weisz, Chu, McLeod, Gordis, & Connor-Smith, 2010). Using a group approach, Barrington *et al.* (2005) randomly assigned youth and their parents (ages 7 to 14 years) to CBT ($n = 28$) or Usual Care (UC, $n = 26$) in CMHCs in Australia. UC included family therapy, play therapy, supportive therapy, psychodynamic therapy, and non-CBT eclectic approaches. Therapists were non-randomly assigned to treatment conditions. Only therapists with at least 2 years' post-doctoral training and experience in CBT were assigned to this condition. Therapists with minimal training in CBT and a preference for treatment approaches other than CBT were assigned to UC.

Overall, CBT did not produce superior treatment effects compared to UC. Rather, youth improved significantly in both CBT and UC from pre- to post-treatment on all the study's measures, with no significant differences between conditions. Measures included diagnostic recovery rates of all anxiety disorders (61% CBT; 50% UC; primary anxiety diagnoses were not reported), youth-rated RCMAS and SCAS, parent-rated SCAS, as well as teacher rating scales. There continued to be no statistically significant differences between CBT and UC at 12-month follow-up on anxiety diagnoses recovery rates (74% CBT; 68% UC), as well as on any of the youth, parent, and teacher rating scales. Of further note is that most clinicians did not complete 12 treatment sessions in the first 3 months as per the CBT protocol. Moreover, the majority of children (78%) were still in therapy 3 months after the first treatment session and 66% had terminated therapy at 6 months.

Southam-Gerow *et al.* (2010) randomized youth (ages 8 to 15 years) seeking treatment at six public, urban, CMHCs to CBT ($n = 24$) or UC ($n = 24$). UC included family therapy, psychodynamic therapy, and client-centered approaches. Therapists were randomly assigned to either CBT ($n = 18$) or UC ($n = 21$). CBT therapists received a 1-day, 6-hour training in CBT. Therapists assigned to UC used treatments they were accustomed to using in practice.

Similar to Barrington *et al.* (2005), Southam-Gerow *et al.* (2010) found a failure of CBT to produce superior treatment effects relative to UC treatment. Again, youth improved in both CBT and UC on all the study's measures. Specifically no statistically significant differences were found between conditions on diagnostic recovery rates of the primary anxiety disorder (CBT 66.7%; UC 73.7%), youth-rated STAIC-Trait, and parent-rated STAIC-Trait, CBCL-I, and CBCL-A/D. Interestingly, a higher proportion of youth in UC (41%) received concurrent services (e.g., a second therapist, school-based services) compared to youth in CBT (0%). Perhaps there was thus a "built-in dose" difference favoring UC over CBT (Weisz, Southam-Gerow, Gordis, Connor-Smith, Chu, & Langer, 2009). The use of concurrent services in UC perhaps means that CBT was in fact the more effective intervention, as it was unnecessary to supplement CBT with concurrent services. Another possibility is that 6 hours of training is insufficient for adequately training therapists in CBT. Nevertheless, such short training sessions are probably more common than not in CMHCs.

Also relevant here is that these trials, similar to most of the efficacy trials, failed to use a measurement and analytic strategy that allowed for intent to treat analyses (e.g., Little & Yau, 1998). This strategy would follow all participants initially enrolled in the study independent of whether they completed treatment. In this way statistical comparisons can be made between treatment completers and treatment non-completers to allow for determining whether there are any biases. If there are such biases, then conclusions about treatment effects would need to be drawn accordingly.

Clearly, both Barrington *et al.* (2005) and Southam-Gerow *et al.* (2010) have produced provocative findings because they raise questions about the superiority of CBT to UC in CMHCs. They await further study and replication, especially with larger samples to ensure sufficient power to detect significant differences, as well as to disentangle the other issues raised above.

Predictors, moderators, mediators, and processes of treatment outcome

The literature on predictors, moderators, mediators, and processes of treatment outcome was sparse at the time the first treatment chapter was written for the first edition of this volume. This state of the literature made sense at the time, as there was more urgency to first obtain empirical evidence for treatment efficacy. As efficacy evidence has accumulated, attention has shifted in recent years toward research designs that integrate features of basic treatment efficacy research with features of treatment prediction, moderation, mediation, and therapeutic process research.

Moderators and predictors of treatment outcome

At the time of the Silverman and Berman (2001) review, there were scant studies on moderators and predictors of treatment outcome. For example, we mentioned our own "in press" study, since published (Berman, Weems, Silverman, & Kurtines, 2000), which found the strongest predictor of treatment outcome was parental depression, with other predictors including other parental symptoms (e.g., fear, hostility) and children's self-ratings of depression and trait anxiety.

A few studies have since been conducted that investigated variables as potential moderators and/or predictors of treatment outcome. Bodden *et al.* (2008) and Kendall *et al.* (2008) both examined parent anxiety as a moderator. Bodden *et al.* (2008) found ICBT to be superior to CBT/P at post-treatment and at 3-month follow-up when parents had an anxiety disorder. Bodden *et al.* (2008) suggested these findings may reflect parental anxiety impeding the transfer of control of CBT skills from parents to child, a notion suggested earlier by Silverman and Kurtines (1996) and Ginsburg, Silverman, and Kurtines (1995). Kendall *et al.* (2008), on the other hand, found CBT/P to be superior to ICBT at 12-month follow-up when fathers, but not mothers, had an anxiety disorder.

Bodden *et al.* (2008) and Alfano, Pina, Villalta, Beidel, Ammerman, and Crosby (2009) (summarized below) examined youth's age as a moderator; neither found that treatment outcome was moderated by age. Alfano *et al.* (2009) also found outcome was not moderated by youth's depressive symptoms.

Although these studies are valuable, future studies designed specifically to test for moderation (rather than post hoc) are needed to fully evaluate the potentially important relations between hypothesized moderators and treatment in a more theoretically guided manner. This would hopefully also lead to the design of studies with sufficient power from the onset to evaluate fully for moderators. This is important given the likelihood that past efforts to discern moderators were insufficiently powered to do so, as relatively large sample sizes are needed to detect moderator effects.

Several studies have examined predictors of treatment outcome – that is, variables accounting for outcome irrespective of treatment condition. Youth's age has not been found to predict treatment outcome (e.g., Kendall *et al.*, 2008; Ollendick *et al.*, 2009) with one exception: Bodden *et al.* (2008) found younger children improved more than older children, based on anxiety disorder diagnoses as the outcome. Ollendick *et al.* (2009) also found youth sex to be a significant predictor: girls responded significantly better than boys to OST than EST at 6-month follow-up but not at post-treatment. The reasons for the different timing effects were not explained, but are deserving of replication and further study.

Within Liber, Van Widenfelt, Goedhart, Utens, Van Der Leeden, and Markus (2008), the authors examined fathers' and mothers' emotional warmth, rejection, overprotection, anxiety symptoms, and depression symptoms as predictors. Fathers' rejection and depression symptoms predicted poor treatment outcome, as did mothers' emotional warmth. Given it is counter-intuitive that mothers who display emotional warmth have children who fare worse in treatment, Liber, Van Widenfelt, Goedhart, *et al.* (2008) suggest that perhaps emotionally warm mothers are likely to engage in excessive reassurance seeking, which is perceived by their children as warmth. This interesting possibility speaks to the importance of using measures that differentiate between related constructs of interest, as well as the need to consider the possibility that diverse sources hold different perspectives in their views of a given construct.

Also in examining parental anxiety as a predictor of treatment outcome, Bodden *et al.* (2008) found that the presence of anxiety disorders in one or both parents predicted the presence of anxiety disorder diagnoses in youth at post-treatment and follow-up. Kendall *et al.* (2008) found that the presence of anxiety disorders in mothers, but not fathers, predicted the presence of the primary anxiety disorder diagnosis in youth at follow-up. Finally, Liber, Van Widenfelt, Van Der Leeden, Goedhart, Utens, and Treffers (2010) and Ollendick, Öst, Reuterskiöld, and Costa (2010) examined comorbidity as a predictor. Comorbidity significantly predicted treatment outcome in Liber, Van Widenfelt, *et al.* (2010), but not in Ollendick *et al.* (2010). Methodological differences in the definition of treatment outcome between the two studies – ADIS-C/P diagnoses in Liber, Van Widenfelt, *et al.* (2010), targeted phobia CSRs in Ollendick *et al.* (2010) – may explain the discrepant findings.

Although these predictor studies are all valuable additions to the treatment literature, similar points we raised above regarding moderators hold here as well. Additionally, as researchers continue to routinely examine theoretically meaningful variables as predictors of treatment outcome, careful consideration must be given to the statistical and methodological approaches. Indeed, statistical and methodological differences largely account for the discrepant findings in most studies, in our view. For instance, in some studies predictors of interest were examined in relation to residual chance scores, which have limitations (Hageman & Arrindell, 1993).

Finally, it will be important to know whether predictors and moderators are relevant only for a particular treatment or are relevant for multiple treatments (Kazdin, 2008). Future child anxiety trials also would benefit from using "treatment matching" models, which are designed to examine moderators of multiple treatments. Such research would reveal whether children with certain characteristics benefit most from one type of treatment and whether children with different characteristics benefit most from another treatment. Such treatment matching or prescriptive treatments have been conducted with children using single-case designs in the area of anxiety (Eisen & Silverman, 1991) including anxious children with school-refusal behavior (Kearney & Silverman, 1990). Further studies are needed that examine treatment matching and other methods for tailoring treatments to individual child and family. These are the kinds of issues that also align well with the US National Institute of Mental Health strategic plan's emphasis on "personalized treatment."

Treatment mediators

Mediation relates to *how* therapeutic change is produced. Knowing not just whether treatment change is produced, but how it is produced, is the cornerstone of advancing theoretical understanding about mechanisms of change (e.g., Kazdin & Nock, 2003; La Greca, Silverman, & Lochman, 2009). Mediation research also has the potential to lead to improved clinical care. This is because having an understanding of what needs to be changed provides the clinician with the flexibility to be adaptable to variations in patients' problems, contexts, or conditions. By having empirical knowledge of the main treatment procedure(s) responsible for producing successful treatment outcomes, clinicians can ensure that effective treatment procedure(s) are in fact being delivered to the child or adolescent client (Silverman & Hinshaw, 2008).

Only recently has mediation been investigated in the child and adolescent anxiety treatment area. We summarize below the work where mediation and/or processes of change were the main foci of the study, not secondary or exploratory mediation analyses (e.g., Wood *et al.*, 2009). We further note that although the studies summarized represent important contributions to the field, they are limited in that the measurement strategies did not include session by session assessments. This thereby precluded the ability to draw inference regarding temporality (i.e., change in mediator preceded the change in outcome), a necessary condition for mediation analyses. We are in the process of writing up a mediation treatment outcome strategy that employed this more intensive measurement approach. We have another trial currently in progress.

Cognitive variables as treatment mediators

Treadwell and Kendall (1996) evaluated the mediating role of negative self-statements, positive self-statements, and state-of-mind (SOM: Schwartz & Garamoni, 1986; i.e., the proportion of positive versus negative self-statements) ratios in youth anxiety. The sample consisted of 151 youth (ages 8 to 13 years); 71 of the youth were clinic-referred and were included in the mediational analysis; the remaining 80 youth were community volunteers with normal levels of anxiety, internalizing and externalizing problems, and depression as measured by standardized measures, whose data were not included in the mediation analysis. Significant pre- to post-treatment improvements were observed in negative self-statements, positive self-statements, and SOM ratios for the treated clinic youth. In terms of treatment mediators, negative self-statements, but not positive self-statements, mediated youth self-ratings of anxiety outcome, but not parent or teacher outcome ratings. Changes in the SOM ratio also mediated treatment outcome. In an independent study, Kendall and Treadwell (2007) essentially replicated the findings of Treadwell and Kendall (1996).

Parent variables as treatment mediators

Silverman *et al.*'s (2009) CBT/P condition targeted three types of parent variables: (1) parental positive/negative behaviors toward the child, (2) conflict in the parent–youth dyadic relationship, and (3) parental anxiety. Of interest was to examine preliminarily the directionality of effects (i.e., parent to child, child to parent, or bidirectionality). The results are the first to provide evidence suggesting that reciprocal influence between youth anxiety and parenting variables is theoretically plausible. For several reasons, the evidence for child-to-parent influence was somewhat stronger than the more traditional view of either parent-to-child influence or bidirectional influence.

First, there were no significant differences in youth anxiety for a treatment intervention that directly targeted the parent variables (CBT/P) as compared with a treatment intervention that did not (CBT). If youth responses are consequents of parent responses, this should not be the case. Second, in the intervention that targeted only youth anxiety (i.e., CBT), all three of the parent variables showed statistically significant improvement and the magnitude of the effects were comparable to the CBT/P condition. This is consistent with the assumption that changes in youth anxiety produce changes in parent anxiety. Third, structural equation modeling analyses showed that changes in youth anxiety from pre-treatment to post-treatment were related to changes in parent anxiety during this same time period. Although the causal direction of this association is ambiguous, the results were consistent with a lagged effect that linked changes in youth anxiety from pre-treatment to post-treatment to improved parental negative behaviors at follow-up – one of the three parent variables examined.

Relatedly, because of its focus on processes of change in parent conditions, Khanna and Kendall (2009) focused on discerning which, if any, components of PT in CBT contributed to positive treatment outcome. The PT techniques considered were parental anxiety management, transfer of control from therapist to parent to child over child's coping, communication skills training, and contingency management training. The data used were from Kendall *et al.* (2008). An observational code book was developed in which each PT was rated for quantity (i.e., presence, duration in seconds) and quality using a five-point rating scale.

Therapists teaching of parental anxiety management and transfer of control contributed to improved child functioning based on C-GAS ratings, but not improved youth anxiety. Therapists teaching of communication skills training and contingency management training did not contribute to any child improvement. Although these findings shed some preliminary light on the effects of specific PT techniques, as Khanna and Kendall (2009) point out, it is unknown whether parents actually used these specific PT techniques out of session, thereby resulting in (i.e., mediating) positive treatment outcome. They also do not touch on the directionality issues, raised by Silverman *et al.* (2009). Future mediation studies are needed to pursue this possibility.

Peer variables as treatment mediators

Alfano *et al.* (2009) is the only study to evaluate mediators of treatment outcome in the behavioral treatment of SOP, Social Effectiveness Training for Youth (SET-C), in a sample of 88 youths (ages 7 to 17 years). The data were derived from two previously published randomized clinical trials (Beidel *et al.*, 2000, $n = 31$; Beidel *et al.*, 2007, $n = 57$). The peer variables targeted in SET-C were the peer–youth relationship and youth social skills behaviors. The quality of the peer–youth relationship was measured using the Loneliness Scale (LS: Asher & Wheeler, 1985), which measures the degree to which youth feel isolated by their peers and socially dissatisfied. Youth social skills behaviors were measured by behavioral observations in which children were rated by trained observers while they engaged in social evaluative tasks. Results revealed that only changes in youth-reported loneliness mediated treatment outcome for only one of the study's main outcome measures (i.e., SPAI). Social skills did not mediate treatment outcome with any of the study's main outcome measures.

Treatment processes

The reader is referred to a recent review by Fjermestad, Haugland, Heiervang, and Öst (2009) on child and adolescent anxiety studies that have investigated treatment process. Our focus here is on those studies that emanated from the randomized clinical trials we summarized in this chapter.

The therapeutic alliance

The therapeutic alliance has been the focus of recent attention in the child and adolescent anxiety area. The therapeutic alliance is a broad term used to characterize the relationship between client and therapist, their collaboration on treatment assignments and goals, and the bond that develops over the course of treatment (e.g., Horvath & Bedi, 2002). The therapeutic alliance is viewed to be one important feature of treatment that may help to explain treatment outcome, perhaps over and beyond the active ingredients of a given treatment approach.

Two studies (Chiu, McLeod, Har, & Wood, 2009; Liber, McLeod, et al., 2010) examined in-session child–therapist alliance in relation to mid- and post-treatment outcome. The data were derived from the earlier trials of Wood et al. (2006) and Liber, Van Widenfelt, Goedhart, et al. (2008), respectively. The child–therapist alliance was assessed in both studies using the Therapy Process Observational Coding System for Child Psychotherapy – Alliance Scale (TPOCS-A: B. D. McLeod, unpublished data), which measures the child–therapist relationship and the child's participation in therapeutic activities. Chiu et al. (2009) found that a strong child–therapist alliance early in treatment did not predict post-treatment outcome. However, a strong child–therapist alliance early in treatment did predict youth anxiety symptom reduction at mid-treatment as rated by parents. Alliance shifts, or improvements in the child–therapist alliance between early treatment sessions and later treatment sessions, also predicted significant youth anxiety symptom reduction at post-treatment as rated by parents.

In contrast to Chiu et al. (2009), Liber, McLeod, et al. (2010) did not find that child–therapist alliance early in treatment predicted anxiety symptom reduction by mid-treatment. Also unlike Chiu et al., Liber et al. did not find that alliance shifts predicted post-treatment outcome. Interestingly, however, a strong child–therapist alliance early in treatment was related to better diagnostic outcomes in ICBT than in GCBT. Liber, McLeod, et al. (2010) suggest that perhaps other non-specific processes, such as group cohesion, facilitate recovery of youth anxiety disorders in GCBT.

These two studies highlight the complexities involved in studying the therapeutic alliance in youth anxiety treatment outcome. For example, neither study allows us to rule out alternative explanations, including: (1) a strong child–therapist alliance and child participation are consequences of youth anxiety reduction, (2) a bidirectional relation exists between child–therapist alliance and youth anxiety reduction, or (3) both (1) and (2), depending on other moderator and mediator variables contained within a particular nomological network. Further, these studies highlight that the timing of outcome assessment may influence the strength of the relation with the alliance (given the different findings at mid- and post-treatment); different treatment approaches (individual, group) may yield different relations; the source of the rater of the alliance (e.g., child, parent) may matter; and that limited sample sizes may yield insufficient power to detect some relations. More theory driven studies employing intensive measurement of the child–therapist alliance and anxiety symptoms are needed to further disentangle these complex issues.

In another study on the therapeutic alliance, which focused on the influence of exposure on the alliance, Kendall *et al.* (2009) developed two interestingly plausible, though, opposing, propositions: (1) therapist prescribed exposure tasks are associated with ruptures in the child–therapist therapeutic alliance because the child is being asked to confront anxiety-evoking situations; or (2) therapist prescribed exposure tasks are associated with enhancements in the child–therapist therapeutic alliance because the child is improving as a result of these exposures, and the alliance ruptures can be remedied within sessions.

To address these two propositions and using data from Kendall *et al.*'s (2008) trial, Kendall *et al.* (2009) examined changes in the child–therapist alliance between and within treatment conditions, before and after, the introduction of exposure tasks in CBT/P, in comparison to ESA/P, which contained no exposures. The child–therapist alliance was assessed using the Therapeutic Alliance Scale (TASC: Shirk & Saiz, 1992). Using growth curve modeling, results indicated that child–therapist alliance ratings increased during the sessions leading up to the introduction of exposures and remained stable thereafter. More importantly, alliance ratings for the sessions following the introduction of exposures were not significantly different between ESA/P and CBT/P, suggesting that exposure tasks are not associated with ruptures in child–therapist alliance. These findings were consistent across therapist, youth, mother, and father ratings of alliance, further suggesting their robustness. Future studies are needed to replicate these findings and determine whether conclusions hold when changes in the child–therapist alliance are examined using other CBT formats.

Specific treatment processes

Safety behaviors are theorized as playing a central role in maintaining debilitating anxiety and its disorders (Salkovskis, 1991). Safety behaviors can include direct avoidance of situations, or escape from situations, as well as subtle avoidance. Safety behaviors are thought to be used by individuals with anxiety disorders because the individuals attribute usage to the prevention or minimization of a feared outcome. (Salkovskis, 1991). A corollary of this notion is that individuals who engage in safety behaviors fare worse in treatment.

To begin to examine this possibility, Hedtke, Kendall, and Tiwari (2009) used post-hoc behavior observation ratings (on a six-point scale) during youth exposure tasks conducted during Kendall *et al.* (2008) to compare the effects of youths' usage of safety-seeking behavior and youths' usage of coping behavior on treatment outcome. Findings showed that youths' usage of safety behaviors significantly predicted poor treatment outcome, based on clinician ratings of severity and global functioning, and father ratings of youth anxiety symptoms. Coping behavior during in-session exposures did not predict treatment outcome. Further, safety-seeking behavior increased during exposure sessions; coping behavior remained stable.

The findings of Hedtke *et al.* (2009) are suggestive of an exciting future scenario: Individuals' usage of safety behaviors is an individual, child–person variable that is relatively easily modifiable; and such modification might lead to enhanced treatment outcome including among "treatment-resistant" patients. Adult research evidence supports this possibility. Wolitzky and Telch (2009) found in adult patients that exposure coupled with actions incompatible with safety behaviors was superior to exposure alone.

Summary of studies

Our update in this chapter shows that much progress has been made in child and adolescent anxiety treatment research in moving beyond WLC conditions. More studies have since been conducted that have investigated the efficacy of CBT relative to credible comparison control conditions that targeted not only phobias, but other anxiety disorders, and that utilized not only an individual approach, but also a group approach, a computerized approach, and that involved parents (Hudson *et al.*, 2009; Kendall *et al.*, 2008; Khanna & Kendall, 2010; Ollendick *et al.*, 2009). Nevertheless, this update continues to reveal mixed evidence regarding whether CBT outperforms education support, as findings are inconsistent across measures, informants, and assessment timing. CBTs outperformed credible comparison control conditions most often on diagnostic recovery rates and CSRs at post-treatment and follow-up (Hudson *et al.*, 2009; Kendall *et al.*, 2008; Khanna & Kendall, 2010; Ollendick *et al.*, 2009), not on youth and parent rating scales of youth anxiety and fear (e.g., Kendall *et al.*, 2008; Ollendick *et al.*, 2009).

In considering the role of parents, Silverman and Berman (2001) concluded that the efficacy of ICBT can be enhanced by involving parents in the treatment process, but further investigations are needed regarding how parents can enhance treatment. Subsequent reviews (e.g., Barmish & Kendall, 2005; Creswell & Cartwright-Hatton, 2007; Silverman *et al.*, 2008) have reached similar conclusions. This latest update continued to find underwhelming evidence that adding parents produces significant enhanced treatment effects. Most studies (i.e., Bodden *et al.*, 2008; Kendall *et al.*, 2008; Silverman *et al.*, 2009) did not provide support for the enhanced effects of parent/family involvement in the youth's treatment. When significant enhanced effects were found, they were generally inconsistent across informants and time (Wood *et al.*, 2006).

The present study also showed that advances have been made in comparing CBT delivered using individual or group approaches, with both approaches being efficacious. That CBT is similarly efficacious when administered in a group format puts to rest concerns that the presence of other children may dampen the therapist–child relationship, may tax therapist resources, and may create a context for negative modeling to occur (Silverman, Kurtines, Ginsburg, Weems, Lumpkin, *et al.*, 1999).

This update highlights several new topics of research that had not yet been addressed at the time of the writing of Silverman and Berman (2001). There now exists empirical support for the long-term effects of CBT and the potential utility of Internet-based and computer-assisted CBTs. There now also exists preliminary evidence showing that combined CBT and pharmacological treatment is superior to either treatment alone, though both CBT and medication are superior to placebo. Considerable more work, however, is needed on this front, as also noted by Pelligrino *et al.* (Chapter 17, this volume).

Another advance since Silverman and Berman (2001) is that two effectiveness studies are now available showing that CBT is feasible and works in CMHCs. However, there is an absence of evidence demonstrating CBT's superiority to UC. This is clearly an issue of large concern, as efforts to implement CBT for anxiety disorders in children in CMHCs could well be dampened if there is no evidence that CBT is superior to what occurs normally in CHMCs. As noted, though, the limited power of these studies and the lack of full experimental procedures hinder full embracing of these findings. Progress in studying predictors, moderators, mediators, and processes of treatment has been made.

Relating to moderation, when trials have examined the effects of CBT for minority youth, we noted in the beginning of this chapter that positive effects have been obtained. Nevertheless, more work is needed on this front to better evaluate ethnicity, as well as culture or race, as potential moderators. Additionally, participants have been composed of ethnic minorities that are highly acculturated (Pina *et al.*, 2003). When the field does move toward working with less acculturated groups, there will be a need to conduct the necessary psychometric testing to ensure measurement equivalence (see Pina, Little, Knight, & Silverman, 2009, for a demonstration).

In summary, there remains much work to be done to move the child and adolescent treatment area forward with regard to confirming the evidence base, as well as in developing evidence-based explanations of treatment. In light of all the exciting new knowledge that will likely be produced and unearthed over the next decade, we are thrilled by the prospect of providing the next treatment update for the third edition of this volume.

References

Achenbach, T. M. (1991). *Manual for the Child Behavior Checklist/4–18.* Burlington, VT: University of Vermont Department of Psychiatry.

Achenbach, T. M. & **Edelbrock, C.** (1986). *Manual for the Teacher Report Form.* Burlington, VT: University of Vermont Department of Psychiatry.

Alfano, C. A., Pina, A. A., Villalta, I. K., Beidel, D. C., Ammerman, R. T., & **Crosby, L. E.** (2009). Mediators and moderators of outcome in the behavioral treatment of childhood social phobia. *Journal of the American Academy of Child and Adolescent Psychiatry*, **48**, 945–953.

American Psychiatric Association (1994). *Diagnostic and Statistical Manual of Mental Disorders*, 4th edn. Washington, DC: American Psychiatric Association.

Asher, S. R. & **Wheeler, V. A.** (1985). Children's loneliness: a comparison of rejected and neglected peer status. *Journal of Consulting and Clinical Psychology*, **53**, 500–505.

Barmish, A. & **Kendall, P. C.** (2005). Should parents be co-clients in cognitive–behavioral therapy for anxious youth? *Journal of Clinical Child and Adolescent Psychology*, **34**, 569–581.

Barrett, P. M. (1998). Evaluation of cognitive–behavioral group treatments for childhood anxiety disorders. *Journal of Clinical Child Psychology*, **27**, 459–468.

Barrett, P. M., Dadds, M. R., & **Rapee, R. M.** (1996). Family treatment of childhood anxiety: a controlled trial. *Journal of Consulting and Clinical Psychology*, **64**, 333–342.

Barrett, P. M., Duffy, A. L., Dadds, M. R., & **Rapee, R. M.** (2001). Cognitive–behavioral treatment of anxiety disorders in children: long-term (6-year) follow-up. *Journal of Consulting and Clinical Psychology*, **69**, 135–141.

Barrington, J., Prior, M., Richardson, M., & **Allen, K.** (2005). Effectiveness of CBT versus standard treatment for childhood anxiety disorders in a community clinic setting. *Behaviour Change*, **22**, 29–43.

Beidel, D. C., Turner, S. M., & **Morris, T. L.** (1995). A new inventory to assess childhood social anxiety and phobia: The Social Phobia and Anxiety Inventory for Children. *Psychological Assessment*, **7**, 73–79.

Beidel, D. C., Turner, S. M., & **Morris, T. L.** (2000). Behavioral treatment of childhood social phobia. *Journal of Consulting and Clinical Psychology*, **68**, 1072–1080.

Beidel, D. C., Turner, S. M., Sallee, F. R., Ammerman, R. T., Crosby, L. A., & Pathak, S. (2007). SET-C versus fluoxetine in the treatment of childhood social phobia. *Journal of the American Academy of Child and Adolescent Psychiatry*, **46**, 1622–1632.

Beidel, D. C., Turner, S. M., & Young, B. J. (2006). Social effectiveness therapy for children: five years later. *Behavior Therapy*, **37**, 416–425.

Beidel, D. C., Turner, S. M., Young, B., & Paulson, A. (2005). Social effectiveness training for children: three-year follow-up. *Journal of Consulting and Clinical Psychology*, **73**, 721–725.

Berman, S. L., Weems, C. F., Silverman, W. K., & Kurtines, W. M. (2000). Predictors of outcome in exposure-based cognitive and behavioral treatments for phobic and anxiety disorders in children. *Behavior Therapy*, **31**, 713–731.

Bird, H. R., Shaffer, D., Fisher, P., Gould, M. S., Staghezza, B., & Chen, J. Y. (1993). The Columbia Impairment Scale (CIS): pilot findings on a measure of global impairment for children and adolescents. *International Journal of Methods in Psychiatric Research*, **3**, 167–176.

Birmaher, B., Khetarpal, S., Brent, D., Cully, M., Balach, L., Kaufman, J., et al. (1997). The Screen for Child Anxiety Related Emotional Disorders (SCARED): scale construction and psychometric properties. *Journal of the American Academy of Child and Adolescent Psychiatry*, **36**, 545–553.

Bodden, D. H. M., Bögels, S. M., Nauta, M. H., de Hann, E., Ringrose, J., Abbelboom, C., et al. (2008). Child versus family cognitive–behavioral therapy in clinically anxious youth: an efficacy and partial effectiveness study. *Journal of the American Academy of Child and Adolescent Psychiatry*, **47**, 1384–1394.

Cartwright-Hatton, S., Roberts, C., Chitsabesan, P., Fothergill, C., & Harrington, R. (2004). Systematic review of the efficacy of cognitive behaviour therapies for childhood and adolescent anxiety disorders. *British Journal of Clinical Psychology*, **44**, 421–436.

Chiu, A. W., McLeod, B. D., Har, K. H., & Wood, J. J. (2009). Child–therapist alliance and clinical outcomes in cognitive behavioral therapy for child anxiety disorders. *Journal of Child Psychology and Psychiatry*, **50**, 751–758.

Cobham, V. E., Dadds, M. R., & Spence, S. H. (1998). The role of parental anxiety in the treatment of childhood anxiety. *Journal of Consulting and Clinical Psychology*, **66**, 893–905.

Cobham, V. E., Dadds, M. R., Spence, S. H., & McDermott, B. (2010). Parental anxiety in the treatment of childhood anxiety: a different story three years later. *Journal of Clinical Child and Adolescent Psychology*, **39**, 410–420.

Compton, S. N., Walkup, J. T., Albano, A. M., Piacentini, J. C., Birmaher, B., Sherrill, J. T., et al. (2010). Child/Adolescent Anxiety Multimodal Study (CAMS): rationale, design, and methods. *Child and Adolescent Psychiatry and Mental Health*, **1**, 5–15.

Creswell, C. & Cartwright-Hatton, S. (2007). Family treatment of child anxiety: outcomes, limitations and future directions. *Clinical Child and Family Psychological Review*, **3**, 232–252.

Eisen, A. R. & Silverman, W. K. (1991). Treatment of an adolescent with bowel movement phobia using self-control therapy. *Journal of Behavior Therapy and Experimental Psychiatry*, **22**, 45–51.

Fjermestad, K. W., Haugland, B. S. M., Heiervang, E., & Öst, L. G. (2009). Relationship factors and outcome in child anxiety treatment studies. *Clinical Child Psychology and Psychiatry*, **14**, 195–214.

Flannery-Schroeder, E. C. & Kendall, P. C. (2000). Group and individual cognitive–behavioral treatments for youth with anxiety disorders: a randomized clinical trial. *Cognitive Therapy and Research*, **24**, 251–278.

Ginsburg, G. S., Silverman, W. K., & Kurtines, W. M. (1995). Family involvement in treating children with phobic and anxiety disorders: a look ahead. *Clinical Psychology Review*, **15**, 457–473.

Goodman, R. (1997). The Strengths and Difficulties Questionnaire: a research note. *Journal of Youth Psychology and Psychiatry*, **38**, 581–586.

Guy, W. & Bonato, R. (eds.) (1970). *CGI: Clinical Global Impressions.* Chevy Chase, MD: National Institute of Mental Health.

Hageman, W. J. & Arrindell, W. A. (1993). A further refinement of the reliable change (RC) index by improving pre–post difference score: introducing RCID. *Behaviour Research and Therapy*, **31**, 693–700.

Hedtke, K. A., Kendall, P. C., & Tiwari, S. (2009). Safety-seeking and coping behavior during exposure tasks with anxious youth. *Journal of Clinical Child and Adolescent Psychology*, **38**, 1–15.

Horvath, A. O. & Bedi, R. P. (2002). The alliance. In: J. C. Norcross (ed.) *Psychotherapy Relationships that Work: Therapist Contributions and Responsiveness to Patients*, pp. 37–69. New York: Oxford University Press.

Hudson, J. L., Rapee, R. M., Deveney, C., Schniering, C. A., Lyneham, H. J., & Bovopoulous, N. (2009). Cognitive behavioral treatment versus an active control for children and adolescents with anxiety disorders: a randomized trial. *Journal of the American Academy of Child and Adolescent Psychiatry*, **48**, 533–544.

In-Albon, T. & Schneider, S. (2007). Psychotherapy of childhood anxiety disorders: a meta-analysis. *Psychotherapy and Psychosomatics*, **76**, 15–24.

James, A., Soler, A., & Weatherall, R. (2005). Cognitive behavioral therapy for anxiety disorders in children and adolescents. *Cochrane Database of Systematic Reviews*, **4**, CD004690.

Kazdin, A. E. (2008). Evidence-based treatment and practice: new opportunities to bridge clinical research and practice, enhance the knowledge base, and improve patient care. *American Psychologist*, **63**, 146–159.

Kazdin, A. E. & Nock, M. (2003). Delineating mechanisms of change in child and adolescent therapy: methodological issues and research recommendations. *Journal of Child Psychology and Psychiatry*, **44**, 1116–1129.

Kearney, C. A. & Silverman, W. K. (1990). A preliminary analysis of a functional model of assessment and treatment for school refusal behavior. *Behavior Modification*, **14**, 340–366.

Kendall, P. C. (1994). Treating anxiety disorders in children: results of a randomized clinical trial. *Journal of Consulting and Clinical Psychology*, **62**, 200–210.

Kendall, P. C. & Southam-Gerow, M. A. (1996). Long-term follow-up of a cognitive–behavioral therapy for anxiety-disordered youth. *Journal of Consulting and Clinical Psychology*, **64**, 724–730.

Kendall, P. C. & Treadwell, K. R. H. (2007). The role of self-statements as a mediator in treatment for youth with anxiety disorders. *Journal of Consulting and Clinical Psychology*, **75**, 380–389.

Kendall, P. C., Comer, J., Marker, C., Creed, T., Puliafico, A., Hughes, A., et al. (2009). In-session exposure tasks and therapeutic alliance across the treatment of childhood anxiety disorders. *Journal of Consulting and Clinical Psychology*, **77**, 517–525.

Kendall, P. C., Flannery-Schroeder, E., Panichelli-Mindel, S. M., Southam-Gerow, M., Henin, A., & Warman, M. (1997). Therapy for youth with anxiety disorders: a second randomized clinical trial. *Journal of Consulting and Clinical Psychology*, **65**, 366–380.

Kendall, P. C., Hudson, J. L., Gosch, E., Flannery-Schroeder, E., & Suveg, C. (2008). Cognitive–behavioral therapy for anxiety disordered youth: a randomized clinical trial evaluating youth and family modalities. *Journal of Consulting and Clinical Psychology*, **76**, 282–297.

Kendall, P. C., Safford, S., Flannery-Schroeder, E., & Webb, A. (2004). Child anxiety treatment: outcomes in adolescence and impact on substance use and depression at 7.4 year follow-up. *Journal of Consulting and Clinical Psychology*, **72**, 276–287.

Khanna, M. S. & Kendall, P. C. (2009). Exploring the role of parent training in the treatment of childhood anxiety. *Journal of Consulting and Clinical Psychology*, **77**, 981–986.

Khanna, M. S. & Kendall, P. C. (2010). Computer-assisted cognitive behavioral therapy for child anxiety: results of a randomized clinical trial. *Journal of Consulting and Clinical Psychology*, **78**, 737–745.

King, N. J., Tonge, B. J., Heyne, D., Pritchard, M., Rollings, S., Young, D., *et al.* (1998). Cognitive–behavioral treatment of school-refusing children: a controlled evaluation. *Journal of the American Academy of Child and Adolescent Psychiatry*, **37**, 395–403.

Kovacs, M. (1992). *Children's Depression Inventory Manual.* North Tonawanda, NY: Multi-Health Systems, Inc.

La Greca, A. M., Silverman, W. K., & Lochman, J. E. (2009). Moving beyond efficacy and effectiveness in child and adolescent intervention research. *Journal of Consulting and Clinical Psychology*, **77**, 373–382.

Last, C. G., Hansen, C., & Franco, N. (1998). Cognitive–behavioral treatment of school phobia. *Journal of the American Academy of Child and Adolescent Psychiatry*, **37**, 404–411.

Liber, J. M., Van Widenfelt, B. M., Van Der Leeden, A. J. M., Goedhart, A. W., Utens, E. M. W. J., & Treffers, P. D. A. (2010). The relation of severity and comorbidity to treatment outcome with cognitive behavioral therapy for childhood anxiety disorders, *Journal of Abnormal Child Psychology*, **38**, 683–694.

Liber, J. M., McLeod, B. D., Van Widenfelt, B. M., Goedhart, A. W., Van Der Leeden, A. J. M., Utens, E. M. W. J., *et al.* (2010). Examining the relation between the therapeutic alliance, treatment adherence, and outcome of cognitive behavioral treatment for children with anxiety disorders. *Behavior Therapy*, **41**, 172–186.

Liber, J. M., Van Widenfelt, B. M., Goedhart, A. W., Utens, E. M. W. J., Van Der Leeden, A. J. M., & Markus, M. T. (2008). Parenting and parental anxiety and depression as predictors of treatment outcome for childhood anxiety disorders: has the role of fathers been underestimated? *Journal of Clinical Child and Adolescent Psychology*, **37**, 747–758.

Liber, J. M., Van Widenfelt, B. M., Utens, E. M. W. J., Ferdinand, R. F., Van Der Leeden, A. J. M., & Van Gastel, W. (2008). No differences between group versus individual treatment of childhood anxiety disorders in a randomized clinical trial. *Journal of Child Psychology and Psychiatry*, **49**, 886–893.

Little, R. J. & Yau, L. H. Y. (1998) Statistical techniques for analyzing data from prevention trials: treatment of no-shows using Rubin's causal model. *Psychological Methods*, **3**, 147–159.

Manassis, K., Avery, D., Butalia, S., & Mendlowitz, S. L. (2004). Cognitive–behavioral therapy with childhood anxiety disorders: functioning in adolescence. *Depression and Anxiety*, **19**, 209–216.

Manassis, K., Mendlowitz, S. L., Scapillato, D., Avery, D., Fiksenbaum, L., Freire, M., *et al.* (2002). Group and individual cognitive behavioral therapy for childhood anxiety disorders: a randomized trial. *Journal of the American Academy of Child and Adolescent Psychiatry*, **41**, 1423–1430.

March, J. S., Parker, J. D. A., Sullivan, K., Stallings, P., & Conners, C. K. (1997). The Multidimensional Anxiety Scale for Children (MASC): factor structure, reliability, and validity. *Journal of the American Academy of Child and Adolescent Psychiatry*, **36**, 554–565.

March, S., Spence, S. H., & Donovan, C. L. (2008). The efficacy of an Internet-based cognitive–behavioral therapy intervention for child anxiety disorders. *Journal of Pediatric Psychology*, **34**, 474–487.

Mendlowitz, S. L., Manassis, K., Bradley, S., Scapillato, D., Miezitis, S., & Shaw, B. F. (1999). Cognitive–behavioral group treatments in childhood anxiety disorders: the role of parental involvement. *Journal of the American Academy of Child and Adolescent Psychiatry*, **38**, 1223–1229.

Nevo, G. A. & Manassis, K. (2009). Outcomes for treated anxious children: a critical review of long-term follow-up studies. *Depression and Anxiety*, **26**, 650–660.

Ollendick, T. H. (1983). Reliability and validity of the Revised Fear Survey Schedule for Children (FSSC-R). *Behaviour Research and Therapy*, **21**, 685–692.

Ollendick, T. H., Öst, L.-G., Reuterskiöld, L., & Costa, N. (2010). Comorbidity in youth with specific phobias: impact of comorbidity on treatment outcome and the impact of treatment on comorbid disorders. *Behaviour Research and Therapy*, **48**, 827–831.

Ollendick, T. H., Öst, L.-G., Reuterskiöld, L., Costa, N., Cederlund, R., & Sirbu, C. (2009). One-session treatment of specific phobias in youth: a randomized clinical trial in the USA and Sweden. *Journal of Consulting and Clinical Psychology*, **77**, 504–516.

Öst, L., Svensson, L., Hellström, K., & Lindwall, R. (2001). One-session treatment of specific phobia in youth: a randomized clinical trial. *Journal of Consulting and Clinical Psychology*, **69**, 814–824.

Pahl, K. M. & Barrett, P. M. (2010). Interventions for anxiety disorders in children using group cognitive–behavioral therapy with family involvement. In: J. R. Weisz & A. E. Kazdin (eds.) *Evidence-Based Psychotherapies for Children and Adolescents*, pp. 61–79. New York: Guilford Press.

Pina, A. A., Little, M., Knight, G. P., & Silverman, W. K. (2009). Cross-ethnic measurement equivalence of the RCMAS in Hispanic/Latino and European American youth with anxiety disorders. *Journal of Personality Assessment*, **91**, 58 – 61.

Pina, A. A., Silverman, W. K., Fuentes, R. M., Kurtines, W. M., & Weems, C. F. (2003). Exposure-based cognitive–behavioral treatment for phobic and anxiety disorders: treatment effects and maintenance for Hispanic/Latino relative to European-American youths. *Journal of the American Academy of Child and Adolescent Psychiatry*, **42**, 1179–1187.

Rapee, R. M., Schniering, C. A., & Hudson, J. L. (2009). Anxiety disorders during childhood and adolescence: origins and treatment. *Annual Review of Clinical Psychology*, **5**, 335–365.

Reynolds, C. R. & Richmond, B. O. (1978). What I think and feel: a revised measure of children's manifest anxiety. *Journal of Abnormal Child Psychology*, **6**, 271–280.

RUPP Anxiety Study Group (2002). The Pediatric Anxiety Rating Scale (PARS): development and psychometric properties. *Journal of the American Academy of Child and Adolescent Psychiatry*, **41**, 1061–1069.

Saavedra, L. M., Silverman, W. K., Morgan-Lopez, A. A., & Kurtines, W. M. (2010). Cognitive behavioral treatment for childhood anxiety disorders: long-term effects on anxiety and secondary disorders in young adulthood. *Journal of Child Psychology and Psychiatry*, **51**, 924–934.

Salkovskis, P. M. (1991). The importance of behavior in the maintenance of anxiety and panic: a cognitive account. *Behavioural Psychotherapy*, **19**, 6–19.

Schniering, C. A. & Rapee, R. M. (2002). Development and validation of a measure of youth's automatic thoughts: the Youth's Automatic Thoughts Scale. *Behaviour Research and Therapy*, **40**, 1091–1109.

Schwartz, R. M. & Garamoni, G. L. (1986). A structural model of positive and negative states of mind: asymmetry in the internal dialogue. In: P. C. Kendall (ed.) *Advances in Cognitive–Behavioral Research and Therapy*, vol. 5, pp. 1–62. New York: Academic Press.

Shirk, S. R. & Saiz, C. C. (1992). Clinical, empirical and developmental perspectives on the therapeutic relationship in child psychotherapy. *Development and Psychopathology*, **4**, 713–728.

Silverman W. K. & Albano, A. M. (1996). *Anxiety Disorders Interview Schedule for DSM-IV: Child and Parent Versions*. New York: Oxford University Press.

Silverman, W. K. & Berman, S. L. (2001). Psychosocial interventions for anxiety disorders in children: status and future directions. In: W. K. Silverman & P. D. A. Treffers (eds.) *Anxiety Disorders in Children and Adolescents: Research, Assessment and Intervention*, pp. 313–334. Cambridge, UK: Cambridge University Press.

Silverman, W. K. & Hinshaw, S. P. (2008). The second Special Issue on evidence-based psychosocial treatments for children and adolescents: a ten-year update. *Journal of Clinical Child and Adolescent Psychology*, **37**, 1–7.

Silverman, W. K. & Kurtines, W. M. (1996). *Anxiety and Phobic Disorders: A Pragmatic Approach*. New York: Plenum Press.

Silverman, W. K. & Ollendick, T. H. (2005). Evidence-based assessment of anxiety and its disorders in children and adolescents. *Journal of Clinical Child and Adolescent Psychology*, **34**, 380–411.

Silverman, W. K., Kurtines, W. M., Ginsburg, G. S., Weems, C. F., Lumpkin, P. W., & Carmichael, D. H. (1999). Treating anxiety disorders in children with group cognitive–behavioral therapy: a randomized clinical trial. *Journal of Consulting and Clinical Psychology*, **67**, 995–1003.

Silverman, W. K., Kurtines, W. M., Ginsburg, G. S., Weems, C. F., Rabian, B., & Serafini, L. T. (1999). Contingency management, self-control, and education support in the treatment of childhood phobic disorders: a randomized clinical trial. *Journal of Consulting and Clinical Psychology*, **67**, 675–687.

Silverman, W. K., Kurtines, W. M., Jaccard, J., & Pina, A. A. (2009). Directionality of change in youth anxiety treatment involving parents: an initial examination. *Journal of Consulting and Clinical Psychology*, **77**, 474–485.

Silverman, W. K., Pina, A. A., & Viswesvaran, C. (2008). Evidence-based psychosocial treatments for phobic and anxiety disorders in children and adolescents. *Journal of Clinical Child and Adolescent Psychology*, **37**, 105–130.

Southam-Gerow, M., Weisz, J. R., Chu, B. C., McLeod, B. D., Gordis, E. B., & Connor-Smith, J. K. (2010). Does cognitive behavioral therapy for youth anxiety outperform usual care in community clinics? An initial effectiveness test. *Journal of the American Academy of Child and Adolescent Psychiatry*, **49**, 1043–52.

Spence, S. H. (1998). A measure of anxiety symptoms among children. *Behaviour Research and Therapy*, **36**, 545–566.

Spence, S. H., Holmes, J. M., March, S., & Lipp, O. V. (2006). The feasibility and outcome of clinic plus internet delivery of cognitive–behavior therapy for childhood anxiety. *Journal of Consulting and Clinical Psychology*, **74**, 614–621.

Spielberger, C. D. (1973). *Preliminary Test Manual for the State-Trait Anxiety Inventory for Children*. Palo Alto, CA: Consulting Psychologists Press.

Treadwell, K. R. H. & Kendall, P. C. (1996). Self-talk in youth with anxiety disorders: states of mind, content specificity, and treatment outcome. *Journal of Consulting and Clinical Psychology*, **64**, 941–950.

Walkup, J. T., Albano, A. M., Piacentini, J., Birmaker, B., Compton, S. N., Sherrill, J. T., *et al.* (2008). Cognitive behavioral therapy, sertraline, or a combination in childhood anxiety. *New England Journal of Medicine*, **359**, 2753–2766.

Weisz, J. R., Southam-Gerow, M. A., Gordis, E. B., Connor-Smith, J. K., Chu, B. C., & Langer, D. A. (2009). Cognitive–behavioral therapy versus usual clinical care for youth depression: an initial test of transportability to community clinics and clinicians. *Journal of Consulting and Clinical Psychology*, **77**, 383–396.

Wolitzky, K. B. & Telch, M. J. (2009). Augmenting in vivo exposure with fear antagonistic actions: a preliminary test. *Behavior Therapy*, **40**, 57–71.

Wood, J. J., McLeod, B. D., Piacentini, J. C., & Sigman, M. (2009). One year follow-up of family versus child CBT for anxiety disorders: exploring the roles of child age and parental intrusiveness. *Child Psychiatry and Human Development*, **40**, 301–316.

Wood, J. J., Piacentini, J. C., Southam-Gerow, M. A., Chu, B., & Sigman, M. (2006). Family cognitive behavioral therapy for child anxiety disorders. *Journal of the American Academy of Child and Adolescent Psychiatry*, **45**, 314–321.

Index